# 1998
# YEAR BOOK OF
# CARDIOLOGY®

# Statement of Purpose

## The YEAR BOOK Service

The YEAR BOOK series was devised in 1901 by practicing health professionals who observed that the literature of medicine and related disciplines had become so voluminous that no one individual could read and place in perspective every potential advance in a major specialty. In the final decade of the 20th century, this recognition is more acutely true than it was in 1901.

More than merely a series of books, YEAR BOOK volumes are the tangible results of a unique service designed to accomplish the following:

- to *survey* a wide range of journals of proven value
- to *select* from those journals papers representing significant advances and statements of important clinical principles
- to provide *abstracts* of those articles that are readable, convenient summaries of their key points
- to provide *commentary* about those articles to place them in perspective

These publications grow out of a unique process that calls on the talents of outstanding authorities in clinical and fundamental disciplines, trained literature specialists, and professional writers, all supported by the resources of Mosby, the world's preeminent publisher for the health professions.

## The Literature Base

Mosby and its editors survey more than 1,000 journals published worldwide, covering the full range of the health professions. On an annual basis, the publisher examines usage patterns and polls its expert authorities to add new journals to the literature base and to delete journals that are no longer useful as potential YEAR BOOK sources.

## The Literature Survey

The publisher's team of literature specialists, all of whom are trained and experienced health professionals, examines every original, peer-reviewed article in each journal issue. More than 250,000 articles per year are scanned systematically, including title, text, illustrations, tables, and references. Each scan is compared, article by article, to the search strategies that the publisher has developed in consultation with the 270 outside experts who form the pool of YEAR BOOK editors. A given article may be reviewed by any number of editors, from one to a dozen or more, regardless of the discipline for which the paper was originally published. In turn, each editor who receives the article reviews it to determine whether the article should be included in the YEAR BOOK. This decision is based on the article's inherent quality, its probable usefulness to readers of that YEAR BOOK, and the editor's goal to represent a balanced picture of a given field in each volume of the YEAR BOOK. In addition, the editor indicates when to include figures and tables from the article to help the YEAR BOOK reader better understand the information.

Of the quarter million articles scanned each year, only 5% are selected for detailed analysis within the YEAR BOOK series, thereby assuring readers of the high value of every selection.

## The Abstract

The publisher's abstracting staff is headed by a seasoned medical professional and includes individuals with training in the life sciences, medicine, and other areas, plus extensive experience in writing for the health professions and related industries. Each selected article is assigned to a specific writer on this abstracting staff. The abstracter, guided in many cases by notations supplied by the expert editor, writes a structured, condensed summary designed so that the reader can rapidly acquire the essential information contained in the article.

## The Commentary

The YEAR BOOK editorial boards, sometimes assisted by guest commentators, write comments that place each article in perspective for the reader. This provides the reader with the equivalent of a personal consultation with a leading international authority—an opportunity to better understand the value of the article and to benefit from the authority's thought processes in assessing the article.

## Additional Editorial Features

The editorial boards of each YEAR BOOK organize the abstracts and comments to provide a logical and satisfying sequence of information. To enhance the organization, editors also provide introductions to sections or individual chapters, comments linking a number of abstracts, citations to additional literature, and other features.

The published YEAR BOOK contains enhanced bibliographic citations for each selected article, including extended listings of multiple authors and identification of author affiliations. Each YEAR BOOK contains a Table of Contents specific to that year's volume. From year to year, the Table of Contents for a given YEAR BOOK will vary depending on developments within the field.

Every YEAR BOOK contains a list of the journals from which papers have been selected. This list represents a subset of the more than 1,000 journals surveyed by the publisher and occasionally reflects a particularly pertinent article from a journal that is not surveyed on a routine basis.

Finally, each volume contains a comprehensive subject index and an index to authors of each selected paper.

# The 1998 Year Book Series

**Year Book of Allergy, Asthma, and Clinical Immunology:** Drs. Rosenwasser, Borish, Boguniewicz, Nelson, Routes, and Spahn

**Year Book of Anesthesiology and Pain Management®:** Drs. Tinker, Abram, Chestnut, Roizen, Rothenberg, and Wood

**Year Book of Cardiology®:** Drs. Schlant, Collins, Gersh, Graham, Kaplan, and Waldo

**Year Book of Chiropractic®:** Dr. Lawrence

**Year Book of Critical Care Medicine®:** Drs. Parrillo, Balk, Calvin, Franklin, and Shapiro

**Year Book of Dentistry®:** Drs. Meskin, Berry, Jeffcoat, Leinfelder, Roser, Summitt, and Zakariasen

**Year Book of Dermatologic Surgery®:** Drs. Greenway, Barrett, Papadopoulos, and Whitaker

**Year Book of Dermatology®:** Dr. Thiers

**Year Book of Diagnostic Radiology®:** Drs. Osborn, Groskin, Dalinka, Maynard, Pentecost, Rebner, Ros, Smirniotopoulos, and Young

**Year Book of Drug Therapy®:** Drs. Lasagna and Weintraub

**Year Book of Emergency Medicine®:** Drs. Wagner, Dronen, Davidson, King, Niemann, and Roberts

**Year Book of Endocrinology®:** Drs. Bagdade, Braverman, Horton, Kannan, Landsberg, Molitch, Morley, Nathan, Odell, Poehlman, Rogol, and Ryan

**Year Book of Family Practice®:** Drs. Berg, Bowman, Davidson, Dexter, and Scherger

**Year Book of Gastroenterology®:** Drs. Aliperti and Fleshman

**Year Book of Geriatrics and Gerontology®:** Drs. Burton, Beck, Ostwald, Rabins, Reuben, Roth, Shapiro, and Whitehouse

**Year Book of Hand Surgery®:** Drs. Amadio and Hentz

**Year Book of Hematology®:** Drs. Spivak, Bell, Ness, Quesenberry, Wiernik, and Horowitz

**Year Book of Infectious Diseases:** Drs. Keusch, Barza, Bennish, Poutsiaka, Skolnik, and Snydman

**Year Book of Medicine®:** Drs. Cline, Frishman, Jett, Klahr, Malawista, Mandell, McCallum, and Utiger

**Year Book of Neonatal and Perinatal Medicine®:** Drs. Fanaroff, Maisels, and Stevenson

**Year Book of Nephrology, Hypertension, and Mineral Metabolism:** Drs. Schwab, Bennett, Emmett, Hostetter, Kumar, and Toto

**Year Book of Neurology and Neurosurgery®:** Drs. Bradley and Gibbs

**Year Book of Nuclear Medicine®:** Drs. Gottschalk, Blaufox, Neumann, Strauss, and Zubal

**Year Book of Obstetrics, Gynecology, and Women's Health:** Drs. Mishell, Herbst, and Kirschbaum

**Year Book of Occupational and Environmental Medicine®:** Drs. Emmett, Frank, Gochfeld, and Hessl

**Year Book of Oncology®:** Drs. Ozols, Eisenberg, Glatstein, Loehrer, and Tallman

**Year Book of Ophthalmology®:** Drs. Wilson, Augsburger, Cohen, Eagle, Grossman, Laibson, Maguire, Nelson, Penne, Rapuano, Sergott, Spaeth, Tipperman, Ms. Gosfield, and Ms. Salmon

**Year Book of Orthopedics®:** Drs. Morrey, Beauchamp, Currier, Tolo, Trigg, and Swiontkowski

**Year Book of Otolaryngology–Head and Neck Surgery®:** Drs. Paparella and Holt

**Year Book of Pathology and Laboratory Medicine®:** Drs. Raab, Cohen, Olson, Sirgi, and Stanley

**Year Book of Pediatrics®:** Dr. Stockman

**Year Book of Plastic, Reconstructive, and Aesthetic Surgery®:** Drs. Miller, Bartlett, Garner, McKinney, Ruberg, Salisbury, and Smith

**Year Book of Psychiatry and Applied Mental Health®:** Drs. Talbott, Ballenger, Frances, Lydiard, Meltzer, Schowalter, and Tasman

**Year Book of Pulmonary Disease®:** Drs. Jett, Maurer, Ryu, Strollo, and Wenzel

**Year Book of Rheumatology®:** Drs. Panush, Hadler, LeRoy, Liang, Reichlin, Simon, and Weinblatt

**Year Book of Sports Medicine®:** Drs. Shephard, Drinkwater, Eichner, Torg, Alexander, and Mr. George

**Year Book of Surgery®:** Drs. Copeland, Bland, Deitch, Eberlein, Howard, Luce, Seeger, Souba, and Sugarbaker

**Year Book of Thoracic and Cardiovascular Surgery®:** Drs. Ginsberg, Wechsler, and Williams

**Year Book of Urology®:** Drs. Andriole and Coplen

**Year Book of Vascular Surgery®:** Dr. Porter

# 1998
# The Year Book of CARDIOLOGY®

Editor in Chief

## Robert C. Schlant, M.D.

*Professor and Chairman, Emory University School of Medicine; Chief of Cardiology, Grady Memorial Hospital, Atlanta, Georgia*

Editors

## John J. Collins, Jr., M.D.

*Chief, Division of Cardiovascular Surgery, Brigham and Women's Hospital, Boston, Massachusetts*

## Bernard J. Gersh, M.B., Ch.B., D.Phil., F.R.C.P.

*Chief, Division of Cardiology; W. Procter Harvey Teaching Professor of Cardiology, Georgetown University Medical Center, Washington, D.C.*

## Thomas P. Graham, M.D.

*Director of Pediatric Cardiology; Ann and Monroe Carell Family Professor of Pediatrics, Vanderbilt University Medical Center, Nashville, Tennessee*

## Norman M. Kaplan, M.D.

*Professor of Internal Medicine, University of Texas Southwestern Medical Center, Dallas, Texas*

## Albert L. Waldo, M.D.

*The Walter H. Pritchard Professor of Cardiology and Professor of Medicine, Case Western Reserve University; Director, Clinical Cardiac Electrophysiology Program, University Hospitals of Cleveland, Cleveland, Ohio*

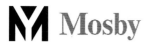 Mosby

St. Louis  Baltimore  Boston  Carlsbad  Naples  New York  Philadelphia  Portland  London
Madrid  Mexico City  Singapore  Sydney  Tokyo  Toronto  Wiesbaden

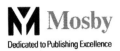

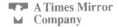

*Publisher:* Theresa Van Schaik
*Developmental Editor:* Jacquelyn M. Leonard
*Manager, Periodical Editing:* Kirk Swearingen
*Manuscript Editor:* Pat Costigan
*Project Supervisor, Production:* Joy Moore
*Production Assistant:* Laura Bayless
*Manager, Literature Services:* Idelle L. Winer
*Illustrations and Permissions Coordinator:* Chidi C. Ukabam

**1998 EDITION**
**Copyright © 1998 by Mosby, Inc.**

Printed in the United States of America
Composition by Reed Technology and Information Services, Inc.
Printing/binding by Maple-Vail

Editorial Office:
Mosby, Inc.
11830 Westline Industrial Drive
St. Louis, MO 63146
Customer Service: customer.support@mosby.com
                www.mosby.com/Mosby/CustomerSupport/index.html
series.editorial@mosby.com

International Standard Serial Number: 0145-4145
International Standard Book Number: 0-8151-7539-6

# Table of Contents

# Journals Represented

Mosby and its editors survey more than 1,000 journals for its abstract and commentary publications. From these journals, the editors select the articles to be abstracted. Journals represented in this YEAR BOOK are listed below.

ASAIO Journal
American Heart Journal
American Journal of Cardiology
American Journal of Clinical Nutrition
American Journal of Clinical Pathology
American Journal of Epidemiology
American Journal of Hematology
American Journal of Hypertension
American Journal of Public Health
American Journal of Roentgenology
American Journal of the Medical Sciences
Anesthesia and Analgesia
Annals of Emergency Medicine
Annals of Internal Medicine
Annals of Surgery
Annals of Thoracic Surgery
Archives of Family Medicine
Archives of Internal Medicine
British Journal of Anaesthesia
British Journal of General Practice
British Medical Bulletin
British Medical Journal
Canadian Journal of Anaesthesia
Cancer
Cardiology in Review
Chest
Circulation
Diabetes
European Heart Journal
Heart
Hypertension
Journal of Cardiac Failure
Journal of Cardiac Surgery
Journal of Cardiovascular Electrophysiology
Journal of Cardiovascular Surgery
Journal of Clinical Epidemiology
Journal of Clinical Investigation
Journal of Clinical Pharmacology
Journal of Developmental and Behavioral Pediatrics
Journal of General Internal Medicine
Journal of Hypertension
Journal of Pediatrics
Journal of Thoracic and Cardiovascular Surgery
Journal of Urology
Journal of the American College of Cardiology
Journal of the American Geriatrics Society
Journal of the American Medical Association

Lancet
Mayo Clinic Proceedings
Medicine
Medicine and Science in Sports and Exercise
New England Journal of Medicine
PACE-Pacing and Clinical Electrophysiology
Pediatric Nephrology
Pediatrics
Progress in Cardiovascular Diseases
Scandinavian Cardiovascular Journal
Stroke
Texas Heart Institute Journal
Trends in Cardiovascular Medicine

## STANDARD ABBREVIATIONS

The following terms are abbreviated in this edition: acquired immunodeficiency syndrome (AIDS), cardiopulmonary resuscitation (CPR), central nervous system (CNS), cerebrospinal fluid (CSF), computed tomography (CT), deoxyribonucleic acid (DNA), electrocardiography (ECG), health maintenance organization (HMO), human immunodeficiency virus (HIV), intensive care unit (ICU), intramuscular (IM), intravenous (IV), magnetic resonance (MR) imaging (MRI), and ribonucleic acid (RNA).

## NOTE

The YEAR BOOK OF CARDIOLOGY is a literature survey service providing abstracts of articles published in the professional literature. Every effort is made to assure the accuracy of the information presented in these pages. Neither the editors nor the publisher of the YEAR BOOK OF CARDIOLOGY can be responsible for errors in the original materials. The editors' comments are their own opinions. Mention of specific products within this publication does not constitute endorsement.

To facilitate the use of the YEAR BOOK OF CARDIOLOGY as a reference tool, all illustrations and tables included in this publication are now identified as they appear in the original article. This change is meant to help the reader recognize that any illustration or table appearing in the YEAR BOOK OF CARDIOLOGY may be only one of many in the original article. For this reason, figure and table numbers will often appear to be out of sequence within the YEAR BOOK OF CARDIOLOGY.

# Introduction

This 1998 YEAR BOOK OF CARDIOLOGY is 38th in the series. Each of your six editors has carefully selected articles that he felt were important and clinically relevant in the various fields of cardiology. An editor has provided appropriate comments on each article.

All of the editors again thank the staff at Mosby, Inc., for their assistance, understanding, and patience.

Robert C. Schlant, M.D.

# 1 Noncoronary Heart Disease in Adults

## Introduction

For this section I have selected 59 articles. This includes four articles on congenital heart disease in adults, 18 on valvular heart disease, 14 on myocarditis and cardiomyopathy, 15 on heart failure, and eight miscellaneous noncoronary heart disease topics. Each article has been selected to provide practicing clinical cardiologists with information relevant to the care of patients that might be encountered in clinical practice, either today or in the future. As noted, many of the studies are preliminary and require confirmation before the results should be accepted and applied.

Robert C. Schlant, M.D.

## Congenital Heart Disease

**Atrial Septal Defect in Adults: Cardiopulmonary Exercise Capacity Before and 4 Months and 10 Years After Defect Closure**
Helber U, Baumann R, Seboldt H, et al (Eberhard-Karls-Universität, Tübingen, Germany)
*J Am Coll Cardiol* 29:1345–1350, 1997                                                    1–1

*Background.*—Individuals with atrial septal defect are often asymptomatic early in life, but may have physical underdevelopment, plus a higher rate of respiratory infections and cardiopulmonary symptoms and complications as adults or older adults. Many adults do not report limited exercise capacity, in spite of significant volume overloading. Closure of defects with significant left-to-right shunting has been performed in adults, although there is no information from controlled, follow-up studies of adults treated surgically vs. medically.

*Methods.*—There were 31 adult patients who had closure of atrial septal defect. The mean patient age at operation was 39.9 years. Mean left-right shunt was 9.6 L/min, mean pulmonary/systemic flow ratio was 2.8, and mean pulmonary artery pressure was 18.2 mm Hg. A bicycle ergometer was used for cardiopulmonary exercise testing. Peak oxygen uptake, anaerobic threshold, performance at anaerobic threshold, and maximal performance in relation to these variables were determined in control subjects. Ventilatory function at rest was determined by vital capacity, maximal voluntary ventilation, and forced expiratory volume in 1 second.

*Results.*—Preoperatively, a moderate reduction in ventilatory function at rest to 75% to 85% was seen. At 4 months, no significant improvement was seen, but at 10 months, ventilatory function at rest had normalized. Preoperatively, cardiopulmonary exercise capacity was significantly reduced to 50% to 60%. At 4 months, it was only slightly higher, but at 10 years, it had improved significantly and normalized.

*Discussion.*—These findings suggest that surgical treatment is superior to medical treatment in terms of long-term survival and prevention of functional limitations because of heart failure. Long-term improvement in cardiopulmonary exercise capacity can be achieved. Cardiopulmonary exercise testing is an important method of detecting functional impairment.

▶ This excellent study was performed in 31 patients with a mean age of 40 years (range 19 to 56). It is noteworthy that the mean pulmonary artery pressure was only 18.2 ± 6.2 mm Hg. This article emphasizes the importance of diagnosing and correcting atrial septal defect in adults.

**R.C. Schlant, M.D.**

## Late (Five to Nine Years) Follow-up After Balloon Dilation of Valvular Pulmonary Stenosis in Adults

Teupe CHJ, Burger W, Schräder R, et al (Univ of Frankfurt, Germany)
*Am J Cardiol* 80:240–242, 1997                                        1–2

*Introduction.*—The treatment of choice for children with pulmonary stenosis is balloon valvuloplasty. In adults, pulmonary stenosis is a rare condition, but those with a transvalvular gradient of more than 50 mm Hg at rest should be treated because the condition can lead to right ventricular hypertrophy and failure. The long-term follow-up of adult patients with pulmonary stenosis having balloon valvuloplasty is described.

*Methods.*—There were 24 adult patients with congenital pulmonary stenosis who had transluminal balloon valvuloplasty. Before valvuloplasty, they had an invasive measure peak gradient of 48 to 149 mm Hg. At follow-up at 4.5 to 9 years after valvuloplasty, 14 of 24 patients were re-examined; there were 9 women and 5 men ranging in age from 19 to 65 years. Right-sided heart catheterization and color- and continuous wave-Doppler echocardiography were performed in all 14 patients at follow-up.

*Results.*—At follow-up, the peak gradients obtained by cardiac catheterization were 24 to 48 mm Hg (Fig 1). There was persistent improvement of 1 to 2 functional classes at follow-up, and no clinical symptoms were seen at all in 13 of 14 patients. Dyspnea with a high level of physical exercise was seen in 1 patient. There were 3 patients with a peak-to-peak gradient of more than 100 mm Hg before dilatation due to narrowing of

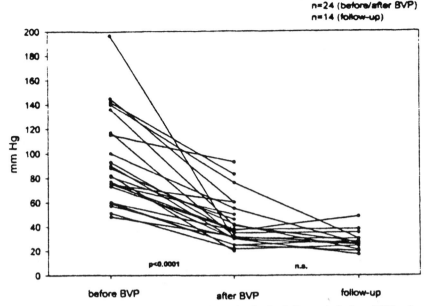

FIGURE 1.—Transvalvular gradient before and immediately after balloon valvuloplasty (BVP) and at follow-up (Reprinted by permission of the publisher from Teupe CHJ, Burger W, Schrader R, et al: Late (Five to Nine Years) Follow-Up After Balloon Dilation of Valvular Pulmonary Stenosis in Adults. *Am J Cardiol* 80:240–242, 1997. Copyright 1997 by Excerpta Medica, Inc.)

the right ventricular outflow tract as a result of muscular hypertrophy. Within the first 3 months after dilatation, all these patients showed further decrease in the gradient. At 9 years after balloon valvuloplasty, all patients had an excellent long-term result. Severe pulmonary insufficiency is rare and occurs more often after surgical relief of stenosis than after balloon valvuloplasty.

*Conclusion.*—In adults, balloon valvuloplasty of pulmonary stenosis is highly effective and associated with excellent long-term outcome. This method should be the first-line treatment of pulmonary stenosis in adults, and the lower complication rate of balloon valvuloplasty versus surgical treatment should be taken into account.

▶ This study adds more support to the use of balloon dilatation to treat adults with pulmonary stenosis. In many laboratories in the United States, this procedure is performed by the pediatric cardiologist, who usually has more experience with the procedure than most adult interventional cardiologists.

**R.C. Schlant, M.D.**

## Clinical Factors Associated With Calcific Aortic Valve Disease

Stewart BF, Siscovick D, Lind BK, et al (Univ of Washington, Seattle; Univ of California Irvine, Orange; Georgetown Univ, Washington, DC; et al)
*J Am Coll Cardiol* 29:630–634, 1997                                    1–3

*Background.*—Degenerative aortic valve disease is apparently not an inevitable consequence of aging. It may be associated with specific clinical factors. The prevalence of aortic sclerosis and stenosis in the elderly was determined and the clinical factors associated with degenerative aortic valve disease identified in the current study.

*Methods and Findings.*—Data on 5,201 persons aged 65 years and older enrolled in the Cardiovascular Health Study were analyzed. Twenty-six percent had aortic valve sclerosis, and 2% had aortic valve stenosis. Sclerosis was discovered in 37% of those aged 75 years and older, and stenosis in 2.6%. Clinical factors independently correlated with degenerative aortic valve disease were age, associated with a 2-fold increase in risk for each 10-year increase in age; male sex, with a 2-fold excess risk; smoking with a 35% increase in risk; and a history of hypertension with a 20% increase in risk (Table 3). Height and high lipoprotein(a) and low-density lipoprotein cholesterol levels were also significant variables.

*Conclusions.*—This study identified several clinical factors associated with degenerative aortic valve disease. A greater understanding of the cellular and molecular mechanisms involved in the pathogenesis of degenerative aortic valve disease and the risk factors for this disease may result in interventions that prevent or delay the progression of disease. Studies determining whether controlling risk factors can prevent aortic valve disease also appear to be warranted.

▶ This report lends support to an impression held by a number of individuals for 10 to 20 years that calcific aortic valve disease is often related to the

TABLE 3.—Clinical Factors Associated With Aortic Stenosis or Sclerosis by Stepwise Multiple Logistic Regression

| Variable | p Value | Odds Ratio | 95% Confidence Limits |
|---|---|---|---|
| Age | <0.001 | 2.18* | 2.15, 2.20 |
| Male gender | <0.001 | 2.03 | 1.7, 2.5 |
| Lp(a) | <0.001 | 1.23† | 1.14, 1.32 |
| Height (cm) | 0.001 | 0.84‡ | 0.75, 0.93 |
| History of hypertension | 0.002 | 1.23 | 1.1, 1.4 |
| Present smoking | 0.006 | 1.35 | 1.1, 1.7 |
| LDLc (mg/dl) | 0.008 | 1.12† | 1.03, 1.23 |

\* ± 75th vs. 25th percentile.
† ± 10-year increase.
‡ ± 10-unit increase.
*Abbreviations: LDLc,* low-density lipoprotein cholesterol; *Lp(a),* lipoprotein (a).
(Reprinted with permission from the American College of Cardiology [*Journal of the American College of Cardiology,* 1997, Vol. 29, No. 3, pp 630–635].)

common clinical risk factors for atherosclerosis. On the basis of this paper and a number of others, it would not be premature to implement lowering risk factor in patients who have aortic valve sclerosis and even possibly in those who have a family history of calcific aortic valve disease. Even if this avoided a fraction of the patients moving on to severe calcific aortic valve stenosis, it would be worthwhile.

**R.C. Schlant, M.D.**

---

**Prospective Study of Asymptomatic Valvular Aortic Stenosis: Clinical, Echocardiographic, and Exercise Predictors of Outcome**
Otto CM, Burwash IG, Legget ME, et al (Univ of Washington, Seattle)
*Circulation* 95:2262–2270, 1997                                        1–4

---

*Objective.*—Recent evidence suggests that interventions can slow or prevent progression of valvular aortic stenosis. There are few data on the rate of hemodynamic progression or predictors of outcome in asymptomatic patients. Results were presented of a prospective study of asymptomatic adults, using annual clinical, echocardiographic, and exercise data to determine the rate of hemodynamic progression of valvular aortic stenosis

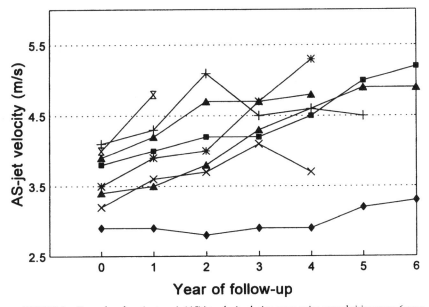

**FIGURE 1.**—Examples of aortic stenosis (*AS*) jet velocity during prospective annual visits over a 6-year period in 8 patients with asymptomatic AS, showing the marked individual variability in the rate of hemodynamic progression. (Courtesy of Otto CM, Burwash IG, Legget ME, et al: Prospective study of asymptomatic valvular aortic stenosis: Clinical, echocardiographic, and exercise predictors of outcome. *Circulation* 95:2262–2270. Reproduced with permission of *Circulation*. Copyright 1997, American Heart Association.)

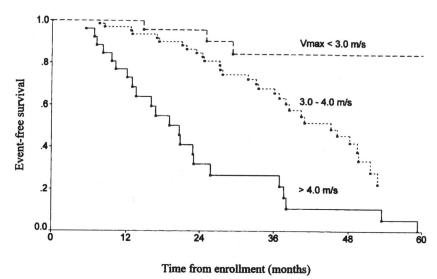

**Time from enrollment (months)**

FIGURE 4.—Cox regression analysis showing event-free survival in groups defined by aortic jet velocity at entry (*P* less than 0.0001 by log-rank test). *Abbreviation*: *Vmax*, peak flow velocity. (Courtesy of Otto CM, Burwash IG, Legget ME, et al: Prospective study of asymptomatic valvular aortic stenosis: Clinical, echocardiographic, and exercise predictors of outcome. *Circulation* 95:2262–2270. Reproduced with permission of *Circulation*. Copyright 1997, American Heart Association.)

and the relationship between hemodynamic severity and symptom onset, and to identify predictors of clinical outcome.

*Methods.*—Between September 1989 and April 1995, primary care physicians or cardiologists referred 123 patients (37 women), aged 22 to 84 years, with asymptomatic valvular aortic stenosis for annual clinical examination, Doppler echocardiography, functional status questionnaire, and an exercise treadmill stress test. Using maximal Bruce protocol treadmill testing, aortic jet velocity, left ventricular outflow tract velocity, and diameter at baseline and immediately after exercise were determined for 104 patients able to exercise. Clinical end points were death or aortic valve surgery. Patients were followed for an average of 2.5 years.

*Results.*—Aortic jet velocity increased by 0.32 m/sec/yr and mean gradient by 7 mm Hg/yr; valve area decreased by 0.12 cm²/yr. The rate of individual hemodynamic progression varied considerably (Fig 1). Of the 274 exercise tests performed, there was a fall in systolic blood pressure of greater than 10 mm Hg in 25 patients (9%) and a greater than 2 mm–ST depression persisting for more than 5 minutes in 4 (2%). Exercise tests were terminated prematurely for fatigue or shortness of breath (60% of patients), leg discomfort (28%), angina (3%), lightheadedness (1%), and fall in blood pressure or arrhythmias (8%). There were 8 deaths (4 of cardiac causes) at an average of 32 months and 48 aortic valve surgeries. Event-free survivals at 1, 3, and 5 years were 93%, 62%, and 26%, respectively. Univariate predictors of outcomes included baseline jet velocity, mean gradient, valve area, and functional status score. Duration of exercise was not predictive of outcome. Multivariate predictors of clinical outcome included only baseline jet velocity, functional status score, and rate in change of jet velocity. Patients with a jet velocity of greater than 4.0 m/sec at baseline had only a 21% probability of survival at 2 years (Fig 4).

*Conclusion.*—Aortic jet velocity at baseline, functional status score, and rate of change of jet velocity are predictors of clinical outcome in patients with asymptomatic valvular aortic stenosis.

▶ The conclusions of this excellent article make good clinical and hemodynamic sense. We should now apply the results of this study in our follow-up of patients with valvular aortic stenosis.

**R.C. Schlant, M.D.**

## Valvular Heart Disease

**Angina Pectoris in Patients With Aortic Stenosis and Normal Coronary Arteries: Mechanisms and Pathophysiological Concepts**
Julius BK, Spillman M, Vassalli G, et al (Univ Hosp, Zurich, Switzerland)
*Circulation* 95:892–898, 1997                                                     1–5

*Introduction.*—In the absence of associated coronary artery, there is a 40% incidence of angina pectoris in patients with aortic stenosis. Angina pectoris is a typical symptom in these patients. Unbalanced myocardial oxygen supply and demand may be the cause of the pathophysiological mechanisms of angina. A reduction in coronary flow reserve may explain this phenomenon in part. Hemodynamic factors and myocardial perfusion were evaluated in patients with angina pectoris and severe aortic stenosis to better understand the pathogenesis of angina pectoris in the absence of coronary artery disease.

*Methods.*—There were 61 patients with severe aortic stenosis and without significant coronary artery disease and 33 controls who were patients with atypical chest pain and angiographically normal arteries. There were 32 patients with angina pectoris and 29 without angina pectoris. In 59 patients and in 22 controls, quantitative coronary angiography was performed. The coronary sinus thermodilution technique was used to determine coronary flow reserve in 29 patients and 7 controls.

*Results.*—A lower left ventricular muscle mass, an increased left ventricular peak systolic pressure, and increased wall stress were seen in patients with angina pectoris when compared to those without angina pectoris. Patients with angina pectoris had smaller vessels of the left coronary artery and lower coronary flow reserve than those without angina pectoris. Patients with angina pectoris had inadequate left ventricular hypertrophy with an increased wall stress, which was not seen in patients without angina pectoris.

*Conclusion.*—In the absence of coronary artery disease, myocardial ischemia in patients with severe aortic stenosis can occur and appears to be due to inadequate left ventricular hypertrophy with high systolic and diastolic wall stress and a reduced coronary flow reserve. It is still unclear what is the cause of inadequate left ventricular hypertrophy. During high

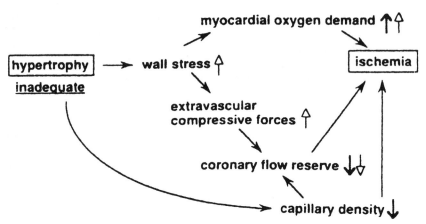

FIGURE 5.—Pathophysiology of myocardial ischemia in angina pectoris+ patients. Left ventricular hypertrophy tends to normalize left ventricular wall stress, but in the presence of inadequate hypertrophy, wall stress is elevated. This leads to an increase in myocardial oxygen consumption and augmentation of extravascular compressive forces. As a result, coronary flow reserve is reduced. Because of left ventricular hypertrophy, diffusion distance is increased and capillary density is decreased. Mechanisms in the presence of inadequate hypertrophy are shown by open arrows. (Courtesy of Julius BK, Spillman M, Vassalli G, et al: Angina pectoris in patients with aortic stenosis and normal coronary arteries: mechanisms and pathological concepts. *Circulation* 95:892–898, 1997.)

flow situations, such as exercise, inadequate left ventricular hypertrophy with small coronary arteries and reduced coronary flow reserve may explain the occurrence of subendocardial ischemia (Fig 5).

▶ Angina pectoris is one of the major components of the classic triad of symptoms in patients with aortic stenosis. In many patients it is in part due to associated coronary artery disease. In other patients it is due to a combination of marked left ventricular hypertrophy, elevated left ventricular diastolic pressure, and impaired left ventricular relaxation. All of these are exaggerated in the presence of tachycardia and some with increased age. The results of the present study suggest that in some patients an inadequate left ventricular hypertrophy may contribute to the angina pectoris.

**R.C. Schlant, M.D.**

---

**Comparison of Age, Gender, Number of Aortic Valve Cusps, Concomitant Coronary Artery Bypass Grafting, and Magnitude of Left Ventricular-Systemic Arterial Peak Systolic Gradient in Adults Having Aortic Valve Replacement for Isolated Aortic Valve Stenosis**
Stephan PJ, Henry AC III, Hebeler RF Jr, et al (Baylor Univ, Dallas)
*Am J Cardiol* 79:166–172, 1997                                                                1–6

---

*Objective.*—Only recently have the features of excised aortic valves been studied. The structure of excised aortic valves in isolated aortic valve stenosis is correlated with age, sex, number of aortic valve cusps, concomitant coronary artery bypass grafting, and magnitude of left ventricular-systemic arterial peak systolic gradient.

*Methods.*—Records of 115 patients having aortic valve replacement for stenosis at Baylor University Medical Center between January 1993 and August 1995 were reviewed. Patients with mitral valve dysfunction were excluded.

*Results.*—Patients under 65 years of age had a significantly higher incidence of congenitally malformed valves than patients 65 years of age or older (75% vs. 41%) and a significantly lower percentage of 3-cuspid valves (21% vs. 59%). Significantly more men than women (57% vs. 43%) had a larger aortic valve area (0.72 vs. 0.62 cm²). The 45% of patients (34 men and 18 women) having concomitant coronary artery bypass grafting (CABG) had smaller average left ventricular–to–systemic arterial peak systolic pressure gradients (46 mm Hg) than patients not having CABG (64 mm Hg). Patients with unicuspid or bicuspid valves were significantly more likely to have pressure gradients of 50 mm Hg or less across the valve, significantly more likely to undergo CABG, and significantly higher valve areas than patients with tricuspid valves (0.76 vs. 0.58 cm²). Patients with congenitally malformed valves (49%) were significantly younger than patients with tricuspid valves (68 vs. 73 years).

*Conclusion.*—Half the patients undergoing aortic valve replacement for stenosis had congenitally malformed valves, were significantly more likely to have pressure gradients of 50 mm Hg or less across the valve, and significantly more likely to undergo CABG.

▶ It is of interest that in the 87 patients 65 years of age or older, 41% had congenitally malformed (bicuspid) valves, compared with 75% of those under 65 years. One of the many lessons in this article is that in older patients, calcific aortic stenosis can still be caused by congenital bicuspid aortic valves.

**R.C. Schlant, M.D.**

---

**M-mode Echocardiography in Aortic Stenosis: Clinical Correlates and Prognostic Significance After Valve Replacement**
Lund O, Nielsen TT, Emmertsen K, et al (Aarhus Univ, Denmark)
*Scand Cardiovasc J* 31:17–23, 1997                                      1–7

---

*Purpose.*—Relatively few studies have examined the links between the echocardiographic, clinical, and hemodynamic findings in patients with aortic stenosis (AS). None have identified the echocardiographic variables associated with a poor prognosis after aortic valve replacement (AVR) for AS. The findings at M-mode echocardiography were correlated to preoperative clinical and hemodynamic variables, and echocardiographic risk factors were sought for mortality after AVR in patients with AS.

*Methods.*—The study included 250 patients undergoing AVR for AS. All patients underwent M-mode echocardiography within 6 months before the operation. The follow-up averaged 3 years, and there were 22 deaths within 30 days and 23 late deaths. The clinical correlates and prognostic significance of the echocardiographic findings were analyzed.

*Results.*—As New York Heart Association functional class, cardiothoracic index, and left ventricular (LV) failure increased, so did LV end-diastolic diameter index (EDDI) and end-systolic diameter index and LV muscle mass. The same factors were related to decreased fractional shortening. Patients with a high peak-to-peak systolic aortic valve gradients and LV end-systolic pressures had small LV dimensions, increased fractional shortening, and increased posterior wall thickness (PWTh). Early mortality was independently predicted by an EDDI of 20 mm/m$^2$ or less and an increasing PWTh. Fractional shortening was normal or supranormal in patients with an EDDI of 20 mm/m$^2$ or less. Five-year survival rates were 81% for patients with PWTh values of 13 or less, 94% for those with PWTh values of 14 to 17, and 85% for those with PWTh values of 18 mm or greater. This was the only factor independently related to long-term survival. Patients who had angina pectoris without coronary artery disease had very high PWTh values. Those with below-normal EDDI values had poor outcomes with regard to AVR; before AVR, this group was characterized by poor LV contraction and congestive heart failure. Although LV hypertrophy was the major risk factor, myocardial ischemia caused by coronary artery disease in low-grade hypertrophy and hypertrophy itself were confounding factors. The postoperative reversibility of moderate or severe LV hypertrophy after AVR was another potential confounder.

*Conclusions.*—The clinical, hemodynamic, and prognostic significance of M-mode echocardiographic findings in patients with AS are reported. The results underscore the adverse influence of abnormal LV diastolic performance. M-mode echocardiography is an important initial method to use for the evaluation of AS. However, because it cannot reliably predict prognosis on its own, it must be combined with other studies.

▶ I think the main conclusion of this study is the significant limitations of M-mode echocardiography in the evaluation of aortic valve stenosis. In most laboratories, transesophageal echocardiography has become the usual method of estimating the severity of aortic valve disease. Because many patients have to have coronary arteriography to rule out concurrent coronary artery disease, the results of transesophageal echocardiography are often compared with the dynamics at cardiac catheterization.

**R.C. Schlant, M.D.**

## Comparison of Multiplane and Biplane Transesophageal Echocardiography in the Assessment of Aortic Stenosis

Kim K-S, Maxted W, Nanda NC, et al (Univ of Alabama, Birmingham)
*Am J Cardiol* 79:436–441, 1997                                    1–8

*Introduction.*—In patients with aortic stenosis, the accuracy of multiplane transesophageal echocardiography (TEE) was compared with the more conventional biplane technique in the direct assessment of aortic valve area.

*Methods.*—There were 145 patients ranging in age from 19 to 91 with aortic stenosis who had transthoracic echocardiography, left and right heart catheterization, and intraoperative transesophageal echocardiography over 18 months. There were 81 patients studied with a multiplane transducer and 64 patients with the biplane approach.

*Results.*—In all 81 patients, short-axis images of the aortic valve were adequate for measuring the aortic valve area in the multiplane technique, but only in 56 of 64 patients (88%) were the images of the aortic valve adequate for measuring the aortic valve area in the biplane technique. There was a higher correlation coefficient for the aortic valve area determined by multiplane transesophageal echocardiography than in the biplane technique. For bicuspid valves, correlations were higher than for tricuspid valves.

*Conclusion.*—In the direct evaluation of aortic valve area in patients with aortic stenosis, the superiority of the multiplane technique was demonstrated over the biplane technique and the transthoracic echocardiography technique. Views with the biplane transducer were frequently through an oblique axis, resulting in a less reliable determination of the true valve orifice. All modes of assessing aortic valve area were superior in patients with bicuspid aortic valves than in those with tricuspid valves. Multiplane TEE is semi-invasive and requires patients to have mild sedation and at least 4 to 6 hours of fasting. The procedure is contraindicated for patients who cannot have transesophageal intubation.

▶ This study demonstrates the superiority of multiplane TEE in the direct evaluation of aortic valve area in patients with aortic stenosis. In contrast, Bernard et al.[1] found that plane imagery of aortic valve area by TEE was difficult and less accurate than the continuity equation for assessing the severity of aortic stenosis.

**R.C. Schlant, M.D.**

*Reference*

1. Bernard Y, Meneveau N, Vuyllemenot A, et al. Planimetry of aortic valve area using multiplane transesophageal echocardiography is not a reliable method for assessing severity of aortic stenosis. *Heart* 78:68–73, 1997.

## Utility of Stress Testing in Valvular Aortic Stenosis

Munt BI, Otto CM (Univ of Washington, Seattle)
Cardiol Rev 5:55–62, 1997

1–9

*Objective.*—Stress testing, performed carefully, may provide useful additional information in selected patients with valvular aortic stenosis. This article reviews exercise physiology, safety, and the potential clinical utility of exercise and pharmacologic stress testing in patients with valvular aortic stenosis.

*Exercise Physiology.*—In adults with aortic stenosis, exercise increases heart rate, but exercise tolerance is diminished. Increases in blood pressure, ejection fraction, and cardiac output are smaller than in normal controls. Transaortic pressure gradients and valve area increase. The increase in valve area may be a measure of the degree of stenosis.

*Risk and Complications of Stress Testing.*—In approximately 500,000 stress tests, there was 1 death from a progressive decrease in systolic blood pressure. Complications—usually ventricular tachycardia or a fall of 25 mm Hg or greater in systolic blood pressure—occurred at moderately low work loads and heart rates. The patient's diagnostic information and current symptom status should be studied carefully, preferably by performing Doppler echocardiography before stress testing is considered.

*Clinical Utility.*—Exercise testing may clarify equivocal symptoms such as angina, exertional dizziness, exercise intolerance, or symptoms of heart failure. Doppler echocardiography can be used to evaluate functional status. Patients with moderate aortic stenosis should be limited to low-intensity sports. Exercise testing can also detect significant coronary artery disease, present in 30% to 50% of patients having valve replacement, because these patients typically have false positive electrocardiographic responses to exercise. Thallium-201 exercise scintigraphy has a high sensitivity but relatively low specificity for detecting coronary artery disease. Technetium-99 sestamibi imaging has a sensitivity and specificity of 92% and 71%, respectively, for detecting coronary artery disease in patients with aortic stenosis. There are no studies on the use of stress echocardiography for detecting coronary artery disease in patients with aortic stenosis. Potentially, it is possible to distinguish those patients who would or would not benefit from valve replacement, using dobutamine echocardiography to measure the increased transvalvular volume flow rate induced by stress as an indication of the degree of stenosis.

*Conclusion.*—The value of stress testing in patients with valvular aortic stenosis is limited by the lack of definitive data. Ongoing studies are evaluating the relationship of stress testing to symptom status and the ability to detect coronary artery disease and to evaluate the degree of aortic stenosis and left ventricular systolic dysfunction.

▶ I would agree with the authors that the exact role of stress testing in patients with aortic stenosis remains incompletely defined. Although stress testing has been used for some time in Europe in pediatric patients and in adults, the potential hazards have limited its applicability in most patients with aortic stenosis. We have seldom found it necessary. We await further studies with great interest.

**R.C. Schlant, M.D.**

---

**Aortic Valve Replacement for Aortic Stenosis With Severe Left Ventricular Dysfunction: Prognostic Indicators**
Connolly HM, Oh JK, Orszulak TA, et al (Mayo Clinic and Mayo Found, Rochester, Minn)
*Circulation* 95:2395–2400, 1997                                              1–10

---

*Objective.*—Although aortic valve replacement for aortic stenosis in patients with severe left ventricular dysfunction carries an increased risk, little information is available regarding the clinical outcome of these patients. Prognostic indicators of operative and long-term risk of aortic valve replacement in these patients were retrospectively investigated.

*Methods.*—Between 1985 and 1992, 154 consecutive patients (47 women), aged 32 to 93 years, with aortic stenosis and left ventricular systolic dysfunction, underwent aortic valve replacement. The ejection fraction (EF), determined from 2-dimensional echocardiography for 141 patients, averaged 27%, the mean gradient was 44 mm Hg, aortic valve area averaged 0.61 cm $^2$, and average cardiac output was 4.1 L/min. Coronary artery bypass grafting was also performed in 78 patients. Potential risk factors, operative mortality, overall survival, and the relationship of preoperative EFs to postoperative values were determined.

*Results.*—The 30-day mortality rate was 9% (14 patients). Significant predictors of early mortality were decreased preoperative mean gradient and prior myocardial infarction. During the median 1.2-year follow-up, another 36 patients died, 11 of them of noncardiac causes (Fig 1). Marked coronary artery disease (CAD) and a lower preoperative cardiac output significantly decreased survival, according to multivariate analysis. Overall 5-year survival (58%) was significantly greater for patients without marked CAD than for patients with marked CAD (69% vs. 39%). Functional status, recorded for 106 patients, was severely symptomatic in 89% before surgery and severely symptomatic in 7% after surgery. New York Heart Association functional class improved by at least 1 class in 88% of patients. After surgery, EF improved in 76% of 140 patients in whom it was preoperatively assessed.

*Conclusion.*—Aortic valve replacement for aortic stenosis in patients with severe left ventricular dysfunction carried an acceptable risk. Preexisting CAD and mean aortic gradients were predictors of survival. Pre-existing CAD and cardiac output were related to long-term survival. Most patients had improvement in symptoms and EF.

▶ In this study, 51% of the patients had simultaneous coronary artery bypass surgery. It is still extremely difficult to know when to recommend

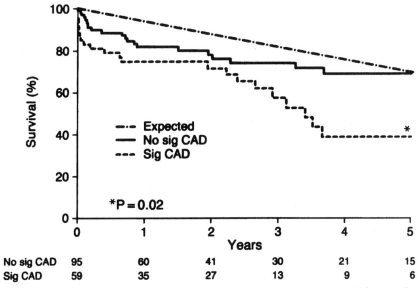

FIGURE 1.—Kaplan-Meier survival curve for patients with aortic stenosis and reduced left ventricular function with and without significant (*sig*) coronary artery disease (*CAD*) (2-vessel disease or greater or left main CAD) in comparison with expected survival. Number of patients alive at each point is shown on the *x axis*. (Courtesy of Connolly HM, Oh JK, Orszulak TA, et al: Aortic valve replacement for aortic stenosis with severe left ventricular dysfunction: Prognostic indicators. *Circulation* 95:2395–2400. Reproduced with permission of *Circulation*. Copyright 1997, American Heart Association.)

surgery in patients without CAD who have estimated aortic valve areas that are small but who have only a very small gradient with significantly diminished left ventricular function. In many patients it is neccessary to take into consideration not only the estimated valve area, but also the ventricular function and stroke volume. Occasionally, a myocardial biopsy may help to determine the cause of the substantial left ventricular dysfunction.

**R.C. Schlant, M.D.**

## Aortic Valve Replacement in Patients 80 Years of Age and Older: Survival and Cause of Death Based on 1100 Cases: Collective Results From the UK Heart Valve Registry

Asimakopoulos G, Edwards M-B, Taylor KM (Hammersmith Hosp, London)
*Circulation* 96:3403–3408, 1997                                1–11

*Objective.*—As the population ages, the number of patients 80 years of age and older undergoing aortic valve replacement (AVR) is increasing. There are few reports evaluating outcome in these patients. The survival and cause of death after AVR in patients 80 years of age and older was evaluated by analyzing data extracted from the United Kingdom Heart Valve Registry (UKHVR).

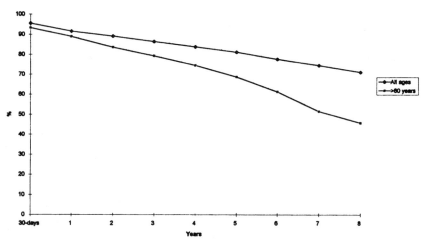

FIGURE 2.—Actuarial survival in patients undergoing aortic valve replacement: 80 years of age and older vs. all ages. (Courtesy of Asimakopoulos G, Edwards M-B, Taylor KM: Aortic valve replacement in patients 80 years of age and older. Survival and cause of death based on 1100 cases: Collective results from the UK Heart Valve Registry. *Circulation* 96:3403–3408. Reproduced with permission from *Circulation.* Copyright 1997, American Heart Association.)

*Methods.*—Actuarial survival, 30-day mortality, and cause of death were established using UKHVR data on 1100 patients (55.5% female), aged 80 to 93 years, who underwent AVR between January 1986 and December 1995. Patients were followed for an average of 38.9 months. Predictors of survival were determined.

*Results.*—The 30-day mortality rate (6.6%) was similar for men and women 80 years of age and older, and most deaths resulted from cardiac causes. The 30-day mortality rate for patients in all age groups was significantly lower (4.3%) (Fig 2). After 30 days, most deaths resulted from malignancy, stroke, and pneumonia. Overall actuarial survivals at 1, 3, 5, and 8 years were 89%, 79.3%, 68.7%, and 45.8%. Men had a significantly lower survival rate than women (male-female hazard ratio, 1.3); however, this was probably expected because men have a shorter life expectancy than women. Bioprosthetic valves were used in 969 patients (88%) and mechanical valves in 131 patients (12%). There was no significant 30-day mortality rate difference between groups. Bioprosthetic valves are recommended for this older population because they do not require lifetime anticoagulation and a slower rate of structural deterioration. Limitations of the study include the unknown number of patients who had concomitant coronary artery bypass grafting and the unknown preoperative clinical status of the patients.

*Conclusion.*—The selection criteria for this age group results in a satisfactory 30-day outcome and a moderate medium-term survival period.

▶ These results from the UKHVR represent 1 of the largest reported series of patients 80 years of age and older undergoing aortic valve replacement. Considering the age of the patients and their co-morbid conditions, the results are quite striking, and, they confirm previous studies from the United States and Europe. It should be noted that the range in patient age was 80 to 93 years and that 55.5% of the patients were female. Unfortunately, we do not have good data on how many of the patients may have had concurrent coronary artery bypass surgery, and we do not have good data on the patients' symptoms.

R.C. Schlant, M.D.

---

**Optimizing Timing of Surgical Correction in Patients With Severe Aortic Regurgitation: Role of Symptoms**
Klodas E, Enriquez-Sarano M, Tajik AJ, et al (Mayo Clinic and Mayo Found, Rochester, Minn)
*J Am Coll Cardiol* 30:746–752, 1997                                      1–12

---

*Objective.*—There is no general agreement on the timing of aortic valve replacement for aortic regurgitation (AR), primarily because of the lack of definitive long-term studies of postsurgical outcome. The outcome of patients who underwent surgical correction of severe isolated AR between 1980 and 1989 was examined.

*Methods.*—Surgical correction (N = 9) or replacement (N = 280) in AR was performed on patients with grade III or IV regurgitation. Patients having associated aortic stenosis or concomitant mitral or tricuspid valve repair or replacement were excluded. There were 161 functional class I/II patients (86 women), with an average age of 50 years), and 128 functional class III/IV patients (70 women) with an average age of 61 years. Patients were followed until 1994 or death. The effect of preoperative features on postoperative survival was assessed.

*Results.*—Class III/IV patients were more likely than class I/II patients to be female and older and to have a higher creatinine level, hypertension, diabetes mellitus, myocardial infarction, and significant coronary artery disease. They were also more likely to require concomitant coronary artery bypass grafting at the time of aortic valve replacement. Mortality rates for class I/II and class III/IV patients were 1.2% and 7.8%, respectively. Class I/II patients had significantly higher 5- and 10-year survival rates than class III/IV patients (Fig 1). Postoperative survival in class I/II patients was similar to that of age- and sex-matched controls, whereas survival in class III/IV patients was significantly worse. Preoperative symptom status was the only significant independent predictor of postoperative mortality (OR, 5.5) and long-term postoperative survival (hazard ratio, 1.81) according to multivariate analysis.

*Conclusion.*—In patients with severe AR, functional class III/IV symptoms increase postoperative mortality and decrease long-term survival. The presence of class II symptoms should be a strong inducement for performing surgical correction.

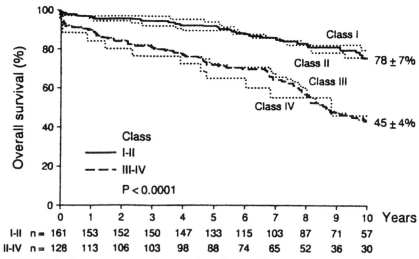

FIGURE 1.—Long-term postoperative survival stratified according to preoperative symptoms. Patients with functional class III or IV symptoms experienced significantly worse survival than patients with class I or II symptoms. (Reprinted with permission from the American College of Cardiology courtesy of Klodas E, Enriquez-Sarano M, Tajik AJ, et al: Optimizing timing of surgical correction in patients with severe aortic regurgitation: Role of symptoms. *J Am Coll Cardiol* 30:746–752, 1997).

▶ Most previous studies of patients with AR have emphasized changes found at cardiac catherization or on echocardiography. This paper clearly shows that severe class III or class IV symptoms are independent risk factors for immediate and long-term postoperative mortality. When evaluated by echocardiography, an end-systolic left ventricular diameter of 55 mm or greater is generally a good indication for aortic valve replacement. In a longitudal study of 127 patients with aortic regurgitation, Padial[1] found that both mild and severe aortic regurgitation represented a progressive disease. It was significant that there appeared to be more progression in patients with more severe aortic regurgitation.

**R.C. Schlant, M.D.**

*Reference*

1. Padial LR, Oliver A, Vivaldi M, et al. Doppler echocardiographic assessment of progression of aortic regurgitation. *Am J Cardiol* 80:306–314, 1997.

## Echocardiographic Assessment of Commissural Calcium: A Simple Predictor of Outcome After Percutaneous Mitral Balloon Valvotomy

Cannan CR, Nishimura RA, Reeder GS, et al (Mayo Clinic and Mayo Found, Rochester, Minn)

*J Am Coll Cardiol* 29:175–180, 1997                                             1–13

*Introduction.*—Percutaneous mitral balloon valvotomy is performed in patients with severely symptomatic mitral stenosis, but its immediate success rate and long-term outcome depend on the underlying mitral valve morphologic characteristics. A low mitral valve "score," based on leaflet thickening, calcification, mobility, and degree of subvalvular fusion (Abascal score) appears to predict immediate success and a low rate of restenosis. Not all patients with a low score, however, do well, and some with higher mitral valve scores have a good outcome. The predictive value of the presence or absence of calcium in mitral valve commissures by 2-dimensional echocardiography was examined in 149 patients.

*Methods.*—The study group consisted of consecutive patients who underwent percutaneous mitral balloon valvotomy at the Mayo Clinic between September 1987 and June 1995. They were evaluated retrospectively for mitral valve morphology scores determined at baseline echocardiography and for calcification in each of the medial and lateral commissures. Patients were contacted by telephone every 6 months, and most were seen yearly for clinical follow-up. End points at follow-up were death, New York Heart Association functional class, repeat percutaneous mitral balloon valvotomy, and mitral valve replacement.

*Results.*—The average patient age was 54.6, and the mean follow-up period was 1.8 years. Compared with patients with an Abascal score >8, there was a trend toward improved survival and freedom from repeat procedures at 36 months among patients with an Abascal score of 8. There was a significant difference in outcome, however, between patients with and without commissural calcium (Fig 2). Survival at 36 months free of death, repeat valvotomy, or mitral valve replacement was 80% in those without commissural calcium vs. 40% in those with commissural calcium. In a model with Abascal score and commissural calcification and their interaction, the only significant variable was calcification.

*Discussion.*—Commissural splitting is the dominant mechanism by which mitral valve stenosis is relieved by percutaneous mitral balloon valvotomy, and the presence of commissural calcium is a strong predictor of outcome after this procedure. This simple determination can help to identify patients who would benefit from percutaneous mitral balloon valvotomy and predict survival and the need for repeat valvotomy or mitral valve replacement after the procedure.

▶ Percutaneous mitral balloon valvotomy is now the procedure of choice in patients who have appropriate findings by echocardiography and who are

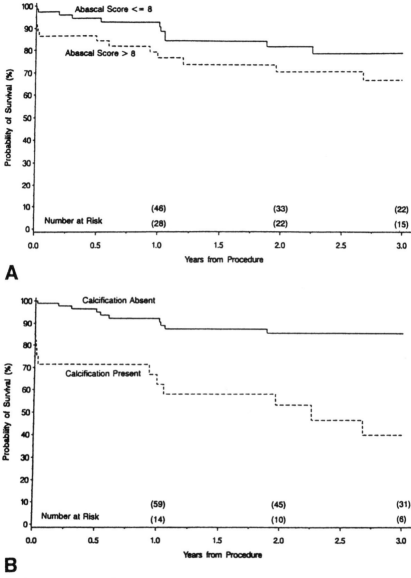

**FIGURE 2.—A,** actuarial survival curves with freedom from death, mitral valve replacement or repeat percutaneous mitral balloon valvuloplasty for patients with Abascal scores ≤8 (*solid line*) or >8 (*dashed line*) (p = NS). **B,** actuarial survival curves with freedom from death, mitral valve replacement or repeat valvuloplasty for patients without commissural calcium (*solid line*) versus those patients with calcium in a commissure (*dashed line*) (P < 0.001). (Courtesy of Cannan CR, Nishimura RA, Reeder GS, et al: Echocardiographic assessment of commissural calcium: A simple predictor of outcome after percutaneous mitral balloon valvotomy. *J Am Coll Cardiol* 29:175–180, 1997. Reprinted with permission from the American College of Cardiology [*Journal of the American College of Cardiology*, 1997, vol. 29, pages 175–180]).

seen at centers with physicians who have experience and special skills in performing this procedure.[1, 2]

**R.C. Schlant, M.D.**

*References*

1. Bahl VK, Chandra S, Jhamb DK, et al: Balloon mitral valvotomy: comparison between antegrade Inoue and retrograde non-transeptal techniques. *Eur Heart J* 18:1765–1770, 1997.
2. Orrange SE, Kawanishi DT, Lopez BM, et al: Actuarial outcome after catheter balloon commissurotomy in patients with mitral stenosis. *Circulation* 95:382–389, 1997.

---

**Valvular Heart Disease Associated With Fenfluramine-Phentermine**
Connolly HM, Crary JL, McGoon MD, et al (Mayo Clinic and Mayo Found, Rochester, Minn)
*N Engl J Med* 337:581–588, 1997                                              1–14

---

*Background.*—Fenfluramine and phentermine are prescription medications that have been individually approved by the Food and Drug Administration (FDA) as appetite suppressants for the treatment of obesity. Although not approved by the FDA for use in combination, these drugs are frequently prescribed together to reduce the dosages of each agent required and thereby lower side effects. In 1996, the total number of prescriptions for these agents exceeded 18 million in the United States alone. This article describes 24 cases of unusual valvular disease in patients taking fenfluramine-phentermine.

*Study Design.*—All patients were identified during the course of routine evaluation. Because more patients with similar clinical features were identified and an association was suspected, other physicians were consulted about cases in their own practices.

*Findings.*—A group of 24 women were identified with unusual valvular morphology and regurgitation by echocardiography, approximately 1 year after the initiation of fenfluramine-phentermine therapy. Pulmonary hypertension was detected in 8 of these women. Cardiac surgical intervention was required in 5 patients. At operation, the heart valves were observed to have a glistening white appearance. Histopathologic findings included plaquelike encasement of the leaflets and chordal structures with intact valve architecture (Figs 3 and 4). These features were similar to those seen in carcinoid or ergotamine-induced valve disease.

*Conclusions.*—These cases suggest that the combination of fenfluramine-phentermine commonly prescribed in the United States as an appetite suppressant may be associated with valvular heart disease. Prospective studies will be required to validate this observation. The mechanism of injury and the frequency of the association have not been determined. Nevertheless, patients considering drug treatment for obesity should be informed of the potential serious adverse effects of this drug combination.

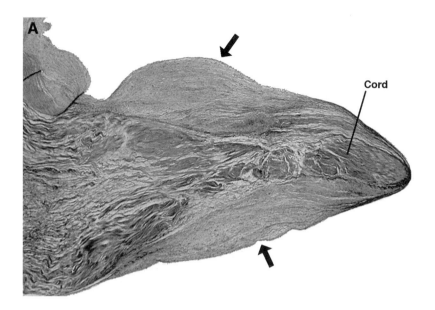

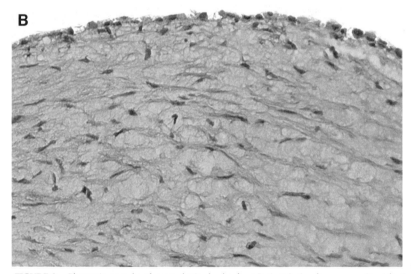

FIGURE 3.—Photomicrographs of resected mitral valve from Patient 2. **A,** a low-power view (elastic–van Gieson stain, ×36) shows intact valve architecture with "stuck-on" plaques (*arrows*). **B,** a high-power view (hematoxylin and eosin, ×360) shows proliferative myofibroblasts in an abundant extracellular matrix. (Reprinted by permission of The New England Journal of Medicine, from Connolly HM, Crary JL, McGoon MD, et al: Valvular heart disease associated with fenfluramine-phentermine. *N Engl J Med* 337:581–588, 1997. Copyright 1997, Massachusetts Medical Society. All rights reserved.)

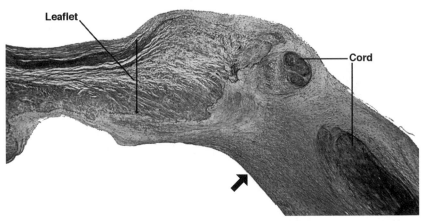

**FIGURE 4.**—Photomicrograph of resected mitral valve from Patient 3. A low-power view (elastic–van Gieson stain, ×36) shows intact leaflet and tendinous cord, with encasement by proliferative plaque (*arrow*). (Reprinted by permission of The New England Journal of Medicine, from Connolly HM, Crary JL, McGoon MD, et al: Valvular heart disease associated with fenfluramine-phentermine. *N Engl J Med* 337:581–588, 1997. Copyright 1997, Massachusetts Medical Society. All rights reserved.)

▶ This is one of the seminal reports of a possible relationship between the appetite suppressants fenfluramine-phentermine and valvular heart disease. In a letter to the editor in the same issue, Graham and Green from the Food and Drug Administration reported an additional 28 patients.[1]

Further studies are necessary to determine whether there is a real relationship between taking the two medications to control weight and the development of predominantly mitral, aortic, and tricuspid valve disease and to determine its mechanism. The use of fenfluramine and phentermine has previously been reported to be associated with fatal pulmonary hypertension.[2]

**R.C. Schlant, M.D.**

*References*

1. Graham DJ, Green L: Further cases of valvular heart disease associated with fenfluramine-phentermine (letter). *N Engl J Med* 337:635, 1997.
2. Mark EJ, Patalas ED, Chang HT, et al: Fatal pulmonary hypertension associated with short-term use of fenfluramine and phentermine. *N Engl J Med* 337:602–606, 1997.

## Prevention of Bacterial Endocarditis: Recommendations by the American Heart Association

Dajani AS, Taubert KA, Wilson W, et al (American Heart Association, Dallas, Tex; American Dental Association, Chicago; Infectious Diseases Society of America, Alexandria, Va; et al)
*JAMA* 277:1794–1801, 1997
1–15

*Introduction.*—Although relatively uncommon, endocarditis is a life-threatening disease and prevention is very important. Persons with underlying structural cardiac defects who develop bacteremia with organisms likely to cause endocarditis are the most likely to develop endocarditis. Guidelines for the prevention of bacterial endocarditis have been updated, but they are not intended as the standard of care or as a substitute for clinical judgment. These new recommendations are an update of the 1990 recommendations and incorporate opinions voiced by national and international experts at endocarditis meetings.

*Methods.*—The American Heart Association appointed an ad hoc writing group with liaison members representing the American Dental Association, the Infectious Diseases Society of America, the American Society for Gastrointestinal Endoscopy, and the American Academy of Pediatrics. They analyzed relevant literature regarding procedure-related endocarditis, results of prophylactic studies in animal models of endocarditis, in vitro susceptibility data of pathogens causing endocarditis, and retrospective analyses of human endocarditis patients in terms of antibiotic prophylaxis usage patterns and apparent prophylaxis failures.

*Changes.*—The major changes in the guidelines emphasize that most cases of endocarditis are not attributed to an invasive procedure: that based on potential outcome, endocarditis develops, cardiac conditions are stratified into high-, moderate-, and negligible-risk categories; prophylaxis recommendations are more clearly specified in procedures that may cause bacteremia; for patients with mitral valve prolapse, an algorithm was developed to more clearly define when prophylaxis is recommended; the initial amoxicillin dose for oral or dental procedures is reduced to 2 g, and a follow-up antibiotic dose is no longer recommended for oral or dental procedures; for penicillin-allergic individuals, erythromycin is no longer recommended, but clindamycin and other alternatives, are offered; and the prophylactic regimens have been simplified for gastrointestinal or genitourinary procedures.

*Conclusion.*—The changes were instituted to improve practitioner and patient compliance, approach more uniform worldwide recommendations, reduce cost and potential gastrointestinal adverse effect, and define when prophylaxis is or is not recommended.

▶ These updated guidelines should be known and available to all health care providers.

**R.C. Schlant, M.D.**

## Role of Echocardiography in Evaluation of Patients With *Staphylococcus aureus* Bacteremia: Experience in 103 Patients

Fowler VG Jr, Li J, Corey GR, et al (Duke Univ, Durham, NC)
*J Am Coll Cardiol* 30:1072–1078, 1997                    1–16

*Objective.*—Infective endocarditis (IE) is difficult to diagnose in patients with *Staphylococcus aureus* bacteremia (SAB). Because transesophageal echocardiography (TEE) is superior to transthoracic echocardiography (TTE) for diagnosing IE, TEE may be diagnostically and prognostically useful in patients with SAB. The relative values of TTE and TEE for detecting IE was evaluated prospectively in a cohort of 103 consecutive patients with SAB.

*Methods.*—Between September 1, 1994 and January 1, 1996, TTE and TEE were performed in 103 patients at Duke University Medical Center. Patients had fever and at least 1 positive blood culture. Patients were followed for 12 weeks.

*Results.*—The source of bacteremia was identified in 94% of patients. Predisposing heart disease was found in 41% of patients, but only 7% had clinical evidence of IE. Five had peripheral emboli and 2 had murmurs. Four patients had a history of IE. Transthoracic echocardiography revealed anatomical abnormalities in 33 patients, was indeterminate in 19, and positive for vegetations in 7. Transesophageal echocardiography was significantly more sensitive than TTE in identifying vegetations. Transesophageal echocardiography also found 2 abscesses, 1 perforation, and 1 new valvular regurgitation undetected by TTE. Infective endocarditis diagnosis based on TTE findings was possible in 7 patients for a sensitivity of 32% and a negative predictive value of 81%. Infective endocarditis diagnosis based on TEE findings was positive in 19 patients (73%) for a sensitivity of 100% and a specificity of 99%. Infection was cured in 77% of patients with IE and in 75% of patients without IE. Significantly more patients with IE than patients without IE died (15% vs. 1.3%). Treatment failure occurred in 19% of patients wih IE and in 13% of patients without IE.

*Conclusion.*—Infective endocarditis is common in patients with SAB and results in increased mortality. Transesophageal endocardiography is more sensitive and specific than TTE for diagnosing IE and detecting other complications.

▶ We would agree to the authors' conclusion that TEE is now part of the early evaluation of virtually all patients with SAB. It is often the best way to diagnose IE.

**R.C. Schlant, M.D.**

### Role of Transthoracic and Transesophageal Echocardiography in Predicting Embolic Events in Patients With Active Infective Endocarditis Involving Native Cardiac Valves

De Castro S, Magni G, Beni S, et al ("La Sapienza" Univ of Rome; Tufts Univ, Boston)

*Am J Cardiol* 80:1030–1034, 1997                                                    1–17

*Objective.*—The role of echocardiography in predicting embolic events is controversial. The introduction of transesophageal echocardiography (TEE) and transthoracic echocardiography (TTE) has improved detection of vegetations and lesions. Whether the distinctive characteristics of vegetative lesions detected by TTE and TEE predict embolic risk was examined in a review of echocardiograms of 75 patients with a diagnosis of acute infective endocarditis.

*Methods.*—Two experienced echocardiographers without knowledge of the patients' clinical histories independently evaluated the site, length, width, mobility, and echodensity of vegetations shown on TTE and TEE and compared them with subsequent embolic events. Subsequent embolic events were defined by an independent investigator blinded to echocardiographic findings. Interobserver agreement was compared statistically.

*Results.*—Of 57 patients, 25 (44%) had at least 1 embolic event involving peripheral arteries (N = 10), CNS (N = 8), lungs (N = 6), and coronary artery (N = 1). Patients with and without emboli did not differ with regard to age, sex, site of valve involvement, predisposing factors, pathogen involved, need for surgery, or death. Rheumatic fever was the most common predisposing factor (N = 19). Transthoracic echocardiography and TEE detected vegetations in 46 of 57 and in 54 of 57 patients, respectively (Table 4). Transesophageal echocardiography detected 8 vegetations in addition to the 46 detected by TTE. Vegetation size was not predictive of an embolic event. Observers agreed on the presence of vegetations in 86% of TTE reviews and in 91% of TEE reviews.

TABLE 4.—Comparison Between Morphologic Characteristics of Vegetations Detected by Transthoracic and Transesophageal Echocardiography and Risk of Embolism

| Features | TTE | | TEE | |
|---|---|---|---|---|
| | Emboli | No Emboli | Emboli | No Emboli |
| L (mm) | 13.1 ± 4.5 | 12.0 ± 6.0 | 14.7 ± 5.0 | 13.7 ± 5.4 |
| W (mm) | 4.0 ± 0.9 | 4.3 ± 2.1 | 4.4 ± 1.9 | 4.6 ± 1.7 |
| Mobility | 18 (72%) | 21 (65%) | 20 (80%) | 26 (81%) |
| Low echogenicity | 10 (40%) | 7 (22%) | 9 (36%) | 10 (31%) |

*Note:* Emboli refers to patients with subsequent embolic events (N = 25); Low echogenicity refers to patients with low echogenicity vegetations; No Emboli refers to patients with no subsequent embolic events (N = 32).

*Abbreviations: TTE,* transthoracic echocardiography; *TEE,* transesophageal echocardiography; *L,* length of vegetation; *W,* width of vegetation.

(Reprinted by permission of the publisher from De Castro S, Magni G, Beni S, et al: Role of transthoracic and transesophageal echocardiography in predicting embolic events in patients with active infective endocarditis involving native cardiac valves. *American Journal of Cardiology* 80:1030–1034, copyright 1997 by Excerpta Medica, Inc.)

*Conclusion.*—Neither TTE or TEE can be used to predict subsequent embolic events on the basis of observed vegetation characteristics in patients with infective endocarditis.

▶ There are a number of studies that have shown a correlation between the size of a vegetation in the likelihood of an embolic event. On the other hand, there have also been several studies that, like this one, have not found any good correlation. At present, I am inclined to think that there is a correlation, but it is rather weak.

**R.C. Schlant, M.D.**

---

**Fungal Prosthetic Valve Endocarditis in 16 Patients: An 11-Year Experience in a Tertiary Care Hospital**
Melgar GR, Nasser RM, Gordon SM, et al (Cleveland Clinic Found, Ohio)
*Medicine* 76:94–103, 1997                                                       1–18

---

*Objective.*—Mortality from fungal prosthetic heart valve endocarditis (PVE) is higher than from bacterial prosthetic heart valve endocarditis and relapses are not uncommon. A review of 16 patients with fungal PVE at the Cleveland Clinic Foundation and a report of a patient who survived 3 episodes of *Candida parapsilosis* PVE were presented, and 5 illustrative cases were discussed.

*Methods.*—Between January 1985 and March 1996, 6,661 prosthetic heart valves were implanted. Sixteen patients experienced 19 episodes of fungal PVE presenting as a variety of manifestations. Patients were followed for from 5 months to 16 years.

*Results.*—The average age of the 16 patients (31% female) was 51 years (range, 27 to 71 years). Predisposing factors for fungal PVE included central IV catheter (50%), previous bacterial endocarditis (38%), prolonged antibiotics (25%), total parenteral nutrition (12%), and immunosuppression (12%). Biologic prostheses accounted for 71% of the cases of fungal PVE and valves in the aortic position for 76%. *Candida* spp. caused 14 of 16 infections. The interval between valve replacement and infection onset ranged from 8 days to 3.4 years. The most common manifestations of infection were fever (83%), new regurgitative murmur (47%), major embolic events (32%), and lower extremity embolism (16%). Transesophageal echocardiography was more sensitive than transthoracic echocardiography (100% vs. 60%) in detecting lesions. Patients were treated with amphotericin B and reoperated. Seven patients experienced major embolic complications. One patient died before surgery. Two patients had 3 relapses as many as 9 years after the previous episode. Ten patients were still alive at a median follow-up of 4.5 years.

*Conclusion.*—Patients with fungal PVE should be followed long term because of the risk of relapse.

▶ The results of this study are very sobering. Of particular note is the greater sensitivity of transesophageal echocardiography compared with transthoracic echocardiography in detecting lesions caused by fungal PVE. The best results were obtained in patients who had valve replacement surgery plus amphotericin B. It was noted that late relapses could occur up to 9 years after the preceding episode.

**R.C. Schlant, M.D.**

**Surgical Treatment of Endocarditis**
Moon MR, Stinson EB, Miller DC (Stanford Univ, Calif)
*Prog Cardiovasc Dis* 40:239–264, 1997                                     1–19

*Objective.*—The indications for surgical intervention, various treatment options, and the expected long- and short-term outcome after valve replacement in patients with valve endocarditis were discussed.

*Indications.*—Indications include severe congestive heart failure. Patients with persistent sepsis require surgical intervention, although a positive valve culture or gram stain at surgery predicts a poor long-term outcome (Table 1). Patients with streptococcal native valve endocarditis can be cured with antibiotics. Transesophageal echocardiography can rule out deep tissue infection or microabscesses, and transthoracic echocardiography can be used to detect progressive valve dysfunction. Peripheral emboli arising from vegetations require emergency surgical intervention. Vegetations without emboli should not automatically trigger emergency surgery. In 13% of patients having an embolic event during treatment, 14% had vegetations, 11% had no vegetations, and 15% had an indeterminate vegetation status. Vegetation size was not a predictor of an embolic event and the presence of vegetations after clinical healing was not pre-

TABLE 1.—Micro-organisms Responsible for Native and Prosthetic Valve Endocarditis

|  | Native Valve (%) | Early Prosthetic (<2 mo) (%) | Late Prosthetic (>2 mo) (%) |
|---|---|---|---|
| Streptococcus | 65 | 5 | 35 |
| α-hemolytic | 35 | <5 | 25 |
| Group D | 25 | <5 | <5 |
| Staphylococcus | 25 | 50 | 30 |
| Aureus | 23 | 20 | 10 |
| Epidermitis | <5 | 30 | 20 |
| Gram-negative bacillus | <5 | 20 | 10 |
| Fungus | <5 | 10 | 5 |

Adapted with permission of The McGraw-Hill Companies from Durack DT: Infective and noninfective endocarditis, in Schlant RC, Alexander RW, (eds): *Hurst's The Heart,* ed 8. San Francisco, McGraw-Hill, 1994, pp 1681–1709.
(Courtesy of Moon MR, Stinson EB, Miller DC: Surgical treatment of endocarditis. *Prog Cardiovasc Dis* 40:239–264, 1997).

dictive of late complications in the absence of valve dysfunction. Surgery when cerebral embolization is present increases the risk of hemorrhage, and a single embolus without a large, mobile vegetation does not necessarily require surgery. If the infection can be controlled without leading to congestive heart failure, surgery should be postponed for 2 or 3 weeks, or after a hemorrhagic brain infarct, as long as possible. Extravalvular extension of the infective process can be identified echocardiographically with a sensitivity and specificity of 85% when certain valve characteristics are observed or when conduction disturbances are present. Surgical intervention should be considered if a first degree block persists or extends to a second or third degree block. Progressive renal dysfunction requires surgical intervention because of attendant glomerulonephritis in 22% to 24% of patients.

*Results.*—Mortality after surgical treatment of native valve endocarditis (NVE) was 12%, and after prosthetic valve endocarditis (PVE) was 25%. Ten-year survival rates were 44% to 70% for NVE and 24% to 55% for PVE. Surgical techniques were described for patients with mitral valve endocarditis, aortic valve endocarditis, and tricuspid valve endocarditis. A minimum of 4 to 6 weeks of species-specific antibiotic treatment is recommended. For patients with positive intraoperative cultures, at least an additional 4 to 6 weeks of antibiotic therapy is recommended, especially in patients with PVE.

*Conclusion.*—The indications for surgery change as more is learned about endocarditis and about the procedures used to treat infections. Techniques and strategies must be constantly re-evaluated.

▶ As I read this article, I noted that little attention was paid to acute endocarditis in drug addicts or to the problem of endocarditis of the triscupid valve. In the past, some surgeons have excised the triscupid valve in what was thought to be curative surgery. Unfortunately, virtually all of these patients later had to have tricuspid prosthetic valves inserted.

**R.C. Schlant, M.D.**

---

**Guidelines for Management of Left-sided Prosthetic Valve Thrombosis: A Role for Thrombolytic Therapy**
Lengyel M, Fuster V, Keltai M, et al (Hungarian Inst of Cardiology, Budapest; Mount Sinai Med Ctr, New York; Semmelweis Med School, Budapest, Hungary, et al)
*J Am Coll Cardiol* 30:1521–1526, 1997                    1–20

---

*Objective.*—Because the use of thrombolysis for left-sided prosthetic valve thrombosis increases the risk of cerebral thromboembolism, its use in low-risk patients is controversial. A consensus conference was convened to formalize guidelines for management of left-sided aortic and mitral prosthetic valve thrombosis that take into account the patient's functional class, left ventricular function, and overall operative risk.

TABLE 2.—Contraindications to Thrombolysis

Absolute contraindications
  Active internal bleeding
  History of hemorrhagic stroke
  Recent cranial trauma or neoplasm
  Blood pressure > 200/120 mm Hg
  Diabetic hemorrhagic retinopathy
Relative contraindications
  Recent (within 10 days) gastrointestinal bleeding
  Recent (within 10 days) puncture of noncompressible vessels
  Recent (within 2 mo) nonhemorrhagic stroke
  Infective endocarditis
  Uncontrolled severe hypertension
  Large thrombus in left atrium or on prosthesis
  Recent (within 2 wk) major operation or trauma
  Known bleeding diathesis
  Previous exposure to streptokinase or APSAC (contraindication to reuse
    any streptokinase-containing agent)

*Abbreviation: APSAC,* anistreplase (anisoylated plasminogen streptokinase activator complex).
(Reprinted with permission from the American College of Cardiology, courtesy of Lengyel M, Fuster V, Keltai M, et al: Guidelines for management of left-sided prosthetic valve thrombosis: A role for thrombolytic therapy. *J Am Coll Cardiol* 30:1521–1526, 1997).

*Diagnosis of Left-Sided Prosthetic Valve Thrombosis.*—Doppler echocardiography is used to assess hemodynamic variables.

*Indications and Contraindications for Thrombolysis.*—Thrombolytic treatment is recommended for critically ill patients in functional class III or IV when surgery is contraindicated. Patients in functional class I or II have a relatively low surgical mortality rate compared with an embolic risk of 12% to 17% from thrombolysis. In 1 study of 32 functional class I or II patients, thrombolytic therapy had an 88% success rate. The lowest surgical mortality rate in a similar group was 5%. Thrombolysis is contraindicated under certain circumstances (Table 2).

*Thrombolytic Agent, Dosage Duration, and Monitoring of Treatment.*—Streptokinase (250,000-U bolus administered in 30 minutes followed by an infusion of 100,000 U/hr and urokinase (4,400 U/kg/hr) are the most commonly used and least expensive fibrinolytic agents. Duration of administration can be determined using Doppler echocardiography to monitor hemodynamic improvement.

*Management of Complications.*—Therapy should be continued until a peripheral embolism is dissolved. Persistent symptoms require embolectomy. Thrombolytic therapy should be stopped if stroke symptoms appear. Computed tomography can be used to rule out brain hemorrhage. Minor bleeding can be controlled by pressure at the site. Bleeding can be reversed with fresh frozen plasma or factor VII therapy. Concurrent anticoagulant treatment is not recommended.

*Conclusion.*—Standard recommendations call for anticoagulation at an international normalized ratio of between 2.5 and 3.5, followed by aspirin, heparin, or warfarin for high-risk patients with left-sided prosthetic valve thrombosis. Doppler echocardiography should be performed monthly for the first 6 months and at 6-month intervals thereafter.

▶ It should be emphasized that these excellent consensus recommendations suggest the use of thrombolytic therapy only for patients who have a high surgical risk for valve replacement or for patients with a contraindication to operation. There is about a 12% to 17% risk of arterial embolism associated with thrombolytic therapy.

**R.C. Schlant, M.D.**

**Circulating Cardiac-specific Autoantibodies as Markers of Autoimmunity in Clinical and Biopsy-proven Myocarditis**
Caforio ALP, and the Myocarditis Treatment Trial Investigators (St George's Hosp Med School, London; Padua Univ, Italy)
*Eur Heart J* 18:270–275, 1997                                                    1–21

*Objective.*—Dilated cardiomyopathy may be an autoimmune disease. Because myocarditis precedes dilated cardiomyopathy in some patients, clinical and experimental attributes imply that, in these patients, myocarditis and dilated cardiomyopathy may represent the acute and chronic stages of a progressive autoimmune disease of the myocardium. Indirect immunofluorescence and α-myosin–specific enzyme-linked immunosorbent assay (ELISA) were used to detect cardiac autoantibodies in sera from Myocarditis Treatment Trial patients.

*Methods.*—At least 4 biopsy specimens of endomyocardium were obtained from each of 53 patients (35 males) with an average age of 42 years, 24 of whom were given a diagnosis of myocarditis (Dallas criteria). Serum samples from patients, 270 normal controls, and 186 ischemic patients were tested by indirect immunofluorescence. Atrial tissue from patients and 203 normal controls was analyzed for anti-α-myosin antibodies using ELISA.

*Results.*—Cardiac autoantibodies (3 organ-specific, 5 cross-reactive 1 type, and 5 cross-reactive 2 type) were detected significantly more frequently in patients with myocarditis ($n = 13$) than in ischemic patients ($n = 11$) or controls ($n = 24$). Immunoglobulin G autoantibodies were found in all positive sera. Significantly more Dallas-positive than ischemic patients or controls had autoantibodies (33% vs. 6%, and 9%, respectively). More patients with myocarditis had abnormally high anti-α-myosin antibody levels compared with ischemic patients or controls (17% vs. 4% vs. 2%). Eighteen patients with myocarditis (34%) had positive immunofluorescence and/or abnormal ELISA results. The proportions of antibody-positive patients were similar in Dallas-negative and Dallas-positive groups. There was no correlation between antibody status and biopsy specimen features.

*Conclusion.*—The incidence of immune-mediated myocarditis in this study was 30%. Both Dallas-negative and Dallas-positive groups had similar proportions of antibody positive patients. Immunohistology techniques, autoantibody testing, and viral genome detection should be used to identify patients with autoimmune endocarditis.

▶ Results of this paper add significantly to the large number of studies suggesting that patients with myocarditis may have autoimmune mechanisms that result in dilated cardiomyopathy. Unfortunately, none of the studies has been clearly definitive. Another article in support of this hypothesis reports on a recent study by Arbustini et al.[1]

**R.C. Schlant, M.D.**

*Reference*

1. Arbustini E, Grasso M, Porcu E, et al: Enteroviral RNA and virus-like particles in the skeletal muscles of patients with idiopathic dilated cardiomyopathy. *Am J Cardiol* 80:1188–1193, 1997.

**Cardiac Autoantibodies in Dilated Cardiomyopathy Become Undetectable With Disease Progression**
Caforio ALP, Goldman JH, Baig MK, et al (St George's Hosp Med School, London; Univ of Padua, Italy)
*Heart* 77:62–67, 1997                                                          1–22

*Objective.*—Cardiac autoantibodies are detected in about one third of patients with dilated cardiomyopathy and in 15% to 20% of symptom-free relatives. Prospective antibody testing was performed in patients with dilated cardiomyopathy at diagnosis and at follow-up to determine the relationship of antibody to disease status.

*Methods.*—Immunofluorescence antibody testing was performed at diagnosis and at 1 to 74 months' follow-up in 110 patients (85 males), with an average age of 44 years, with dilated cardiomyopathy and in 301 control patients with cardiac disease other than dilated cardiomyopathy. Anti-α-myosin antibody titers were measured by enzyme-linked immunosorbent assay in 57 of the patients with dilated cardiomyopathy, 203 healthy controls, and 92 patients with coronary artery disease. Maximal symptom-limited exercise testing was performed in 71 patients who had demonstrated consistent maximal oxygen consumption.

*Results.*—Cardiac autoantibodies were significantly less common at follow-up (10%) than at baseline (25%). Mean anti-α-myosin antibody titers were significantly lower at follow-up (0.24) than at baseline (0.30). At baseline, 24% of patients with cardiomyopathy had abnormally high antibody titers, whereas at follow-up only 14% had abnormally high antibody titers. The 43 patients with normal results at baseline also had normal results at follow-up. Organ-specific antibody was detected in 28 patients with dilated cardiomyopathy (25%), whereas cross-reactive 1 type cardiac antibody was detected in 18 patients with dilated cardiomyopathy (16%). The proportion of patients with milder symptoms and greater exercise capacity was higher in those patients with organ-specific antibodies (25 patients or 89%) than in patients with cross-reactive antibodies (10 patients or 55%).

*Conclusion.*—Organ-specific autoantibodies become undetectable as the disease progresses. Detection of these antibodies at diagnosis may provide a marker of early disease. Patients with the antibody present at diagnosis had milder symptoms than did patients with cross-reactive 1 type antibody.

▶ This study provides additional support for the autoimmune mechanism in idiopathic dilated cardiomyopathy. It's noteworthy that only about 25% of the patients had positive antibodies at the time of diagnosis and that this significantly decreased during the period of follow-up of approximately 14 months. Ultimately, of course, it is hoped that one can diagnose and prevent the progression of the autoimmune myocardial damage.

**R.C. Schlant, M.D.**

## Myocarditis and Cardiomyopathy

### Cardiac Troponin T in Patients With Clinically Suspected Myocarditis
Lauer B, Niederau C, Kühl U, et al (Universitätsklinik für Kardiologie, Leipzig, Germany; Universität Düsseldorf, Germany; Universitätsklinikum Benjamin Franklin, Berlin; et al)
*J Am Coll Cardiol* 30:1354–1359, 1997                    1–23

*Objective.*—There is no screening variable that detects myocardial cell damage in patients with suspected myocarditis. Recently, an assay has been developed to detect cardiac troponin T (cTnT), an isoform specific to cardiac tissue. An investigation was conducted to determine whether measurement of serum levels of cTnT can provide sensitive evidence of myocardial damage in patients with clinically suspected myocarditis and whether increased levels of cTnT correlate with histologic and immunohistologic findings in endomyocardial biopsy specimens.

*Methods.*—Endomyocardial biopsy specimens were obtained from 80 patients (28 female), age 12–85 years, with suspected myocarditis and analyzed histologically and immunohistologically. Serum levels of cTnT, creatine kinase, and the MB isoform of CK were measured.

*Results.*—Serum levels of cTnT were elevated in 28 patients (35%), 26 of whom were given an immunohistologic and/or histologic diagnosis of myocarditis, Myocarditis was diagnosed in 23 patients (44%) with normal cTnT levels. Mean cTnT levels were significantly higher in patients with myocarditis than in those without (0.59 vs. 0.04 ng/mL). The sensitivity, specificity, positive predictive value, negative predictive value, and effectiveness of the cTnT assay for the histologic detection of myocarditis were 53%, 94%, 93%, 56%, and 69%, respectively. Histologic analysis showed myocarditis in 5 patients, all of whom had elevated cTnT levels, but did not show myocarditis in the remaining 23 with elevated cTnT levels. Immunohistologic analysis revealed myocarditis in 49 patients

(61%), including the 5 patients with positive histology, and no myocarditis in 31 (39%). Immunohistologic analysis was positive for myocarditis in 26 of 28 patients with elevated cTnT levels. In the 52 patients with normal cTnT levels, 23 patients (44%) had immunohistologic evidence of myocarditis, and 29 patients (56%) did not. The sensitivity, specificity, positive predictive value, negative predictive value, and effectiveness of the immunohistologic detection of myocarditis were 53%, 94%, 93%, 56%, and 69%, respectively.

*Conclusion.*—Serum cTnT levels can provide a measure of myocardial damage in some patients with suspected myocarditis and are highly predictive of myocarditis. Immunohistologic analysis appears to be a better diagnostic tool than histologic analysis for detection of myocardial damage from myocarditis.

▶ With the increased use of measurements of cTnT to diagnose recent acute myocardial infarction, it is important to recognize that cTnT can also be elevated by myocarditis. It has also been noted that myocarditis can cause elevations of cardiac troponin I.[1]

**R.C. Schlant, M.D.**

*Reference*

1. Smith SC, Ladenson JH, Mason JW, et al: Elevations of cardiac troponin I associated with myocarditis: Experimental and clinical correlates. *Circulation* 95:163–168, 1997.

---

**Viral Infection of the Myocardium in Endocardial Fibroelastosis: Molecular Evidence for the Role of Mumps Virus as an Etiologic Agent**
Ni J, Bowles NE, Kim Y-H, et al (Baylor College of Medicine, Houston)
*Circulation* 95:133–139, 1997                                    1–24

---

*Objective.*—Endocardial fibroelastosis (EFE) is usually found in children who are seen with signs of congestive heart failure. Idiopathic EFE has been thought to be secondary to viral myocarditis, although there has been little direct evidence of viral infection. A link has recently been established between mumps myocarditis and cardiomyopathy. The polymerase chain reaction was used to identify the viral genome in the myocardium of patients with myocarditis and dilated cardiomyopathy.

*Methods.*—Myocardial autopsy specimens obtained from 29 children, aged 26 weeks to 7 years, with EFE and congestive heart failure and from 65 control patients with congenital heart disease ($n = 53$) and hypertrophic cardiomyopathy ($n = 12$), were subjected to reverse transcriptase-polymerase chain reaction for detection of genomic nucleic acid of enterovirus, adenovirus, mumps, cytomegalovirus, parvovirus, influenza, and herpes simplex virus.

*Results.*—Mumps viral DNA was identified in 21 patients (72%), with 16 having viral RNA corresponding to the *P* gene, 8 with sequences of the

*NP* gene, and 3 with sequences of both. The remaining 8 patients carried adenovirus. Enterovirus was identified in 1 control patient.

*Conclusion.*—In this study, more than 70% of patients with viral myocarditis carried the mumps virus genome. All patients died. Endocardial fibroelastosis appears to be a consequence of mumps virus–induced myocarditis.

▶ This study shows the relationship between the common mumps virus and possible virus infection of the myocardium. A recent study from Japan presented evidence that there was a relationship between hepatitis C virus and the development of dilated cardiomyopathy.[1]

**R.C. Schlant, M.D.**

*Reference*

1. Okabe M, Fukuda K, Arakawa K, et al: Chronic variant myocarditis associated with hepatitis C virus infection. *Circulation* 96:22–24, 1997.

---

**Persistence of Restrictive Left Ventricular Filling Pattern in Dilated Cardiomyopathy: An Ominous Prognostic Sign**
Pinamonti B, Zecchin M, Di Lenarda A, et al (Univ of Trieste, Italy)
*J Am Coll Cardiol* 29:604–612, 1997                                  1–25

---

*Objective.*—Whereas the restrictive filling pattern (RFP) characterized on Doppler echocardiography by a shortened transmitral E-wave deceleration time (EDT), is associated with a poor prognosis in patients with dilated cardiomyopathy (DCM), there is little information on the RFP changes during the course of the disease. The clinical and prognostic implications of the change in left ventricular (LV) filling pattern in DCM were evaluated.

*Methods.*—Doppler echocardiography was performed at baseline, after 3 months of treatment, and after 1 and 2 years of follow-up in a consecutive series of 110 patients with DCM (89 men) with an average age of 40 years. Patients with significant coronary stenosis and myocarditis were excluded. On the basis of Doppler LV filling pattern at baseline and at 3-month follow-up, patients with persistent RFP (EDT at baseline and at 3 months of less than 115 msec) were classified as group 1A ($n = 24$), patients with reversible RFP (EDT less than 115 msec at baseline and more than 115 msec at 3 months) were classified as group 1B ($n = 29$), and patients with non-RFP (EDT more than 115 msec at baseline and at 3 months) were classified as group 2 ($n = 57$).

*Results.*—At 3 months, there was a significant improvement in most clinical and Doppler parameters in all groups, but it was significantly more common in group 1B patients (46% at 1 year and 67% at 2 years) and in group 2 patients (40% at 1 year and 55% at 2 years) compared with group A (12% at 1 year and 0% at 2 years). The 1-, 2-, and 4-year survivals of patients with persistent RFP were significantly lower in group 1A (65%,

46%, and 13%, respectively) than in group 1B (100%, 100%, 96%, respectively) and group 2 (100%, 100%, and 97%, respectively). Significantly more group 1A patients than group 1B or 2 patients died or underwent heart transplantation. Whereas the sensitivity of baseline RFP was good, the 3-month RFP was significantly more specific and accurate.

*Conclusion.*—Whereas DCM patients with persistent RFP have high mortality and heart transplantation rates at 3 months, patients with reversible RFP improve and have a significantly higher survival rate. The change in LV filling over time with drug therapy predicts outcome in patients with DCM.

▶ Substantial data now document the poor prognosis of a "restrictive" LV filling pattern on Doppler echocardiography. I think we should be using this method fairly routinely to identify patients with cardiomyopathy who are at high risk.

**R.C. Schlant, M.D.**

---

**Idiopathic Giant-Cell Myocarditis—Natural History and Treatment**
Cooper LT, for the Multicenter Giant Myocarditis Study Group Investigators
(Univ of California, San Diego; Stanford Univ, Calif)
*N Engl J Med* 336:1860–1866, 1997                                      1–26

---

*Background.*—Idiopathic giant-cell myocarditis is rare and often fatal. The natural history of this disorder and the effects of treatment were determined in the current study using a multicenter database.

*Methods and Findings.*—Data were obtained on 63 patients with idiopathic giant-cell myocarditis seen at cardiovascular centers worldwide (Fig 3). The patients were 33 men and 30 women (mean age 42.6 years). Eighty-eight percent were white; 5%, black; 5%, Southeastern Asian or Indian; and 2%, Middle Eastern. Seventy-five percent of the patients presented with congestive heart failure; 14%, ventricular arrhythmia; and 5%, heart block. In some patients, however, the initial symptoms resembled those of acute myocardial infarction. Autoimmune disorders were also present in 19% of the patients. The rate of death or cardiac transplantation was 89%. Median survival was only 5.5 months from symptom onset. Mean survival was 12.3 months among the 22 patients treated with corticosteroids and cyclosporine, azathioprine, or a combination of the latter 2 drugs, compared with 3 months among the 30 patients given no immunosuppressive therapy. Twenty-six percent of the 34 patients undergoing heart transplantation had a giant-cell infiltrate in the transplanted heart, 1 of whom died of recurrent giant-cell myocarditis.

*Conclusions.*—Giant-cell myocarditis occurs in relatively young, primarily healthy adults. Without cardiac transplantation, patients usually die of heart failure and ventricular arrhythmia. Although fatal disease may recur, transplantation is the treatment of choice for most patients.

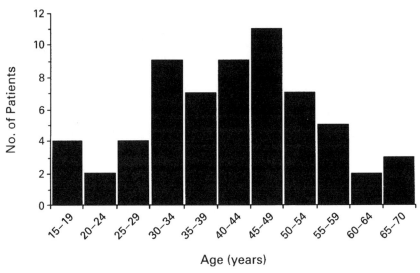

Age (years)

**FIGURE 3.**—Age at the time of onset of symptoms in 63 patients with giant-cell myocarditis. (Reprinted by permission of The New England Journal of Medicine, from Cooper LT, for the Multicenter Giant Myocarditis Study Group Investigators: Idiopathic giant-cell myocarditis — natural history and treatment. *N Engl J Med* 336:1860–1866, 1997. Copyright 1997, Massachusetts Medical Society. All rights reserved.)

▶ Most of us have never diagnosed idiopathic giant-cell myocarditis. Accordingly, it behooves us to try to become familiar with the findings in this study. This is particularly important because transplantation appears to be the treatment of choice.

**R.C. Schlant, M.D.**

---

**Spectrum of Alcohol-induced Myocardial Damage Detected by Indium-111–Labeled Monoclonal Antimyosin Antibodies**
Ballester M, Martí V, Carrió I, et al (Hosp de la Santa Creu i Sant Pau, Barcelona; Hosp Vall d'Hebrón, Barcelona)
*J Am Coll Cardiol* 29:160–167, 1997                                           1–27

---

*Objective.*—The impact of short- and long-term alcohol consumption on the myocardium was evaluated by studying the binding of $^{111}$In-labeled monoclonal antibodies that bind to myocardium only when the sarcolemma is disrupted and the intracellular myosin is exposed, indicating irreversible myocyte damage.

*Methods.*—Antimyosin antibody studies were performed in 56 patients (2 women), aged 25 to 73 years, with alcohol-induced dilated cardiomyopathy (group I); 15 male alcoholics, aged 29 to 45 years (group II); and 6 healthy fasting male volunteers, aged 20 to 32 years, before and after consuming 1.2 g/kg of alcohol in 30 minutes for 3 days (group III). Electrocardiographic, echocardiographic, and Doppler scans were performed. Monoclonal antimyosin antibody studies were performed 48 hours after injection of 2.0 mCi of $^{111}$In chloride.

*Results.*—Group I patients had consumed an average of 123 g/day of alcohol for an average of 21 years for a total intake of 914 kg. The average duration of heart disease symptoms was 46 months, the mean left ventricular end-diastolic diameter was 71 mm, and the mean ejection fraction was 28%. The prevalence and intensity of antimyosin uptake and heart-lung ratio (HLR) were significantly higher in the 28 active consumers (75% and 1.75, respectively), than in the 28 past consumers (32% and 1.49, respectively). Cessation of alcohol consumption and HLR were significantly inversely related. At restudy of 19 of 28 active consumers who stopped drinking showed a significantly improved left ventricular ejection fraction (from 30% to 43%), an unchanged diastolic diameter, and a reduction in HLR (from 71 to 67 mm). Parameters were unchanged in former consumers. Group II patients had consumed an average of 156 g of alcohol for an average of 17 years for a total alcohol intake of 978 kg. The mean left ventricular diastolic diameter was 46 mm and the ejection fraction averaged 77%. The HLR averaged 1.44, but uptake was shown in only 3 patients. The prevalence of antimyosin uptake was higher in the older members of group I, despite the higher daily dose of alcohol consumption in group II. No uptake was shown in group III controls.

*Conclusion.*—Patients with alcoholic-induced dilated cardiomyopathy who stop drinking have improved function and reduced or repaired myocardial damage. Antibody uptake varies both in patients with and those without cardiac involvement, suggesting a difference in susceptibility to alcohol. Short-term alcohol consumption does not appear to cause myocardial damage.

▶ This study documents improved ventricular function associated with alcohol withdrawal. Guillo et al.[1] also documented an improved long-term prognosis in patients with alcoholic cardiomyopathy and severe heart failure after total abstinence. Whereas there is now strong evidence that patients with alcoholic cardiomyopathy should abstain from all alcohol, for other patients, a very low level of alcohol intake appears to protect from coronary disease.[2]

**R.C. Schlant, M.D.**

*References*

1. Guillo P, Mansourati J, Maheu B, et al: Long-term prognosis of patients with alcoholic cardiomyopathy and severe heart failure after total abstinence. *Am J Cardiol* 79:1276–1278, 1997.
2. Klatsky AL, Armstrong MA, Fredman GD. Red wine, white wine, liquor, beer, and risks for coronary artery disease hospitalization. *Am J Cardiol* 80:416–420, 1997.

### Arrhythmogenic Right Ventricular Cardiomyopathy: A Still Underrecognized Clinic Entity

Thiene G, Basso C, Danieli GA, et al (Univ of Padua, Italy)
*Trends Cardiovasc Med* 7:84–90, 1997                          1–28

*Introduction.*—Arrhythmogenic right ventricular cardiomyopathy (ARVC) is one of the most frequent causes of electrical instability resulting in cardiac arrest and sudden death among young people. It is characterized by a thinning of the right ventricle (RV) and replacement of myocardium with a fatty or fibrofatty infiltrate. The etiology is unknown. It is not accompanied by significant cardiomegaly. Most patients with fibrofatty infiltration have inflow aneurysms in the inferior wall, severe atrophy, focal myocarditis, and myocardial thinning and scarring. Patients with transmural fatty infiltration of the RV free wall with scattered residual monocytes usually have a normal or thickened wall with no scarring or aneurysms. In almost half the patients, extension to the left ventricle can be shown, and 20% have interventricular septum involvement.

*Clinical Picture, Diagnosis, and Natural History.*—The pattern of ventricular tachycardia with left bundle branch block is characteristic of ARVC. Noninvasive radiologic methods provide the clearest demonstration of the RV, with MRI and myocardial scintigraphy allowing visualization of some of the manifestations of ARVC. The course of the disease runs from a concealed phase, in which sudden death may occur, through an overt electrical disorder phase characterized by ventricular arrhythmias and imminent cardiac arrest, to cardiomegaly and biventricular pump failure.

*Genetics.*—Arrhythmogenic right ventricular cardiomyopathy can be inherited as an autosomal dominant or autosomal recessive trait with loci on chromosomes 1 and 14.

*Etiopathogenesis.*—The disease has been postulated to be a developmental defect of the myocardium, a (probably genetic) metabolic or ultrastructural disorder, or the result of an injury and repair inflammatory process. Findings support the hypothesis that ARVC is a disease of the heart muscle with progressive loss of myocardial cells and replacement by fatty infiltrates.

*Research Perspectives.*—Research studies are examining the possibility that progressive disappearance of myocardial tissue is the result of apoptosis occurring not only in infancy, as in the normal heart, but also in childhood and adulthood.

▶ Some patients with this condition have responded well to catheter ablation of the arrhythmogenic focus in the RV. Other patients have had recurrence after ablation. In some patients, there has been some apparent involvement of the left ventricle as well as the right.

**R.C. Schlant, M.D.**

### Natural History of Hypertrophic Cardiomyopathy: A Benign or Progressive Disorder?

Spirito P, Maron BJ (Ospedala Sant'Andrea, La Spezia, Italy; Minneapolis Heart Inst Found, Minn)

*Cardiol Rev* 5:312–316, 1997                                    1–29

*Introduction.*—Hypertrophic cardiomyopathy (HCM) is usually an autosomal dominant disease characterized by left ventricular hypertrophy. In most cases, it is diagnosed using 2-dimensional echocardiography in the absence of other systemic or cardiac diseases.

*Perspectives on Natural History.*—The heterogeneity of the clinical course of HCM is the major obstacle to the assessment of prognosis; patients are sometimes asymptomatic throughout life, some have severe symptoms of heart failure, and others die suddenly and unexpectedly. Preliminary data on 274 patients with HMC showed an annual mortality rate of 1.3% over an average follow-up of 9 years, a mortality rate similar to that of the general population.

*Patients at High Risk.*—Although most patients with HCM have a benign clinical course, patients who have survived a cardiac arrest, patients with episodes of sustained ventricular tachycardia, and young patients with a malignant family history are at high risk and require aggressive therapy to prevent sudden death (Fig 1).

*Patients at Low Risk.*—The absence of variables with a high negative-predictive accuracy can be used to develop a profile of low-risk asymptomatic or mildly symptomatic patients. These patients should not engage in intense athletic activities.

*Conclusion.*—Although most patients with HCM will have a benign clinical course, some asymptomatic patients are at high risk of sudden death and must be identified and treated aggressively.

▶ Because of the marked variation in the pathophysiology of HCM, it has been difficult to obtain a good natural history. The reported natural history of HCM was probably biased because of tertiary referral bias. In many patients, however, the actual natural history is much more benign.

**R.C. Schlant, M.D.**

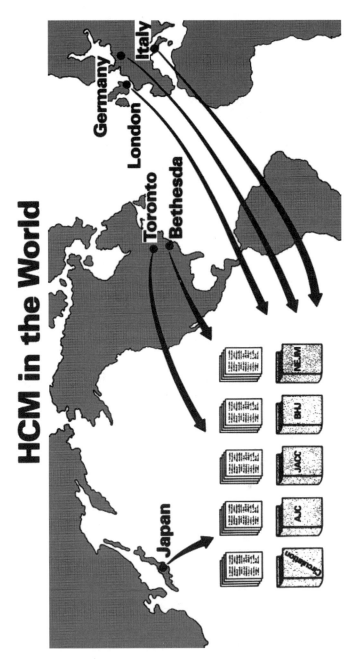

FIGURE 1.—Illustrative diagram shows the unique referral network for patients with hypertrophic cardiomyopathy (*HCM*). Severely symptomatic and/or high risk patients with HCM are referred to a relatively small number of tertiary HCM centers throughout the world. These same centers publish most of the studies on HCM. Inevitably, the literature reflects the clinical features of a highly selected and small proportion of the overall HCM population and, thus projects a distorted image of the disease. *Abbreviations: AJC*, American Journal of Cardiology; *BHJ*, British Heart Journal; *JACC*, Journal of the American College of Cardiology; *NEJM*, New England Journal of Medicine. (From Spirito P, Maron BJ: Natural history of hypertrophic cardiomyopathy: A benign or progressive disorder? *Cardiol Rev* 5:312–316, 1997. Courtesy of Maron BJ and Spirito P: Impact of patient selection biases in the perception of hypertrophic cardiomyopathy and its natural history. *Am J Cardiol* 72:970–972, 1993. Copyright 1993 by Excerpta Medica, Inc.)

### Septal Myectomy in Hypertrophic Obstructive Cardiomyopathy: Late Results With Stress Echocardiography

Göl MK, Emir M, Keleş T, et al (Türkiye Yüksek İhtisas Hosp, Ankara, Turkey)
*Ann Thorac Surg* 64:739–745, 1997                                    1–30

*Objective.*—Hypertrophic obstructive cardiomyopathy (HOCM) is characterized by a primary hypertrophy of cardiac muscle with increased systolic but impaired diastolic function. Patients with HOCM who have mild symptoms or have more than 50 mm Hg systolic left ventricular outflow tract (LVOT) gradients usually are treated surgically with septal myectomy/myotomy. The functional capacity of surgically treated patients with HOCM patients in late follow-up was assessed by dobutamine stress echocardiography.

*Methods.*—Between 1975 and 1996, 69 patients with HOCM (10 females), ages 6 to 58 years, underwent septal myectomy. Preoperatively 7 patients were classified as New York Heart Association (NYHA) I, 24 as NYHA II, and 38 as NYHA III. Patients were followed for an average of 44 months. There were 3 early deaths. Of 66 survivors, 49 underwent echocardiography and 29 had dobutamine stress testing.

*Results.*—The actuarial survival rate was 95.6%. The mean functional capacity was 1.47. Postoperatively, 37 patients were classified as NYHA I, 27 as NYHA II, and 3 as NYHA III. Three patients were reoperated for aortic valve replacement ($n = 2$) and aortic valve endocarditis ($n = 1$). In the 26 patients who completed the dobutamine stress test, echocardiographic measurements of the interventricular septum thickness decreased significantly from 1.14 to 1.03 cm, subvalvular aortic gradients from 78.4 to 17.9 mm Hg, septum thickness from 1.99 to 1.55 cm, and posterior wall thickness from 1.74 to 1.5 cm.

*Conclusion.*—Septal myectomy is safe and effective long-term for patients with HOCM with significant, refractive LVOT.

▶ I agree with our surgical colleagues from Ankara regarding the value of septal myectomy for patients with HOCM. This probably should be used more frequently in the United States.

**R.C. Schlant, M.D.**

### Dual-chamber Pacing for Hypertrophic Cardiomyopathy: A Randomized, Double-blind, Crossover Trial

Nishimura RA, Trusty JM, Hayes DL, et al (Mayo Clinic and Mayo Found, Rochester, Minn)
*J Am Coll Cardiol* 29:435–441, 1997                                    1–31

*Background.*—Several recent cohort studies have demonstrated that implanting a dual-chamber pacemaker in patients with severely symptomatic hypertrophic obstructive cardiomyopathy can relieve symptoms and reduce the severity of left ventricular outflow tract gradient. However, there have been no randomized, double-blind comparisons of dual-chamber pacing and standard treatment.

*Methods.*—Twenty-one patients with severely symptomatic hypertrophic obstructive cardiomyopathy were enrolled in a double-blind, randomized, crossover trial after baseline studies. Minnesota quality-of-life assessment, 2-dimensional and Doppler echocardiography, and cardiopulmonary exercise testing were done. Nineteen patients completed the protocol and were randomly assigned to dual-chamber paced, dual-chamber sensed, triggered, inhibited (DDD) pacing for 3 months followed by back-up atrial paced, atrial-sensed, inhibited (AAI) pacing for 3 months or to these treatments in the reverse order.

*Findings.*—After DDD pacing, left ventricular outflow tract gradient declined significantly to a mean 55 mm Hg, compared to the mean baseline gradient of 76 mm Hg and of 83 mm Hg after AAI pacing. Quality-of-life scores and exercise duration were improved significantly after DDD pacing compared to baseline but not compared to the back-up AAI arm. Peak oxygen consumption did not differ significantly among the 3 arms. Overall, symptomatic improvement was noted in 63% during DDD pacing and in 42% during AAI pacing. Thirty-one percent had no symptomatic change, and 5% had symptom deterioration during DDD pacing.

*Conclusions.*—Dual-chamber pacing may alleviate symptoms and reduce gradient in patients with hypertrophic obstructive cardiomyopathy. However, symptoms are unaffected or even worsen in some patients. Subjective improvement may also occur after implantation of the pacemaker without the hemodynamic benefit, which suggests a placebo effect.

▶ It appears that the left ventricular outflow tract gradient can be decreased in some patients in association with dual-chamber pacing. At the same time, however, a significant number of patients had no change and even a few had deterioration of symptoms during DDD pacing. Accordingly, I would consider this still to be a experimental form of therapy for patients with severe symptoms in hypertrophic obstructive cardiomyopathy that are unresponsive to medical therapy. Two reports recently found benefit from pacing therapy of patients with hypertrophic obstructive cardiomyopathy.[1, 2]

**R.C. Schlant, M.D.**

*References*

1. Gadler F, Linde C, Guhlin-Dannfelt A, et al: Long-term effects of dual chamber pacing in patients with hypertrophic cardiomyopathy without outflow tract obstruction at rest. *Eur Heart J* 18:636–642, 1997.
2. Kappenberg L, Linde C, Daubert C, et al: Pacing in hypertrophic obstructive cardiomyopathy: A random crossover study. *Eur Heart J* 18:1249–1256, 1997.

**Nonsurgical Septal Reduction for Hypertrophic Obstructive Cardiomyopathy: Outcome in the First Series of Patients**

Knight C, Kurbaan AS, Seggewiss H, et al (Royal Bromptom Hosp, London; Universitatsklinik der Ruhr-Universitat Bochum, Bad Oeynhausen, Germany)

*Circulation* 95:2075–2081, 1997                                        1–32

*Objective.*—Patients with hypertrophic obstructive cardiomyopathy may achieve symptomatic relief with a nonsurgical reduction in septal mass, using a catheter technique to produce an infarct that reduces left ventricular outflow tract obstruction. The immediate hemodynamic effects and the results of echocardiographic evaluation, exercise testing, and symptomatic follow-up for the first 18 patients treated by this technique were reported.

*Methods.*—A PTCA balloon catheter was inserted into each of 18 patients, and 2–5 mL of absolute alcohol was injected into the septal artery and left for 5 minutes. The balloon was deflated and the blockage was confirmed angiographically. If gradient reduction was small, the procedure was repeated on a second and third septal artery. Doppler echocardiography was performed before and after the procedure and 3 months later. Exercise testing and ambulatory monitoring were performed before and 3 months after the procedure.

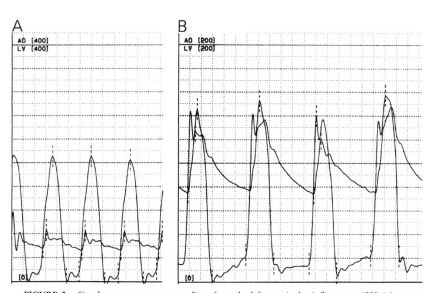

**FIGURE 2.**—Simultaneous pressure recordings from the left ventricular inflow tract (*LV*) (via transseptal catheterization) and aorta (*AO*) (via retrograde catheterization) before (**A**) and after (**B**) septal reduction. The left ventricular outflow tract gradient is abolished by the procedure. (Courtesy of Knight C, Kurbaan AS, Segewiss H, et al: Nonsurgical septal reduction for hypertrophic obstructive cardiomyopathy: Outcome in the first series of patients. *Circulation* 95:2075–2081. Reproduced with permission of *Circulation.* Copyright 1997, American Heart Association.)

*Results.*—The outflow gradient was reduced or eradicated immediately after alcohol injection in the majority of patients (Fig 2). Postprocedurally, the maximal gradient was significantly reduced from 119 mm Hg to 29 mm Hg. The mean gradient was significantly reduced from 67 mm Hg to 25 mm Hg postprocedurally and to 22 mm Hg at 3 months. All patients had chest pain during alcohol injection; 4 patients had heart block and 2 patients had ventricular arrhythmias. Symptoms improved substantially for most patients. Exercise capacity increased nonsignificantly. Whereas the reduction in gradient was maintained at 3 months, left ventricular size was essentially unchanged.

*Conclusion.*—Nonsurgical septal reduction using catheter ablation is a safe and effective technique for reducing left ventricular outflow obstruction in patients with hypertrophic obstructive cardiomyopathy. The technique results in symptomatic and hemodynamic improvement.

▶ This report described 18 patients who were treated with selective intercoronary alcohol injection to induce localized infarction of the ventricular septum. There appeared to be a significant reduction in the left ventricular outflow tract obstruction after the procedure. One concern I would have is that the scar tissue may set up an area likely to produce re-entry ventricular arrhythmias. This procedure is now being performed in a number of selected centers throughout the world. Some patients have had transient complete heart block. A report from Germany described beneficial effects in 10 patients.[1]

**R.C. Schlant, M.D.**

*Reference*

1. Kuhn H, Gietzen F, Leumer C, et al: Induction of sub-aortic septal ischaemia to reduce obstruction in hypertrophic obstructive cardiomyopathy: Studies to develop a new catheter-based concept of treatment. *Eur Heart J* 18:846–851, 1997.

---

**Restrictive Cardiomyopathy**
Kushwaha SS, Fallon JT, Fuster V (Mount Sinai Med Ctr, New York)
*N Engl J Med* 336:267–276, 1997                                                1–33

---

*Introduction.*—Restrictive cardiomyopathy is characterized by increasing ventricular pressure that can affect either the left or right ventricle. The pathogenesis, natural history, and specific findings of restrictive cardiomyopathy, with emphasis on idiopathic restrictive cardiomyopathy, amyloid heart disease, endomyocardial fibrosis, and infiltrative disease were reviewed (Table 1).

*Presentation.*—Symptoms of restrictive cardiomyopathy include dyspnea, peripheral edema, orthopnea, and ascites. Later, heart failure appears. Atrial fibrillation is common.

*Diagnostic Evaluation.*—Constrictive pericarditis should be ruled out. There may be hemodynamic impairment, peripheral edema, ascites, ab-

TABLE 1.—Classification of Types of Restrictive Cardiomyopathy
According to Cause

**Myocardial**
Noninfiltrative
    Idiopathic cardiomyopathy*[5]
    Familial cardiomyopathy[6,7]
    Hypertrophic cardiomyopathy[4]
    Scleroderma[8,9]
    Pseudoxanthoma elasticum[10]
    Diabetic cardiomyopathy[11,12]
Infiltrative
    Amyloidosis*[13,14]
    Sarcoidosis*[15,16]
    Gaucher's disease[17]
    Hurler's disease[18]
    Fatty infiltration[19]
Storage diseases
    Hemochromatosis[20]
    Fabry's disease[21]
    Glycogen storage disease[22,23]
**Endomyocardial**
Endomyocardial fibrosis*[24,25]
Hypereosinophilic syndrome[26]
Carcinoid heart disease[27,28]
Metastatic cancers[29,30]
Radiation*[31]
Toxic effects of anthracycline*[32,33]
Drugs causing fibrous endocarditis[34,35]
    (serotonin, methysergide, ergotamine,
    mercurial agents, busulfan)

*This condition is more likely than the others to be encountered in clinical practice.
(Reprinted by permission of *The New England Journal of Medicine.* Courtesy of Kushwaha SS, Fallon JT, Fuster V: Restrictive cardiomyopathy. *N Engl J Med* 336:267–276, copyright 1997, Massachusetts Medical Society. All rights reserved.)

normal heart sounds, atrial enlargement, low output carotid and peripheral pulse, pulmonary edema, interstitial edema, and pleural effusions. Doppler echocardiography can be diagnostic.

*Distinction Between Restrictive Cardiomyopathy and Constrictive Pericarditis.*—A history of pericarditis or tuberculosis would suggest constrictive pericarditis, as would trauma and radiation therapy. Differences in the results of physical examinations, electrocardiography, echocardiography, Doppler studies, cardiac catheterization, endomyocardial biopsy and CT/MRI are tabulated.

*Treatment.*—Careful use of diuretics to treat venous congestion can avoid hypotension and hypoperfusion. Amiodarone can be used to correct sinus rhythm. Cardioversion to correct atrial fibrillation may cause an abnormal sinus node to fail. A pacemaker may be necessary to correct advanced-conduction system disease. Warfarin is recommended to prevent thrombus formation. Specific therapy, with chemotherapy, is necessary for treatment of the underlying cause of amyloidosis. Corticosteroids and cytotoxic drugs are appropriate for the early stage of endomyocardial fibrosis. Venesection, iron-chelation therapy, or heart and liver transplantation is recommended for hemochromatosis. Heart transplantation may be necessary for patients with refractory symptoms, unless they are caused by systemic disorders.

▶ This is a superb overview of restrictive cardiomyopathy. In previous years, the diagnosis was almost always 1 of occlusion. In contrast, today the diagnosis is more and more an active diagnosis based upon specific medical and laboratory findings.

**R.C. Schlant, M.D.**

**Cardiac Amyloidosis**
Reisinger J, Dubrey SW, Falk RH (Boston Univ)
*Cardiol Rev* 5:317–325, 1997                                    1–34

*Objective.*—A review of types of amyloidosis and their general clinical manifestations, plus a discussion of the etiology, clinical presentation, and treatment of cardiac amyloidosis, was presented.

*Classification.*—Amyloidoses are classified by the nature of the deposited protein fibrils such as immunoglobulin light chains (AL), mutant and normal transthyretin (ATTR), and amyloid protein A (AA).

> *AL (Primary) Amyloidosis.*—This is a late-onset disease affecting virtually all organs and resulting in congestive heart failure in 30% to 50% of patients.
>
> *ATTR (Familial) Amyloidosis.*—This is an autosomal dominant inherited disease characterized by deposition of a mutant form of transthyretin in various organs, usually beginning in the second to fourth decade of life.
>
> *Senile Amyloidosis.*—This is a rare disease that occasionally leads to massive deposition and heart failure.
>
> *Amyloid A (Secondary) Amyloidosis.*—This variant, associated with chronic infection and inflammation, rarely involves the heart.

*Clinical Presentation and Findings.*—Signs and symptoms are of right-sided heart failure solely or predominantly with early diastolic ventricular dysfunction and late systolic dysfunction. Lung, liver, and kidneys may also be involved. Hypertensive patients may experience spontaneous resolution of arterial hypertension.

*Electrocardiography.*—Whereas electrocardiograms may lead to a misleading diagnosis of coronary artery disease, Doppler echocardiography is diagnostic (Fig 5).

*Prognosis.*—AL is far more serious than ATTR, leading to progressive heart failure or sudden death.

*Therapy.*—Symptomatic treatment includes cautious use of diuretics to avoid hypovolemia. Vasodilator drugs, digoxin, calcium channel blockers, and β-blockers are not effective and may worsen the condition. Oral melphalan and prednisone are effective for treating the underlying disease

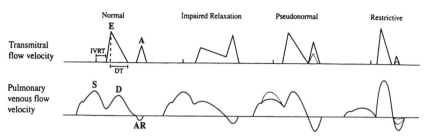

**FIGURE 5.**—Diagram depicts changes in transmitral and pulmonary venous flow velocity tracings that occur with progression of amyloid infiltration in the myocardium. *Dotted lines* in the transmitral flow velocity tracings indicate the effect of progression of restrictive physiology and atrial mechanical dysfunction on the A-wave. In patients with a pseudonormal transmitral Doppler, preserved systolic ventricular function may be associated with a higher systolic pulmonary venous flow velocity (indicated by *dotted line*). Progressive atrial mechanical dysfunction results in a decreasing velocity of the atrial flow reversal (indicated by *dotted line* in the restrictive pattern). *E* indicates transmitral flow velocity in early diastole; *DT* indicates mitral deceleration time; *A* indicates transmitral flow velocity at atrial contraction; *IVRT* indicates isovolumetric relaxation time; *S* shows pulmonary venous flow velocity during ventricular systole; *D* shows pulmonary venous flow velocity during ventricular diastole; and *AR* shows atrial flow reversal in the pulmonary vein at atrial contraction. (Courtesy of Reisinger J, Dubrey SW, Falk RH: Cardiac amyloidosis. *Cardiol Rev* 5:317–325, 1997.)

and achieve a modest increase in survival. Intensive IV melphalan therapy with autologous blood stem cell transplantation has resulted in stabilization of some patients with less-than-severe cardiac involvement. Heart transplantation with posttransplant chemotherapy may be effective. ATTR amyloidosis has been successfully treated by liver and heart transplantation from 1 donor. Aggressive treatment or removal of the source of inflammation in AA amyloidosis may halt progression. Treatment of the familial disease with colchicine prevents amyloidosis.

*Conclusion.*—Cardiac amyloidosis in AL is progressive and fatal. Liver transplantation increases long-term survival in ATTR but not AL patients. Intensive treatment with IV melphalan plus autologous stem cell transplantation can halt progression of AL. Chemotherapy may benefit patients with severe cardiac amyloidosis.

▶ Cardiac amyloidosis is one of the classic causes of restrictive cardiomyopathy. Two other articles have dealt with echocardiographic findings and its prognostic value.[1, 2]

**R.C. Schlant, M.D.**

*References*

1. Dubrey SW, Cha K, Skinner M, et al: Familial and primary (AL) cardiac amyloidosis: Echocardiographically similar diseases with distinctly different clinical outcomes. *Heart* 78:74–82, 1997.
2. Patel AR, Dubrey SW, Mendes LA, et al: Right ventricular dilation in primary amyloidosis: An independent predictor of survival. *Am J Cardiol* 80:486–492, 1997.

### Apoptosis in the Failing Human Heart

Olivetti G, Abbi R, Quaini F, et al (New York Med College, Valhalla; Univ of Parma, Italy; Univ of Udine, Italy; et al)

*N Engl J Med* 336:1131–1141, 1997                    1–35

*Introduction.*—Patients with cardiomyopathy, whether of ischemic or nonischemic origin, have progressive loss of myocytes. Although experimental studies have demonstrated apoptosis in myocytes, it is unknown whether programmed cell death occurs in the human heart as it fails. Apoptosis of myocytes was studied in patients with intractable congestive heart failure.

*Methods.*—Specimens of myocardial tissue from 36 patients who received heart transplants and from 3 who died soon after myocardial infarction, as well as from 11 normal hearts were analyzed. Histochemical and biochemical analyses were performed, as well as a combination of histochemical analysis and confocal microscopy. The analysis also included measurement of the expression of *BCL2* and *BAX*, 2 proto-oncogenes that protect against and promote apoptosis, respectively.

*Results.*—The specimens from patients with heart failure had a 232-fold increase in morphological evidence of myocyte apoptosis. On biochemical assessment, these specimens showed DNA laddering as a marker of apoptosis. Histochemically, the specimens showed DNA-strand breaks in myocyte nuclei; confocal microscopy revealed chromatin condensation and fragmentation. In failing hearts, the percentage of myocytes labeled with *BCL2* was nearly doubled; this finding was confirmed by Western blotting. There was no difference in expression of *BAX*.

*Conclusions.*—During failure, the human heart undergoes myocyte apoptosis. Programmed cell death occurs despite enhanced expression of *BCL2*, which protects cells from apoptosis. This suggests that the overloaded myocardium activates compensatory mechanisms in an attempt to preserve cells. Myocyte apoptosis may play a role in the progression of cardiac dysfunction.

▶ One of the ultimate causes of heart failure is a loss of cardiac myocytes. The programmed death of myocytes (apoptosis) is a probable chronic occurrence in many patients with heart failure. The evidence for apoptosis of cardiac myocytes and its potential role in the progression of heart failure is also reviewed by Feuerstein and colleagues,[1] and Nishigaki et al. found evidence of elevated levels of plasma sFas-L in human heart failure.[2]

**R.C. Schlant, M.D.**

*References*

1. Feuerstein G, Ruffolo RR Jr, Yue T-L: Apoptosis in congestive heart failure. *Trend Cardiovas Med* 7:249–255, 1997.
2. Nishigaki K, Minatoguchi S, Seishima M, et al: Plasma Fas ligand, an inducer of apoptosis and plasma Fas, an inhibitor of apoptosis, in patients with congestive heart failure. *J Am Coll Cardiol* 29:1214–1220, 1997.

**Haemodynamic, Neuroendocrine and Metabolic Correlates of Circulating Cytokine Concentrations in Congestive Heart Failure**
Lommi J, Pulkki K, Koskinen P, et al (Helsinki Univ; Turku Univ, Finland)
*Eur Heart J* 18:1620–1625, 1997                                    1–36

*Objective.*—Some patients with congestive heart failure have increased levels of circulating cytokines. Because the mechanisms responsible for this increased cytokine production are largely unknown, the associations between circulating cytokines and central hemodynamics, neuroendocrine status, and intermediary metabolism were assessed in patients with moderate or severe congestive heart failure (CHF).

*Methods.*—Fasting peripheral and hepatic venous plasma concentrations of tumor necrosis factor-$\alpha$ (TNF-$\alpha$), soluble tumor necrosis factor-receptor II (sTNF-RII), interleukin 6 (IL-6), selected neurohormones, and metabolites were sampled from 44 with CHF patients (28 men) (average age, 56 years) and 14 patients (9 men) without CHF (average age, 53 years) undergoing cardiac catheterization and echocardiography.

*Results.*—Systolic wedge pressure, left ventricular ejection fraction, and distance in a 6-minute walking test were significantly lower in patients with CHF than in patients without CHF (116 vs. 135 beats/min, 39% vs. 54%, and 309 vs. 464 m, respectively). P-noradrenaline and P-Nt-proANP levels were significantly higher in patients with CHF than in patients without (1.8 vs. 1.1 mmol/L and 1.46 vs. 0.44 mmol/L, respectively). Levels of sTNF-RII were significantly higher in patients with CHF than in patients without. Peripheral TNF-$\alpha$ was significantly correlated with 6-minute walking distance ($r = -0.37$). Peripheral IL-6 was significantly correlated with New York Heart Association (NYHA) class ($r = 0.66$), 6-minute walking distance ($r = -0.52$), right atrial pressure ($r = 0.55$), pulmonary artery wedge pressure ($r = 0.50$), and left ventricular ejection fraction ($r = -0.39$). According to multivariate analysis, only right atrial pressure was a significant independent predictor of IL-6. Soluble tumor necrosis factor-receptor II was significantly related to NYHA class.

*Conclusion.*—Plasma levels of TNF-$\alpha$ and sTNF-RII were significantly correlated with exercise tolerance and symptoms of CHF. Levels of IL-6 were related to NYHA class and hemodynamic measures. Right atrial pressure was a predictor of IL-6.

▶ Over the past 5 years, a number of reports have shown an increase of plasma as well as myocardial inflammatory cytokines in patients with advanced heart failure. These appear to be responsible for much of the reversible cardiac depression often seen in such patients. Hopefully, future studies will give us specific agents to block the effects of pro-inflammatory cytokines. Several other recent articles have also dealt with the relationship between cytokines and heart failure.[1–5]

**R.C. Schlant, M.D.**

*References*

1. Shan K, Kurrelmey K, Seta Y, et al: A role of cytokines in disease progression in heart failure. *Curr Opin Cardiol* 12:218–223, 1997.
2. Birks EJ, Yacoub MH: The role of nitric oxide and cytokines in heart failure. *Coronary Artery Dis* 8:389–402, 1997.
3. Mohler ER, Sorensen LC, Ghali JK, et al: The role of cytokines in the mechanism of the action of amlodipine: The PRAISE Heart Failure Trial. *J Am Coll Cardiol* 30:35–41, 1997.
4. Anker SD, Clark AL, Kemp M, et al: Tumor necrosis factor and steroid metabolism in chronic heart failure: Possible relation to muscle wasting. *J Am Coll Cardiol* 30:997–1001, 1997.
5. Matsumori A, Ono K, Nishio R, et al: Modulation of cytokine production and protection against lethal endotoxemia by the cardiac glycoside Ouabain. *Circulation* 96:1501–1506, 1997.

## Heart Failure

**Upregulation of Cell Adhesion Molecules and the Presence of Low Grade Inflammation in Human Chronic Heart Failure**
Devaux B, Scholz D, Hirche A, et al (Max-Planck-Inst, Bad Nauheim, Germany)
*Eur Heart J* 18:470–479, 1997                                    1–37

*Objective.*—Although expression of cell adhesion molecules has been shown in many cardiovascular diseases, their occurrence has seldom been immunohistochemically evaluated. The presence of E-selectin, VCAM-1, PECAM-1, and ICAM-1 as markers of inflammation was evaluated in human hearts failing because of acute myocarditis.

*Methods.*—At transplantation, tissue was taken from hearts of 24 patients (6 women) (average age, 44 years) with end-stage heart failure as a result of myocarditis (N = 6), chronic ischemic heart disease (N = 6), or dilated cardiomyopathy (N = 12). Control tissues were left ventricular biopsy specimens from hearts of 6 patients (5 men) (average age, 35 years) undergoing mitral valve replacement. The tissues were subjected to immunohistochemical analysis, electron microscopy, immunostaining for tumor necrosis factor-α (TNF-α), and Western blot analysis.

*Results.*—PECAM-1 was expressed in the cell membrane of human umbilical vein endothelial cells. Stimulated endothelial cells expressed ICAM-1, E-selectin, and VCAM-1. E-selectin and VCAM-1 were absent in tissue sections. Whereas ICAM-1 was not expressed in all control blood vessels, it was found in all endothelial cells of blood vessels in diseased myocardium and in myocytes bordering areas of inflammation. ICAM-1/PECAM-1 was significantly higher in patients with end-stage heart failure than in controls. CD3 was found in the extracellular space, CD68 in macrophages, CD11a/CD18 in leukocytes, and TNF-α in macrophages of patients but not of controls.

*Conclusion.*—Whatever the cause of heart failure, increased release of cytokines results in chronic low-grade inflammation which can worsen the deterioration in congestive heart failure.

▶ This study clearly documents the fact that many patients with chronic heart failure have upregulation of cell adhesion molecules. The fact that chronic low-grade inflammation occurs in cardiac tissues in patients with dilated cardiomyopathy, myocarditis, or ischemic heart disease suggests that it may play an important role in the pathophysiology of heart failure. If we can learn to decrease the upregulation or else block the effects of the cell adhesion molecules and inflammation, perhaps the natural course of heart failure can be favorably influenced.

**R.C. Schlant, M.D.**

**Prognostic Value of Plasma Endothelin-1 in Patients With Chronic Heart Failure**
Pousset F, Isnard R, Lechat P, et al (Pittié-Salpêtrière Hosp, Paris; Institut Fédératif de Recherche Physiopathologique et Génétique Cardiovasculaire, Paris)
*Eur Heart J* 18:254–258, 1997                                                  1–38

*Objective.*—Activation of neurohormones, such as endothelin-1, contributes to deterioration in congestive heart failure. Persistent high levels in chronic congestive heart failure may be associated with a poor prognosis.

*Methods.*—Plasma endothelin-1 and plasma atrial natriuretic peptide levels were measured by radioimmunoassay and plasma catecholamine levels were measured by a radioenzymatic assay in 120 patients with congestive heart failure (20 females) with a mean ejection fraction of 28%. Their average age was 52 years. There were 21 New York Heart Association (NYHA) class I, 35 class II, 61 class III, and 3 class IV patients. Patients were given a diagnosis of idiopathic heart failure (77%), chronic coronary artery disease (19%), anthracycline-induced cardiomyopathy (1.7%), or aortic regurgitation (2.5%). Patients were followed for an average of 361 days. Survival differences were analyzed statistically.

*Results.*—Fourteen cardiac deaths occurred, and 8 patients underwent heart transplantation. Endothelin-1 levels, NYHA class, atrial natriuretic peptide levels, left ventricular echocardiographic end-diastolic diameter index, noradrenaline concentration, and age were significant predictors of mortality in the Cox proportional-hazard model. A multivariate model confirmed these 6 variables as significant predictors of outcome, but only the endothelin-1 level was significantly associated with outcome. Patients with endothelin-1 levels of more than 5 pg/mL had a significantly higher mortality rate than patients with lower endothelin-1 levels (21% vs. 4%).

*Conclusion.*—Plasma endothelin-1 level was a significant predictor of mortality in patients with mild-to-moderate heart failure.

▶ This study documents the fact that patients with chronic heart failure have elevated levels of plasma endothelin-1 and that such high levels are associated with poor prognosis. Chronic blockade of the endothelin$_A$ receptor appears to improve ventricular myocyte function in rabbits with pacing-induced congestive heart failure.[1]

**R.C. Schlant, M.D.**

*Reference*

1. Spinale FG, Walker JD, Mukherjee R: Concomitant endothelin receptor subtype-A blockade during the progression of pacing induced congestive heart failure in rabbits: Beneficial effects on left ventricular myocyte function. *Circulation* 95:1918–1929, 1997.

### Role of Endogenous Endothelin in Chronic Heart Failure: Effect of Long-term Treatment With an Endothelin Antagonist on Survival, Hemodynamics, and Cardiac Remodeling

Mulder P, Richard V, Derumeaux G, et al (Rouen Univ, France)
*Circulation* 96:1976–1982, 1997                                                    1–39

*Objective.*—Elevated plasma levels of endothelin-1 (ET-1) increase deterioration in patients with chronic heart failure and are a predictor of mortality in these patients. Bosetan is an ET-1 antagonist. A rat study assessed whether chronic treatment with bosetan affects survival, systemic and cardiac hemodynamics, and cardiac remodeling.

*Methods.*—The left coronary arteries of 10-week-old male Wistar rats were ligated. Bosetan (30 mg/kg/day) was then administered for 9 months to 52 infarcted, untreated rats and placebo to 53 infarcted rats. Twelve sham-operated rats served as controls. In another study, 10 infarcted rats were untreated and 12 rats received bosetan (30 or 100 mg/kg/day). Eight sham-operated rats served as controls. Hemodynamic measurements were determined and plasma ET-1 and plasma catecholamines were measured. The left ventricular pressure-volume relationship was determined. Echocardiographic studies were performed. Urinary cyclic quanosine monophosphate (cGMP) was measured. Cardiac morphometry was performed.

*Results.*—After 9 months, survival was significantly higher in the bosetan 100 mg/kg/d group than in the untreated group (65% vs. 47%). Bosetan at 30 mg/kg/day had no effect on survival, hemodynamic variables, or degree of deterioration when compared with placebo. Infarct size was similar in all groups. At 2 and 9 months, bosetan reduced central venous pressure, plasma catecholamines, urinary cGMP, left ventricular collagen density, and left ventricular dilatation. Results of echocardiographic studies showed a reduction in hypertrophy and an increase in contractility of the noninfarcted left ventricular wall after 2 months of bosetan treatment.

*Conclusion.*—Chronic treatment with bosetan at 100 mg/kg/day significantly increased survival in infarcted rats and had beneficial hemodynamic and structural effects.

▶ In this experimental study, the survival of rats with heart failure was significantly improved with chronic treatment with the endothelin receptor antagonist bosetan. This is a very promising adjunctive therapy for heart failure. It may represent a major breakthrough.

**R.C. Schlant, M.D.**

---

**Attenuation of Compensation of Endogenous Cardiac Natriuretic Peptide System in Chronic Heart Failure: Prognostic Role of Plasma Brain Natriuretic Peptide Concentration in Patients With Chronic Symptomatic Left Ventricular Dysfunction**

Tsutamoto T, Wada A, Maeda K, et al (Shiga Univ, Tsukinowa, Seta, Japan)
*Circulation* 96:509–516, 1997                                    1–40

---

*Introduction.*—High plasma levels of atrial natriuretic peptide (ANP), mainly from the atrium, and brain natriuretic peptide (BNP), mainly from the ventricle, are found in patients with congestive heart failure (CHF), and ANP is reported to be a significant prognostic predictor. A study of 85 patients with chronic CHF was conducted to examine the prognostic role of plasma BNP in comparison with plasma ANP and other factors known to be associated with high mortality.

*Methods.*—Patients were 61 men and 24 women with a mean age of 60. All had a left ventricular ejection fraction (LVEJ) of < 45% and were clinically stable on constant doses of diuretics. Causes of heart failure were dilated cardiomyopathy in 41 patients, ischemic heart disease in 41, and hypertensive heart disease in 3. Patients were followed for 2 years for the relationship between severity of CHF and plasma levels of ANP, BNP, cGMP (a biological marker of ANP and BNP), and norepinephrine (NE). Measurements of right atrial pressure, mean pulmonary arterial pressure, and pulmonary capillary wedge pressure (PCWP) were also obtained.

*Results.*—Twenty-five patients died from a cardiac cause during the follow-up period. Plasma levels of ANP, BNP, NE, and cGMP all increased with severity of CHF, but only high levels of plasma BNP and PCWP were significant independent predictors of mortality (relative risk ratios 1.003 and 1.083, respectively). Plasma levels of NE, ANP, and BNP were significantly higher in nonsurvivors than in survivors, but these 2 groups showed no difference in plasma cGMP levels. The plasma BNP concentration was approximately 5-fold higher in nonsurvivors versus survivors, and plasma levels of BNP and cGMP exhibited a significant positive correlation in survivors.

*Discussion.*—In these patients with chronic CHF and left ventricular dysfunction, plasma BNP proved to be more useful than ANP as a prognostic predictor. The level of plasma BNP provides important prognostic information independent of hemodynamic parameters for predicting mortality.

▶ Patients with congestive heart failure have elevated plasma levels of both ANP, which is produced primarily from the atria, and BNP, which is produced primarily from the ventricles. Of the two peptides it appears that BNP is more useful for assessing prognosis of patients with chronic heart failure. The plasma half-life of BNP is longer than that of ANP, and BNP has greater natriuretic and arterial pressure-lowering effects than ANP. Infusion of BNP in patients with impaired left ventricular systolic function of the heart appears to cause favorable hemodynamic changes.[1]

**R.C. Schlant, M.D.**

*Reference*

1. Lainchbury JG, Richard AM, Nicholls MG, et al: The effects of pathophysiological increments in brain natriuretic peptide in left ventricular systolic dysfunction. *Hypertension* 1997;30(part 1):398–404.

---

**Diastolic Dysfunction in Heart Failure**
Brutsaert DL, Sys SU (Univ of Antwerp, Belgium)
*J Card Fail* 3:225–242, 1997                                        1–41

*Background.*—A great deal has been written about diastolic dysfunction and diastolic failure in the face of normal systolic ventricular function. However, largely because of the lack of appropriate definitions, the diagnosis, prevalence, prognosis, and management of diastolic function, dysfunction, and failure remain unclear. A conceptual review of diastolic dysfunction is presented.

*Diastolic Failure.*—The review takes a conceptual approach, viewing the heart as a muscular pump (Fig 1). From this viewpoint, diastole can be said to consist of diastasis and atrial contraction, comparing the last 5% to 15% of ventricular filling. By this definition, diastolic dysfunction and failure can be defined as disease processes that shift the end of the pressure-volume diagram upward. Thus left ventricular (LV) filling pressures increase in a manner disproportionate to the magnitude of LV dilation. The authors suggest that LV diastolic failure is caused by increased resistance to LV filling. Symptoms of pulmonary congestion result from inappropriate upward shift of the diastolic pressure-volume relation. At first, during exercise, this can be termed diastolic dysfunction; later, at rest, it becomes diastolic failure. Causes of diastolic failure are impaired systolic relaxation (Fig 2) and decreased myocardial or ventricular compliance. The diagnosis depends on demonstration of an inappropriate upward shift of the diastolic pressure-volume relation, or of an inappropriate increase in any directly related measurements.

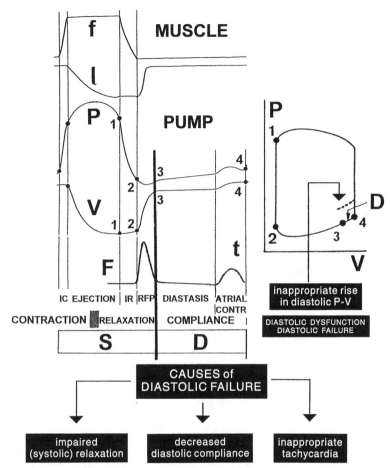

**FIGURE 1.**—Cardiac cycle of the heart as a muscular pump. Comparison of muscle (*f* = force, *l* = length) and pump (*P* = pressure, *V* = volume, *F* = mitral flow). The similarity between the corresponding time (*t*) traces led to the inclusion of isovolumetric relaxation (*IR*) and rapid filling phase (*RFP*) into the relaxation part of systole. As a consequence, diastolic dysfunction or failure can be defined as an inappropriate rise in the diastolic pressure-volume relation during exercise or at rest, respectively. Possible causes of diastolic dysfunction or failure are impaired (systolic) relaxation, decreased diastolic compliance, and inappropriate tachycardia or mismatch of systolic to total duration. (Courtesy of Brutsaert DL, Sys SU: Diastolic dysfunction in heart failure. *J Card Fail* 3:225–242, 1997.)

*Discussion.*—The authors' definition of diastolic failure has important implications for diagnosis and therapy. A low-dose beta blocker is the treatment of choice for patients with symptoms of pulmonary congestion or exercise intolerance involving an inappropriate increase in heart rate. There is a growing emphasis on drugs to improve the passive properties of the myocardium, either by suppressing inappropriate growth of noncontractile tissues or by bringing about regression of myocardial hypertrophy. Though research has been done to develop lusitropic drugs—that is, drugs

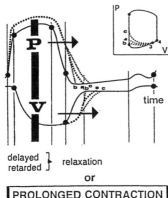
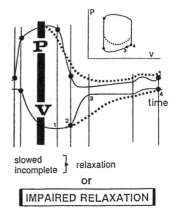

delayed } relaxation
retarded }

or

**| PROLONGED CONTRACTION |**

slowed } relaxation
incomplete }

or

**| IMPAIRED RELAXATION |**

## MODULATION OF SYSTOLIC DURATION
(= dominant, compensatory, physiological)
* *heterometric* autoregulation
  - pressure-volume loading (CL vs RL)
  - stage 1 hypertrophy
* *homeometric* autoregulation
  - neuro-humoral, drugs
    $\oplus$ angiotensin II    $\ominus$ $Ca^{++}$, digitalis
       alpha-agonists      beta-agonists
       vasopressin
  - heart rate
* cardiac **endothelial** autoregulation
  (cytokines, Et, NO, $PGI_2$ , ...)

## MODULATION OF RELAXATION RATE
(= epiphenomenon)

* secondary to changes in systolic duration
* instantaneous changes in relaxation loadings (RL)
* neuro-humoral, heart rate

## CAUSES
* stages 2 and 3 hypertrophy
* ischemia
* ...

## MECHANISMS
* inappropriate *loading*
  - pressure-volume overloading
* inappropriate *inactivation*
  - impaired $Ca^{++}$ homeostasis
    ($Ca_i^{++}$ overload, impaired sarcopl. retic.)
  - impaired affinity of contractile proteins
  - ...
* inappropriate *non-uniformity* of loading and
  inactivation in space and time

FIGURE 2.—Prolonged contraction is not impaired relaxation. *Prolonged* contraction—or delayed onset of relaxation—causes an increase in the duration of systole as indicated by the dotted lines in the pressure (*P*) and volume (*V*) traces on the left. This compensatory and physiologic modulation of systolic duration can result from a number of different heterometric, homeometric ($\oplus$, prolongation; $\ominus$, abbreviation), and cardiac endothelial types of autoregulation. These may be accompanied by substantial but often divergent changes in the relaxation rate (*b* and *c* vs. *a*). *Impaired* relaxation, illustrated by slower (inappropriately decreased rate) and incomplete (inappropriately decreased extent) relaxation (*dotted lines on the right*), is pathologic and leads to diastolic dysfunction or failure. Causes of impaired relaxation can be interpreted in terms of an impaired triple control of relaxation (16, 19), that is, inappropriateness of loading, inactivation, or nonuniformity. *CL*, contraction load; *RL*, relaxation load. (Courtesy of Brutsaert DL, Sys SU: Diastolic dysfunction in heart failure. *J Card Fail* 3:225–242, 1997.)

that would improve impaired relaxation—few studies have looked at their effects on diastolic pressure-volume relations.

▶ This is a superb review of diastolic dysfunction. Unfortunately, the term is probably abused and over diagnosed from echocardiographic studies.

**R.C. Schlant, M.D.**

**Impaired Left Ventricular Diastolic Filling Occurs in Diabetic Patients Without Atherosclerotic Coronary Artery Disease**
Inoue T, Fujito T, Asahi S, et al (Dokkyo Univ, Saitama, Japan)
*Am J Med Sci* 313:125–130, 1997                                                                    1–42

*Objective.*—Diabetic patients sometimes experience angina in the absence of large-vessel atherosclerosis. Left ventricular diastolic function and systolic function were evaluated by left ventriculography in patients with diabetes mellitus who had typical anginal chest pain but whose angiograms showed intact large coronary arteries.

*Methods.*—Left ventriculography was performed in 14 diabetic patients with angina who had exercise-induced ST-T changes on their electrocardiograms (group A) and 10 diabetic patients with angina but without significant ST-T changes. Left ventricular volume, left ventricular end-diastolic volume index, end-systolic volume index, ejection fraction, peak ejection rate, peak filling rate, and time to peak filling rate were calculated and compared with those of control patients without diabetes or cardiac diseases.

*Results.*—Whereas left ventricular systolic function was normal in diabetic patients, left ventricular diastolic filling was impaired (Fig 3). Total time differences for group A (86 msec) was significantly higher than for group B (47 msec) or controls (38 msec).

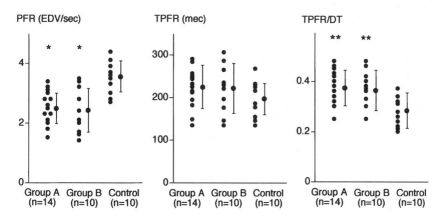

*       P<0.01 vs Control

**       P<0.05 vs Control

FIGURE 3.—The values of global peak filling rate in group A and group B were significantly less than the value in the controls (**left**). The value of the time to peak filling rate was similar among the 3 patient groups (**center**). The ratio of global time to peak filling rate to diastolic time in both group A and group B was higher than the value in the controls (**right**). *Abbreviations: PFR*, peak filling rate; *TPFR*, time to peak filling rate; *TPFR/DT*, ratio of time to peak filling rate to diastolic time. (Courtesy of Inoue T, Fujito T, Asahi S, et al: Impaired left ventricular diastolic filling occurs in diabetic patients without atherosclerotic coronary artery disease. *Am J Med Sci* 313:125–130, 1997.)

*Conclusion.*—In this study, patients with diabetes but without atherosclerotic large-vessel coronary artery disease had impaired left ventricular diastolic filling function.

▶ This study shows that patients with diabetes but without atherosclerotic coronary artery disease of any significance may have abnormalities of left ventricular diastolic filling. This abnormality of diastolic filling is almost certainly worse with tachycardia.

**R.C. Schlant, M.D.**

---

**Effects of Aging on Left Ventricular Relaxation in Humans: Analysis of Left Ventricular Isovolumic Pressure Decay**
Yamakado T, Takagi E, Okubo S, et al (Mie Univ, Tsu, Japan)
*Circulation* 95:917–923, 1997                                    1–43

---

*Objective.*—Whereas left ventricular (LV) systolic function at rest is not affected by aging, early diastolic filling velocity worsens with age, possibly because of a decrease in the rate of LV relaxation. High-fidelity LV pressures were retrospectively analyzed in normal individuals who had undergone diagnostic cardiac catheterization to study whether aging alters ventricular isovolumic relaxation.

*Methods.*—Using a catheter-tipped manometer and biplane left ventriculograms, high-fidelity LV pressures were measured in 55 normal individuals (17 women) age 20–77. The time constant of isovolumic pressure decay was calculated. Two time constants, Tb and Tw, were calculated from 2 different exponentially fitted curves: Tb from a curve fit with a variable asymptote pressure and Tw from a curve fit with a zero asymptote pressure. Left ventricular end-diastolic and end-systolic volume indices, ejection fraction, LV wall thickness, and LV mass were calculated from biplane left ventriculograms.

*Results.*—All LV relaxation constants were independent of age. Whereas LV peak systolic pressure was weakly but significantly correlated with age ($r = 0.47$), LV systolic function, heart rate, LV free-wall thickness, and mass index were age-independent. Multivariate analysis showed no correlation between age and LV relaxation or asymptote pressure.

*Conclusion.*—Left ventricular relaxation is unchanged by aging.

▶ I was very surprised with the results of this study. It is important that the study was a retrospective review from cardiac catheterizations performed over 16 years. Furthermore, no patient over the age of 80 was included. I rather suspect that significant abnormalities of diastolic relaxation and left ventricular filling would be noted with slight tachycardia in elderly patients.

**R.C. Schlant, M.D.**

**The Effect of Digoxin on Mortality and Morbidity in Patients With Heart Failure**
Garg R, and the Digitalis Investigation Group (Mount Sinai Med Ctr, New York)
*N Engl J Med* 336:525–533, 1997                                      1–44

*Background.*—Digoxin is a commonly prescribed drug for treatment of heart failure, but its long-term safety and efficacy are uncertain. Recent studies have shown that discontinuing digoxin in patients with heart failure can worsen functional status, exercise capacity, and left ventricular ejection fraction. The effects of digoxin on hospitalization and mortality rates in patients with heart failure were assessed in a randomized, double-blind, placebo-controlled trial.

*Methods.*—Patients with heart failure and a left ventricular ejection fraction of 0.45 or less were treated with digoxin or placebo, plus angiotensin-converting enzyme inhibitors and diuretics. The median dose of digoxin was 0.25 mg/day. The average follow-up was 37 months. In a substudy of patients with a left ventricular ejection fraction of 0.45 or more, 492 patients were treated with digoxin and 496 were given placebo.

*Results.*—In the main study, mortality was similar in both groups of patients (Fig 1). In patients treated with digoxin, there was a trend toward

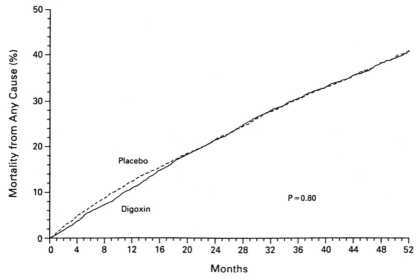

NO. OF PATIENTS AT RISK

| | | | | | | | | | | | | | |
|---|---|---|---|---|---|---|---|---|---|---|---|---|---|
| Placebo | 3403 | 3239 | 3105 | 2976 | 2868 | 2758 | 2652 | 2551 | 2205 | 1881 | 1506 | 1168 | 734 | 339 |
| Digoxin | 3397 | 3269 | 3144 | 3019 | 2882 | 2759 | 2644 | 2531 | 2184 | 1840 | 1475 | 1156 | 737 | 335 |

FIGURE 1.—Mortality in the digoxin and placebo groups. The number of patients at risk at each 4-month interval is shown below the figure. (Reprinted by permission of The New England Journal of Medicine, from Garg R, and the Digitalis Investigation Group: The effect of digoxin on mortality and morbidity in patients with heart failure. *N Engl J Med* 336:525–533, Copyright 1997. Massachusetts Medical Society. All rights reserved.)

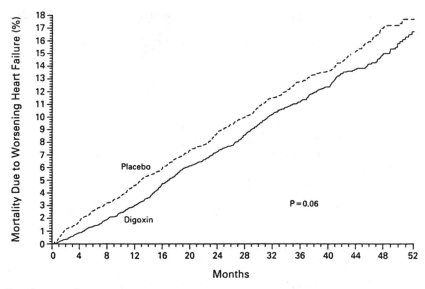

No. of Patients at Risk

| | | | | | | | | | | | | | |
|---|---|---|---|---|---|---|---|---|---|---|---|---|---|
| Placebo | 3403 | 3239 | 3105 | 2976 | 2868 | 2758 | 2652 | 2551 | 2205 | 1881 | 1506 | 1168 | 734 | 339 |
| Digoxin | 3397 | 3269 | 3144 | 3019 | 2882 | 2759 | 2644 | 2531 | 2184 | 1840 | 1475 | 1156 | 737 | 335 |

FIGURE 2.—Mortality resulting from worsening heart failure in the digoxin and placebo groups. The number of patients at risk at each 4-month interval is shown below rhe figure. (Reprinted by permission of The New England Journal of Medicine, from Garg R, and the Digitalis Investigation Group: The effect of digoxin on mortality and morbidity in patients with heart failure. *N Engl J* 336:525–533, Copyright 1997, Massachusetts Medical Society. All rights reserved.)

a lower risk of death from worsening heart failure (Fig 2). Also, in patients treated with digoxin, the hospitalization rate was 6% less than in patients given placebo, and fewer patients were admitted for worsening heart failure (Fig 3). In the substudy, the mortality and hospitalization rates from worsening heart failure were consistent with the rates in the main study.

*Discussion.*—In these patients, digoxin did not affect overall mortality in patients also receiving angiotensin-converting enzyme inhibitors and diuretics, but it lowered the death and hospitalization rates from worsening heart failure. In clinical practice, it is unlikely that digoxin would affect survival rates.

▶ This long-awaited study found digoxin therapy reduced the overall rate of hospitalization and the rate of hospitalization for worsening heart failure. Thus it clearly documents the value of digoxin therapy, even though the study did not document a clear reduction in overall mortality. Other studies of digoxin have shown that digitalis produces an increase of plasma levels of atrial natriuretic peptide and brain natriuretic peptides as well as a significant decrease in plasma renin activity and angiotensin II, aldosterone, and nor-epinephrine levels.[1] Patients with mild heart failure deteriorated clinically

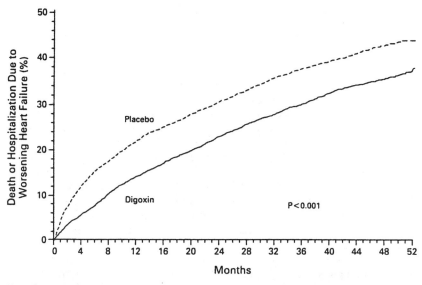

| | | | | | | | | | | | | | |
|---|---|---|---|---|---|---|---|---|---|---|---|---|---|
| Placebo | 3403 | 2915 | 2674 | 2473 | 2328 | 2197 | 2071 | 1954 | 1659 | 1397 | 1111 | 859 | 546 | 250 |
| Digoxin | 3397 | 3120 | 2888 | 2696 | 2544 | 2392 | 2241 | 2115 | 1825 | 1521 | 1188 | 916 | 578 | 255 |

FIGURE 3.—Incidence of death or hospitalization resulting from worsening heart failure in the digoxin and placebo groups. The number of patients at risk at each 4-month interval is shown below the figure. (Reprinted by permission of The New England Journal of Medicine, from Garg R, and the Digitalis Investigation Group: The effect of digoxin on mortality and morbidity in patients with heart failure. *N Engl J Med* 336:525–533, Copyright 1997, Massachusetts Medical Society. All rights reserved.)

after digoxin was withdrawn.[2] I interpret the results to support the use of digoxin in patients with heart failure and normal sinus rhythm.

**R.C. Schlant, M.D.**

*References*

1. Tsutamoto T, Wada A, Maeda K, et al: Digitalis increases brain natriuretic peptides in patients with severe congestive heart failure. *Am Heart J* 134:910–916, 1997.
2. Adams KF, Jr, Gheorghiade M, Uretsky BF. Patients with mild heart failure worsened during withdrawal from digoxin therapy. *J Am Coll Cardiol* 30:42–48, 1997.

## Direct Vascular Effects of Furosemide in Humans

Pickkers P, Dormans TPJ, Russel FGM, et al (Univ of Nijmegen, The Netherlands; Imperial College of Science, Technology, and Medicine, London; Univ of Maastricht, The Netherlands)
*Circulation* 96:1847–1852, 1997 1–45

*Introduction.*—For several years, the standard treatment for heart failure has been the loop-active diuretic furosemide. Arterial vasoconstriction and venous vasodilation have been observed after systemic administration of the drug. Other studies have shown that the drug exerts a direct vasodilator effect on isolated arterial and venous vessels. No studies have examined whether furosemide-induced effects on systemic hemodynamics are the result of a direct or indirect action of the drug on the vasculature in vivo. The genuine direct vascular effects of furosemide on resistance arteries in the forearm and on the dorsa hand vein were thoroughly investigated in healthy individuals with the perfused forearm technique.

*Methods.*—Venous occlusion plethysmography was used to record forearm blood flow in response to infusion of increasing dosages of furosemide into the rachial artery. A linear variable differential transformer was used to measure venous distensibility of a dorsal hand. Five increasing doses of furosemide (1 to 100 μg/min) were administered locally during precontraction with norepinephrine. to determine whether effects were dependent on local prostaglandin or nitric oxide synthesis, additional experiments using local administration of indomethacin or Ng-monomethyl-L-arginine were performed. There was an examination of the effects of systemic administration of furosemide.

*Results.*—During the highest infused dose, local plasma concentrations of furosemide reached a maximum of 234 plus or minus 40 μg/mL, but the ratio of flow in the infused and noninfused arms was not significantly affected. There was a dose-dependent venorelaxation of 18 plus or minus 6% at the first dose of local administration of furosemide to 72 plus or minus 16% at the last dose of local administration of furosemide. Furosemide-induced venorelaxation was almost completely abolished by indomethacin. No effect was seen with Ng-monomethyl-L-arginine. A time-dependent increase of hand vein distensibility was seen with systemic administration of furosemide, reaching 45 plus or minus 11% after 8 minutes.

*Conclusion.*—Even at supratherpeutic concentrations, furosemide does not exert any direct arterial vasoactivity in the human forearm. There was a dose-dependent direct venodilator effect on the dorsal hand vein that appears to be mediated by local vascular prostaglandin synthesis with concentrations estimated to be in the therapeutic range.

▶ This careful study employing forearm blood flow measurements following the infusion of increasing dosages of furosemide into the brachial artery clearly showed a dose-dependent direct venodilator effect on the dorsal hand veins but no direct arterial vasoactivity in the human forearm. Thus, the effects of intravenous furosemide are primarily due to direct venodilatation that may be mediated by local vascular prostaglandin synthesis. In many patients with severe heart failure, it is appropriate to give intravenous furosemide to initiate diuresis. This appears to relieve edema of the GI-tract, which delays and interferes with the diuretic effect of furosemide when given by mouth.

**R.C. Schlant, M.D.**

## Randomised Trial of Losartan Versus Captopril in Patients Over 65 With Heart Failure (Evaluation of Losartan in the Elderly Study, ELITE)

Pitt B, on behalf of ELITE Study Investigators (Univ Hosp, Ann Arbor, Mich; Instituto de Medicina la Paz, Cordoba, Argentina; Innere Medizin-Kardiologie, Krankenhaus Vinzentinum, Ruhpolding, Germany; et al)

*Lancet* 349:747–752, 1997                                                  1–46

*Background.*—Angiotensin-converting enzyme (ACE) inhibitors are useful in the treatment of chronic heart failure and left ventricular dysfunction. However, probably because of their preservation of bradykinin, these drugs (such as captopril) are associated with significant side effects such as cough, angioedema, renal dysfunction, and hypotension. Angiotensin II type 1 receptor antagonists exert their effects without increasing bradykinin levels, and thus these drugs (such as losartan) may avoid the side effects of ACE inhibitors. The safety and efficacy of captopril and losartan were compared in the treatment of heart failure in elderly patients.

*Methods.*—This prospective, double-blind, randomized study involved 722 patients age 65 and older with New York Heart Association class II–IV heart failure, decreased (40% or less) left ventricular ejection fraction, and no history of previous ACE inhibitor use. Patients received 48 weeks of therapy with either captopril (titrated to 50 mg 3 times daily; $n$ = 370) or losartan (titrated to 50 mg once a day; $n$ = 352). End points for discontinuing therapy included a persistent increase in serum creatinine levels of 0.3 mg/dL or more (indicating renal dysfunction); hospitalization for heart failure, myocardial infarction, or angina; worsening of heart failure; hypotension-related symptoms; adverse reaction to the study drugs; and death.

*Findings.*—The 2 groups were similar at baseline with respect to demographics, other drug therapies, and hemodynamic parameters. After treatment, both groups were also similar in the increases in serum creatinine (10.5% in each group) and symptoms related to hypotension. However, the losartan group experienced fewer all-cause deaths (4.8%) than the captopril group (8.7%), primarily because of fewer sudden cardiac deaths in the losartan group. Significantly more patients discontinued therapy or died while taking captopril (30%) than while taking losartan (18.5%).

*Conclusions.*—Neither renal dysfunction nor hospitalizations and deaths because of heart failure were more common with either drug. Similarly, both drugs improved cardiac function after long-term treatment. However, losartan was associated with less all-cause mortality, mainly because of fewer sudden cardiac deaths. Losartan was also associated with fewer drop-outs as a result of drug intolerance. Whether the effects of losartan on reducing cardiac deaths are specific to this drug, or are general to all angiotensin II type 1 receptor antagonists, remains to be determined.

▶ This study in patients aged 65 years and older with systolic left ventricular dysfunction clearly shows the benefit of losartan. Losartan caused persistent increase in serum creatinine about as often as captopril. It may have advantages over ACE inhibitors, which may not produce complete blockade of the effects of angiotensin II. Losartan may be of particular value in patients who have severe cough in response to regular therapy with ACE inhibitors.

R.C. Schlant, M.D.

### Randomised, Placebo-controlled Trial of Carvedilol in Patients With Heart Failure Due to Ischaemic Heart Disease

Krum H, and the Australia/New Zealand Heart Failure Research Collaborative Group (Austin Hosp, Melbourne, Australia)
*Lancet* 349:375–380, 1997                                                      1–47

*Introduction.*—Carvedilol is a β-blocker that has antioxidant and anti-ischemic properties, and has the potential to reduce morbidity and mortality in heart failure. In a previous study of 415 patients with heart failure resulting from ischemic heart disease, carvedilol was administered, and was shown to have improved left ventricular function. The effects of long-term treatment are still unknown, and the follow-up results of these patients for an average of 19 months later were evaluated.

*Methods.*—There was a random assignment of treatment of 415 patients with chronic stable heart failure, with 207 receiving carvedilol and 208 receiving matching placebo. Several measurements were taken at baseline, 6 months, and 12 months, including specific activity scale score, New York Heart Association class, 6-minute walk distance, treadmill exercise duration, left ventricular dimensions, and left ventricular ejection fraction. All deaths, hospital admissions, and episodes of worsening heart failure were documented with the double-blind follow-up for an average of 19 months.

*Results.*—In the carvedilol group compared to the placebo group, left ventricular ejection fraction increased by 5.3% after 12 months, end-diastolic dimension decreased by 1–7 mm, and end-systolic dimension decreased by 3.2 mm. There were no clear changes, however, in the 6-minute walk distance, New York Heart Association class, specific activity scale, or treadmill exercise duration. The rate of death or hospital admission was lower in the carvedilol group than in the placebo group after 19 months, but the frequency of episodes of worsening heart failure was similar.

*Conclusion.*—For at least a year after the start of treatment, the beneficial effects of carvedilol on left ventricular function and size were maintained; however, no extra benefits were demonstrated on symptoms, exercise performance, or episodes of worsening heart failure. After a year of treatment with carvedilol, there was an overall reduction in events resulting in death or hospital admission. To show whether this drug can be recommended as first-line therapy for heart failure, together with angiotensin-converting enzyme inhibitors, trials of several thousand patients and several years must be designed to investigate the effects of carvedilol on survival.

► In this study of 415 patients with chronic stable heart failure resulting from ischemic heart disease, 207 were treated with carvedilol and 208 with matching placebo. Carvedilol apparently had no effect on exercise performance, symptoms, or episodes of worsening heart failure, although it did appear to be associated with an overall reduction in events resulting in death or hospital admission. To date, the studies with carvedilol have been associated with too few deaths to calculate reliably the effect of the drug on survival in patients with heart failure. Hopefully, ongoing studies will provide adequate data regarding the effect of carvedilol upon survival.

**R.C. Schlant, M.D.**

---

**Primary Prevention of Sudden Cardiac Death in Heart Failure: Will the Solution Be Shocking?**
Uretsky BF, Sheahan RG (Univ of Texas, Galveston)
*J Am Coll Cardiol* 30:1589–1597, 1997                    1–48

---

*Introduction.*—In as many as 40% of all patients who suffer from heart failure, sudden cardiac death may occur. Arrhythmia is the major, if not exclusive, cause of sudden death. It is not known what the incidence is of various initiating arrhythmias in sudden cardiac death in heart failure because there are few actual electrocardiographic recordings taken. In the heart failure patient, there is also the possibility that further myocardial necrosis and previous myocardial damage may produce enough pump dysfunction that myocardial failure can occur if sudden death does not (Fig 1). The simplest variable to predict overall survival is the degree of functional impairment, typically classified by the New York Heart Association schema, but there are no indisputably accepted markers to identify the patient with heart failure who is most prone to die suddenly. The current knowledge of sudden cardiac death in heart failure and strategies for primary prevention are reviewed.

*Therapeutic Agents.*—In decreasing mortality in patients with varying degrees of functional impairment, angiotensin converting enzyme inhibitors are used, but the effect of these drugs on sudden cardiac death is less clear, and perhaps has a small effect in preventing sudden cardiac death. Digoxin also seemed to have a low effect on preventing sudden cardiac death in previous studies. No data are found on the effect of diuretic agents on survival in heart failure. Generally, the strategy is to minimize the diuretic dose to a level that allows the patient to be congestion-free as an outpatient. Other agents used have been beta-adrenergic blocking agents, calcium channel blockers, and antiarrhythmic agents.

*Cardioverter-Defibrillator.*—In preventing sudden cardiac death in heart failure patients, most enthusiasm has been generated over the implantable cardioverter-defibrillator, but scientific data are still not available. One study showed that while sudden cardiac death was significantly decreased with the implantable cardioverter-defibrillator, overall mortality was not. The best case scenario for an implantable cardioverter-defibrillator is the patient in functional class II with mortality being decreased by 50%. A

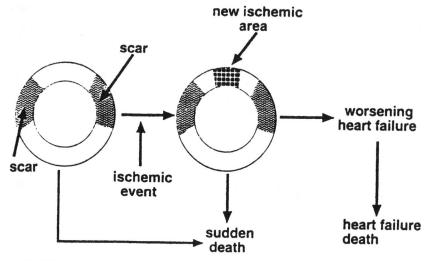

**FIGURE 1.**—In the patient with heart failure from ischemic cardiomyopathy, a small infarction may tip the balance into profound and terminal myocardial failure if the acute ischemic event does not produce a fatal arrhythmia. This possibility must be considered in determining a strategy of sudden death prevention in the individual patient. (Reprinted with permission from the American College of Cardiology from Uretsky BF, Sheahan RG: Primary prevention of sudden cardiac death in heart failure: Will the solution be shocking? *J Am Coll Cardiol* 30:1589–1597, 1997.)

patient in functional class III will have mortality decreased by 30%. In patients in functional class II, 30 life-years will be saved and in patients in class III, 65 life-years will be saved with the cost per life-year saved being about $133,000 for patients in functional class III and $62,000 for those in functional class III.

*Conclusion.*—The greatest benefit in preventing sudden cardiac death occurs in patients with left ventricular dysfunction with mild-to-moderate symptoms, according to data from pharmacologic therapy studies. Drugs become less effective as functional impairment increases. In patients with established heart failure, angiotensin-converting enzyme inhibitors provide only modest, if any protection. Some data support the possibility that beta-blockers and amiodarone decrease the risk of sudden cardiac death. Understanding of the initiating arrhythmias of sudden cardiac death will increase with interrogating electrograms. Approval will soon be granted to newer devices with dual-chamber pacing capabilities. The greatest gain in overall survival from prophylactic implantable cardioverter-defibrillator will occur with less functionally impaired patients with heart failure.

▶ There is a strong possibility that more and more patients with heart failure will be treated with implantable cardioverter-defibrillators. At present, this seems to be the most efficient method of preventing sudden cardiac death. Obviously, there are very significant cost effectiveness questions to be resolved before such therapy can be widely applied.

**R.C. Schlant, M.D.**

**Exercise Training in Patients With Severe Congestive Heart Failure: Enhancing Peak Aerobic Capacity While Minimizing the Increase in Ventricular Wall Stress**
Demopoulos L, Bijou R, Fergus I, et al (Albert Einstein College of Medicine, Bronx, NY)
*J Am Coll Cardiol* 29:597–603, 1997                                                1–49

*Objective.*—Long-term exercise training at conventional work loads (70% of peak aerobic activity) increases cardiac output in patients with severe congestive heart failure. Whether low work load (50% of peak oxygen consumption) exercise programs reverse peripheral abnormalities in these patients is not known. The effects of 12 weeks of low work load exercise training on peak aerobic capacity and hyperemic calf blood flow in patients with severe congestive heart failure and on left ventricular diastolic pressure and wall stress during low and conventional work loads were investigated.

*Methods.*—Sixteen patients (7 women) aged 45–78 years, with congestive heart failure trained 1 hour/day, 4 times/week for 12 weeks. Expired gas was monitored continuously, and limb peak hyperemic blood flow was determined. Left ventricular wall stress was assessed during low levels and conventional levels of exercise in 11 patients (5 women). Echocardiography was performed on all patients at baseline and at the end of the study.

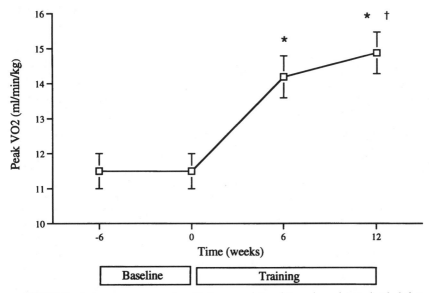

**FIGURE 3.**—Peak oxygen consumption ($V_{O_2}$) measured 6 and 3 weeks and immediately before training and after 6 and 12 weeks of low work load exercise training. \*$P < 0.001$ vs. baseline. †$P < 0.005$ vs. 6 weeks. (Reprinted with permission from the American College of Cardiology, from Demopoulos L, Bijou R, Fergus I, et al: Exercise training in patients with severe congestive heart failure: Enhancing peak aerobic capacity while minimizing the increase in ventricular wall stress. *J Am Coll Cardiol* 29:597–603, 1997.)

*Results.*—Although pulmonary wedge pressure and left ventricular wall stress increased significantly during both low and conventional exercise levels, the increases at low work load levels were substantially less. Peak oxygen consumption increased significantly from 11.5 to 14.0 mL/kg per minute after 6 weeks of training and to 15.0 mL/kg per minute after 12 weeks of training (Fig 3). Peak reactive hyperemia in the calf increased significantly from 19 mL/min at baseline to 32 mL/min at 12 weeks in the calf. Peak reactive hyperemia in the forearm was unchanged. Increases in peak reactive hyperemia were correlated with peak oxygen consumption. Left ventricular end-diastolic volume was unchanged.

*Conclusion.*—Long-term exercise programs at low work loads increase peak aerobic capacity in patients with severe congestive heart failure with smaller increases in left ventricular diastolic wall stress than exercise programs at conventional work loads.

*Clinical Significance.*—Long-term low work load exercise programs benefit patients with severe congestive heart failure by increasing peak aerobic capacity and subjecting the left ventricle to lower wall stress than conventional work load exercise programs.

▶ The usefulness of exercise training of patients with congestive heart failure is well established. In addition to this study, there are at least 10 other publications during 1997 indicating the beneficial effect of exercise training in patients with heart failure.[1–10]

**R.C. Schlant, M.D.**

*References*

1. Hambrecht R, Fiehn E, Jiangtao Y, et al: Effects of endurance training on mitochondrial ultrastructure and fiber type distribution in skeletal muscle of patients with stable chronic heart failure. *J Am Coll Cardiol* 29:1067–1073, 1997.
2. Harrington D, Anker SD, Chua TP, et al: Skeletal muscle function and its relation to exercise tolerance in chronic heart failure. *J Am Coll Cardiol* 30:1758–1764, 1997.
3. Schaufelberger M, Eriksson BO, Grimby G, et al: Skeletal muscle alterations in patients with chronic heart failure. *Eur Heart J* 18:971–980, 1997.
4. Meyer K, Görnandt L, Schwaibold M, et al: Predictors of response to exercise training in severe chronic congestive heart failure. *Am J Cardiol* 80:56–60, 1997.
5. Tyni-Lenné R, Gordon A, Jansson E, et al: Skeletal muscle endurance training improves peripheral oxidative capacity, exercise tolerance, and health-related quality of life in women with chronic congestive heart failure secondary to either ischemic cardiomyopathy or idiopathic dilated cardiomyopathy. *Am J Cardiol* 80:1025–1029, 1997.
6. Belardinelli R, Barstow TJ, Nguyen P, et al: Skeletal muscle oxygenation and oxygen uptake kinetics following constant work rate exercise in chronic congestive heart failure. *Am J Cardiol* 80:1319–1324, 1997.
7. Gordon A, Tyni-Lenné R, Jansson E, et al: Improved ventilation and decreased sympathetic stress in chronic heart failure patients following local endurance training with leg muscles. *Cardiac Failure* 3:3–12, 1997.
8. Kiilavuori K, Sovijärvi A, Näveri H, et al: Effect of physical training on exercise capacity and gas exchange in patients with chronic heart failure. *Chest* 110:985–991, 1996.

9. Meyer K, Samek L, Schwaibold M, et al: Interval training in patients with severe chronic heart failure: Analysis and recommendations for exercise procedures. *Med Sci Sports Exerc* 29:306–312, 1997.
10. Cider Å, Tygesson H, Hedberg M, et al: Peripheral muscle training in patients with clinical signs of heart failure. *Scand J Rehabil Med* 29:121–127, 1997.

---

**Management of Anticoagulation Before and After Elective Surgery**
Kearon C, Hirsh J (McMaster Univ, Hamilton, Ont)
*N Engl J Med* 336:1506–1511, 1997                                    1–50

---

*Objective.*—Questions remain about the perioperative management of patients receiving long-term warfarin therapy. Two competing approaches are an aggressive approach, in which the patient receives IV heparin for 2 days before and after surgery, and a minimalist approach, in which the patients receive no heparin immediately before and after surgery. The expected risks and benefits of these 2 approaches were reviewed.

*Stopping Warfarin.*—If warfarin is stopped 4 days before surgery and resumed as soon as possible afterward, the patient would be expected to have a subtherapeutic international normalized ratio (INR) for 2 days before and 2 days after surgery. However, there will still be partial protection against thromboembolism while the INR remains somewhat elevated. Thus, the thromboembolism risk of stopping warfarin is equivalent to 1 day without anticoagulation before and after surgery. Thromboembolism risk may also be increased by rebound hypercoagulation caused by cessation of warfarin and the prothrombotic effect of surgery. The risk of preoperative arterial and venous thromboembolism and of postoperative venous thromboembolism is comparable to that expected without anticoagulation. However, the risk of postoperative venous thromboembolism will increase greatly. For patients with previous venous thromboembolism, major surgery increases the short-term recurrence risk by more than 100-fold. Anticoagulation produces an 80% reduction in the risk of recurrent venous thromboembolism; a 66% reduction in the risk of arterial thromboembolism in patients with nonvalvular atrial fibrillation; and a 75% reduction in the risk of major thromboembolism in patients with mechanical heart valves.

The risk of bleeding is low if IV heparin is given for 2 days before surgery, but high if heparin is restarted immediately afterward. Giving 2 days of IV heparin will increase the absolute risk of major postoperative bleeding by about 3%. Death will result from recurrent venous thromboembolism in about 6% of cases, from arterial thromboembolism in 20%, and from major postoperative bleeding in 3%.

*Perioperative IV Heparin.*—The risk of postoperative venous thromboembolism is very high for patients with acute venous thromboembolism. Thus, postoperative IV heparin reduces postoperative morbidity in these patients, even though it doubles the risk of bleeding. By 2 or 3 months after the acute episode, however, the risk has dropped sufficiently that preoperative heparin is no longer justified unless other risk factors are present.

Heparin is still indicated postoperatively because of the high risk of postoperative venous thromboembolism. When it has been more than 3 months since the acute venous thromboembolism, prophylactic measures that carry a lower risk of bleeding than IV heparin should be considered. Within 1 month after acute arterial thromboembolism, preoperative IV heparin is indicated. Postoperative heparin is recommended only for patients undergoing minor surgery with a low risk of bleeding. For patients at lower risk of arterial thromboembolism, postoperative IV heparin is more likely to increase morbidity than to reduce it. An alternative approach that has been suggested is outpatient administration of subcutaneous heparin or low-molecular weight heparin. However, this may be impractical and give less predictable results than IV heparin.

*Recommendations.*—If warfarin is withheld the day before surgery, measuring the INR the day before the operation is recommended. This gives the physician the alternative of giving a small dose of vitamin K, if needed. When the INR is less than 2.0, other forms of preoperative and/or postoperative prophylaxis should be considered. If surgery must be performed in the first month after acute venous thromboembolism, give IV heparin preoperatively and postoperatively while the INR is below 2.0. Intravenous heparin may be stopped 6 hours before surgery if the activated partial thromboplastin time is in the therapeutic range. After major surgery, heparin should not be restarted for at least 12 hours, longer if there are signs of bleeding. When restarted, heparin should be given at no more than the expected maintenance infusion rate.

▶ This article should be kept readily available for reference on this problem, which arises very often. The recommendations seem reasonable and very practical.

**R.C. Schlant, M.D.**

---

**Guidelines for Perioperative Cardiovascular Evaluation for Noncardiac Surgery: An Abridged Version of the Report of the American College of Cardiology/American Heart Association Task Force on Practice Guidelines**

Eagle KA, Brundage BH, Chaitman BR, et al (American College of Cardiology)
*Mayo Clin Proc* 72:524–531, 1997                                                    1–51

---

*Introduction.*—Physicians involved in the preoperative, operative, and postoperative care of patients having noncardiac surgery will benefit from a review of these guidelines, which provide a framework for considering cardiac risk of noncardiac surgery. Careful teamwork and communication among patient, primary-care physician, anesthesiologist, surgeon, and medical consultant is necessary. The recommendation is to use a conservative approach in the use of expensive tests and treatments. The preoperative clinical evaluation involves physical examination, initial history, and electrocardiographic assessment, which should focus on identifying potentially serious cardiac disorders. To determine which patients are most likely to benefit from preoperative coronary assessment and treatment, a stepwise bayesian strategy with clinical markers and functional capacity is recommended.

*Steps.*—Eight steps are involved in the stepwise approach to preoperative cardiac assessment. (1) Determine the urgency of noncardiac surgery. (2) Determine whether the patient had coronary revascularization in the past 5 years. (3) Determine whether the patient had coronary evaluation in the past 2 years. (4) Determine whether the patient had an unstable coronary syndrome or a major clinical predictor of risk. (5) Determine whether the patient had intermediate clinical predictors of risk, such as mild angina pectoris or diabetes mellitus. (6) An intermediate risk operation with little likelihood of perioperative death or myocardial infarction is possible in patients without major but with intermediate predictors of clinical risk and with moderate or excellent functional capacity. (7) For patients with neither major nor intermediate predictors of clinical risk and moderate or excellent functional capacity, noncardiac surgery is generally safe. (8) To determine further preoperative management, such as intensified medical therapy, the results of noninvasive testing can be used.

*Assessing Risk.*—The risk of various types of noncardiac surgeries are categorized as high (emergent major operations), intermediate (carotid endarterectomy), or low (endoscopic procedures). Indications for coronary angiography are outlined for class I, class II, and class III patients. Methods of assessing cardiac risk include measuring resting left ventricular function, exercise stress testing, pharmacologic stress testing, ambulatory ECG monitoring, and coronary angiography.

*Conclusion.*—The guidelines also outline the effects of risk assessment strategies on costs and the management of specific preoperative cardiovascular conditions, such as hypertension, valvular heart disease, and myocardial heart disease. Preoperative coronary revascularization is reviewed in regard to coronary artery bypass grafting and coronary artery angioplasty. Anesthetic considerations and intraoperative management includes perioperative pain management, intraoperative nitroglycerin, and transesophageal echocardiography. Perioperative surveillance includes pulmonary artery catheters and intraoperative and post-operative ST-segment monitoring.

▶ These guidelines should be familiar to all physicians who deal with patients during the perioperative phase of noncardiac surgery.

**R.C. Schlant, M.D.**

## Miscellaneous

### A Prospective Study of Risk Factors for Pulmonary Embolism in Women

Goldhaber SZ, Grodstein F, Stampfer MJ, et al (Brigham and Women's Hosp, Boston; Harvard Med School, Boston; Harvard School of Public Health, Boston)
*JAMA* 277:642–645, 1997                                                    1–52

*Background.*—Primary prevention strategies for pulmonary embolism are based on a patient's risk profile. However, few prospective data are available on risk factors in the absence of antecedent cancer, trauma, surgery, or immobilization. Genetic predisposition appears to account for about one fifth of venous thromboembolism cases in women, which implies the existence of many environmental determinants. Risk factors for pulmonary embolism in women were further studied.

*Methods.*—Data were obtained from 112,822 women 30–55 years of age, participating in the Nurses' Health Study between 1976 and 1992. All were free from diagnosed cardiovascular disease or cancer at baseline. Two hundred eighty cases of pulmonary embolism occurred during the 1,619,770 person-years of follow-up. One hundred twenty-five were considered primary, occurring in women with no known antecedent cancer, trauma, surgery, or immobilization.

*Findings.*—A multivariate analysis demonstrated that obesity, cigarette smoking, and hypertension independently predicted pulmonary embolism. Women with a body mass index of 25–28.9 kg/m² had a relative risk (RR) of 1.7. Current smokers of 25–34 cigarettes per day had an age-adjusted RR of 1.8 for primary pulmonary embolism. Those smoking 35 cigarettes a day or more had a RR of 3.4.

*Conclusions.*—Obesity, current cigarette smoking, and hypertension increase the risk for pulmonary embolism. Controlling these risk factors will reduce the risk of pulmonary embolism as well as that for coronary heart disease.

▶ This prospective study indicates that many of the classic risk factors for coronary heart disease such as cigarette smoking, systemic arterial hypertension, and obesity are also associated with increased risk of pulmonary embolism in women. This provides even stronger motivation to decrease these risk factors, particularly in women, but also in men.

**R.C. Schlant, M.D.**

### CT Evaluation of Pulmonary Embolism: Technique and Interpretation

Kuzo RS, Goodman LR (Med College of Wisconsin, Milwaukee)
*AJR* 169:959–965, 1997                                                    1–53

*Introduction.*—It is possible to image the thorax in a short period of time, often during a single breath-hold with the helical and electron beam

CT technology. For the evaluation of suspected pulmonary embolism to the level of the segmental or larger vessels, the helical and electron beam CT are approximately 90% sensitive and 90% specific, according to the results of previous studies. For pulmonary emboli evaluation, CT is being used as a routine clinical tool and has the potential to replace the ventilation-perfusion scan for diagnosing pulmonary embolism. Experience helps distinguish the main subtleties and ambiguities found on CT scan.

> *Technique.*—A test injection is used to estimate circulation time. The main pulmonary artery is located and 10 images are obtained in axial mode over 20 seconds during the injection of 18 mL of full-strength contrast material. A central vein line or a 20-gauge or larger peripheral IV catheter in an antecubital fossa vein is used as the ideal vascular access. Using a 3 mm collimation, a 1.5 mm reconstruction interval, 300 mA, and a pitch of 1.7:1, the diagnostic examination is performed and the patient is scanned in the caudal-to-cranial direction for 12 cm from just above the lower hemidiaphragm to the aortic arch. Using a scan time of 24 seconds, 80 images are obtained. To complete the examination of the entire

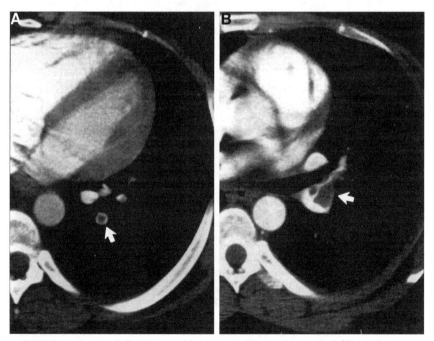

FIGURE 3.—Acute emboli in 26-year-old woman. **A,** CT scan shows central filling defect (*arrow*) within lumen of posterior basal segment artery. **B,** CT scan shows eccentric filling defects (*arrow*) in left interlobar artery with extension into lingular artery. (Courtesy of Kuzo RS, Goodman LR: CT evaluation of pulmonary embolism: Technique and interpretation. *AJR* 169:959–965, 1997.)

chest, the remaining portions of the chest are scanned with 5 mm or 10 mm images.

*Interpretation.*—To interpret CT scans for pulmonary embolism, knowledge of bronchovascular anatomy is essential. A central filling defect outlined by contrast material within the vessel lumen or an eccentric defect that projects into the lumen with an acute angle between the filling defect and vessel wall is the most reliable sign of an acute embolus (Fig 3). Chronic thrombi are represented by filling defects that form a smooth, obtuse angle with the vessel wall. A sign of an acute embolus is complete cutoff of the contrast material opacification of a vessel. Up to 10% of CT scans will be nondiagnostic because of poor contrast opacification or other technical factors. There are some areas where lymphatic tissue can be mistaken for thrombus in an adjacent vessel.

*Diagnosis.*—The most widely used method for the diagnosing pulmonary embolism has been perfusion scintigraphy, but it can only indirectly test for thromboembolic disease. The inability to show most subsegmental emboli is the main shortcoming of CT. In the diagnosis of pulmonary embolism, CT is reasonably accurate and has the potential to become the initial imaging study in workup for suspected thromboembolism. All of the best strategies for cost-effectiveness in diagnosing various pulmonary emboli have included CT. Doppler sonography can be used in instances in which the CT examination findings are negative for pulmonary embolism.

▶ In more and more institutions, CT is being used for the evaluation of patients with suspected embolism, often in place of the ventilation-perfusion scan. In a preliminary study gadolinium-enhanced magnetic resonance angiography of the pulmonary arteries appears to have high sensitivity and specificity for the diagnosis of pulmonary embolism.[1]

**R.C. Schlant, M.D.**

*Reference*

1. Meaney JFM, Weg JG, Chenevert TL, et al: Diagnosis of pulmonary embolism with magnetic resonance angiography. *N Engl J Med* 336:1422–1427, 1997.

---

**A Comparison of Low-molecular-weight Heparin With Unfractionated Heparin for Acute Pulmonary Embolism**
Simonneau G, for the THÉSÉE Study Group (Hôpital Antoine Béclère, Clamart, France; Hôpital Trousseau, Tours, France; et al)
*N Engl J Med* 337:663–669, 1997 1–54

*Introduction.*—Low-molecular weight heparin seems to be at least as effective and safe as standard, unfractionated heparin in the treatment of deep-vein thrombosis. Data are scarce regarding the use of low-molecular weight heparin in the treatment of acute, symptomatic, pulmonary embolism. Six hundred twelve patients with symptomatic pulmonary embolism who did not require thrombolytic therapy or pulmonary embolectomy were randomly assigned to treatment with subcutaneous low-molecular weight heparin given in a fixed dose once daily, or IV unfractionated heparin given in an adjusted dose.

*Methods.*—In both sets of patients, oral anticoagulation therapy was initiated between the first and third days of the start of heparin therapy and was continued for at least 3 months on an open-label basis. Treatments were compared on day 8 and day 90 for major end points: recurrent thromboembolism, major bleeding, and death.

*Results.*—At least 1 end point was reached within the first 8 days of treatment in 9 of 308 (2.9%) patients treated with unfractionated heparin and in 9 of 304 patients treated with low-molecular weight heparin (3.0%). By day 90, these numbers were 22 (7.1%) and 18 (5.9%), respectively. Both treatment groups had similar risks of major bleeding throughout follow-up.

*Conclusion.*—Subcutaneous therapy with low-molecular weight heparin seemed to be as effective and safe as IV unfractionated heparin in the treatment of patients with acute pulmonary embolism.

▶ In this study, 612 patients with symptomatic pulmonary embolism were treated with either adjusted-dose, IV unfractionated heparin or with subcutaneous low-molecular heparin (tinzaparin). The low-molecular weight heparin appeared to be as effective as unfractionated heparin. Although this study was unblinded, there did not appear to be a significant difference in the effects of the 2 forms of heparin. Although most forms of low-molecular weight heparin cost 10–20 times as much as IV unfractionated heparin, fewer tests to monitor the effects of heparin are necessary and, in some instances, outpatient treatment could also substantially reduce costs.

**R.C. Schlant, M.D.**

---

**Association Between Thrombolytic Treatment and the Prognosis of Hemodynamically Stable Patients With Major Pulmonary Embolism: Results of a Multicenter Registry**

Konstantinides S, Geibel A, Olschewski M, et al (Abteilung Innere Medizin III-Kardiologie, Freiburg, Germany; Universitaetsklinik Freiburg, Germany; Universitaetsklinik Gießen, Herz-Zentrum Frankfurt, Germany; et al)

*Circulation* 96:882–888, 1997                                                        1–55

---

*Objective.*—In patients with acute major pulmonary embolism, thrombolytic therapy is commonly used. This treatment can hasten resolution and quickly improve right-sided hemodynamics. However, it is unknown whether these effects translate into improved clinical outcomes for patients who are without severe hemodynamic compromise at presentation. This multicenter trial examined the efficacy and safety of thrombolytic therapy—as an alternative to conventional heparin anticoagulation—for patients with major pulmonary embolism who were in stable hemodynamic condition.

*Methods.*—The analysis included 719 consecutive patients from the Management Strategy and Prognosis of Pulmonary Embolism Registry. All had major pulmonary embolism, as established by clinical, echocardiographic, scintigraphic, and cardiac catheterization criteria. Approximately two-thirds of patients had an acute symptom onset (i.e., within less than 48 hours). At presentation, all patients were in hemodynamically stable condition, with no evidence of cardiogenic shock. One hundred sixty-nine patients received primary thrombolytic therapy within 24 hours of diagnosis. The remaining 550 patients received initial therapy with heparin alone. The study hypothesis was that prompt thrombolytic therapy would lower the risk of death and recurrent pulmonary thromboembolism, with an acceptably low risk of serious bleeding complications.

*Results.*—Thirty-day mortality was 5% in patients receiving thrombolytic therapy vs. 11% in those receiving heparin. Patients with syncope, arterial hypotension, a history of congestive heart failure, and chronic pulmonary disease were more likely to die. However, on multivariate analysis, the only independent predictor of survival was primary thrombolytic therapy: odds ratio 0.46 for in-hospital death, with a 95% confidence interval of 0.21 to 1.00. Recurrent pulmonary embolism occurred in 8% of the thrombolysis group, compared with 19% of the heparin group. However, the rate of major bleeding episodes was 22% with thrombolytic therapy vs. 8% with heparin. Two patients in each group had cerebral hemorrhage, and 1 patient in each group died from a hemorrhagic complication.

*Conclusions.*—For patients with major pulmonary embolism presenting in hemodynamically stable condition, early thrombolytic therapy may lead to improved in-hospital clinical outcomes. Mortality and recurrence rates are lower in patients receiving thrombolytic therapy vs. conventional heparin therapy, although the risk of serious bleeding episodes is somewhat increased. A prospective, randomized trial is needed to define the role of thrombolytic therapy in patients with potentially life-threatening pulmonary embolism but apparent hemodynamic stability.

▶ This study would favor the administration of thrombolytic therapy to patients who have no contraindications, have normal systemic arterial pressure, and have moderate or severe right ventricular dysfunction. At present, one may administer 100 mg of rt-PA as a continuous infusion over a 2-hour period. The risk of intracranial hemorrhage can be lessened by attention to control of hypertension or history of stroke or seizure disorders.

Daniels et al.[1] conducted an overview of 308 patients with pulmonary embolism treated by thrombolysis. They concluded that thrombolytic therapy should commence as soon as possible after diagnosis of pulmonary embolism but that there was still evidence of value of thrombolytic therapy in patients who had symptoms for 6–14 days.

**R.C. Schlant, M.D.**

*Reference*

1. Daniels LB, Parker A, Patel SR, et al: Relation of duration of symptoms with response to thrombolytic therapy in pulmonary embolism. *Am J Cardiol* 80:184–188, 1997.

---

**Atrial Fibrillation Activates Platelets and Coagulation in a Time-dependent Manner: A Study in Patients With Paroxysmal Atrial Fibrillation**
Sohara H, Amitani S, Kurose M, et al (Shinkyo Hosp, Kagoshima, Japan)
*J Am Coll Cardiol* 29:106–112, 1997                                           1–56

---

*Introduction.*—Patients with chronic atrial fibrillation have a higher coagulative state than those with normal sinus rhythm. A risk factor for stroke may be paroxysmal atrial fibrillation, but no studies have examined a change in the coagulative state in patients with paroxysmal atrial fibrillation. Changes in coagulative variables in patients with paroxysmal atrial fibrillation were examined to determine whether the coagulative system is affected by the duration of paroxysmal atrial fibrillation.

*Methods.*—There were 21 patients with paroxysmal atrial fibrillation who had measurements taken of fibrinocoagulation variables taken during atrial fibrillation and 7 days after recovery of sinus rhythm. Positive correlations were seen between beta-thromboglobulin, platelet factor 4, thrombin-antithrombin II complex, and fibrinogen and the duration of atrial fibrillation. At 12 hours after the occurrence of paroxysmal atrial fibrillation, these variables increased significantly. Ten patients had paroxysmal atrial fibrillation that lasted less than 12 hours, and 11 patients had paroxysmal atrial fibrillation that lasted more than 12 hours. The control group was formed by 9 age-matched healthy participants.

*Results.*—In the paroxysmal atrial fibrillation group that lasted more than 12 hours, the levels of beta-thromboglobulin and platelet factor 4 were significantly higher, and thrombin-antithrombin III complex and fibrinogen levels were higher but not significantly higher than the patients who had paroxysmal atrial fibrillation for less than 12 hours. In activated partial thromboplastin time, D-dimer or plasmin inhibitor complex, there were no significant differences between the 2 groups.

*Conclusion.*—Platelet aggregation and coagulation are enhanced by atrial fibrillation, and the duration of atrial fibrillation influences the coagulation and platelet aggregation. Twelve hours after the occurrence of atrial fibrillation, the acceleration of platelet activity and coagulation occurred.

▶ This study presents good evidence that atrial fibrillation itself enhances platelet aggregation and coagulation. This was also shown in a study of 60 patients with nonrheumatic atrial fibrillation.[1] A third study showed some activation of the hemostatic mechanisms after pharmacologic cardioversion of acute nonvalvular atrial fibrillation.[2]

**R.C. Schlant, M.D.**

*References*

1. Pongratz G, Brandt-Pohlmann M, Henneke K-H, et al: Platelet activation in an embolic and pre-embolic status of patients with nonrheumatic atrial fibrillation. *Chest* 111:929–933, 1997.
2. Oltrona L, Broccolino M, Merlini PA, et al: Activation of the hemostatic mechanism after pharmacological cardioversion of acute nonvalvular atrial fibrillation. *Circulation* 95:2003–2006, 1997.

---

**Primary Pulmonary Hypertension: Improved Long-term Effects and Survival With Continuous Intravenous Epoprostenol Infusion**
Shapiro SM, Oudiz RJ, Cao T, et al (Harbor-Univ of California, Los Angeles; St Mary's Med Ctr, Long Beach, Calif; Fourth Military Med Univ, Xi'an, People's Republic of China, et al)
*J Am Coll Cardiol* 30:343–349, 1997                                   1–57

---

*Introduction.*—It is difficult to manage patients with primary pulmonary hypertension because there are few effective therapies. The disease often progresses with increasing pulmonary vascular resistance and pressures, right heart failure, dyspnea, and decreasing functional status. Many agents have been studied in the past 3 decades as potential therapies for primary pulmonary hypertension. A recent agent is epoprostenol, a prostacyclin analogue, which demonstrated short-term benefits in a previous study and sustained benefits after 1 year. The drug's effect on pulmonary artery pressure and cardiac output is not known. Patients with primary pulmonary hypertension were examined using Doppler-echocardiography to determine whether adequate hemodynamic measurements could be taken and to evaluate changes in pulmonary artery pressures and cardiac function in patients treated with continuous infusion of epo.

*Methods.*—Right heart catheterization and Doppler-echocardiography were performed on patients with primary pulmonary hypertension and New York Heart Association functional class III or IV symptoms of congestive heart failure to measure the maximal systolic pressure gradient between the right ventricle and right atrium and cardiac output. A comparison was made between Doppler-echocardiography data and catheterization data. Doppler-echocardiography was used to follow-up patients long term. Eighteen of 69 patients who received epoprostenol were followed up for more than 330 days.

*Results.*—A significant reduction was seen, in the maximal systolic pressure gradient between the right ventricle and right atrium the pressure decreased from 84.1 plus or minus 24.1 to 62.7 plus or minus 18.2. Improved survival was seen in study patients when compared to historical controls. The 1-year survival for the study patients was 80%, the 2-year survival was 76%, and the 3-year survival was 49%. The controls had a 10-month survival of 88%, a 20-month survival of 56%, and a 30-month survival of 47%.

*Conclusion.*—A decrease in pulmonary artery pressure is seen in patients receiving continuous infusion of epo for treatment of primary pulmonary hypertension. Improved long-term survival was seen in patients receiving epo therapy compared to those who did not, according to long-term follow-up results. The predicted improved outcomes were based on shorter follow-up periods.

▶ This study documents improvement in hemodynamics and possibly survival of patients with primary pulmonary hypertension treated with continuous infusions of epoprostenol for up to 700 days. Similar benefit was reported by Hinderlitter et al.[1] In a superb review of primary pulmonary hypertension, Rubin recommended such therapy for patients who do not respond to oral calcium-channel-blocker therapy.[2]

**R.C. Schlant, M.D.**

*References*

1. Hinderlitter AL, Willis PW IV, Barst RJ, et al: Effects of long-term infusion of prostacyclin (epoprostenol) on echocardiographic measures of right ventricular structure and function in primary pulmonary hypertension. *Circulation* 95:1479–1486, 1997.
2. Rubin LJ: Primary pulmonary hypertension. *N Engl J Med* 336:111–117, 1997.

---

**Cocaine-induced Myocardial Ischemia and Infarction: Pathophysiology, Recognition, and Management**
Pitts WR, Lange RA, Cigarroa JE, et al (Univ of Texas, Dallas)
*Prog Cardiovasc Dis* 40:65–76, 1997                                    1–58

---

*Introduction.*—Among patients seeking care in hospital emergency departments, cocaine remains the most commonly used illicit drug, costing $80 million in hospital admissions per year. The effects of cocaine are mediated systemically through alterations in synaptic transmission. By blocking the presynaptic reuptake of norepinephrine and dopamine, cocaine produces an excess of these neurotransmitters at the postsynaptic receptor site and acts as a powerful sympathomimetic agent.

*Ischemia and Infarction.*—A combination of increased myocardial oxygen demand in the setting of limited or fixed supply, marked coronary arterial vasoconstriction, and enhanced platelet aggravations and thrombus formation seem to cause the pathophysiology of cocaine-related myocardial ischemia and infarction. By blocking the presynaptic reuptake of norepinephrine and dopamine, cocaine produces central and peripheral adrenergic stimulation Both α- and β-adrenergic receptors are found in coronary arteries, and α-adrenergic receptor stimulation causes vascular smooth muscle contraction whereas β-adrenergic stimulation induces the

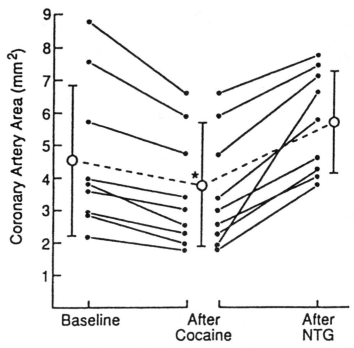

FIGURE 4.—Cross-sectional areas of nondiseased coronary arterial segments at baseline (*left*), after cocaine (*center*), and after nitroglycerin (NTG) (*right*). Each line represents the data from 1 patient. Mean values plus or minus 1 SD are displayed. Coronary arterial area was reduced by cocaine, and this decrease was alleviated by nitroglycerin. *$P$ less than 0.05 in comparison to baseline and nitroglycerin. (Reprinted with permission from the *American College of Cardiology* [Journal of the *American College of Cardiology,* 18:581–586, 1991.] From Brogan WC III, Lange RA, Kim AS, et al: Alleviation of cocaine-induced coronary vasoconstriction by nitroglycerin. *J Am Coll Cardiol* 18:581–586, 1991. Courtesy of Pitts WR, Lange RA, Cigarroa JE, et al: Cocaine-induced myocardial ischemia and infarction: pathophysiology, recognition and management. *Prog Cardiovas Dis* 40:65–76, 1997.)

opposite effect. α-Adrenergic stimulation seems to mediate the cardiovascular effects of cocaine because they are reversed by phentolamine. In patients with cocaine intoxication, β-adrenergic blockers should be avoided because it may increase the magnitude of cocaine-induced myocardial ischemia. Delayed or recurrent coronary arterial vasoconstriction can occur in the setting of cocaine use and is likely due to the effects of its major metabolites. The effects of cocaine may be more pronounced in arterial segments narrowed by atherosclerosis because cocaine induces coronary arterial vasoconstriction in a manner similar to exercise. Those at greater risk of having an ischemic event in response to cocaine are patients with atherosclerotic coronary artery disease.

*Other Substances.*—Cocaine-induced vasoconstriction may be potentiated by other substances used simultaneously, such as cigarettes. Concomitant cigarette smoking exacerbates the deleterious effects of cocaine on myocardial oxygen supply. The metabolic requirement of the heart for oxygen is substantially increased, and the diameter of diseased coronary

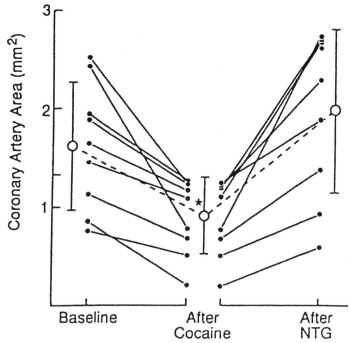

**FIGURE 5.**—Cross-sectional areas of diseased coronary arterial segments at baseline (*left*) and after administration of cocaine (*center*) and nitroglycerin (NTG) (*right*). Each line represents the data from 1 patient. Mean values plus or minus 1 SD are displayed. Coronary arterial area was reduced by cocaine, and this decrease was alleviated by nitroglycerin. *P less than 0.05 in comparison with baseline and nitroglycerin. (Reprinted with permission from the *American College of Cardiology* [Journal of the *American College of Cardiology*, 18:581–586, 1991.] From Brogan WC III, Lange RA, Kim AS, et al: Alleviation of cocaine-induced coronary vasoconstriction by nitroglycerin. *J Am Coll Cardiol* 18:581–586, 1991. Courtesy of Pitts WR, Lange RA, Cigarroa JE, et al: Cocaine-induced myocardial ischemia and infarction: pathophysiology, recognition and management. *Prog Cardiovas Dis* 40:65–76, 1997.)

arterial segments are simultaneously deceased, potentially resulting in more intense myocardial ischemia. Ethanol is also abused simultaneously with cocaine. The combination of the two may increase the determinants of myocardial oxygen demand and simultaneously diminish supply, and the combination may lead to the production of a metabolite which induces marked coronary arterial vasoconstriction leading to myocardial ischemia, infarction, sudden death. or all of these.

*Conclusion.*—Cocaine-induced increase in systemic arterial pressure may be reversed by intravenous labetalol, but labetalol does not alleviate cocaine-induced coronary arterial vasoconstriction. Nitroglycerin or verapamil have been shown to reverse cocaine-induced hypertension and coronary arterial vasoconstriction in patients with cocaine-associated chest pain. In nondiseased and diseased coronary arterial segments, sublingual nitroglycerin abolished the vasoconstriction (Fig 4, Fig 5). Cocaine-induced coronary arterial vasoconstriction can be effectively alleviated with nitroglycerin given in a dose sufficient to reduce mean systemic arterial pressure 10% to 15%.

▶ The group at the University of Texas Southwestern Medical Center have been leaders in the study of cocaine upon the cardiovascular system. Their recommendations appear physiologically sound and are clinically effective. I would heartily endorse their recommendations for treating patients with cocaine-related chest pain.

**R.C. Schlant, M.D.**

---

**Color Duplex Ultrasonography in the Diagnosis of Temporal Arteritis**
Schmidt WA, Kraft HE, Vorpahl K, et al (Clinic of Rheumatology, Berlin; Klinikum Buch, Berlin)
*N Engl J Med* 337:1336–1342, 1997                                    1–59

---

*Introduction.*—Biopsy of the temporal artery is usually recommended to confirm the clinical diagnosis of temporal arteritis, but the procedure may lead to complications, and false negative findings can occur if the biopsy is taken from an area without lesions. Patients with clinically suspected active temporal arteritis or polymyalgia rheumatica were studied prospectively to assess the value of color duplex US in diagnosing temporal arteritis.

*Methods.*—Thirty patients met at least 3 of the 5 criteria for temporal arteritis. Biopsy was performed in 27 patients and yielded positive findings in 21, negative findings in 4, and insufficient material for analysis in 2. Symptoms of both temporal arteritis and polymyalgia rheumatica were present in 16; 2 had symptoms of temporal arteritis alone and 2 had symptoms of polymyalgia rheumatica alone. Thirty-seven patients met 3 criteria for polymyalgia rheumatica, and 15 patients with negative histologic findings received a diagnosis other than temporal arteritis or polymyalgia rheumatica. Controls were 30 patients with rheumatoid arthritis but no signs of temporal arteritis. Two color duplex US studies performed in each case were read before the biopsies.

*Results.*—In patients with temporal arteritis, the diameter of the artery wall was significantly larger than in the other groups. The US studies of 22 (73%) patients with temporal arteritis showed a dark halo around the lumen of the temporal arteries, and the halos disappeared after corticosteroid treatment (mean 16 days). Stenoses or occlusions of temporal artery segments were present in 80% of patients; 93% had stenoses, occlusions, or a halo. None of the US studies of patients without temporal arteritis showed a halo, but stenoses or occlusions were observed in 7%. The interrater agreement was 95% for each of the 3 types of abnormalities identified at US.

*Conclusion.*—Color duplex US visualizes characteristic signs of temporal arteritis with a sensitivity and specificity (Table 2) that may provide a diagnosis without the need for temporal artery biopsy. A dark halo is the

TABLE 2.—Sensitivity and Specificity of Duplex Ultrasonography of the Temporal
Arteries for the Diagnosis of Temporal Arteritis and to Confirm Histologic Findings

| FINDING | DIAGNOSIS* | | CONFIRMATION OF HISTOLOGIC FINDINGS† | |
|---|---|---|---|---|
| | SENSITIVITY positive tests/total (%) | SPECIFICITY negative tests/total (%) | SENSITIVITY positive tests/total (%) | SPECIFICITY negative tests/total (%) |
| Halo | 22/30 (73) | 82/82 (100) | 16/21 (76) | 24/26 (92) |
| Stenosis or occlusion | 24/30 (80) | 76/82 (93) | 18/21 (86) | 23/26 (88) |
| Halo, stenosis, or occlusion | 28/30 (93) | 76/82 (93) | 20/21 (95) | 22/26 (85) |

*Thirty patients had temporal arteritis, and 82 patients had been given other diagnoses.
†Twenty-one patients had positive histologic findings, and 26 patients had negative histologic findings (4 in the temporal arteritis group, 7 in the group with polymyalgia rheumatica, and 15 with other diagnoses).
(Reprinted by permission of the New England Journal of Medicine, from Schmidt WA, Kraft HE, Vorpahl K, et al: Color duplex ultrasonography in the diagnosis of temporal arteritis. *N Engl J Med* 337:1336–1342, Copyright 1997, Massachusetts Medical Society. All rights reserved.)

most specific sign; patients with strong clinical evidence of temporal arteritis but no clear halo should still undergo biopsy.

▶ Giant-cell (temporal) arteritis is a disease most often found in middle-aged and older individuals. Among the vascular complications are loss of vision, stroke, occlusions of the arteries of the arm and neck (aortic arch syndrome), or even rupture of the thoracic aorta. The use of color duplex US as a method of examining blood vessels for evidence of giant-cell arteritis appears to be eminently valuable. Temporal artery biopsy is the standard procedure but is associated with some complications. As stated in the accompanying editorial, a combination of US findings may prove a highly sensitive indicator of the presence or absence of vasculitis and would help in making decisions about whether or not to perform a temporal artery biopsy.[1]

**R.C. Schlant, M.D.**

*Reference*

1. Hunder GG, Weyand CM: Sonography and giant-cell arteritis (editorial). *N Engl J Med* 337:1385–1386, 1997.

# 2 Coronary Heart Disease

## Acute Myocardial Infarction

### Introduction

The articles selected for this edition of the Year Book reflect the spectrum of new developments in the management of acute and chronic coronary artery disease.

The field of acute reperfusion in myocardial infarction remains active, as does the pharmacology of the acute ischemic syndromes, with the emphasis on new antithrombotics and platelet inhibitors. Interventional techniques for both the coronary and the peripheral vasculature continue to proliferate. In this respect, emerging randomized trials of different devices, in addition to comparisons of percutaneous transluminal coronary angioplasty (PTCA) vs. coronary bypass surgery, are providing a growing body of objective evidence from which comparisons of efficacy can be made.

Reference is made to several articles which illustrate socioeconomic and racial differences in the use of therapies and their outcomes. These include studies in which the outcomes with PTCA and devices are correlated with both operator and institutional volumes.

Prior epidemiologic studies clarified the role of the traditional risk factors in coronary artery disease; recent data continue to emphasize the powerful effect of fisk-factor reduction upon the natural history of coronary disease. Increasingly, we are identifying strong associations between coronary disease and "non-traditional" risk factors such as homocysteine. Much attention has also been drawn to the role of inflammation and the genesis of atherosclerosis—this will surely continue to be a focus of intense interest in the coming years.

In summary, as we struggle to adapt to changes in the *delivery of health care*, it is encouraging to note that the pace of scientific advance accelerates.

**Bernard J. Gersh, M.B., Ch.B., D.Phil., F.R.C.P.**

## Early Thrombolytic Treatment in Acute Myocardial Infarction: Reappraisal of the Golden Hour

Boersma E, Maas ACP, Deckers JW, et al (Erasmus Univ, Rotterdam, The Netherlands)
*Lancet* 348:771–775, 1996                                              2–1

*Background.*—The ability of fibrinolytic therapy to reduce the rate of death from acute myocardial infarction is strongly related to the time from the start of symptoms to the start of treatment. However, whether a further significant reduction can be achieved with very early treatment—within 2 to 3 hours after the start of treatment—remains open to debate. Previously reported data were reanalyzed in an attempt to tell whether very early thrombolytic therapy can achieve additional benefits in patients with acute myocardial infarction.

*Methods.*—The analysis considered data on 50,246 patients from 22 large, randomized, placebo-controlled trials of fibrinolytic therapy. Of these, 5,762 patients were randomly assigned within the first 2 hours after symptom onset and another 10,435 between 2 and 3 hours. The data were analyzed to assess the relation between delay to treatment and short-term mortality rate, that is, up to 35 days.

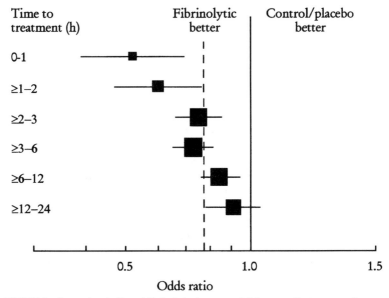

FIGURE 3.—Proportional effect of fibrinolytic therapy on 35-day mortality rate according to treatment delay. Odds ratios, plotted with 95% confidence intervals on a log scale, are significantly different over the 6 groups (Breslow-Day test, $p = 0.001$). Areas of black squares proportional to amount of statistical information. (Courtesy of Boersma E, Maas ACP, Deckers JW, et al: Early thrombolytic treatment in acute myocardial infarction: reappraisal of the golden hour. *Lancet* 348:771–775, 1996. Copyright by The Lancet, Ltd.)

*Results.*—Giving fibrinolytic therapy within the first hour after symptom onset saved 65 lives per 1,000 patients treated. This compared to 37 per 1,000 for patients treated from 1 to 2 hours, 26 per 1,000 from 2 to 3 hours, and 29 per 1,000 from 3 to 6 hours. The reduction in mortality rate was 44% for patients treated within 2 hours compared with 20% for those treated after 2 hours (Fig 3). A nonlinear equation better explained the relation between treatment delay and mortality rate reduction than did a nonlinear regression equation.

*Conclusions.*—In acute myocardial infarction, fibrinolytic therapy is significantly more beneficial when given within 2 hours after symptom onset than when it is given later. Steps are needed to meet the challenges posed by very early fibrinolytic therapy, such as increasing public awareness of the need for immediate medical attention and enhancing early diagnosis. Avoiding unnecessary treatment delays will improve the chances of survival for patients with suspected myocardial infarction.

▶ This article is based on a complex analysis of 22 trials of 50,246 patients treated with fibrinolytic drugs for presumed acute myocardial infarction. The conclusions do, however, bear repeated emphasis: "time is of the essence." These data reaffirm the concept of the "golden hour." The window of great opportunity probably extends to 3 hours.[1] Thereafter, thrombolytic therapy remains of benefit, but the challenge is to initiate treatment within 2 to 3 hours of symptom onset. How to achieve this is more difficult and requires increasing public awareness, more rapid diagnosis both in and out of the hospital,[2] shortening the hospital door-to- needle time, and, in some regions, the use of prehospital thrombolytic therapy.[3]

**B.J. Gersh, M.B., Ch.B., D.Phil., F.R.C.P.**

*References*

1. Gersh BJ, Anderson JL: Thrombolysis in myocardial salvage: results of clinical trials in the animal paradigm—paradoxical predictable? *Circulation* 88:296–306, 1993.
2. Bouten MJM, Simoons ML, Hartman JAM, et al: Prehospital thrombolysis with alteplase (rt-PA) in acute myocardial infarction. *Eur Heart J* 13:925–931, 1992.
3. Great Group: Feasibility, safety and efficacy of domiciliary thrombolysis by general practitioners: Grampien region, early anistreplase trial. *BMJ* 305:548–553, 1992.

---

**Difference in Countries' Use of Resources and Clinical Outcome for Patients With Cardiogenic Shock After Myocardial Infarction: Results From the GUSTO Trial**

Holmes DR Jr, for the GUSTO-I Investigators (Mayo Clinic, Rochester, Minn; Duke Univ, Durham, NC; Universitaire Ziekenhuizen Leuven, Belgium; et al)
*Lancet* 349:75–78, 1997                                                     2–2

---

*Objective.*—More invasive and aggressive cardiologic procedures are used in the United States than in other countries. It is uncertain how this fact translates into improved outcomes, especially for high-risk patients.

TABLE 2.—Use of Interventions and Medications by Geographical Location

| Intervention | USA (n=1891) | Other countries (n=1081) | p* |
|---|---|---|---|
| Cardiac catheterisation | 1092 (58%) | 253 (23%) | <0·001 |
| IABP | 652 (35%) | 80 (7%) | <0·001 |
| Right-heart catheterisation | 1074 (57%) | 236 (22%) | <0·001 |
| Ventilatory support | 1021 (54%) | 405 (38%) | <0·001 |
| CABG | 295 (16%) | 43 (4%) | <0·001 |
| PTCA | 483 (26%) | 82 (8%) | <0·001 |
| Inotropic agent | 1850 (98%) | 998 (93%) | <0·001 |
| β-blocker | 1024 (54%) | 410 (38%) | <0·001 |
| Aspirin | 1768 (94%) | 1016 (94%) | 0·610 |

*Data on types of interventions used for some patients were not available; differences between geographical locations were assessed only for patients whose data were available.
(Courtesy of Holmes DR Jr, for the GUSTO-I Investigators: Difference in countries' use of resources and clinical outcome for patients with cardiogenic shock after myocardial infarction: Results from the GUSTO trial. *Lancet* 349:75–78, 1997. Copyright by The Lancet Ltd.)

Resource utilization and clinical outcomes were compared for patients with cardiogenic shock in the United States vs. other countries.

*Methods.*—Data for the study were drawn from the GUSTO-I trial. The analysis included 3,692 patients with cardiogenic shock after myocardial infarction: 1,891 treated in the United States and 1,081 treated elsewhere. In the study protocol, the patients were randomly assigned to receive combinations of streptokinase, heparin, and accelerated tissue-plasminogen activator. The attending physician made all further patient management decisions. The interventions under question were pulmonary artery catheterization, cardiac catheterization, intravenous inotropic agents, ventilatory support, intraaortic balloon counterpulsation (IABP), percutaneous transluminal coronary angioplasty (PTCA), and coronary artery bypass grafting. Thirty-day all-cause mortality rate was the main outcome measure.

*Results.*—Median age was 68 years for patients treated in the United States vs. 70 years for those treated elsewhere. American patients were also less likely to have anterior myocardial infarction (49% vs. 53%) and had a shorter mean time to treatment (3.1 vs. 3.3 hr). All aggressive interventions were used more frequently in the United States than elsewhere: 58% vs. 23% for cardiac catheterization, 35% vs. 7% for IABP, 57% vs. 22% for right-heart catheterization, and 54% vs. 38% for ventilatory support (Table 2). Twenty-six percent of patients treated in the United States had PTCA compared with just 8% of those treated elsewhere. Patients in all countries survived longer if they had revascularization (Table 3). Adjusted 30-day mortality rate was 50% for patients treated in the United States vs. 66% for those treated elsewhere. By 1 year, the death rate was 56% for patients treated in the United States vs. 70% for those treated elsewhere, for a hazard ratio of 0.69.

*Conclusions.*—For patients with cardiogenic shock after acute myocardial infarction, mortality rate is lower for those treated in the United States

TABLE 3.—Outcome of Cardiogenic Shock by 30 Days and Type of Revascularization Used

| Intervention | USA | Other countries | p |
|---|---|---|---|
| All patients | | | |
| n | 1891 | 1081 | |
| Deaths by 30 days | 936 (50%) | 711 (66%) | <0·001 |
| CABG | | | |
| n | 295 | 43 | <0·001 |
| Deaths by 30 days | 81 (27%) | 17 (38%) | 0·722* |
| PTCA | | | |
| n | 483 | 82 | <0·001 |
| Deaths by 30 days | 84 (30%) | 39 (48%) | 0·090* |

*Value for differential effect of intervention in patients from United States vs patients from other countries.
(Courtesy of Holmes DR Jr, for the GUSTO-I Investigators: Difference in countries' use of resources and clinical outcome for patients with cardiogenic shock after myocardial infarction: Results from the GUSTO trial. *Lancet* 349:75–78, 1997. Copyright by The Lancet Ltd.)

than for those treated elsewhere. This finding could be related to the more aggressive treatment received by U.S. patients. Selection bias could also play a role.

▶ The most likely explanation for the lower mortality rate among patients with cardiogenic shock treated in the United States is the fact that they undergo aggressive interventions (both diagnostic and therapeutic) more frequently than their counterparts in other countries. Nonetheless, before we automatically give ourselves a congratulatory pat on the back and attribute the better results to the more aggressive use of catheterization and revascularization, we need to take other factors into account, including selection bias. In a large registry study, Hochman et al.[1] showed that the major determinant of a lower mortality rate in patients with cardiogenic shock was selection for cardiac catheterization, irrespective of whether revascularization was performed. Other factors that may account for these geographic differences in outcomes include differences in hospital facilities and attitudes among both physicians and patients toward the treatment of severely ill patients with emergency conditions such as cardiogenic shock.

In summary, it may well be that emergency cardiac catheterization and coronary revascularization is the preferred approach to the treatment of cardiogenic shock in evolving myocardial infarction.[2] Results of ongoing randomized trials should soon be available. Nonetheless, a sobering aspect of these data, emanating from the current era of thrombolysis and acute reperfusion, is the persistently high mortality rate from cardiogenic shock both in the United States and elsewhere. It follows that there is ample room for improvement.

**B.J. Gersh, M.B., Ch.B., D.Phil., F.R.C.P.**

*References*

1. Hochman JS, Boland J, Sleeper JA, et al: Current spectrum of cardiogenic shock and effect of early revascularization on mortality. *Circulation* 91:873–881, 1995.

2. Hibbard MD, Holmes DR, Bailey KR, et al: Percutaneous transluminal coronary angioplasty in patients with cardiogenic shock. *J Am Coll Cardiol* 19:639–646, 1992.

## TNK-Tissue Plasminogen Activator in Acute Myocardial Infarction

Cannon CP, and the TIMI 10A Investigators (Harvard Med School, Boston; West Roxbury VA Med Ctr, Mass; Iowa Heart Ctr, Des Moines; et al)
*Circulation* 95:351–356, 1997                    2–3

*Introduction.*—Many different variants of tissue plasminogen activator (TPA) have been created using genetic engineering techniques. One of these, designated TNK-TPA, has several promising characteristics: slow plasma clearance, high specificity for fibrin, and high resistance to plasminogen activator inhibitor-1. The pharmacokinetics, safety, and efficacy of TNK-TPA were assessed in a pilot study.

*Methods.*—The phase 1 trial included 113 patients with acute myocardial infarction and ST-segment elevation. All patients were seen within 12 hours of symptom onset. All patients received a single dose of TNK-TPA. The dose ranged from 5 to 50 mg, with all doses given over 5–10 seconds. The safety and pharmacokinetic profiles of TNK-TPA were evaluated. Coagulation measures were evaluated to determine the effects of the various doses. Angiograms were evaluated by Thrombolysis in Myocardial Infarction (TIMI) flow grade and TIMI frame count.

*Results.*—Plasma clearance of TNK-TPA was 151 mL/min, compared to 572 mL/min for wild-type TPA. Half-life was 17 and 3.5 minutes, respectively. One hour after TNK-TPA treatment, systemic fibrinogen had fallen by 3% and plasminogen by 13%. Fifty-seven percent of patients receiving the 30 mg dose of TNK-TPA had achieved TIMI grade 3 flow at 90 minutes. Of patients receiving the 50 mg dose, 64% achieved TIMI grade 3 flow. Major bleeding occurred in 6% of patients, usually at a vascular access site.

*Conclusions.*—TNK-tissue plasminogen activator is a promising new thrombolytic agent that warrants further investigation. Its long half-life permits it to be given as a single bolus. It is highly specific for fibrin, achieves a high rate of patency, and has a good safety profile. These preliminary results suggest that TNK-TPA offers more rapid and complete thrombolysis than front-loaded TPA.

▶ Despite the interest in primary angioplasty, the search continues for a new generation of improved thrombolytic agents. It must be accepted that for the majority of patients in the world with an acute myocardial infarction, prompt access to a cardiac catheterization laboratory is not an option.

TNK-tissue plasminogen activator is a promising agent that has a half-life approximately three-fold longer than that of TPA and, consequently, blood levels similar to those of a 90-minute infusion of TPA can be achieved by a single bolus. Moreover, TNK-TPA is markedly more fibrin-specific than TPA, and in animal studies has been found to produce more rapid recanalization and a greater degree of clot lysis than a front-loaded TPA regimen. Whether this will actually translate into improved patency rates and a reduced incidence of hemorrhage in the clinical setting remains to be seen. Nonetheless, these initial results are promising, and the TIMI grade 3 flow achieved by 90 minutes in 64% of patients treated with the higher dose compares favorably with previous data using front-loaded TPA.[1] However, overall infarct-related patency (TIMI grade 2 and TIMI grade 3 flow) was 86% at 90 minutes, which is similar to that reported with front-loaded TPA or the double-bolus TPA regimen. It does suggest that perhaps there is a "ceiling" on *overall* patency that can be achieved with thrombolytic agents, aspirin, or heparin, although it is likely that the most important determinant of mortality is TIMI grade 3 flow. A randomized comparison of TNK-TPA and front-loaded TPA is needed and is currently underway.

**B.J. Gersh, M.B., Ch.B., D.Phil., F.R.C.P.**

*Reference*

1. The GUSTO Angiographic Investigators: The comparative effects of tissue plasminogen activator, streptokinase or both on coronary arterial patency, ventricular function and survival after acute myocardial infarction. *N Engl J Med* 329:1615–1622, 1993.

---

**Improved Outcome of Elderly Patients (≥75 Years of Age) With Acute Myocardial Infarction From 1981–1983 to 1992–1994 in Israel**
Gottlieb S, for the SPRINT and Thrombolytic Survey Groups (Neufeld Cardiac Research Inst, Tel Hashomer, Israel; Bikur Cholim Hosp, Jerusalem)
*Circulation* 95:342–350, 1997                                            2–4

---

*Introduction.*—More and more patients aged 75 years and older are being treated for acute myocardial infarction (AMI). Despite the decline in mortality from AMI and the removal of age as a contraindication to thrombolytic therapy, mortality remains high for elderly patients with AMI. The management, complications, and prognosis of elderly patients treated before and after the introduction of thrombolytic therapy were compared.

*Methods.*—Two groups of patients aged 75 years and older treated for AMI in Israeli coronary care units were studied. One group of 789 patients were treated in 1981–1983, before the availability of reperfusion therapy. The other group consisted of 366 patients treated in 1992–1994, after the introduction of reperfusion therapy. The 2 groups were compared for their characteristics and hospital management. Complications were assessed, as were 30-day and 1-year outcomes.

*Findings.*—A higher percentage of elderly patients were hospitalized in the coronary care units in the 1990s. The 1990s cohort was slightly older than the 1980s cohort and had more non–Q-wave and inferior Q-wave infarctions. One third of the later cohort received reperfusion therapy. The complication rate was lower in the 1990s cohort. Thirty-day mortality was

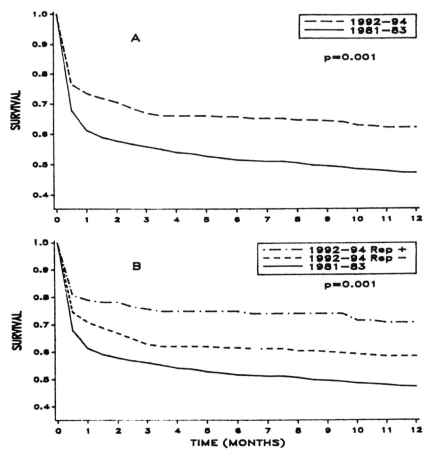

FIGURE 1.—Cumulative 1-year survival curves of patients 75 years of age or older for 1981–1983 vs. 1992–1994 cohorts (A) and 1981–1983 vs. reperfused (*Rep +*) and nonreperfused (*Rep–*) patients in 1992–1994 (B). (Reproduced with permission from Gottlieb S, for the SPRINT and Thrombolytic Survey Groups: Improved outcome of elderly patients (≥75 years of age) with acute myocardial infarction from 1981–1983 to 1992–1994 in Israel. *Circulation* 95:342–350, 1997. Copyright 1997, American Heart Association.)

38% in the 1981–1983 vs. 27% in 1992–1994, odds ratio 0.49. Cumulative 1-year mortality was 52% vs. 38%, respectively, hazard ratio 0.62 (Fig 1). In the later cohort, patients who received reperfusion therapy—i.e., thrombolysis and/or percutaneous transluminal coronary angioplasty, or coronary artery bypass grafting—had the greatest reduction in mortality. However, mortality was also reduced in the nonreperfused patients. Cumulative 1-year mortality was 29% in reperfused patients and 42% in nonreperfused patients, with hazard ratios of 0.45 and 0.60, respectively (Fig 3).

*Conclusions.*—This study documents improved outcomes for elderly patients with AMI over the past decade. The in-hospital complication rate

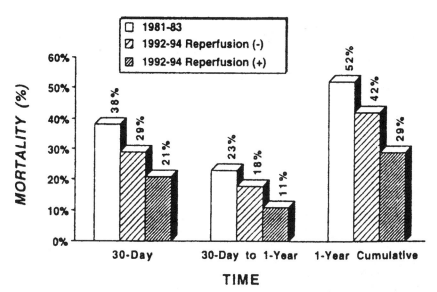

FIGURE 3.—Thirty-day, 30-day to 1-year, and cumulative 1-year total mortality rates in 1981–1983 and for reperfused and nonreperfused patients in 1992–1994. (Reproduced with permission from Gottlieb S, for the SPRINT and Thrombolytic Survey Groups: Improved outcome of elderly patients (≥75 years of age) with acute myocardial infarction from 1981–1983 to 1992–1994 in Israel. *Circulation* 95:342–350, 1997. Copyright 1997, American Heart Association.)

has decreased, and mortality has declined by about 30%, especially in patients undergoing reperfusion therapy. The results suggest that changes in patient management have led to improved outcomes for elderly patients with AMI. Patients aged 75 years or older should receive reperfusion therapy unless otherwise contraindicated.

▶ The increased mortality of AMI associated with increasing age is well documented. The reasons are multifactorial, including a greater prevalence of co-morbidity, more extensive coronary artery disease, preexisting left ventricular dysfunction and hypertrophy, and a greater risk of cardiac rupture, among other factors.[1, 2] This large study from Israel is encouraging, in that mortality in the elderly is declining in conjunction with an increased use of thrombolytic therapy and invasive procedures in the elderly. Although it is well established that the contraindications to thrombolytic therapy are more frequent in the elderly,[3] it would still appear that thrombolytic agents are underutilized in this population, even among the subgroup who are eligible for therapy. Among those who are not, consideration should be given to primary angioplasty.

In any event, this and other studies demonstrate the efficacy of thrombolysis in the elderly, and because the latter are a very high risk subgroup, the overall number of lives saved is greater in the elderly than in younger patients.[4] Among elderly patients who are not candidates for thrombolytic therapy, there is disturbing evidence that other drugs known to be beneficial such as aspirin and beta-blockers are underutilized.[5]

Postdischarge mortality in the elderly is high, particularly among patients older than 70 years. Many of the late deaths are probably the result of ischemia, and this raises the question of whether we should be more aggressive in regard to invasive procedures in the elderly as opposed to being more conservative. Whether such an approach is justified will require further meticulously controlled studies because the implications in terms of costs and periprocedural morbidity and mortality are substantial.

**B.J. Gersh, M.B., Ch.B., D.Phil., F.R.C.P.**

*References*

1. Weaver WD, Litwin PE, Martin JS, et al: Effect of age on use of thrombolytic therapy and mortality in acute myocardial infarction. *J Am Coll Cardiol* 18:657–662, 1991.
2. Smith SC, Gilpin E, Ahnve S, et al: Outlook after acute myocardial infarction in the very elderly compared with that in patients aged 65–75 years. *J Am Coll Cardiol* 16:784–792, 1990.
3. Chaitman BR, Thompson B, Wittry MD, et al: The use of tissue plasminogen activator for acute myocardial infarction in the elderly: Results from Thrombolysis in Myocardial Infarction phase I, open label studies and the Thrombolysis and Myocardial Infarction phase II pilot study. *J Am Coll Cardiol* 14:1159–1165, 1989.
4. Grines CL, DeMaria AN: Optimal utilization of thrombolytic therapy for acute myocardial infarction: Concepts and controversies. *J Am Coll Cardiol* 16:223–231, 1990.
5. Krumholz HM, Radford MJ, Ellerbeck EF, et al: Aspirin in the treatment of acute myocardial infarction in elderly Medicare beneficiaries: Pattern of use and outcome. *Circulation* 92:2841–2847, 1995.

---

### Gender and Acute Myocardial Infarction: Is There a Different Response to Thrombolysis?

Woodfield SL, Lundergan CF, Reiner JS, et al (George Washington Univ, Washington, DC; Univ Community Hosp, Tampa, Fla; Univ of Alberta, Edmonton, Canada; et al)

*J Am Coll Cardiol* 29:35–42, 1997 2–5

---

*Background.*—The mortality rate of women after acute myocardial infarction is believed to be higher than that of men. The effect of gender on the success rate of thrombolytic therapy and on the ventricular response to injury and reperfusion has not been well documented. The effect of gender on early and late infarct-related artery patency and reocclusion after thrombolytic therapy for acute myocardial infarction, left ventricular function in response to injury/reperfusion, and 30-day mortality rate was examined.

*Methods.*—The study group consisted of participants in the Global Utilization of Streptokinase and Tissue Plasminogen Activity for Occluded Coronary Arteries (GUSTO-I) Angiographic Study. Global and regional left ventricular function and patency rates were compared in men and women 90 minutes and 5–7 days after thrombolytic therapy for acute

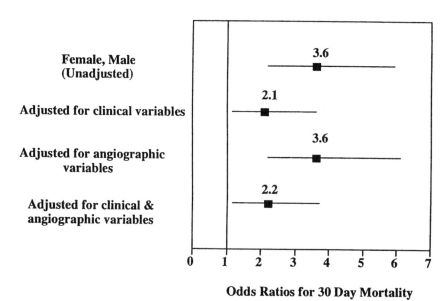

Female, Male
(Unadjusted)

Adjusted for clinical variables

Adjusted for angiographic
variables

Adjusted for clinical &
angiographic variables

**Odds Ratios for 30 Day Mortality**

FIGURE 3.—Effect of gender on 30-day mortality after adjustment for clinical and angiographic variables, or both. The relative ORs (*squares*) and 95% CIs (*horizontal lines*) for mortality are plotted for men vs. women. A ratio greater than 1 denotes higher risk for mortality among women. Clinical variables included age, diabetes, history of previous myocardial infarction, initial heart rate, and initial blood pressure. Angiographic variables included multivessel disease and 90-minute TIMI flow grade. *Abbreviations: OR,* odds ratio; *CI,* confidence interval; *TIMI,* thrombolysis in myocardial infarction. (Reprinted with permission from the American College of Cardiology, from Woodfield SL, Lundergan CF, Reiner JS, et al: Gender and acute myocardial infarction: Is there a different response to thrombolysis? *J Am Coll Cardiol* 29:35–42, 1997.)

myocardial infarction. The effect of gender on infarct-related artery patency, left ventricular function, and 30-day mortality was investigated.

*Results.*—As compared to the men in the study group, the women were significantly older, with more hypertension, diabetes, hypercholesterolemia, heart failure, and shock. The women were also less likely to have smoked, had a previous myocardial infarction, or previous bypass surgery. Ninety-minute patency rates and reocclusion rates were not significantly different for men and women. Women had more recurrent ischemia than men. The 90-minute ejection fraction and the regional ventricular flow were clinically similar in men and women. There were no clinically significant differences in left ventricular function at 5- to 7-day follow-up. The 30-day mortality rate was significantly higher in women than in men. After adjustment for age, diabetes, previous myocardial infarction, initial heart rate, and initial blood pressure, gender remained an independent risk factor for 30-day mortality (Fig 3).

*Conclusions.*—Thrombolytic therapy is equally effective in establishing early patency in the infarct-related artery of both men and women. This implies that thrombolytic therapy remains an effective method of ventricular salvage for patients of either gender. There was no gender-specific difference between male and female myocardium in response to injury and reperfusion. The hyperkinesia of the noninfarct zone was significantly greater in women than in men. Despite these findings, 30-day mortality remained significantly higher for women, even after adjustment for clinical and angiographic variables.

▶ Mortality of acute myocardial infarction in women is generally regarded to be higher than in men even in the reperfusion era.[1] The reasons underlying this consistent increase in mortality are, however, unclear and remain speculative. This study from the GUSTO-I database suggests that patency rates and both global and regional left ventricular function are similar in women and in men, even though there was a significantly higher 30-day mortality rate for women. Part of the difference may be attributable to the higher incidence of hypertension, diabetes, and hypercholesterolemia in the women, among whom there was also a higher incidence of heart failure and shock. On the other hand, even after adjustment for clinical variables, there appeared to be a slight but nonetheless significant *independent* adverse effect of female gender upon survival. One contributing factor may be the slightly higher risk of reocclusion in women, but it is unlikely that this would account for all of the difference.

One should point out that in this study, which is based upon a patient population entered into randomized trials, the use of subsequent coronary revascularization procedures, and by definition, thrombolysis, was equal in the 2 groups. This may not be the case in the community at large in which there is evidence that women (for a variety of reasons) are less likely to receive thrombolytic therapy and subsequent revascularization.[2, 3] One has to conclude that there is much about gender-related differences in morbidity and mortality after acute myocardial infarction that we still do not understand.

**B.J. Gersh, M.B., Ch.B., D.Phil., F.R.C.P.**

*References*

1. ISIS-2 (Second International Study of Infarct Survival) Collaborative Group: Randomized trial of intravenous streptokinase, oral aspirin, both or neither among 17,187 cases of acute myocardial infarction. *Lancet* 2:349–360, 1988.
2. Maynard C, Althouse R, Cerqueira M, et al: Underutilization of thrombolytic therapy in eligible women with acute myocardial infarction. *Am J Cardiol* 68:529–530, 1991.
3. Ayanian JZ, Epstein EM: Differences in the use of procedures between women and men hospitalized for coronary heart disease. *N Engl J Med* 352:221–225, 1991.

### Delayed Hospital Presentation in Patients Who Have Had Acute Myocardial Infarction

Gurwitz JH, McLaughlin TJ, Willison DJ, et al (Harvard Med School, Boston; Univ of Massachusetts, Boston; McMaster Univ, Hamilton, Ont, Canada)
*Ann Intern Med* 126:593–599, 1997                                              2–6

*Introduction.*—In-hospital and long-term mortality have been correlated with time from the onset of symptoms of acute myocardial infarction to hospital presentation. Delayed hospital presentation has been recognized as the largest contributor to postponed treatment of acute myocardial infarction with the advent of the thrombolytic era. A relationship between early treatment and improvements in short-term survival has been demonstrated. To develop appropriate patient-directed educational interventions to reduce delay, the identification of factors contributing to delayed hospital presentation in patients who have had acute myocardial infarction is essential. Patients with acute myocardial infarction at the time of admission to a hospital were evaluated.

*Methods.*—There were 2,409 patients hospitalized in 37 hospitals in a 10-month period who had a retrospective review of their charts. The main outcome measure was hospital presentation that was delayed more than 6

TABLE 3.—Adjusted Odds Ratio Relating Patient Characteristics to Delay of More Than 6 Hours

| Characteristic | Adjusted Odds Ratio (95% CI) |
|---|---|
| Age | |
| <55 years | 1.00 |
| 55–64 years | 0.83 (0.64–1.09) |
| 65–74 years | 0.95 (0.74–1.22) |
| 75–84 years | 1.07 (0.83–1.39) |
| ≥85 years | 1.40 (1.00–1.95)* |
| Sex | |
| Male | 1.00 |
| Female | 1.24 (1.04–1.48) |
| Hypertension | |
| No | 1.00 |
| Yes | 1.21 (1.02–1.44) |
| Mechanical revascularization | |
| No | 1.00 |
| Yes | 0.67 (0.52–0.88) |
| Chest discomfort | |
| No | 1.00 |
| Yes | 0.67 (0.52–0.86) |
| Time of symptom onset† | |
| 6:00 a.m. to 11:59 a.m. | 1.00 |
| Noon to 5:59 p.m. | 1.55 (1.05–2.27) |
| 6:00 p.m. to 11:59 p.m. | 3.07 (2.18–4.33) |
| Midnight to 5:59 a.m. | 3.64 (2.55–5.21) |

*$P = 0.048$
†For patients who arrived at the hospital within 24 hours of symptom onset.
*Abbreviation: CI,* confidence interval.
(Courtesy of Gurwitz JH, McLaughlin TJ, Willison DJ, et al: Delayed hospital presentation in patients who have had acute myocardial infarction. *Ann Intern Med* 126:593–599, 1997.)

hours after symptoms of acute myocardial infarction became apparent. The analysis included age, sex, marital status, living arrangement, location of residence, employment status, health insurance status, median income, presence of chest discomfort, and medical history.

*Results.*—Forty percent of the patients were delayed for more than 6 hours for presentation to the hospital after the onset of their symptoms. Advanced age and female sex were the factors associated with prolonged delay (Table 3). The risks for prolonged delay were significantly reduced by the presence of chest discomfort and a history of mechanical revascularization. During the evening and early morning hours, the risk for delay was greatest. Presentation was more likely to be delayed by patients with a history of hypertension. Emergency medical transport services were used by 42% of patients hospitalized with acute myocardial infarction.

*Conclusion.*—Hospital presentation is often delayed by patients with acute myocardial infarction. The prompt use of emergency medical transport services should be promoted, as should information targeted to elderly persons, women, and persons with cardiac risk factors to reduce the length of delay and to improve the outcomes of patients with acute myocardial infarction.

▶ It is well established that the time from symptom onset to presentation to hospital correlates strongly with the mortality of acute myocardial infarction. In the era of reperfusion, time delays translate into loss of salvageable muscle. The reasons for delay are multifactorial, but patient indecision in seeking medical help is perhaps the most important.[1] It is of interest that women suspected of having acute myocardial infarction are more likely than men to delay presentation. There are several potential explanations, including differences between men and women in age, premorbid conditions, symptoms, social support, and other socioeconomic factors, although even when a multivariate analysis attempted to adjust for these factors, female sex remained an independent predictor of delay.

Programs that are targeted to reducing the delays between symptom onset and presentation have not been very successful in the past, in contrast with the striking reductions achieved in reducing delays from arrival to hospital to treatment.[2] Innovative approaches to reducing patient-related delay are needed and this study would suggest that the elderly and women are prime targets for such intervention. If these new strategies were successful, this could likely exert a powerful effect upon reducing the overall *community* mortality of acute myocardial infarction, given the proved benefit of reperfusion and other therapies that are available in the hospital or, in some countries, in the ambulance.

**B.J. Gersh, M.B., Ch.B., D.Phil., F.R.C.P.**

*References*

1. Meischke H, Ho MT, Eisenberg MS, et al: Reasons patients with chest pain delay or do not call 911. *Ann Emerg Med* 25:193–197, 1995.
2. Weaver WD: Time to thrombolytic therapy; Factors affecting delay and their inference on outcome. *J Am Coll Cardiol* 25:3S–9S, 1995.

**Can We Provide Reperfusion Therapy to All Unselected Patients Admitted With Acute Myocardial Infarction?**
Juliard J-M, Himbert D, Golmard J-L, et al (Hôpital Bichat, Paris; Hôpital Pitié-Salpétrìre, Paris)
*J Am Coll Cardiol* 30:157–164, 1997                                                    2–7

*Introduction.*—Intravenous thrombolysis is of proven benefit during the early hours of acute myocardial infarction, but only a minority of patients receive this treatment because of contraindications, uncertainty of diagnosis, or other reasons. In addition, among those receiving IV thrombolysis, a considerable number fail to achieve Thrombolysis in Myocardial Infarction (TIMI) flow grade 3 patency. The maximal rate of acute TIMI grade 3 patency that could be achieved in unselected patients was determined prospectively in a cohort of 500 consecutive patients.

*Methods.*—The study used a patency-oriented management approach in which 257 patients eligible for thrombolysis received thrombolysis and underwent 90-minute angiography to detect persistent occlusions for treatment with rescue percutaneous transluminal coronary angioplasty (PTCA). Emergency PTCA was attempted in 193 patients with contraindications to thrombolysis, cardiogenic shock, uncertain diagnoses, or who were admitted with ideal conditions for primary PTCA. Thirty-eight patients underwent direct angiography without PTCA and 12 were treated with conventional medical therapy.

*Results.*—The mean age of the cohort was 59 years; 81.4% of patients were men. The average delay between symptom onset and admission to the

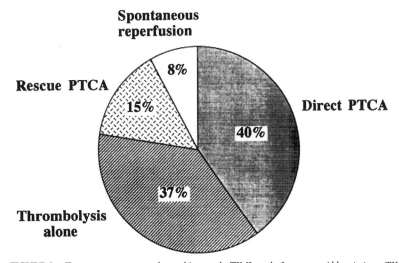

**FIGURE 3.**—Treatment strategy used to achieve early TIMI grade 3 patency. *Abbreviations: TIMI*, Thrombolysis in Myocardial Infarction; *PTCA*, percutaneous transluminal coronary angioplasty. (Reprinted with permission from the American College of Cardiology from Juliard J-M, Himbert D, Golmard J-L, et al: Can we provide reperfusion therapy to all unselected patients admitted with acute myocardial infarction? *J Am Coll Cardiol* 30:157–164, 1997.)

coronary care unit was 184 minutes. Angiographically proven early TIMI grade 3 patency was achieved in 78% of the 98% of patients who received reperfusion therapy. Early TIMI grade 3 was achieved by direct PTCA in 40% of cases, thrombolysis alone in 37%, and rescue PTCA in 15%; 8% of patients experienced spontaneous reperfusion (Fig 3). Forty-seven patients (9.4%) died in the hospital. The mortality rate was increased in patients with TIMI grade 2 (17.5%) and grade 1 or 0 patency (18.8%) compared with those with angiographically proven TIMI grade 3 flow (6.6%). Reocclusion was detected in 27 (7%) of 391 patients with proven early grade 3 patency just before discharge.

*Conclusion.*—The addition of direct and emergency PTCA to IV thrombolysis provides options that allow nearly all patients with myocardial infarction to receive reperfusion therapy. In this cohort of unselected patients, 78% achieved angiographically proven early TIMI grade 3 patency, which is more than twice the rate provided by IV thrombolysis alone.

▶ This series documents an interesting and comprehensive approach to reperfusion therapy in patients with acute myocardial infarction admitted within 6 hours after symptoms. The initial therapy was thrombolysis, unless there were contraindications, which included cardiogenic shock, or unless conditions were "ideal" for primary angioplasty (i.e., the immediate availability of a catheterization laboratory during daytime hours). Mortality in the thrombolysis alone group was low, just as it was (surprisingly so) in patients undergoing rescue PTCA, perhaps because this was dictated by routine 90-minute angiography to evaluate patency as opposed to persistent symptoms or complications after thrombolytic therapy. The high mortality in the primary PTCA group is related to the presence of cardiogenic shock, older age, and the fact that contraindications to thrombolytic therapy defined a higher risk population.

The problem with this approach are the costs involved in undertaking routine angiography 90 minutes after lytic therapy. What would have been the results if angiography was limited to those patients who did not respond clinically to IV thrombolytics?

My own bias is that this kind of approach is the most practical for the majority of institutions, which are not geared to perform primary angioplasty around-the-clock. What we really need are new and improved techniques for the noninvasive assessment of successful reperfusion after IV thrombolytic therapy that would avoid the costs and logistics involved in routine angiography to assess graft patency. The most promising on the horizon are the IV myocardial contrast echocardiographic agents, but their clinical application is a few years away.

**B.J. Gersh, M.B., Ch.B., D.Phil., F.R.C.P.**

**Comparison of Primary Coronary Angioplasty and Intravenous Thrombolytic Therapy for Acute Myocardial Infarction: A Quantitative Review**

Weaver WD, Simes RJ, Betriu A, et al (Henry Ford Health System, Detroit; Natl Health and Med Research Council Clinical Trials Centre, Sydney, Australia; Hosp Clinico y Provincial, Barcelona; et al)
*JAMA* 278:2093–2098, 1997                                                    2–8

*Introduction.*—Direct or primary percutaneous transluminal coronary angioplasty has become more popular and widely used as a means to further improve reperfusion rates since the first comparison of percutaneous transluminal coronary angioplasty and thrombolytic therapy in patients with acute myocardial infarction. One shortcoming of angioplasty is the requirement for consistent and rapid access to a fully equipped and staffed catheterization laboratory. Thrombolysis trials provide strong evidence that delays in the time to treatment lead to a reduction in effectiveness and higher mortality rates, and it is uncertain whether early treatment with angioplasty is as important. The relative effects of primary angioplasty or IV thrombolytic therapy were compared on the rates of death or reinfarction, major bleeding, total stroke, and hemorrhagic stroke.

*Methods.*—Data from all known trials of IV thrombolytic drug therapy vs. direct or primary angioplasty were combined to compare the effects of the 2 treatments. There were 2,606 patients who were randomly assigned to receiving either primary angioplasty or IV thrombolytic therapy. The thrombolytic therapy was either streptokinase, a 3- to 4-hour infusion of tissue-type plasminogen activator, or "accelerated" administration of tissue-type plasminogen activator every 90 minutes.

*Results.*—For the 1,290 patients treated with primary angioplasty, mortality at 30 days or less was 4.4% compared to 6.5% for the 1,316 patients treated with thrombolysis. Among thrombolytic regimens, the effect was similar. A significant reduction in death was not demonstrated in any subgroup. For angioplasty, the rate of death or nonfatal reinfarction was 7.2% and for thrombolytic therapy it was 11.9%. A significant reduction in total stroke was associated with angioplasty at 0.7% compared to thrombolytic therapy at 2%. A significant reduction in hemorrhage stroke was associated with angioplasty at 0.1% compared to thrombolytic therapy at 1.1%.

*Conclusion.*—For treatment of patients with acute myocardial infarction, primary angioplasty appears to be superior to thrombolytic therapy on the basis of outcomes at hospital discharge or 30 days. There may be little advantage of angioplasty over thrombolytic therapy, however, unless the procedural success rates and outcomes for angioplasty are equivalent to those reported in these trials. Before primary angioplasty can be universally recommended as the preferred treatment, data evaluating longer term outcomes, operator experience, and time delay before treatment are needed.

▶ This is a very useful quantitative review of the results of 10 trials and 2,606 patients (including the most recent GUSTO IIb trial). The data are quite persuasive, suggesting that primary percutaneous transluminal coronary angioplasty (PTCA) is the preferred method of reperfusion, particularly in the elderly, in whom the risk of hemorrhagic stroke is substantial.

What is of concern has been the lack of a sustained benefit over PTCA at 6 months or 1 year, at least in some trials.[1] In the GUSTO IIb trial, the initial benefit attributable to PTCA was substantially attenuated. What also needs to be understood is that a very much larger trial of approximately 12,700 patients would be required to demonstrate a 20% relative risk reduction in mortality from PTCA over lytic agents.[2]

Although PTCA may be the preferred method of reperfusion under optimal conditions, there is tremendous heterogeneity in the outcomes from different institutions.[3–5] Moreover, other factors such as the skill and experience of individual operators and institutions; the learning curve of primary angioplasty; the "door-to-balloon time"; the speed of thrombolytic therapy; and, in some cases, the time to presentation may affect outcome. What is clear is that thrombolytic therapy given within the first 70 minutes of an acute myocardial infarction is associated with a strikingly low mortality that may not be bettered by other techniques.[6, 7]

The key is for every individual and institution to analyze their *own* results and not rely upon the experience of the clinical trials or other large centers, in which the procedure may have been performed by enthusiasts with extensive experience in this particular approach to therapy. The next few years will see intensive investigation into newer and better methods of thrombolytic therapy in addition to stents and adjunctive drugs such as the newer platelet inhibitors. What needs to be borne in mind is that we should focus not so much upon the method of reperfusion, but on the efficacy of its delivery, and what may work for some institutions may not work in others.

In summary, "PTCA is great for some" but not for everyone.

**B.J. Gersh, M.B., Ch.B., D.Phil., F.R.C.P.**

*References*

1. The Global Use of Strategies to Open Occluded Coronary Arteries in Coronary Syndromes. GUSTO II Angioplasty Substudy Investigators: A clinical trial comparing primary coronary angioplasty with tissue plasminogen activator for acute myocardial infarction. *N Engl J Med* 336:1621–1628, 1997.
2. Yusuf S, Pogue J: Primary angioplasty compared with thrombolytic therapy for acute myocardial infarction (editorial). *JAMA* 278:2110–2111, 1997.
3. Avery N, Parsons L, Hlatky M, et al: A comparison of thrombolytic therapy with primary coronary angioplasty for acute myocardial infarction. *N Engl J Med* 335:1253–1260, 1996.
4. Jhangiani AH, Jorgensen MB, Mansukhani PW, et al: Community practice of primary angioplasty for myocardial infarction. *J Am Coll Cardiol* 27:62A, 1996.

5. Caputo RP, Lopez JJ, Stoler RC, et al: The effect of institutional experience on the outcome of primary angioplasty for acute MI. *J Am Coll Cardiol* 27:(suppl A) 62A, 1996.
6. Gersh BJ, Anderson JL: Thrombolysis and myocardial salvage: Results of clinical trials and the animal paradigm—paradoxic or predictable? *Circulation* 88:296–306, 1993.
7. Weaver WD, Cerqueira M, Halstrom AP, et al: Prehospital-initiated versus hospital-initiated thrombolytic therapy. *JAMA* 270:1211–1216, 1993.

**Randomized, Double-blind Comparison of Hirulog Versus Heparin in Patients Receiving Streptokinase and Aspirin for Acute Myocardial Infarction (HERO)**

White HD, for the Hirulog Early Reperfusion/Occlusion (HERO) Trial Investigators (Green Lane Hosp, Auckland, New Zealand; Flinders Cardiovascular Centre, Adelaide, South Australia; Heart Ctr of Sarasota, Fla; et al)

*Circulation* 96:2155–2161, 1997                                    2–9

*Introduction.*—In the management of acute myocardial infarction, the administration of aspirin and thrombolytic therapy has been a major advance. Hirulog, a 20-amino acid synthetic peptide that directly inhibits free and clot-bound thrombin, may prevent clot formation and extension and facilitate clot lysis when used in appropriate regimens as an adjuvant during thrombolytic therapy. In patients with acute myocardial infarction receiving streptokinase and aspirin, the safety and efficacy of 2 hirulog regimens for achieving early and complete flow of the infarct-related artery were compared with those of heparin.

*Methods.*—Aspirin and streptokinase were given to 412 patients who had ST-segment elevation, and they were randomly allocated to receive either 60 hours of heparin with a 5,000 U bolus followed by 1,000–1,200 U/hr, low-dose hirulog with a 0.125 mg/kg bolus followed by 0.25 mg/kg$^{-1}$/hr$^{-1}$ for 12 hours then 0.125 mg/kg$^{-1}$/hr$^{-1}$, or high-dose hirulog with a 0.25 mg/kg bolus followed by 0.5 mg/kg$^{-1}$/hr$^{-1}$ for 12 hours then 0.25 mg/kg$^{-1}$/hr$^{-1}$. Patients were evaluated for Thrombolysis In Myocardial Infarction grade 3 flow of the infarct-related artery at 90–120 minutes

*Results.*—With heparin, the Thrombolysis In Myocardial Infarction 3 flow was 35%, with low-dose hirulog it was 46%, and with high-dose hirulog it was 48% (Table 2). By the second day, reocclusion occurred in 1% of the high-dose hirulog group, 5% of the low-dose hirulog group, and in 7% of the heparin group. In 25 patients receiving heparin (17.9%), 19 patients receiving low-dose hirulog (14%), and 17 patients receiving high-dose hirulog (12.5%), death, cardiogenic shock, or reinfarction had occurred by 35 days. In the heparin group, 2 strokes had occurred and in the high-dose hirulog group, 2 occurred, whereas in patients treated with low-dose hirulog, none had occurred. In 28% of the heparin group, 14% of the low-dose hirulog group, and 19% of the high-dose hirulog group, major bleeding occurred, with 40% from the groin site.

TABLE 2.—Thrombolysis In Myocardial Infarction 3 Patency at 90–120 Minutes

| Hours From Symptom Onset | Heparin | Low-Dose Hirulog | High-Dose Hirulog | All Hirulog | Significance Level (2P) All Hirulog vs Heparin | High-Dose Hirulog vs Heparin |
|---|---|---|---|---|---|---|
| 0–3 | 33/64 (52%) [39–61] | 34/61 (56%) [43–68] | 41/59 (70%) [57–80] | 75/120 (63%) [54–71] | .15 | .04 |
| >3–6 | 11/48 (23%) [13–37] | 18/43 (42%) [28–57] | 15/47 (32%) [20–46] | 33/90 (37%) [27–42] | .09 | .33 |
| >6–12 | 4/24 (17%) [6–31] | 7/24 (29%) [15–50] | 6/23 (26%) [12–47] | 13/47 (28%) [17–42] | .31 | .45 |
| All patients | 48/136 (35%) [28–44] | 59/128 (46%) [38–55] | 62/129 (48%) [40–57] | 121/257 (47%) [41–53] | .02 | .03 |

Note: Figures in brackets denote 95% confidence intervals (in percents).
(Reproduced with permission, from White HD, for the Hirulog Early Reperfusion/Occlusion (HERO) Trial Investigators: Randomized, double-blind comparison of hirulog versus heparin in patients receiving streptokinase and aspirin for acute myocardial infarction (HERO). *Circulation* 96:2155–2161, Copyright 1997, American Heart Association.)

*Conclusion.*—In patients treated with aspirin and streptokinase, hirulog was more effective than heparin in producing early patency without increasing the risk of major bleeding. Clinical outcome may be improved with direct thrombin inhibition.

▶ The Achilles heel of reperfusion therapy is reocclusion, and it should be appreciated that the very process of lysis may initiate rethrombosis, through a variety of direct and indirect mechanisms. The direct antithrombins are an attractive new therapeutic option, given the limitations of heparin against clot-bound thrombin and its interactions with platelet factor 4 and other plasma proteins, which in turn reduce its efficacy and introduce an unpredictable dose-response relationship. Initial expectations were not met by the GUSTO IIb and TIMI 9b trials, which demonstrated only a modest benefit from hirudin in patients with acute ischemic syndromes, although there was a greater ease of administration of hirudin with less fluctuation in activated partial thromboplastin time levels.[1, 2]

Is this a case of "paradise lost, or paradise postponed?" I veer toward the latter, and these data from the HERO trial in patients receiving streptokinase are encouraging, as are preliminary data from another trial of patients with unstable angina. Several issues still need to be resolved, including the optimum dose, both initial and maintenance. The potential for severe and fatal bleeding is real and the activated partial thromboplastin time should not exceed 85–90 seconds.

Perhaps the most intriguing unresolved question about the use of these agents is the optimal duration of therapy, to protect against rethrombosis during the period of "endothelial passivation." In the GUSTO IIb and TIMI trials, the initial benefit at 24–48 hours was diminished at 30 days. Similar trends were noted in the FRISC trial of low-molecular weight heparin.[3]

It has been suggested that the minimum duration of antithrombotic therapy is around 30 days. Whether this will turn out to be warfarin, low-molecular weight heparin, a direct antithrombin, or one of the new platelet inhibitors remains to be seen. Either way, I do not believe we have seen the last of the direct antithrombins, which I believe could play a key role in the management of unstable angina and acute myocardial infarction in patients undergoing angioplasty.

**B.J. Gersh, M.B., Ch.B., D.Phil., F.R.C.P.**

*References*

1. The Global Use of Strategies to Open Occluded Coronary Arteries (GUSTO) IIb Investigators: A comparison of recombinant hirudin with heparin for the treatment of acute coronary syndromes. *N Engl J Med* 335:775–782, 1996.
2. Antman EM, for the TIMI 9b Investigators: Hirudin in acute myocardial infarction: Thrombolysis and thrombin inhibition in myocardial infarction (TIMI 9b Trial). *Circulation* 94:911–921, 1996.
3. Fragment During Instability in Coronary Artery Disease (FRISC) Study Group: Low-molecular-weight heparin during instability in coronary artery disease. *Lancet* 347:56–58, 1996.

## Myocardial Infarction—Late Prognosis

**Improved Survival With an Implanted Defibrillator in Patients With Coronary Disease at High Risk for Ventricular Arrhythmia**
Moss AJ, for the Multicenter Automatic Defibrillator Implantation Trial Investigators (Univ of Rochester, NY; Good Samaritan Hosp, Los Angeles; Scripps Mem Hosp, La Jolla, Calif; et al)
*N Engl J Med* 335:1933–1940, 1996                      2–10

*Objective.*—Unsustained ventricular tachycardia in patients with coronary disease carries a 2-year mortality rate of approximately 30%. There is no evidence that antiarrhythmic therapy improves survival rate. Results of a prophylactic trial of high-risk patients with coronary heart disease and asymptomatic unsustained ventricular tachycardia randomly allocated to receive an implantable cardioverter defibrillator or conventional medical therapy were presented (Table 1).

*Methods.*—Of the 196 patients enrolled, 98 were in the transthoracic stratum (45 in the defibrillator group and 53 in the conventional therapy group) and 98 in the transvenous stratum (50 in the defibrillator group and 48 in the conventional therapy group). All patients were in New York Heart Association functional class I, II, or III, and all had an angiographically determined ejection fraction ≤0.35. Patients were seen 1 month after randomization and every 3 months thereafter and were monitored for an average of 27 months. Survival in the 2 groups was compared statistically.

*Results.*—Eleven patients in the conventional therapy group crossed over into the defibrillator group, and 5 patients in the defibrillator group never had a defibrillator implanted. There were 15 deaths in the defibrillator group and 39 in the conventional therapy group (hazard ratio for overall mortality = 0.46) (Fig 2). Antiarrhythmic medications had no significant effect on the hazard ratio.

TABLE 1.—Baseline Characteristics of 196 Randomized Patients*

| CHARACTERISTIC | CONVENTIONAL THERAPY (N = 101) | DEFRIBRILLATOR (N = 95) |
|---|---|---|
| Age (yr)† | 64 ± 9 | 62 ± 9 |
| Sex (M/F)† | 92/8 | 92/8 |
| Cardiac history (%) | | |
| ≥2 prior myocardial infarctions† | 29 | 34 |
| Treatment for ventricular arrhythmias | 35 | 42 |
| NYHA class II or III†‡ | 67 | 63 |
| Treatment for congestive heart failure† | 51 | 52 |
| Treatment for hypertension† | 35 | 48 |
| Insulin-dependent diabetes | 5 | 7 |
| Cigarette smoking (any time) | 73 | 79 |
| Coronary bypass surgery† | 44 | 46 |
| Coronary angioplasty | 27 | 17 |
| Implanted pacemaker | 7 | 2 |
| Interval of ≥6 mo between most recent myocardial infarction and enrollment (%)† | 76 | 75 |
| Cardiac findings at enrollment (%) | | |
| Pulmonary congestion§ | 20 | 18 |
| Blood urea nitrogen >25 mg/dl (8.92 mmol/liter)† | 21 | 22 |
| Cholesterol >200 mg/dl (5.17 mmol/liter) | 49 | 41 |
| Left bundle-branch block† | 8 | 7 |
| Ejection fraction† | 0.25 ± 0.07 | 0.27 ± 0.07 |
| Qualifying unsustained ventricular tachycardia (no. of consecutive beats) | 9 ± 10 | 10 ± 9 |
| Electrophysiologic study (%) | | |
| Initial induction | | |
| Monomorphic ventricular tachycardia | 91 | 87 |
| Polymorphic ventricular tachycardia | 7 | 7 |
| Ventricular fibrillation | 2 | 6 |
| Induction after antiarrhythmic challenge¶ | | |
| Monomorphic ventricular tachycardia | 94 | 92 |
| Polymorphic ventricular tachycardia | 5 | 7 |
| Ventricular fibrillation | 1 | 1 |

*Plus-minus values are means ± SD.
†This variable was preselected for inclusion in the Cox regression analyses.
‡NYHA denotes New York Heart Association.
§Pulmonary congestion was defined radiographically as mild, moderate, or severe.
¶Rhythms were electrophysiologically induced after antiarrhythmic challenge with procainamide.
(Courtesy of Moss AJ, for the Multicenter Automatic Defibrillator Implantation Trial investigators: Improved survival with an implanted defibrillator in patients with coronary disease at high risk for ventricular arrhythmia. N Engl J Med 335:1933–1940, 1996. Reproduced by permission of The New England Journal of Medicine. Copyright 1997, Massachusetts Medical Society. All rights reserved.)

*Conclusion.*—Implanted defibrillators significantly improve survival in patients with previous myocardial infarction and left ventricular dysfunction who are at risk for unsustained ventricular tachycardia.

▶ The last issue of the 1996 *New England Journal of Medicine* saw the publication of a trial that has extraordinary implications for clinical practice and the economics of health care. At first glance, the trial demonstrates a very impressive benefit of the implantable cardioverter defibrillator over drug therapy in patients with asymptomatic nonsustained or unsustained ventricular tachycardia after myocardial infarction. The implications for clinical prac-

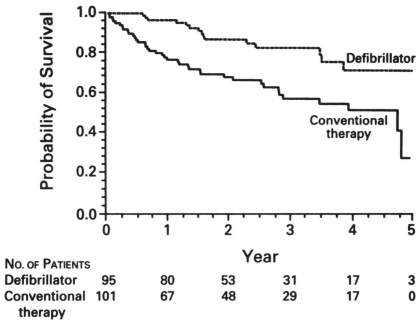

No. OF PATIENTS

| | Year | | | | |
|---|---|---|---|---|---|
| | 0 | 1 | 2 | 3 | 4 | 5 |
| Defibrillator | 95 | 80 | 53 | 31 | 17 | 3 |
| Conventional therapy | 101 | 67 | 48 | 29 | 17 | 0 |

FIGURE 2.—Kaplan-Meier analysis of the probability of survival according to assigned treatment. The difference in survival between the two treatment groups was significant ($P = 0.009$). (Courtesy of Moss AJ, for the Multicenter Automatic Defibrillator Implantation Trial investigators: Improved survival with an implanted defibrillator in patients with coronary disease at high risk for ventricular arrhythmia. *N Engl J Med* 335:1933–1940, 1996. Reproduced by permission of *The New England Journal of Medicine*. Copyright 1997, Massachusetts Medical Society. All rights reserved.)

tice are that all patients with significant left ventricular dysfunction after myocardial infarction (ejection fraction <0.35) should undergo ambulatory monitoring and in the event that unsustained ventricular tachycardia is documented, an invasive electrophysiologic study followed by implantation of an implantable cardioverter defibrillator among patients in whom ventricular tachycardia or ventricular fibrillation is induced and not suppressed by intravenous procainamide.

A thoughtful editorial by Friedman and Stevenson highlights several concerns about adopting a national policy without additional information.[1] The trial population comprises a high-risk group with an ejection fraction of <0.35 and inducible arrhythmias that do not respond to intravenous procainamide. We need more data on those patients who were not inducible and among those who were inducible but suppressible. Is this the majority of patients with unsustained ventricular tachycardia or not? What about patients with lesser degrees of left ventricular dysfunction, for example, ejection fractions ranging from 0.40–0.50. Moreover, the group treated with "conventional therapy" who faired poorly in this trial needs further definition in the light of current knowledge. Another question is to what extent were the adverse outcomes the result of the use of class IA antiarrhythmics, which have been largely and appropriately discredited in the late 1990s, and was amiodarone used appropriately and in sufficient patients?

Nonetheless, this was not an easy trial to perform, and the investigators should be commended for providing us with new information. I do believe that this trial will result in a more intensive search for unsustained ventricular tachycardia in patients with left ventricular dysfunction after myocardial infarction and a higher use of invasive electrophysiologic studies and implantable cardioverter defibrillators, which is appropriate given the data from MADIT. However, before a comprehensive strategy can be defined toward all asymptomatic postinfarct patients, we must await the results of the MUSTT Trial, which is currently in its follow-up phase.[2] Moreover, for patients who have survived an out-of-hospital cardiac arrest (excluded from MADIT), other trials are ongoing.

MADIT focuses on the electrophysiologic approach to patients with asymptomatic unsustained ventricular tachycardia and left ventricular dysfunction after myocardial infarction. A different approach is to intensify our efforts to prevent left ventricular dysfunction—namely, the earlier administration of acute reperfusion therapy and to more patients. This, in turn, will likely result in fewer patients with left ventricular dysfunction and unsustained ventricular tachycardia (the MADIT population) and will soften the economic impact of the results of this important trial, in addition to providing better outcomes for an increasing number of our patients.

**B.J. Gersh, M.B., Ch.B., D.Phil., F.R.C.P.**

*References*

1. Friedman PL, Stevenson WG: Unsustained ventricular tachycardia—to treat or not to treat. *N Engl J Med* 335:1984–1985, 1996.
2. Buxton AE, Fisher JD, Josephson ME, et al: Prevention of sudden death in patients with coronary artery disease: The Multicenter Unsustained Tachycardia Trial [MUSTT]. *Prog Cardiovasc Dis* 36:215–226, 1993.

---

**Beta Blockers Prevent Cardiac Death Following a Myocardial Infarction: So Why Are So Many Infarct Survivors Discharged Without Beta Blockers?**
Viskin S, Barron HV (Univ of California, San Francisco)
*Am J Cardiol* 78:821–822, 1996                                    2–11

---

*Objective.*—β-blockers dramatically reduce mortality rates and incidence of sudden cardiac death in patients with myocardial infarction. Unfortunately, many of these patients are not treated with these drugs. The reasons and clinical applications for this undertreatment were discussed.

*Discussion.*—Although as many as 80% of infarct survivors could receive β-blockers, only about 50% actually do. Approximately 3,000 additional lives could be saved annually by such treatment. Impaired left ventricular function, use of diuretics, the presence of peripheral vascular disease, diabetes mellitus, and advanced age have been considered reasons to avoid prescribing β-blockers. β-blockers are prescribed for 65% of those with preserved left ventricular function but only for 30% of those with impaired left ventricular function, possibly because of physicians' fears of precipitating heart failure. However, studies show the incidence of heart failure precipitation among patients treated with β-blockers was similar to that of placebo-treated patients. Data suggest that β-blockers may actually prevent heart failure. Parameters from large prospective trials that correlate with infarcts indicate a reduction in mortality rate for patients treated with β-blockers compared with those receiving placebo. Nonselective β-blockers may exacerbate diabetes mellitus but may also reduce mortality rate from myocardial infarction, which is high in patients with diabetes. In randomized trials, the use of β-blockers did not result in deterioration of peripheral vascular disease. Concern about the use of β-blockers in the elderly seems to be misplaced. Most trials suggest that older patients actually benefit more from the use of β-blockers than do younger patients. Survival rate is improved at higher than normal doses, but clinical doses may also be effective.

*Conclusion.*—There is a difference between the information that has been generated from clinical studies and what is practiced with regard to the use of β-blockers in patients with myocardial infarction and diabetes, peripheral vascular disease, or left ventricular impairment or who are elderly.

▶ This is a useful editorial that points out that one of the few drugs that has been unequivocally shown to improve prognosis in postinfarct survivors is markedly underutilized in clinical practice.[1] The authors point out why the presence of an impaired left ventricular ejection fraction, diabetes, peripheral vascular disease, and older age should not be viewed as absolute contraindications to the use of β-blockers. In fact, many of these patients may have the most to gain from such therapy because they are at higher risk to begin with. In my own practice, I always start in the hospital with drugs that have a short half-life and switch to longer-acting preparations at a later stage. The individualization of therapy and careful surveillance of the patient are the keys to management. β-Blockers work and are well tolerated in the majority—the least we can do is to use what has unquestionably been shown to be effective.

**B.J. Gersh, M.B., Ch.B., D.Phil., F.R.C.P.**

*Reference*

1. The Beta-Blocker Pooling Project Research Group. The Beta-Blocker Pooling Project (BBPP): subgroup findings from randomized trials in post infarction patients. *Eur Heart J* 9:8–16, 1988.

### Adverse Outcomes of Underuse of β-Blockers in Elderly Survivors of Acute Myocardial Infarction

Soumerai SB, McLaughlin TJ, Spiegelman D, et al (Harvard Med School, Boston; Harvard School of Public Health, Boston; Brigham and Women's Hosp, Boston)

*JAMA* 277:115–121, 1997         2–12

*Purpose.*—β-Blocker treatment is highly effective in reducing cardiovascular mortality rates and reinfarction after acute myocardial infarction (AMI). There are few data on how many and which patients receive β-blockers, however, especially among elderly patients living in the community. Levels, determinants, and outcomes of β-blocker treatment among elderly survivors of AMI were studied.

*Methods.*—The retrospective study used Medicare and drug claims data covering the years 1987 to 1992. It included a cohort of 5,332 elderly patients who survived for 30 days after AMI. Of these, 3,737 met eligibility requirements for β-blocker treatment. The analysis looked at the use of β-blockers and calcium-channel blockers in the first 90 days after hospital discharge. Mortality and cardiac hospital readmission rates were evaluated for the 2-year period after discharge, with adjustment for sociodemographic and baseline risk variables. Factors associated with underuse of β-blockers, and the consequences of that underuse, were assessed. The relative risk (RR) of survival in patients taking β-blockers was compared with those from previously reported randomized, controlled trials.

*Results.*—Throughout the period studied, just 21% of patients received β-blocker therapy. After AMI, prescription rates were nearly 3 times higher for calcium-channel blockers as for β-blockers. Older patients and those taking calcium-channel blockers were less likely to receive β-blockers. Mortality rate was significantly reduced (RR 0.57) for patients receiving β-blockers after adjustment for other survival predictors. β-Blockers significantly improved survival in all age groups—including those aged 85 years or older—as reported in the elderly subgroups of previous trials. Patients taking β-blockers were also less likely to be readmitted to the hospital (RR 0.78). The risk of death was doubled (RR 1.98) for patients receiving a calcium-channel blocker rather than a β-blocker. This was not because of any adverse effect of calcium-channel blockers, but rather because they were used instead of β-blockers.

*Conclusions.*—β-Blockers are not prescribed to elderly survivors of AMI as often as they should be, which leads to higher rates of adverse outcomes. β-Blockers can extend survival even for patients older than 75 years, who have been excluded from previous randomized, controlled trials. One reason for β-blocker underuse may be the mistaken belief that these drugs are potentially harmful for patients with left ventricular dysfunction or diabetes. The study is limited by the lack of information on lifestyle risk factors and on patients who may have received β-blockers in the hospital but stopped taking them before discharge.

▶ I expect that the underutilization of β-blockers in this study is an overestimate for several reasons. First, the study does not take into account patients in whom the drug may have been started in the hospital and then discontinued, patients who are judged to be at low risk and as such were thought not to require β-blockers (a subgroup that was not identified a priori in the all-encompassing randomized trials), or subgroups of patients with other contraindications that were not identified by the database. Nonetheless, we cannot ignore the major discomforting message of this paper, and these data support prior studies.[1, 2]

β-Blockers, a drug for which abundant evidence exists to show their benefit in postinfarct survivors, are markedly underutilized, particularly in comparison with the calcium-channel blockers, in which evidence supporting a benefit is scanty.

The issue is not confined to β-blockers in postinfarct patients. It relates to our apparent failure to speedily translate the information from randomized trials and the research community into the clinical arena and the hands of practitioners—in particular, primary care physicians.[3] We would all like to feel that we practice "evidence-based" medicine, but how do we keep up with the evidence in the era of the information explosion? An editorial by Felch and Scanlon[3] argues persuasively for a radical change in the paradigm of continuing medical education. We need to alter methods of disseminating information in addition to our abilities to absorb and integrate this wealth of data into our daily practice. However, there is a need to develop methods of monitoring the impact of new technologies and strategies on clinical practice behavior. Although this paper is at first glance a disappointing analysis of clinical practice patients, it does identify a problem, and there are grounds for optimism in that the boundaries between research and its applications into the clinical arena are slowly being broken down.

**B.J. Gersh, M.B., Ch.B., D.Phil., F.R.C.P.**

*References*

1. Kennedy HL, Rosenson RS: Physician use of beta-adrenergic blocking therapy: a changing perspective. *JACC* 547:547–552, 1995.
2. Ellerbeck EF, Jencks SF, Radford MJ, et al: Quality of care for Medicare patients with acute myocardial infarction: four-state pilot study from the Cooperative Cardiovascular Project. *JAMA* 273:1509–1514, 1995.
3. Felch WC, Scanlon DM: Bridging the gap between research and practice: the role of continuing medical education [editorial]. *JAMA* 277:155–156, 1997.

### Ventricular Dysfunction and the Risk of Stroke After Myocardial Infarction

Loh E, Sutton MSJ, Wun CC, et al (Univ of Pennsylvania, Philadelphia; Univ of Texas, Houston; Montreal Heart Inst; et al)
*N Engl J Med* 336:251–257, 1997                                                       2–13

*Introduction.*—Stroke is a known early complication of myocardial infarction. The long-term risk of stroke after myocardial infarction, and how it relates to the extent of left ventricular dysfunction, remains to be determined. The effects of reduced left ventricular ejection fraction on stroke risk after myocardial infarction were assessed. Other potential risk factors were examined as well.

*Methods.*—The study used prospectively collected data on 2,231 patients who had left ventricular dysfunction after surviving acute myocardial infarction. The patients were drawn from the randomized, controlled Survival and Ventricular Enlargement (SAVE) trial. The patients were followed up for a mean of 42 months, with stroke risk factors analyzed by univariate and multivariate analysis. In addition to left ventricular ejection fraction, potential risk factors analyzed included age, anticoagulant therapy, thrombolytic therapy, and captopril therapy.

TABLE 1.—Baseline Clinical Characteristics of Patients Who Subsequently Had Stroke and Those Who Did Not*

| Characteristic | With Stroke (N = 103) | Without Stroke (N = 2128) | P Value† |
|---|---|---|---|
| Age — yr | 63 ± 9 | 59 ± 11 | <0.001 |
| LVEF — % | 29 ± 7 | 31 ± 7 | 0.01 |
| Male sex — no. (%) | 83 (81) | 1758 (83) | NS |
| History of diabetes — no. (%) | 30 (29) | 462 (22) | 0.08 |
| History of hypertension — no. (%) | 44 (43) | 793 (37) | NS |
| Current smoking — no. (%) | 46 (45) | 879 (41) | NS |
| Previous myocardial-infarction — no. (%) | 42 (41) | 750 (35) | NS |
| Atrial fibrillation or flutter — no. (%) | 17 (16) | 210 (10) | 0.03 |
| Anticoagulant therapy — no. (%) | 39 (38) | 593 (28) | 0.03 |
| Aspirin use — no. (%) | 47 (46) | 1263 (59) | <0.01 |
| Location of infarction — no. (%) | | | |
| Anterior Q-wave | 59 (57) | 1170 (55) | NS |
| Inferior Q-wave | 18 (17) | 376 (18) | NS |
| Anterior and inferior Q-wave | 11 (11) | 250 (12) | NS |
| Non–Q-wave | 8 (8) | 208 (10) | NS |
| Other | 7 (7) | 124 (6) | NS |
| Thrombolytic therapy — no. (%) | 25 (24) | 744 (35) | 0.03 |

*Plus-minus values are means ± SD. Characteristics are listed as assessed at the time of randomization.
†*p* Values were calculated by the two-sample *t* test for age and left ventricular ejection fraction and by the chi-square test for the other variables. *NS*, Not significant.
(Courtesy of Loh E, Sutton MSJ, Wun CC, et al: Ventricular dysfunction and the risk of stroke after myocardial infarction. *N Engl J Med* 336:251–257, 1997. Reprinted by permission of *The New England Journal* of Medicine. Copyright 1997, Massachusetts Medical Society. All rights reserved.)

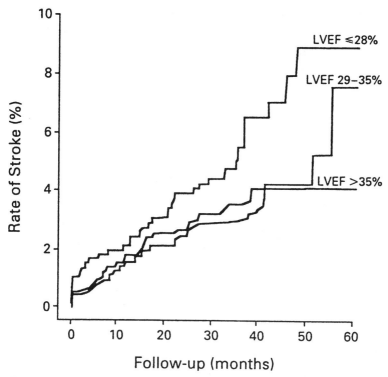

**FIGURE 2.**—Cumulative rate of stroke in the SAVE trial according to left ventricular ejection fraction. (Courtesy of Loh E, Sutton MSJ, Wun CC, et al: Ventricular dysfunction and the risk of stroke after myocardial infarction. *N Engl J Med* 336:251–257, 1997. Reprinted by permission of *The New England Journal* of Medicine. Copyright 1997, Massachusetts Medical Society. All rights reserved.)

*Results.*—During follow-up, 4.6% of patients had a fatal or nonfatal stroke at a 15% rate of stroke per year of follow-up. The estimated overall 5-year stroke rate was 8.1%. Mean ejection fraction was 29% in patients with stroke versus 31% in those without. Mean age was 63 versus 59 years, respectively (Table 1). Reduced ejection fraction was a significant risk factor for stroke—for each 5% decrease in ejection fraction, stroke risk increased by 18% (Fig 2). Older age and not receiving aspirin or anticoagulant therapy were also significant risk factors. When postinfarction ejection fraction was ≤28%, the risk of stroke was 1.86, relative to patients with ejection fractions of >35%. Stroke risk was unaffected by thrombolytic or captopril therapy.

*Conclusions.*—Stroke risk is elevated in the 5 years after myocardial infarction. Independent risk factors are reduced ejection fraction and older age. Anticoagulant therapy may have a protective effect at all strata of ejection fraction. Future studies should assess whether aspirin provides as much protection against stroke as warfarin does.

▶ In this study, confined to postmyocardial infarction survivors with an ejection fraction of ≤40%, the risk of stroke during follow-up was 1.5% per year. This rate is probably slightly higher than the risk of major bleeding on coumadin, if one uses the randomized trials of patients with nonrheumatic atrial fibrillation as a yardstick.[1, 2] Stroke rates were, however, substantially higher among patients with an ejection fraction of ≤35%.

The implications for coumadin therapy are obvious, and in this nonrandomized study both coumadin and aspirin were associated with a reduced risk of stroke. If the postulated mechanisms are embolic from thrombi in a dilated left ventricle or left atrium, the apparent benefit of aspirin is not readily explicable.

This study raises many questions. Is coumadin alone preferable to aspirin alone, or would a combination of the two be more effective? What is the effective range of international normalized ratio values, and are they similar to the target international normalized ratio values in patients with atrial fibrillation or prosthetic valves? What are the risks vs the benefits of anticoagulation in older patients, and over what range of ejection fractions? Pending more definitive data, the case for long-term anticoagulation in postinfarct survivors with significant left ventricular dysfunction is persuasive.

**B.J. Gersh, M.B., Ch.B., D.Phil., F.R.C.P.**

*Reference*

1. Atrial Fibrillation Investigators. Risk factors for stroke and efficacy for antithrombotic therapy in atrial fibrillation. Analysis of pooled data from five randomized controlled trials. *Arch Intern Med* 154:1449–1457, 1994.
2. Stroke Prevention in Atrial Fibrillation Investigators. Bleeding during antithrombotic therapy for atrial fibrillation. *Arch Intern Med* 156:409–416, 1996.

---

**Randomised Trial of Effect of Amiodarone on Mortality in Patients With Left-ventricular Dysfunction After Recent Myocardial Infarction: EMIAT**
Julian DG, for the European Myocardial Infarct Amiodarone Trial Investigators (Netherhall Gardens, London; St George's Hosp; Sanofi Recherche, Montpellier, France; et al)
*Lancet* 349:667–674, 1997                                    2–14

---

*Introduction.*—In survivors of acute myocardial infarction, ventricular arrhythmias are one of the main causes of death. After many studies of antiarrhythmic drugs that block the sodium-channel showed no efficacy in suppressing arrhythmias and preventing death in survivors of myocardial infarction, the European Myocardial Infarct Amiodarone Trial (EMIAT) was conducted. Amiodarone and β-adrenergic blocking agents showed promise as antiarrhythmic drugs. A large trial of amiodarone in survivors of myocardial infarction at increased risk of death was conducted. The

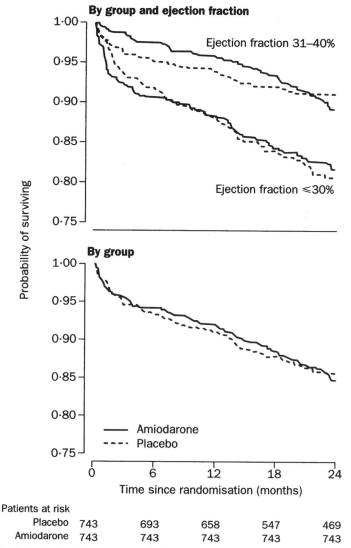

**FIGURE 2.**—Kaplan-Meier estimates of all-cause mortality by group and ejection fraction. (Courtesy of Julian DG: Randomised trial of effect of amiodarone on mortality in patients with left-ventricular dysfunction after recent myocardial infarction: EMIAT. *Lancet* 349:667–674, 1997. Copyright The Lancet Ltd. 1997.)

main entry criterion was the presence of depressed left-ventricular ejection fraction, which has been shown to be the single most powerful independent predictor of mortality, including sudden death.

*Methods.*—The effect of amiodarone on all-cause mortality, cardiac mortality, and arrhythmic death was studied in 1,486 survivors of myocardial infarction with depressed left-ventricular function of 40% or less in a randomized, placebo-controlled double-blind trial. Analyses of on-treatment (efficacy) and intention-to-treat were conducted. Patients were divided into 2 groups with 743 in the amiodarone group and 743 in the placebo group. They were followed up for a median of 21 months.

*Results.*—Between the 2 groups, there was no difference in all-cause mortality with 103 deaths in the amiodarone group and 102 in the placebo group (Fig 2). There was no difference in cardiac mortality in the 2 groups. There was a 35% risk reduction in arrhythmic deaths in the amiodarone group. In the amiodarone group, there were more deaths from non-arrhythmic cardiac and noncardiac causes than in the placebo group. The risk of death was significantly increased by a history of myocardial infarction.

*Conclusion.*—The systematic prophylactic use of amiodarone in all patients with depressed left-ventricular function after myocardial infarction was not supported by these findings. The use of amiodarone in patients for whom anti-arrhythmic therapy is indicated, however, was supported by the lack of proarrhythmia and the reduction in arrhythmic death.

▶ This large randomized trial, in addition to the Canadian Amiodarone Myocardial Infarction Arrhythmia Trial (CAMIAT) reported in the same issue of the journal[1]demonstrates the safety of amiodarone, unlike other anti-arrhythmic agents. Moreover, there is evidence from trials of amiodarone in heart failure, that the drug may be beneficial in patients with congestive heart failure not attributable to ischemic heart disease. Nonetheless, in the European Myocardial Infarct Amiodarone Trial (EMIAT), there was no benefit on overall mortality despite a reduction in arrhythmic death. The CAMIAT demonstrated a nonsignificant reduction in overall mortality, and the conclusion was drawn that the drug is effective in reducing arrhythmic death and resuscitative ventricular fibrillation.

I would argue that a total *overall mortality* is the only valid end point, given the well-known difficulties involved in classifying arrhythmic death, whether this be defined by an individual or by a committee. One can conclude that amiodarone is the drug of choice after a myocardial infarction or in patients with left-ventricular dysfunction who are to be treated with an anti-arrhythmic agent—primarily patients with symptomatic ventricular arrhythmias, or perhaps very frequent or complex nonsustained ventricular tachycardia—although the definition of the latter is uncertain. On the other hand, these studies do not support the use of amiodarone for all patients with left-ventricular dysfunction after myocardial infarction, irrespective of the presence or absence of premature ventricular extrasystoles. We do have other therapies that are of proven benefit in the postinfarct setting, e.g., beta-blockers or angiotensin-converting enzyme inhibitors. It therefore comes as a surprise that such drugs are used in only approximately 50% of patients in both EMIAT and CAMIAT.

**B.J. Gersh, M.B., Ch.B., D.Phil., F.R.C.P.**

*Reference*

1. Cairns JA, Connolly SJ, Roberts R, et al: Randomised trial with outcome after myocardial infarction in patients with frequent or repetitive ventricular premature depolarization: CAMIAT. *Lancet* 349:675–682), 1997.

**Attenuation of Unfavorable Remodeling by Exercise Training in Postinfarction Patients With Left Ventricular Dysfunction: Results of the Exercise in Left Ventricular Dysfunction (ELVD) Trial**
Giannuzzi P, for the ELVD Study Group (Rehabilitation Inst of Veruno, Italy)
*Circulation* 96:1790–1797, 1997                                                    2–15

*Introduction.*—The impact of a long-term physical training program on left ventricular size and function was evaluated in patients with systolic dysfunction after myocardial infarction in a multicenter, randomized study. Although patients who have had infarctions are advised to start an exercise program, the effects of such a program on the remodeling process have not been defined.

*Methods.*—Patients were enrolled in the multicenter Exercise in Left Ventricular Dysfunction trial. After baseline evaluations, they were randomized to physical training or to a control group. All patients had ejection fractions of less than 40% after a first Q-wave myocardial infarction. The exercise program consisted of 30-minute bicycle ergometry 3 times a week. Those in the training intervention returned to the laboratory every 2 weeks so that a new level of exercise could be tested and prescribed. The target heart rate was 80% of that achieved at peak incremental exercise.

TABLE 4.—Left Ventricular Function and Remodeling

| | | Training Group (n=39) | Control Group (n=38) |
|---|---|---|---|
| EDV, mL/m² | Pre | 93 ± 28 | 94 ± 26* |
| | Post | 92 ± 28 | 99 ± 27 |
| ESV, mL/m² | Pre | 61 ± 22 | 62 ± 20* |
| | Post | 57 ± 23 | 67 ± 23 |
| EF, % | Pre | 34 ± 5 | 34 ± 5* |
| | Post | 38 ± 8 | 33 ± 7 |
| WMA, % | Pre | 49 ± 8 | 50 ± 10* |
| | Post | 44 ± 10 | 51 ± 12 |
| Reg Dil, % | Pre | 43 ± 18 | 47 ± 18* |
| | Post | 45 ± 26 | 57 ± 22 |

*Note:* Values are mean plus or minus standard deviation.
*$P < 0.01$ interaction.
*Abbreviations: Pre,* initial study; *Post,* final study (after 6 months); *EDV,* end-diastolic volume; *ESV,* end-systolic volume; *EF,* ejection fraction; *WMA,* wall motion abnormalities; *Reg Dil,* regional dilatation.
(Courtesy of Giannuzzi P, for the ELVD Study Group: Attenuation of unfavorable remodeling by exercise training in postinfarction patients with left ventricular dysfunction: Results of the Exercise in Left Ventricular Dysfunction (ELVD) trial. *Circulation* 96:1790–1797, 1997. Reproduced with permission from *Circulation.* Copyright 1997, American Heart Association.)

*Results.*—Seventy-six men and 4 women were enrolled in the study but 2 withdrew, which left 39 in the training group and 38 in the control group. The 2 groups were similar in baseline clinical data, infarct size, and other relevant variables. The heart rate at rest was similar for exercise and control groups at entry and final evaluation. After 6 months, only the exercise group demonstrated a significant increase in work capacity (from a mean of 4.462 to 5.752 kilopond-meters). The work capacity in controls was essentially unchanged (mean, 4.375 to 4.388 kilopond-meters). Left ventricular volumes increased in the control group but not in the training group. The mean ejection fraction improved in the exercise group (from 34% to 38%) but was slightly reduced in the control group (from 34% to 33%) (Table 4).

*Conclusion.*—Cardiac rehabilitation exercise after an acute myocardial infarction is known to have a beneficial effect on exercise tolerance and symptoms, but its impact on ventricular function and remodeling has not been established. This study, specifically designed to address this question, suggests that exercise can prevent the progression of left ventricular dysfunction.

▶ The clinical and psychological benefits of cardiac rehabilitation on risk factor reduction and the quality of life in patients with coronary artery disease and survivors of myocardial infarctions are not in dispute. Exercise cardiac rehabilitation programs have also been successfully expanded to include patients with congestive heart failure; however, with regard to patients who have had anterior infarcts and reduced left ventricular ejection fractions and in whom left ventricular remodeling and the late development of congestive heart failure is frequent, there have been reports suggesting that exercise training may be deleterious.[1] This Italian study is the first prospective, randomized trial specifically designed to address whether regular exercise affects left ventricular function (ventricular remodeling) in survivors of infarctions. The results are very encouraging and should dispel the perception raised by prior studies that regular exercise in this setting may be harmful. In this study, during a 6-month period, exercise training attenuated the remodeling process and improved left ventricular function in some patients, and the significant increase in work activity was accompanied by an improvement in psychological and quality-of-life indices.

What are the explanations? One can only speculate, but a reduction in left ventricular wall stress via peripheral adaptive mechanisms and perhaps a favorable modification of the coronary circulation, leading to increased myocardial perfusion, may have played a role. In addition, the increase in vagal tone and the reduction in sympathetic activity that is accompanied by a reduced heart rate and reduced vasoconstriction (or other beneficial sequelae of exercise) may have a favorable effect on myocardial oxygen demands and ventricular remodeling.

I wish health care programs would take notice of the fact that cardiac rehabilitation after a myocardial infarction is beneficial in many ways and may even turn out to be cost-effective.

**B.J. Gersh, M.B., Ch.B., D.Phil., F.R.C.P.**

*Reference*

1. Jugdutt BI, Michorowski BL, Kappagoda CT: Exercise training after anterior Q wave myocardial infarction: Importance of regional left ventricular function and topography. *J Am Coll Cardiol* 12:362–372, 1988.

# Unstable Angina

### Production of C-Reactive Protein and Risk of Coronary Events in Stable and Unstable Angina

Haverkate F, for the European Concerted Action on Thrombosis and Disabilities Angina Pectoris Study Group (Royal Postgraduate Med School, London)
*Lancet* 349:462–466, 1997                                                2–16

*Purpose.*—The inflammation associated with atherosclerotic lesions has been linked to activation and proliferation of certain types of cells, production of cytokines and growth factors, complement activation and deposition, and the presence of inflammatory mediators. Patients with severe unstable angina who had enhanced production of the acute-phase reactant C-reactive protein (CRP) reportedly have a poor prognosis. The acute-phase responses of CRP and of serum amyloid A protein (SAA) were investigated in patients with unstable or stable angina.

*Methods.*—The study included 2,121 patients with various forms of angina: 1,030 unstable, 743 stable, and 348 atypical. In each patient, new automated, ultrasensitive enzyme immunoassays were used to measure plasma concentrations of CRP and SAA. The results were correlated with known coronary risk factors and coronary events over 2 years' follow-up.

*Results.*—A coronary event occurred during follow-up in 75 patients: 41 with unstable angina, 29 with stable angina, and 5 with atypical angina. For the former 2 groups, the baseline CRP concentration was significantly correlated with risk of coronary event. Patients with unstable or stable angina whose CRP concentration was in the 5th quintile were at double the risk of coronary events (Fig). One third of the coronary events recorded occurred in patients whose CRP concentration was in the 5th quintile, i.e., greater than 3.6 mg/L. Factors significantly and positively associated with CRP were age, smoking, body mass index, triglyceride level, extent of coronary stenosis, history of myocardial infarction, and lower ejection fraction. There was no link between SAA concentration and coronary event risk.

*Conclusions.*—Patients with unstable or stable angina who have an elevated plasma CRP concentration are at elevated risk of later coronary events. The elevations of CRP seen in this population are within the range previously considered normal and are probably not the result of myocardial necrosis. Sensitive assays for CRP measurement may be able to provide useful prognostic information before the patient has even had any

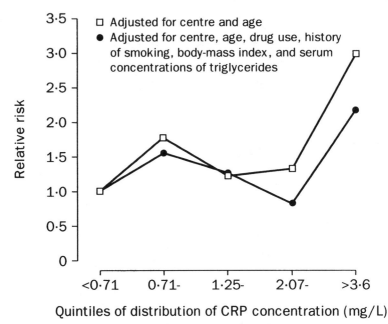

FIGURE.—Relative risk of coronary events by quintiles of distribution of C-reactive protein concentration. *Abbreviation*: CRP, C-reactive protein. (Courtesy of Haverkate F, for the European Concerted Action on Thrombosis and Disabilities Angina Pectoris Study Group: Production of C-reactive protein and risk of coronary events in stable and unstable angina. *Lancet* 349:462–466, 1997. Copyright by The Lancet Ltd., 1997.)

symptoms. Concentration of SAA, another acute-phase reactant, is unrelated to the coronary event rate.

▶ The acute-phase response is a nonspecific phenomenon, but the association between the increased production of CRP and subsequent coronary events among patients without evidence of necrosis (many of whom also had stable angina) extends prior data in patients with unstable angina.[1] The explanations are not well understood, but these findings provide further tantalizing, although circumstantial, evidence in favor of the inflammatory theory of atherosclerosis, plaque rupture, and thrombosis. An alternative explanation is that increased CRP concentrations are a marker of inflammation or infection elsewhere in the body which may in turn lead to atherogenesis.[2] Is there currently a clinical role for testing of CRP in patients with coronary disease or risk factors for coronary disease? At this stage, I would say not, but this study does point in an interesting direction for future research.

**B.J. Gersh, M.B., Ch.B., D.Phil., F.R.C.P.**

*References*

1. Liuzzo G, Biasucci LM, Gallimore JR et al: The prognostic value of C-reactive protein in serum amyloid A-protein in severe unstable angina. *N Engl J Med* 331:417–424,1994.
2. Mendall MA, Patel P, Ballan L, et al: C-reactive protein in its relation to cardio-vascular risk factors: A population-based cross-sectional study. *BMJ* 312:1061–1065, 1996.

---

**Troponin T Identifies Patients With Unstable Coronary Artery Disease Who Benefit From Long-term Antithrombotic Protection**
Lindahl B, for the Fragmin in Unstable Coronary Artery Disease (FRISC) Study Group (Univ Hosp, Uppsala, Sweden)
*J Am Coll Cardiol* 29:43–48, 1997                                        2–17

---

*Objective.*—Dalteparin (Fragmin), a low–molecular-weight heparin, reduces the number of new cardiac events in patients with unstable coronary artery disease (CAD). Because patients with even slightly elevated troponin T levels are at increased risk for new cardiac events, risk stratification of patients with unstable CAD is important in devising the most beneficial and cost-effective therapeutic approach. Results were presented regarding a double-blind, placebo-controlled, randomized study prospectively evaluating the effect of low–molecular-weight heparin on patients with different levels of troponin T and its relationship to long-term vs. short-term treatment benefits.

*Methods.*—Troponin T levels were measured in a subgroup of 971 patients consisting of men over 40 years of age and postmenopausal women from the Fragmin in Unstable Coronary Artery Disease (FRISC) study. They had been hospitalized within 72 hours of an episode of chest pain. Patients received either placebo (n = 488) or a twice daily injection of 120 U/kg of body weight of dalteparin (n = 483) for 5 to 7 days followed by a once daily dose of 7,500 U for 5 weeks. After release, patients were followed at 6 weeks and 5 to 6 months. Death and nonfatal myocardial infarction (MI) were recorded and compared statistically between groups.

*Results.*—The short-term (6 day) MI and death rates were significantly higher in the placebo group (4.7%) than in the dalteparin group (1.7%). By day 40, the MI and death rates were significantly higher in the placebo group (10.9%) than in the dalteparin group (6.8%). After 150 days, there was no significant difference in MI and death rates between groups. The short-term MI and death rates in the dalteparin group were lower at all troponin T tertiles. By day 40, there was a decreased death and MI rate in patients in the second and third troponin T tertiles (Table 2).

*Conclusion.*—Determination of troponin T levels in patients with unstable CAD soon after admission for chest pain identifies those who would benefit from prolonged treatment with dalteparin.

TABLE 2.—Effect of Dalteparin on the Rate of Death or Myocardial Infarction in Relation to Troponin T Level at Inclusion

| Troponin T (placebo/dalteparin) | Death/MI, Day 6 | | | Death/MI, Day 40 | | | Death/MI, Day 150 | | |
|---|---|---|---|---|---|---|---|---|---|
| | Placebo [no. (%)] | Dalteparin [no. (%)] | RR (95% CI) | Placebo [no. (%)] | Dalteparin [no. (%)] | RR (95% CI) | Placebo [no. (%)] | Dalteparin [no. (%)] | RR (95% CI) |
| <0.1 µg/liter (170/157) | 4 (2.4) | 0 (0) | p = 0.12 | 8 (4.7) | 9 (5.7) | 1.22 (0.48–3.1) | 10 (5.9) | 14 (8.9) | 1.52 (0.69–3.31) |
| ≥0.1 µg/liter (318/326) | 19 (6.0) | 8 (2.5) | 0.41 (0.18–0.92) | 45 (14.2) | 24 (7.4) | 0.52 (0.32–0.83) | 65 (20.4) | 52 (16.0) | 0.78 (0.56–1.09) |

*Abbreviations: CI*, confidence interval; *MI*, myocardial infarction; *RR*, relative risk.
(Reprinted by permission from the American College of Cardiology, courtesy of Lindahl B, for the Fragmin in Unstable Coronary Artery Disease (FRISC) Study Group: Troponin T identifies patients with unstable coronary artery disease who benefit from long-term antithrombin protection. *J Am Coll Cardiol* 29:43–48, 1997.)

► This paper is interesting on 2 accounts. First, this substudy is part of the double-blind, randomized FRISC trial of patients with unstable angina. These data confirm the promise of low–molecular-weight heparin (dalteparin sodium) as an antithrombotic agent. Low–molecular-weight heparin acts mainly by inhibiting factor Xa which is a key agent in the formation of thrombin.[1] Moreover, the ability to use low–molecular-weight heparin over the "long term" avoids the problem of "rebound" after heparinization and allows time for the plaque fissure, which triggered the acute event initially, to heal.

The second interesting aspect of this study is the proposed role of troponin T elevation in identifying a subgroup of patients in whom prolonged antithrombotic treatment—e.g., with dalteparin—is beneficial. The results of this study are actually quite impressive and the multivariate analysis does demonstrate an interaction between treatment and favorable outcomes in patients with elevated troponin T levels, whereas there appeared to be no long-term protective effect of low–molecular-weight heparin in patients with very low or undetected levels of troponin T. I would emphasize, however, that the drug is beneficial in the short term in both groups.

Does this mean that in every patient with unstable angina, troponin T levels should be measured and used to identify a group who require long-term therapy? This is premature, and one needs to determine whether elevated troponin T levels are, in themselves, predictors, *over and above* other indicators of high risk. For instance, although there were no statistically significant differences in clinical characteristics between the 2 groups, it does appear that patients with elevated troponin T levels had a higher incidence of both ST-segment depression and T-wave inversion and were much more likely to have a diagnosis of non–Q wave myocardial infarction, whereas those with low troponin T levels nearly all had a diagnosis of unstable angina. What also needs to be determined is whether troponin T levels add prognostic information to an exercise test.

In any event, this is a useful study which highlights the promise of low–molecular-weight heparin and emphasizes, again, that the key to the management of unstable angina is risk stratification. Those patients at increased risk based upon troponin T levels, Holter ST-segment monitoring, exercise testing, thallium scintigraphy, etc., are candidates for cardiac catheterization and revascularization—or perhaps other, more powerful forms of medical therapy such as low–molecular-weight heparin.

**B.J. Gersh, M.B., Ch.B., D.Phil., F.R.C.P.**

*Reference*

1. Eriksson B, Soderberg K, Widlund L, et al: A comparative study of three low-molecular weight heparins and unfractionated heparin [UH] in healthy volunteers. *Thromb Haemost* 73:398–401, 1995.

### A Comparison of Low-molecular-weight Heparin With Unfractionated Heparin for Unstable Coronary Artery Disease

Cohen M, for the Efficacy and Safety of Subcutaneous Enoxaparin in Non–Q-Wave Coronary Events Study Group (Allegheny Univ, Philadelphia; Hôpital St Sacrement, Quebec; Instituto de Cardiologia y Cirugia, Buenos Aires, Argentina; et al)

*N Engl J Med* 337:447–452, 1997                                    2–18

*Introduction.*—Standard therapy for patients hospitalized with unstable angina or non–Q-wave myocardial infarction consists of IV unfractionated heparin plus oral aspirin. Because of the substantial failure rate of this treatment, a randomized trial was conducted to assess the efficacy of low–molecular weight heparins in this setting. Previous trials have documented the advantages of the low–molecular weight heparins, including their more predictable anticoagulant effect.

*Methods.*—Patients were enrolled from October 1994 to May 1996 at 176 centers in the United States, Canada, South America, and Europe. The double-blind study assigned 3,171 patients to receive either enoxaparin (1 mg/kg of body weight administered subcutaneously twice daily) or continuous IV unfractionated heparin. Patients were treated for at least 48 hours, to a maximum of 8 days. The primary outcome was the composite triple end point of death, myocardial infarction (or reinfarction), or recur-

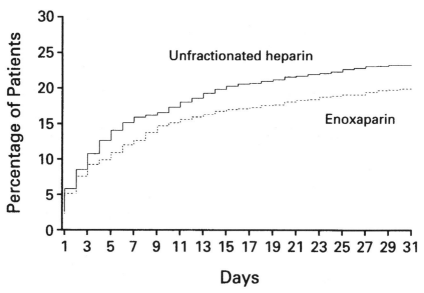

FIGURE 1.—Kaplan-Meier plots of the time to a first event over a period of 30 days for the composite end point of death, myocardial infarction, or recurrent angina. (Reprinted by permission of *The New England Journal of Medicine* from Cohen M, for the Efficacy and Safety of Subcutaneous Enoxaparin in Non–Q-Wave Coronary Events Study Group. A comparison of low-molecular-weight heparin with unfractionated heparin for unstable coronary artery disease. *N Engl J Med* 337:447–452. Copyright 1997, Massachusetts Medical Society. All rights reserved.)

rent angina at 14 days of follow-up. Data on coronary end points were collected during a period of 30 days. The targeted activated partial-thromboplastin time was 55–85 sec.

*Results.*—The 2 treatment groups were similar in baseline variables. Assigned therapies were initiated within 12 hours of randomization in 96% of patients, and both trial therapies were continued for a median of 2.6 days. At 14 days, patients randomized to enoxaparin had a significantly lower risk of death, myocardial infarction, or recurrent angina (16.6%) than those randomized to unfractionated heparin (19.8%). The risk of this composite end point continued to be significantly lower (Fig 1) in the enoxaparin group at 30 days (19.8% vs. 23.3%). Enoxaparin treatment was also associated with a significantly less frequent need for revascularization procedures but a significantly higher incidence of bleeding overall.

*Conclusion.*—Enoxaparin plus aspirin was a more effective antithrombotic therapy than unfractionated heparin plus aspirin for patients hospitalized with unstable angina or non–Q-wave myocardial infarction. The risk of death, myocardial infarction, or recurrent angina was significantly reduced at both 14 and 30 days in patients randomized to enoxaparin. Minor bleeding was the only adverse effect reported for enoxaparin.

▶ The use of heparin in the acute coronary syndromes is standard and logical, given the abundant evidence of coronary thrombosis as the pathophysiologic common denominator in the majority of patients. Unfractionated or "conventional" heparin has many drawbacks, including a wide variability in its anticoagulant efficacy and its relative inefficacy in platelet-rich thrombi. The former is illustrated by the large proportion of patients whose activated partial thromboplastin times (APTTs) were outside the desired therapeutic range.

The narrow risk–benefit ratio of unfractionated heparin has stimulated interest in the search for better alternatives, including the direct antithrombins (hirudin and hirulog) and low–molecular weight heparins. The latter have a higher bioavailability, are less subject to binding to plasma and tissue proteins, are more resistant to the effect of platelets, and exert a more durable and predictable therapeutic effect and a much more pronounced effect on thrombin generation via factor Xa. Low-molecular weight heparins are easy to administer, can be given subcutaneously once or twice per day, and obviate the need for laboratory monitoring of the aPTT.

These advantages have been translated into a rapid acceptance of its use in outpatients with deep-vein thrombosis.[1] This study by Cohen et al. certainly implies the superiority of the low–molecular weight heparin, enoxaparin, in patients with unstable angina, particularly with regard to the end points of recurrent angina and myocardial infarction; however, there was no difference in overall mortality, although the trial was not powered to answer the latter alone. These data are in contrast to another recent but smaller trial of a different low–molecular weight heparin that did not demonstrate a benefit over unfractionated heparin.[2] Moreover, another phase 3 trial of enoxaparin pointed toward a higher rate of hemorrhaging, particularly in older patients with smaller body masses.[3]

In summary, the drug is promising, but there are many questions to be answered with regard to its mechanisms of action, appropriate doses, and the efficacy of other low–molecular weight heparins, which have different molecular weights, different rates of plasma clearance, and different spectrums of anti-factor Xa and antithrombin activity.[4] One thing is for sure: conventional heparin and aspirin are under siege—the direct antithrombins, newer platelet inhibitors, and the low–molecular weight heparins will remain very much in the news in the near future.

**B.J. Gersh, M.B., Ch.B., D.Phil., F.R.C.P.**

*References*

1. Levine M, Gent M, Hirsh J, et al: A comparison of low-molecular-weight heparin administered primarily at home with unfractionated heparin administered in the hospital for deep-vein thrombosis. *N Engl J Med* 334:677–681, 1996.
2. Klein W, Buchwald A, Hillis SE, et al: Comparison of low-molecular-weight heparin with unfractionated heparin acutely and with placebo for 6 weeks in the management of unstable coronary artery disease: Fragmin in Unstable Coronary Artery Disease Study (FRIC). *Circulation* 96:61–68, 1997.
3. The Thrombolysis in Myocardial Infarction (TIMI) 11A Trial Investigators: Dose-ranging trial of enoxaparin for unstable angina: Results of TIMI 11A. *J Am Coll Cardiol* 29:1474–1482, 1997.
4. Armstrong PW: Heparin in acute coronary disease—Requiem for a heavyweight? (editorial). *N Engl J Med* 337:492–494, 1997.

---

**Emergency Room Triage of Patients With Acute Chest Pain by Means of Rapid Testing for Cardiac Troponin T or Troponin I**

Hamm CW, Goldmann BU, Heeschen C, et al (Univ Hosp Eppendorf, Hamburg, Germany)
*N Engl J Med* 337:1648–1653, 1997                                    2–19

---

*Background.*—Patients seen in the emergency department with acute chest pain may have no clear evidence of evolving myocardial infarction. Both ECGs and serial measurements of creatine kinase and its MB isoenzyme are often nondiagnostic, and patients may be unnecessarily hospitalized or sent home inappropriately. A prospective study examined the value of bedside tests for cardiac troponin T and troponin I as indicators of myocardial injury.

*Methods.*—Eligible patients came to the emergency department with acute anterior, precordial, or left-sided chest pain lasting 12 hours or less that was unexplained by local trauma or chest film abnormalities. None had ST-segment elevation on their ECGs. The 773 patients who met entry criteria had a mean age of 62 years; 465 were men. All had blood collected for testing with newly developed bedside kits that provide troponin T and troponin I status within 15–20 minutes. Testing was performed on arrival

**TABLE 1.**—Numbers of Deaths and Nonfatal Acute Myocardial Infarctions Occurring in the Hospital and Within 30 Days After Discharge, According to Troponin Status

| EVENT | TROPONIN I– POSITIVE (N=171) | TROPONIN I– NEGATIVE (N=602) | TROPONIN T– POSITIVE (N=123) | TROPONIN T– NEGATIVE (N=650) |
|---|---|---|---|---|
| Death in hospital | 11 | 0 | 9 | 2 |
| Acute myocardial infarction in hospital | 9 | 0 | 7 | 2 |
| Death after discharge | 8 | 1 | 7 | 2 |
| Acute myocardial infarction after discharge | 4 | 1 | 4 | 1 |
| All events | 32 | 2 | 27 | 7 |

(Reprinted by permission of *The New England Journal of Medicine* from Hamm CW, Goldmann BU, Heeschen C, et al: Emergency room triage of patients with acute chest pain by means of rapid testing for cardiac troponin T or troponin I. *N Engl J Med* 337:1648–1653. Copyright 1997, Massachusetts Medical Society. All rights reserved.)

and at 4 or more hours later. Patients were followed up for 30 days after hospital discharge for cardiac events.

*Results.*—Routine measurements of creatine kinase activity within 24 hours after arrival yielded a final diagnosis of acute myocardial infarction in 47 patients (6%). Diagnoses in the remaining patients were unstable angina (315), stable angina (121), acute heart failure (15), pulmonary embolism (12), and myocarditis (5); 258 patients had no evidence of coronary heart disease. Overall, 63% of patients were admitted to the hospital, and 29% were admitted to the ICU. Troponin T tests were positive in 16% of patients, and troponin I tests were positive in 22%. Among those with evolving myocardial infarction, troponin T tests were positive in 94% and troponin I tests were positive in 100%. Fewer patients with unstable angina had at least 1 positive troponin T test (22%) or at least 1 positive troponin I test (36%). There were 20 deaths and 14 nonfatal myocardial infarctions during the follow-up period (Table 1). Event rates in patients with negative tests were quite low (1.1% for troponin T and 0.3% for troponin I).

*Conclusion.*—Bedside tests for cardiac-specific troponins were strong, independent predictors of cardiac events in patients with acute chest pain but no ST-segment elevation. Negative troponin T and troponin I results allow patients to be safely discharged; those with at least 1 positive result should be admitted for further evaluation.

▶ The evaluation of patients with chest pain in the emergency department is often a clinical dilemma with huge economic implications, given the approximately 5 million patients a year who come to emergency departments with chest pain.[1] Although the decision in patients with chest pain and ST-segment elevation is fairly clear-cut, as it is in many patients with significant ST-segment depression, a majority of patients have a normal or nondiagnostic ECG. A number of these patients will eventually have a myocardial infarction yet are inappropriately sent home.[2] On the other hand, the economic impact of unnecessary hospitalization to "rule out" myocardial infarction is also substantial.

This useful, large German study demonstrates the sensitivity of troponin T and troponin I using a bedside test kit that can produce a qualitative result within 15–20 minutes. The results are encouraging, both with regard to the sensitivity and specificity and in the light of the excellent prognosis of patients with troponin-negative status who are presumably candidates for early discharge. Nonetheless, there are several caveats that apply. First of all, studies such as this need to be repeated by others. Second, one should never place complete reliance on a test, and, in a patient with a convincing clinical history, with or without ECG changes, I would be cautious about excluding coronary disease on the basis of a negative troponin T level. Third, as pointed out in the accompanying editorial by Hlatky,[1] the authors took care to obtain at least 2 negative samples, and the second was at least 6 hours after the onset of chest pain; so perhaps a single value could result in a false-negative test. Finally, one must point out that, among patients with ST-segment depression and negative troponin T or troponin I values, there was nonetheless a 2.8% to 1.4% rate of death from myocardial infarction in the ensuing 30 days, which is not trivial. Nonetheless, although mindful of these caveats, one has to accept that troponin levels are a useful addition to the armamentarium with which to evaluate acute ischemic syndromes in the emergency department.

**B.J. Gersh, M.B., Ch.B., D.Phil., F.R.C.P.**

*References*

1. Hlatky MA: Evaluation of chest pain in the emergency department (editorial). *N Engl J Med* 337:1687–1689, 1997.
2. Lee TH, Rovan GW, Weisberg MC, et al: Clinical characteristics and natural history of patients with acute myocardial infarction sent home from the emergency room. *Am J Cardiol* 60:219–224, 1987.

---

**Long-term Protection From Myocardial Ischemic Events in a Randomized Trial of Brief Integrin β3 Blockade With Percutaneous Coronary Intervention**
Topol EJ, for the EPIC Investigator Group (Cleveland Clinic Found, Ohio; Baylor College of Medicine, Houston; Florida Heart Group, Orlando; et al)
*JAMA* 278:479–484, 1997                                                    2–20

---

*Introduction.*—The frequency of coronary renarrowing, resulting in the need for repeat procedures or bypass surgery, is the major limitation of percutaneous coronary intervention by 1 year of follow-up in nearly half of the patients. Stenting has been shown to be the only intervention that has significantly reduced the rate of recurrence, and many pharmacologic agents have failed to reduce restenosis or improve long-term clinical outcomes. Abciximab is a monoclonal antibody fragment directed against the

$\beta_3$ integrin and has been shown to reduce clinical recurrence at 6 months in a previous study. Clinical follow-up was performed 2.5 years after the index percutaneous coronary revascularization procedure in patients who had coronary angioplasty and were administered abciximab to determine whether the effects of abciximab would continue beyond 6 months.

*Methods.*—There were 2,099 high-risk patients having coronary angioplasty who were randomly assigned to receive an abciximab bolus of 0.25 mg/kg followed by infusion at 10 µg/min for 12 hours, abciximab bolus of 0.25 mg/kg followed by placebo infusion, or placebo bolus followed by placebo infusion. Follow-up occurred up to 3 years.

*Results.*—In 41.1% of those receiving abciximab bolus plus infusion, composite end points occurred at 3 years. In 47.4% of those receiving abciximab bolus only and in 47.2% of those receiving placebo only, composite end points occurred at 3 years. In 6.8% of those receiving abciximab bolus plus infusion, 8.0% of those receiving abciximab bolus only, and 8.6% of those receiving placebo, death occurred. In 10.7% of those receiving abciximab bolus plus infusion, 12.2% of those receiving abciximab only, and 13.6% of those receiving placebo, myocardial infarction occurred. In 34.8% of those receiving abciximab bolus plus infusion, 38.6% of those receiving abciximab bolus only, and 40.1% receiving placebo, revascularization occurred. Death occurred in 5.1% of those receiving abciximab bolus plus infusion, 9.2% of those receiving abciximab only, and 12.7% of those receiving placebo among those with refractory unstable angina or evolving myocardial infarction. As periprocedural creatine kinase levels increased, death rates increased.

*Conclusion.*—Outcomes are improved as long as 3 years after coronary angioplasty with abciximab bolus with infusion given at the time of the procedure.

▶ Although the Evaluation of Platelet IIb/IIIa-Inhibition for Prevention of Ischemic Complication (EPIC)[1] and EPILOG[2] trials demonstrated a reduction in clinical events at 30 days in patients with acute ischemic syndromes undergoing percutaneous transluminal coronary angioplasty, what was particularly intriguing was the 23% reduction in clinical recurrences at 6 months.[1, 2]

This follow-up study demonstrates a sustained benefit at 2.5 years upon each of the end points of death, myocardial infarction, and repeat revascularization. This is somewhat surprising given the relatively brief duration of the original infusion (12 hours) and the natural history of coronary artery disease, which is characterized by disease progression and recurrent events from new lesions and in different vessels. What is particularly fascinating in this study is the divergence of the mortality curves after approximately a year, demonstrating a higher mortality in patients treated with a bolus compared to the bolus plus infusion. This is particularly evident in high-risk patients with unstable angina and evolving myocardial infarction. One explanation for a sustained benefit after a relatively brief period of infusion may stem from the dual action of abciximab consisting of the abciximab antibody *Fab* fragment against the IIb/IIIa integrin and another integrin, mainly the vitronectin receptor. A blockade of the latter may have an additional beneficial effect upon smooth muscle cell migration, the fibrinolytic pathway, and thrombin generation.

This is a fascinating area, which raises the possibility that the new generation of platelet inhibitors may have the ability to stabilize atherosclerotic coronary disease. A logical outcome of this is the development of the oral GP IIb/IIIa receptor blockers, and I would expect that we would hear a great deal about this approach in the coming years. Nonetheless, the introduction of oral platelet inhibitors as a new class of therapeutic agents is not a simple matter by any means, because it appears that they may have a very steep dose-response curve and fatal bleeding is the price that could potentially be paid. Further questions that need be answered include the optimum dose and methods of monitoring the dose and patient-specific dose adjustments. In the event that monitoring is desirable, we still do not know what end point should be monitored—whether this be plasma levels of the drug, the intensity of receptor blockade, or the effect of the drug on platelet function such as the bleeding time. Moreover, there are problems with many of the assays currently available.[3] The answers to these multiple questions will come from very carefully designed clinical trials. The specific objective of assessing not only the expense and the effort involved in developing techniques of monitoring the efficacy of the IIb/IIIa inhibitors, but also whether this could be justified in terms of safety and improved therapeutic efficacy will not be achieved by one large megatrial.

**B.J. Gersh, M.B., Ch.B., D.Phil., F.R.C.P.**

*References*

1. Topol EJ, Califf RM, Weisman HF, et al: Randomized trial of coronary intervention with antibody against platelet IIb/IIIa integrin for reduction of clinical restenosis; Results at six months. *Lancet* 343:881–886, 1994.
2. The EPILOG Investigators: Platelet glycoprotein IIb/IIIa receptor blockade and low-dose heparin during percutaneous coronary revascularization. *N Engl J Med* 336:1689–1696, 1997.
3. Coller BS: GP IIb/IIIa antagonists; Pathophysiologic and therapeutic insights from studies of c7E3 Fab. *Thromb Haemost* 78:730–735, 1997.

# Epidemiology and Risk Factors

## Plasma Homocysteine and Cardiovascular Disease Mortality

Alfthan G, Aro A, Gey KF (Natl Public Health Inst, Helsinki; Univ of Bern, Switzerland)
*Lancet* 349:397, 1997                                    2–21

*Objective.*—Patients with inherited homocysteinuria are at risk of early vascular disease and thromboembolism. Plasma homocysteine (Hcy) is an independent risk factor for cardiovascular disease (CVD). Reported mean plasma Hcy values in healthy subjects vary widely, from 6 μmol/L in Japan to 13 μmol/L in South Africa. The reasons for these differences are unknown. Differences in plasma total Hcy concentrations in various coun-

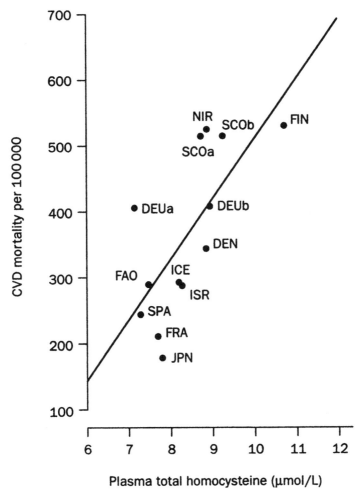

**Plasma total homocysteine (μmol/L)**

**FIGURE.**—Relationship between plasma total homocysteine concentration and mortality from all cardiovascular diseases according to World Health Organization data. Points represent mean plasma homocysteine concentrations of 20 men. Mortality data for Faroe Islands taken from Iceland. *Abbreviations*: *DEUa*, Germany, Schleiz; *DEUb*, Germany, Cottbus; *SPA*, Spain, Barcelona; *FAO*, Faroe Islands; *FRA*, France, Toulouse; *JPN*, Japan, Okinawa; *ISR*, Israel, Tel Aviv; *ICE*, Iceland, Reykjavik; *SCOa*, Scotland, Aberdeen; *SCOb*, Scotland, Glasgow; *DEN*, Denmark, Glostrup; *NIR*, Northern Ireland, Belfast; *FIN*, Finland, Kuopio. (Courtesy of Alfthan G, Aro A, Gey KF: Plasma homocysteine and cardiovascular disease mortality. *Lancet* 349:397, copyright 1997, The Lancet Ltd.)

tries were assessed, together with the possible associations with mortality from CVD.

*Methods.*—The analysis included heparinized plasma samples from healthy men participating in a large World Health Organization study. Samples from 20 men in each of 13 areas around the world were analyzed. High-performance liquid chromatography fluorimetry was performed to measure plasma total Hcy concentration. All samples were obtained according to the same protocol.

*Results.*—The lowest mean value was in Germany (7 μmol/L), whereas the highest was in Finland (11 μmol/L). Some areas had a very high proportion of elevated plasma total Hcy values (Iceland, Denmark, and Scotland) as reflected by high standard deviations. The mean plasma Hcy was significant related to CVD mortality, which was highest in Finland and Northern Ireland (Fig).

*Conclusion.*—The geographic differences in plasma total Hcy concentrations are real, and not the result of differing sampling and assay procedures between reports. Plasma Hcy may play an important role in the variation in CVD among different populations. Increased plasma Hcy may be a risk factor for CVD.

▶ The evidence that increased levels of plasma Hcy constitute a risk factor for CVD continues to mount, and a trial of folate supplementation is, to my mind, overdue.[1] One explanation for the association lies in the in vitro observation that Hcy is cytotoxic to endothelial cells and is able to promote low-density lipoprotein oxidation.

**B.J. Gersh, M.B., Ch.B., D.Phil., F.R.C.P.**

*Reference*

1. Malinow MR: Plasma homocyst(e)ine: A risk factor for arterial occlusive diseases. *J Nutr* 126:1238S–1243S, 1996.

---

**The Recent Decline in Mortality From Coronary Heart Disease, 1980–1990: The Effect of Secular Trends in Risk Factors and Treatment**
Hunink MGM, Goldman L, Tosteson ANA, et al (Harvard Med School, Boston; Univ of Groningen, The Netherlands; Univ of California, San Francisco; et al)
*JAMA* 277:535–542, 1997                                        2–22

---

*Background.*—Coronary heart disease is still the major cause of morbidity and mortality in the United States, even though the incidence of and death rate from coronary disease have been decreasing in recent decades. Possible explanations for this are the effect of risk factor reductions in decreasing the incidence of coronary disease and event rates in patients with existing coronary heart disease, and improved treatment of current patients with coronary disease. It is unclear to what extent each of these factors has affected mortality rates. A computer simulation model was designed by the coronary heart disease policy model research group to replicate *Vital Statistics of the United States 1980* and has been updated for 1986. The model was used to determine if secular trends in risk factors and treatment can account for the decrease in mortality rates from coronary disease between 1980 and 1990.

*Methods.*—Data from the medical literature, health surveys, clinical trials, and U.S. statistics were collected. A computer simulation state-transition model of individuals between ages 35 and 84 years was developed to predict the death rate from coronary heart disease.

*Results.*—In 1990, the actual death rate from coronary heart disease in the United States was 34% lower than would have been predicted if risk factor levels, case-fatality rates, and event rates in individuals with and without coronary disease were the same as in 1980. After secular changes in these factors were included in the model, the predicted death rate from coronary disease for 1990 was within 3% of the actual death rate, and 92% of the decrease was accounted for. Primary prevention accounted for 25% of the decrease, secondary reduction of risk factors in patients with coronary heart disease accounted for 29% of the decrease, and other improvements in treatment of patients with coronary disease accounted for 43% of the decrease.

*Discussion.*—Primary and secondary reductions in risk factors account for 50% of the decrease in mortality rates from coronary heart disease in the United States between 1980 and 1990. More than 70% of the overall decline in the death rate has been among current patients with coronary heart disease.

▶ Although the methodology of this paper, which used a computer simulation model, is complex, the results are encouraging in regard to the decline in coronary heart disease mortality but are also sobering and somewhat provocative in relation to the increased prevalence of coronary heart disease from 1980 to 1990. It would appear that primary prevention in patients without documented coronary artery disease is clearly beneficial in reducing the overall mortality rate from coronary heart disease, but the bulk of the mortality decline is attributable to patients with already established coronary heart disease. Approximately half of the decline in this group is from risk factor reductions (secondary prevention) and approximately 40% from improvements in treatments other than risk factor reduction. To what extent this reflects coronary revascularization vs drug and other therapeutic interventions is unclear.[1]

In summary, it would appear that there has been a decline in the incidence of coronary heart disease (although this is not universally accepted), but the mortality rate, particularly the acute coronary heart disease death rate, has declined quite strikingly. What this means is that one can expect little change or even an increase in the prevalence of coronary artery disease, and this may be seen primarily in an elderly population. The economic implications of this trend are obvious, and we have to accept that the enormous burden that coronary artery disease imposes on this country continues despite improvements in some areas. The net result, however, is that patients with coronary heart disease live longer, causing a shift toward a more chronic form of the disease in older patients.

**B.J. Gersh, M.B., Ch.B., D.Phil., F.R.C.P.**

*Reference*

1. McGovern PG, Fulsom AR, Sprafka JM, et al: Trends in survival of hospitalized myocardial infarction patients between 1970 and 1986: The Minnesota Heart Survey. *Circulation* 85:172–179, 1992.

**Coronary Artery Calcium in Acute Coronary Syndrome: A Comparative Study of Electron-beam Computed Tomography, Coronary Angiography, and Intracoronary Ultrasound in Survivors of Acute Myocardial Infarction and Unstable Angina**

Schmermund A, Baumgart D, Görge G, et al (Univ Clinic Essen, Germany; Mayo Clinic and Found, Rochester, Minn; Univ Witten/Herdecke, Mülheim an der Ruhr, Germany; et al)
*Circulation* 96:1461–1469, 1997                    2–23

*Introduction.*—Coronary atherosclerotic plaque formation is almost invariably associated with coronary artery calcium. A tool for noninvasive detection of calcium formation is electron-beam CT, as patients with little or no coronary artery calcium detected by this procedure may have a small chance of having clinically manifest coronary syndromes over the course of 1–2 years when compared to those with high calcium burdens. A subgroup of patients seen with acute coronary syndromes may not have coronary artery calcium but this has not been specifically examined. The detection of calcified atherosclerotic plaques by electron-beam CT in patients with acute coronary syndromes was evaluated. In survivors of acute myocardial infarction or unstable angina, electron-beam CT was compared with coronary angiography.

*Methods.*—There were 118 patients with previous myocardial infarction or unstable angina with a mean age of $57\pm11$ years who had electron-beam CT performed. For the definition of coronary artery calcium, a standard protocol requiring CT density greater than 130 Hounsfield units in an area of $1.03$ mm$^2$ or greater was used.

*Results.*—Moderate to severe coronary artery disease was found by coronary angiography in 110 patients, with 8 patients having either mildly stenotic plaques at a single site or nonatherosclerotic causes of the unstable coronary syndrome. A positive result of electron-beam CT was found in 105 of 110 patients (96%) with moderate to severe angiographic disease but in only 1 of the 8 other patients (13%). Patients with positive results on electron-beam CT were significantly older ($58\pm10$ years) than patients with negative results ($46\pm12$ years) who also were actively smoking.

*Conclusion.*—Identifiable coronary calcium is seen by electron-beam CT in the vast majority of patients with acute coronary syndrome and at least moderate angiographic disease. Minimal or no atherosclerotic plaque formation is found in those patients with negative electron-beam CT results, who tend to be active cigarette smokers and younger.

▶ What was not surprising in this study is the high incidence of coronary calcification in the vast majority of patients with vulnerable atherosclerotic plaque. This is consistent with previous studies, demonstrating the excellent prognostic value of coronary calcification using electron-beam CT.[1]

Nonetheless, there is a substantial group of patients seen with acute myocardial infarction who have had premature rupture of a vulnerable plaque with relatively little underlying plaque burden or pre-existing stenosis. This study emphasizes that many of these patients may have been missed by prescreening electron-beam CT before the acute clinical event. There is no doubt that electron-beam CT is a highly sensitive technique, but its lack of specificity argues against its role for routine screening purposes. What is also not known is the predictive value of a negative electron-beam CT result, particularly in younger patients and active smokers, in whom premature plaque rupture with relatively little fixed coronary stenosis may be present.

**B.J. Gersh, M.B., Ch.B., D.Phil., F.R.C.P.**

*Reference*

1. Arad Y, Sparado LA, Goodman K, et al: Predictive value of electron-beam computed tomography of the coronary artery; 19–Month follow-up of 1173 asymptomatic subjects. *Circulation* 93:1951–1953, 1996.

---

**Prospective Study of Effect of Switching From Cigarettes to Pipes or Cigars on Mortality From Three Smoking Related Diseases**
Wald NJ, Watt HC (Wolfson Inst of Preventive Medicine, London)
*BMJ* 314:1860–1863, 1997                                    2–24

---

*Introduction.*—Men who smoke only pipes or cigars tend not to inhale tobacco smoke while those who smoke cigarettes do tend to inhale the smoke. Because of this difference, pipe and cigar smokers are at lower risk of the main smoking-related diseases, but smokers who switch from cigarettes to pipes or cigars tend to maintain their inhaling habits. It is uncertain how much the inhaling habit negates the potential health benefits associated with smoking cigars or pipes rather than cigarettes. The extent to which cigarette smokers who switch to cigars or pipes alter their risk of dying of lung cancer, ischemic heart disease, or chronic obstructive lung disease was estimated.

*Methods.*—There were 21,520 men during a 7-year period aged 35–64 years who gave a detailed history of smoking, including self-reported inhaling habits. Blood samples were collected and carboxyhemoglobin saturation and other factors such as serum cholesterol were measured. The group was divided into current pipe or cigar smokers who had switched from smoking cigarettes at least 20 years before entry, pipe or cigar smokers who were current smokers and had never smoked cigarettes, cigarette smokers who did not smoke cigars or pipes, former smokers, and lifelong nonsmokers. The number of deaths from the 3 smoking-related

TABLE 3.—Relative Mortality (With 95% Confidence Intervals) According to Smoking Group for the 3 Specific Diseases Compared With Mortality Among Lifelong Nonsmokers

| Smoking group at entry | Total No of men | Ischaemic heart diseases | | Lung cancer | | Chronic obstructive lung diseases | | All three diseases | | All cases mortality | |
|---|---|---|---|---|---|---|---|---|---|---|---|
| | | Relative mortality | No of deaths | Relative mortality | No of deaths | Relative mortality | No of deaths | Relative mortality | No of deaths | Relative mortality | No of deaths |
| Lifelong non-smoker | 6539 | 1.00 | 125 | 1.00 | 7 | 1.00 | 1 | 1.00 | 133 | 1.00 | 346 |
| Former cigarette smoker, stopped smoking over 20 years before entry | 1465 | 1.05 (0.77 to 1.45) | 59 | 1.01 (0.26 to 3.91) | 3 | † | 1 | 1.07 (0.79 to 1.45) | 63 | 1.11 (0.92 to 1.34) | 162 |
| Pipe/cigar smoker, never smoked cigarettes (non-switchers) | 1309 | 0.98 (0.67 to 1.44) | 33 | 3.19* (1.07 to 9.50) | 6 | † | 1 | 1.11 (0.78 to 1.59) | 40 | 1.23 (0.99 to 1.75) | 113 |
| Pipe/cigar smoker, switched from cigarettes over 20 years before entry (switchers) | 522 | 1.29 (0.88 to 1.99) | 25 | 8.64* (3.19 to 23.3) | 9 | † | 1 | 1.68* (1.16 to 2.45) | 35 | 1.33 (1.03 to 1.73) | 69 |
| Current cigarette smoker | 4182 | 2.27* (1.81 to 2.84) | 193 | 16.4* (7.55 to 44.2) | 77 | 29.5* (3.96 to 220) | 20 | 3.13* (2.55 to 3.84) | 290 | 2.26 (1.97 to 2.58) | 540 |

*$P < 0.05$ compared with mortality in lifelong nonsmokers.
†Too few deaths to give reliable estimate.

(Courtesy of Wald NJ, Watt HC: Prospective study of effect of switching from cigarettes to pipes or cigars on mortality from three smoking related diseases. *BMJ* 314:1860–1863, 1997. Acknowledgment to BMJ Publishing Group.)

diseases—lung cancer, ischemic heart disease, and chronic obstructive lung disease—among the various categories of smokers were evaluated.

*Results.*—Less tobacco was smoked by pipe and cigar smokers who had switched from cigarettes (8.1 g/day) more than 20 years before entry to the study than cigarette smokers (20 g/day), but they had the same consumption as cigar and pipe smokers who had never smoked cigarettes (8.1g). Higher carboxyhemoglobin saturation was seen among former cigarette smokers who switched to pipe and cigar smoking (1.2%) when compared to those who never smoked cigarettes (1.0%), indicating that more tobacco smoke was inhaled by the former cigarette smokers. Those who switched to pipe and cigar smoking had a 51% higher risk of dying of the 3 smoking-related diseases than those who never smoked cigarettes and a 68% higher risk than lifelong nonsmokers (Table 3). They also had a 56% higher risk than those who quit smoking altogether more than 20 years before entry into the study. Their risk was 46% lower, however, than those who continued smoking cigarettes.

*Conclusion.*—Changing to cigars or pipes may be a better alternative to continuing to smoke cigarettes for cigarette smokers who have difficulty in giving up smoking altogether. The reduction in the quantity of tobacco smoked causes much of the effect, and some of the effect is the result of less inhaling. Pipe and cigar smokers who have never smoked cigarettes have a lower risk than cigarette smokers who switch to pipe and cigar smoking. Lifelong nonsmokers or former smokers have a lower risk than all pipe and cigar smokers.

▶ Some of the lessening in risk resulting from switching from cigarettes to pipes or cigars is attributable to the quantity of tobacco smoked and inhaling less. Nonetheless, the risk of dying of the 3 smoking-related diseases (lung cancer, ischemic heart disease, and chronic obstructive lung disease) was 68% higher than that of lifelong nonsmokers and 61% higher than cigar or pipe smokers who had never smoked cigarettes. The best option is not to smoke, or at least give up altogether. Failing that, a pipe or the cigar is a better alternative than continued cigarette smoking.

**B.J. Gersh, M.B., Ch.B., D.Phil., F.R.C.P.**

---

**Submissiveness and Protection From Coronary Heart Disease in the General Population: Edinburgh Artery Study**
Whiteman MC, Deary IJ, Lee AJ, et al (Univ of Edinburgh, Scotland)
*Lancet* 350:541–545, 1997                                                  2–25

---

*Introduction.*—An increased risk of coronary heart disease has been associated with type A personalities, which are characterized by a wish to do too much in too little time, competitiveness, frustration, and aggression. Another study found that the trait of submissiveness-low self-confidence was independent of hostility. The Bedford-Foulds Personality Deviance Scales define a submissive person as one who prefers to stay in the

TABLE 3.—Mean (SE) Submissiveness and Hostility Scores by Coronary Heart Disease Category in Men and Women

| | Myocardial Infarction Non-fatal | | Fatal | | All | | Angina | |
|---|---|---|---|---|---|---|---|---|
| | Yes | No | Yes | No | Yes | No | Yes | No |
| **Men** | | | | | | | | |
| Number of men | 57 | 611 | 25 | 643 | 80 | 588 | 48 | 620 |
| Submissiveness score | 17·70 (0·40) | 18·88 (0·15)* | 19·32 (0·69) | 18·76 (0·15) | 18·19 (0·37) | 18·86 (0·16) | 18·63 (0·54) | 18·80 (0·15) |
| Hostility score | 17·98 (0·46) | 17·38 (0·13) | 17·48 (0·64) | 17·73 (0·13) | 17·88 (0·38) | 17·37 (0·13) | 17·79 (0·50) | 17·46 (0·12) |
| **Women** | | | | | | | | |
| Number of women | 28 | 642 | 8 | 662 | 34 | 636 | 41 | 629 |
| Submissiveness score | 18·18 (0·86) | 20·76 (0·17)† | 22·12 (1·47) | 20·64 (0·17) | 18·94 (0·77) | 20·75 (0·17)‡ | 21·59 (0·71) | 20·58 (0·17) |
| Hostility score | 16·71 (0·60) | 17·29 (0·13) | 17·00 (1·18) | 17·27 (0·13) | 16·68 (0·55) | 17·29 (0·13) | 17·56 (0·53) | 17·26 (0·13) |

Note: Individuals were excluded from scale calculations if all items were not completed (which left 774 men and 740 women); those with history of angina or myocardial infarction at baseline are excluded (142 men, 89 women); an individual may appear in more than one category.

*P = 0.023.
†P = 0.002.
‡P = 0.019 for differences between those with and without relevant coronary heart disease event.

(Courtesy of Whiteman MC, Deary IJ, Lee AJ, et al: Submissiveness and protection from coronary heart disease in the general population: Edinburgh Artery Study. Lancet 350:541–545. Copyright 1997 by The Lancet Ltd.)

background and let others lead and dominate; the trait is related to self-confidence and a lack of self-assurance. Whether the risk of coronary heart disease was related to the independent trait of submissiveness was assessed.

*Methods.*—There were 809 men and 783 women aged 55–74 years who were administered the Bedford-Foulds Personality Deviance Scales at baseline. For 5 years, the participants were followed up for cardiovascular events, which were defined by the American Heart Association and ascertained from the Information and Statistics Division of the Scottish Office Home and Health Department, United Kingdom National Health Service Central Register, general practitioners, second examination at the end of follow-up, and questionnaires sent annually to the participants.

*Results.*—Nonfatal myocardial infarctions occurred in 56 men (7%) and 28 women (3.06%) during follow-up. Fatal myocardial infarctions occurred in 25 men (3.01%) and 8 women (1.0%). Angina pectoris developed in 48 men (5.09%) and 41 women (5.02%). Men and women who did not have a nonfatal myocardial infarction had mean submissiveness scores that were significantly higher. In women only, submissiveness remained independently associated with risk of myocardial infarction in multiple logistic regression models. An increase of 1 SD in submissiveness was associated with a decreased risk of nonfatal myocardial infarction and, to a lesser extent, total myocardial infarction (Table 3).

*Conclusion.*—Particularly in women, the personality trait of submissiveness may be protective against nonfatal myocardial infarction. The complicated effects of personality on development of coronary heart disease need to be better understood.

▶ The finding that submissiveness protects against myocardial infarction is complicated and difficult to interpret. It is not just an example of "the meek shall inherit the earth." In the Western collaborative group study, a reduction in mortality was noted among men who are submissive, but a trend in the opposite direction was noted among Whitehall civil servants in the United Kingdom.[1] Among baboons and monkeys, submissiveness or subordination does not appear to be beneficial.[2] Although the data are not clear-cut to say the least, the relationship between various patterns of behavior, including personality types A and B, hostility and submissiveness, and the cardiovascular system, is always of interest and controversial. It is likely that these personality traits do not exert their impact in isolation but in concert with other factors, e.g., working, social class, and social instability, and control of a professional and social environment.

**B.J. Gersh, M.B., Ch.B., D.Phil., F.R.C.P.**

*References*

1. Bosma H, Marmot MG, Hemingway H, et al: Low job control and risk of coronary heart disease in Whitehall II (Prospective cohort) Study. *BMJ* 314:558–565, 1997.
2. Sapolsky RM: Social subordinance as a marker of hypercortisolism: Some unexpected subtleties. *Ann NY Acad Sci* 771:626–639, 1995.

## Percutaneous Transluminal Coronary Angioplasty/Devices

**Fish Oils and Low-molecular-weight Heparin for the Reduction of Restenosis After Percutaneous Transluminal Coronary Angioplasty: The EMPAR Study**
Cairns JA, for the EMPAR Collaborators (McMaster Univ, Hamilton, Ont, Canada; Univ of Ottawa, Ont, Canada; Univ of Western Ontario, Canada; et al)
*Circulation* 94:1553–1560, 1996                                             2–26

*Background.*—Restenosis continues to be a major problem after percutaneous transluminal coronary angioplasty, with 6-month restenosis rates of >40%. Previous reports have suggested that taking large amounts of fish oil (n-3 fatty acids) may help to reduce the rates of restenosis and coronary events. Another possibly useful intervention is low-molecular-weight heparin (LMWH), which reduces cellular proliferation and restenosis in experimental systems. These 2 interventions were studied for their ability to reduce the rate of restenosis after percutaneous transluminal coronary angioplasty (PTCA).

*Methods.*—The study included 814 patients at 4 Canadian hospitals who were scheduled for PTCA. The patients were randomly assigned to receive fish oil (n-3 fatty acids, 5.4 gm/day, or placebo). Treatment started a median of 6 days before PTCA and continued for 18 weeks. Six hundred fifty-three patients had at least one successfully dilated lesion at the time of sheath removal. They were randomly assigned in a 2 × 2 factorial design to receive 6 weeks of treatment with LMWH, 30 mg SC bid, or standard therapy (no injections). Follow-up quantitative coronary angiography was performed and interpretable in 96% of these groups.

*Results.*—Restenosis rates per patient were 46.5% for the n-3 group, 45% for the placebo group, 46% for the LMWH group, and 39% for the control group. On a per-lesion basis, the rates were 40%, 39%, 38%, and 40%, respectively. Mean angiographic luminal diameters at follow-up were 1.12 mm with n-3, 1.10 mm with placebo, 1.12 mm with LMWH, and 1.10 with standard treatment (Figure). Rates of early discontinuation were 15% with n-3 or placebo and 21% with LMWH. Rates of ischemic events were comparable among groups. Although bleeding was a more common problem with LMWH, it was usually mild and rarely led to discontinuation of therapy. Patients receiving n-3 had more gastrointestinal side effects than did those receiving placebo.

*Conclusions.*—Neither fish oil nor LMWH can reduce the rate of restenosis after PTCA. Combined with previous results, the findings suggest that further studies of fish oil for the reduction of PTCA restenosis are unwarranted. The evidence suggests that LMWH is unlikely to have any beneficial effect either.

▶ Theoretical animal studies and prior smaller trials suggested that fish oils may be of benefit in reducing restenosis.[1] Moreover, documentation that

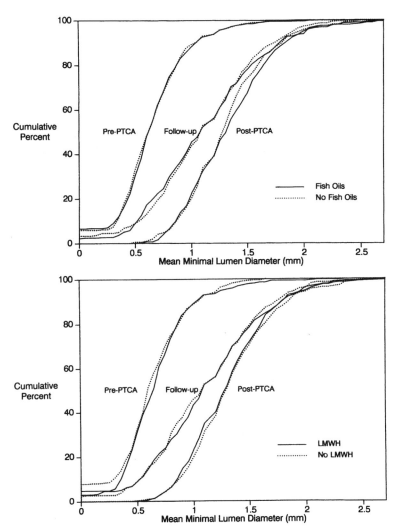

**FIGURE.**—Cumulative frequency distribution curves of the mean minimal lumen diameters of lesions undergoing visually successful PTCA measured before PTCA, immediately after PTCA, and at follow-up. *Top*, Fish oils and placebo groups; *bottom*, LMWH and control groups. (Courtesy of Cairns JA, for the EMPAR Collaborators: Fish oils and low-molecular-weight heparin for the reduction of restenosis after percutaneous transluminal coronary angioplasty: The EMPAR study. *Circulation* 94:1553–1560, 1996. Reproduced with permission. Copyright American Heart Association.)

LMWH can reduce the cellular proliferation that causes smooth muscle cell hyperplasia and restenosis in animal models prompted this large trial.[2] The EMPAR trial provides yet more emphatic evidence that pharmacologic interventions are of little value in reducing restenosis, which remains the "Achilles heel" of PTCA.

**B.J. Gersh, M.B., Ch.B., D.Phil., F.R.C.P.**

*References*

1. Dehmer GJ, Popma JJ, Van der Berg EK, et al: Reduction in the rate of early restenosis after coronary angioplasty by a diet supplemented with n3 fatty acids. *N Engl J Med* 319:733–740, 1988.
2. Guyton RJ, Rosenberg RD, Clowes AW, et al: Inhibition of rat arterial smooth muscle proliferation by heparin: in vivo studies with anticoagulant and non-anticoagulant heparin. *Circ Res* 46:625–634, 1990.

**Coronary Angioplasty Volume-Outcome Relationships for Hospitals and Cardiologists**
Hannan EL, Racz M, Ryan TJ, et al (State Univ of New York, Albany; Boston Univ; Mid America Heart Inst, Kansas City, Mo; et al)
*JAMA* 279:892–898, 1997                                                    2–27

*Objective.*—Many studies have examined the association between adverse outcomes of various procedures and the volume of procedures performed by the physician or hospital. However, none of these studies have looked at the relationship between volume and outcomes for percutaneous transluminal angioplasty (PTCA). Outcomes of PTCA were analyzed for their relationship to various measures of provider volume.

*Methods.*—The study included data on 62,670 patients undergoing PTCA. All patients were discharged from New York State hospitals after PTCA from 1991 through 1994. The indicators of volume analyzed were annual hospital volume and annual cardiologist volume. The outcomes studied were in-hospital mortality and same-stay coronary artery bypass grafting (CABG).

*Results.*—For the overall cohort, in-hospital mortality was 0.90% and the rate of CABG surgery during the same hospitalization was 3.43%. Risk-adjusted in-hospital mortality was 0.96% for patients having PTCA at low-volume hospitals, i.e., those performing less than 600 procedures per year. Risk-adjusted same-stay CABG rate for this group of patients was 3.92%. For patients whose PTCA was performed by low-volume cardiologists—those performing less than 75 procedures per year—in-hospital mortality was 1.03% and same-stay CABG rate was 3.93. The same-stay CABG rate was 2.99 for patients whose PTCA was performed by a cardiologist who performed 75–174 procedures per year at hospitals with a volume of 600–999 procedures per year. For patients at these middle-volume hospitals whose cardiologists performed 175 or more procedures per year, same-stay CABG rate was 2.84%.

*Conclusions.*—The outcomes of PTCA are significantly affected by the volume of procedures performed at a given hospital and by a given cardiologist. Mortality and same-stay CABG rates are elevated for patients whose cardiologist performs less than 75 procedures per year. Mortality is significantly increased for hospitals with an annual volume of less than 600. The results suggest that minimum provider volumes for maintenance of competence should be set even higher than recommended by the recent

American College of Cardiology and American Heart Association guidelines.

▶ The volume-outcome relationship is a highly controversial and at times emotional area that has major implications for patterns of reimbursement. This study from New York State is the fourth to show a relationship between operator and institutional volume and outcomes after PTCA, although (as discussed) it would have been helpful to have had additional data on the rates of acute myocardial infarction.[1, 2]

The ideal "minimum" number of procedures will continue to be a subject of heated debate. This study pointed toward even higher minimum provider volumes than were recommended by the recent guideline of the American College of Cardiology and the American Heart Association.[3] These guidelines are currently being revised, and it would be helpful to have further data comparing results among operators performing less than 50 procedures per year, 50–75 procedures, and more than 75 procedures per year. What is also difficult to quantify in these studies is the role of operator experience, which I would expect would be an important component of a favorable outcome. Another issue relates to the results from a low-volume operator in a high-volume institution, or vice versa, but this study did not demonstrate an interaction between the two, suggesting that there is evidence that neither hospital PTCA volume nor cardiologist PTCA volume has such a protective effect that outcomes cannot be improved by simultaneously optimizing the other volume measure. In other words, even if operator volume was in an optimal range, there still appears to be an independent effect of low institutional volume and vice versa. This is certainly not the last we will hear of this particular issue.

**B.J. Gersh, M.B., Ch.B., D.Phil., F.R.C.P.**

*References*

1. Jollis JG, Peterson ED, DeLong ER, et al: The relationship between the volume of coronary angioplasty procedures in hospitals treating medicare beneficiaries and short-term mortality. *N Engl J Med* 331:1625–1629, 1994.
2. Ritchie JL, Phillips KA, Luft HS: Coronary angioplasty; Statewide experience in California. *Circulation* 88:2735–2743, 1993.
3. (The American College of Cardiology/American Heart Association Task Force on Assessment of Diagnostic and Therapeutic Cardiovascular Procedures (Subcommittee on Percutaneous Transluminal Angioplasty): Guidelines for percutaneous transluminal coronary angioplasty. *J Am Coll Cardiol* 12:2033–2054, 1993.

### Prognostic Implication of Creatine Kinase Elevation Following Elective Coronary Artery Interventions

Kong TQ Jr, Davidson CJ, Meyers SN, et al (Northwestern Univ, Chicago)
JAMA 277:461–466, 1997      2–28

*Introduction.*—Some patients will have a rise in serum creatine kinase (CK) after elective coronary artery procedures. The prognostic importance of an elevation in CK occurring after percutaneous transluminal angioplasty (PTCA) is unknown. Late cardiac mortality was compared in patients who did and those who did not have an increase in CK after PTCA.

*Methods.*—The retrospective study included 373 patients who had undergone elective PTCA. The case patients were 253 consecutive patients whose total CK and CK-MB rose after PTCA. The controls were 120 patients who did not have CK elevations. The 2 groups underwent PTCA at about the same time and using the same equipment. They were compared for in-hospital and late cardiac mortality, subsequent myocardial infarction, and a combined end point of cardiac mortality or myocardial infarction. Both groups were followed up for longer than 3.5 years.

*Results.*—The 2 groups were comparable in terms of age, sex, extent of coronary artery involvement, left ventricular function, and number of lesions treated. The case patients tended to have more complex target lesions, were more likely to have lesions in degenerated saphenous vein grafts, and were more likely to have occluded target vessels. The patients with postprocedural CK elevations showed a significant increase in cardiac mortality. On stratification by peak CK elevation, cardiac mortality was increased for patients with intermediate elevations (1.5–3.0 times normal) and high elevations (more than 3 times normal). The main predictors of increased cardiac mortality on multivariate analysis were higher peak CK level and lower ejection fraction. Each 100 U/L increase in CK carried a 1.05 relative risk of cardiac death.

*Conclusions.*—Elevation of CK after PTCA is an independent prognostic factor for cardiac death. The findings reflect the difficulty of performing percutaneous procedures in patients with previous bypass operations, especially those with lesions in saphenous vein grafts. More study is needed to determine whether new treatment strategies can alter the long-term prognosis of patients with postprocedural CK elevation.

▶ This case-control study, which is prospective and included all consecutive patients with enzyme elevations after transcatheter procedures, provides the strongest evidence to date that an elevation in CPK-MB fraction (even if mild) is an independent predictor of an increased mortality. Although some studies have tended to discount this finding,[1] others have stated a higher cardiac mortality during extended follow-up than those who did not have such elevations.[2] In the majority of cases with CK elevations, this was accompanied by periprocedural complications such as transient vessel closure, side branch occlusion, or coronary embolism, but in approximately 30% of patients, there was no obvious cause for the rise in cardiac markers.

Although the multivariant analysis suggested that an elevation in CPK was an independent predictor of mortality, the relative risk was relatively minor (1.05 with 95% confidence intervals of 1.03–1.08), and it may well be that elevations in CPK are a *marker* of more severe and extensive disease, which in turn is responsible for the increase in mortality.[3] An alternative explanation for the higher mortality is that this is the end-result of *necrosis* at the time of the procedure, and certainly the higher the CPK rise, the greater the mortality. What is also evident from this study are the problems involved in performing percutaneous interventions in patients who have undergone bypass surgery, particularly for lesions involving saphenous vein grafts. Ohman and Tardiff's thoughtful editorial suggests that it probably is worthwhile to monitor CPK prospectively after percutaneous interventions, and in patients with uncomplicated procedures who have a rise in enzymes, it may be prudent to observe them more closely during the period of late follow-up. Whether this in fact will alter long-term prognosis remains to be determined, and it may well be that CPK elevations are a marker of higher risk but there is not much we can do about it. It also will be of interest to investigate the role of troponin elevations in this setting.

**B.J. Gersh, M.B., Ch.B., D.Phil., F.R.C.P.**

*References*

1. Kugelmass AD, Cohen BJ, Mascucci M, et al: Elevation of the creatine kinase myocardial isoform following otherwise successful directional coronary atherectomy and stenting. *Am J Cardiol* 74:748–754, 1994.
2. Abdelmeguid AE, Topol EJ, Whitlow PL, et al: Significance of mild transient release of creatine kinase-MB fraction after percutaneous coronary intervention. *Circulation* 94:1528–1536, 1996.
3. Ohman EM, Tardiff BE: Peri-procedural cardiac marker elevation after percutaneous coronary artery revascularization, importance and implications (editorial). *JAMA* 277:495–497, 1997.

---

**Relationship Between HLA-C Locus and Restenosis After Coronary Artery Balloon Angioplasty**
Watanabe Y, Yamada N, Yokoi H, et al (Juntendo Univ, Tokyo; Univ of Tokyo)
*JAMA* 277:983–984, 1997                                                             2–29

---

*Background.*—Percutaneous transluminal coronary angioplasty (PTCA) improves the prognosis of patients with coronary stenosis, but causes severe injury to the arterial wall. This injury causes a cascade of cellular reactions to occur, including the release of many cytokines and growth factors that are secreted by the cells of the arterial wall after injury. This cascade triggers proliferation of vascular smooth muscle cells and extracellular matrix expansion in the intima, and can lead to restenosis within 6 months. This restenotic process may be influenced by the immune system of the patient. Human leukocyte antigens (HLAs) play an important role in the immune response. The relationship between the HLA loci and restenosis after PTCA was investigated.

*Methods.*—The HLA phenotypes were investigated in blood samples obtained from 65 patients who underwent PTCA at Juntendo University Hospital, Tokyo, Japan, between October 1994 and June 1995. There were 58 men and 7 women in the study group. Standard balloon angioplasty was performed on each patient, followed by selective coronary arteriography at 6 months. Restenosis was defined as at least 50% stenosis in the affected artery.

*Results.*—The HLA phenotypes of the patients in this study group were not significantly different from those of the Japanese population as a whole. The patients with and without restenosis were not significantly different in age, plasma lipid levels, glucose tolerance, or body mass index. There were significantly fewer cases of restenosis after PTCA among patients with the HLA-Cw1 locus and significantly more among patients with the Cw3 locus. There was no other significant correlation to any other HLA loci.

*Conclusions.*—Studies of the HLA loci from patients who had PTCA have indicated an association between restenosis and the HLA-C locus. This suggests that the HLA-C locus may be associated with the process of vascular response to injury after PTCA. Typing of HLA may be useful as a prognostic factor in restenosis after PTCA.

▶ The pathophysiologic hallmark of restenosis is reactive proliferation of vascular smooth muscle cells and increased extracellular matrix in the intima, although other responses are being identified with increasing frequency. It would appear that there are multiple cytokines and growth factors which are secreted by cells in response to injury, which in turn are involved in the pathophysiology of restenosis.

Some aspects of the process may be related to a genetically determined immune response, and the identification of specific HLA antigens provides further support for this. It is possible that the HLA-C locus may be responsible for some aspects of the process of vascular repair after PTCA. The authors suggest that this may be a useful prognostic factor for restenosis, but I believe that the importance of this paper lies not so much in its clinical application, but in identifying a new direction for research into the mechanisms of restenosis. Is there a particular HLA-C gene product that initiates an immune reaction, and if so, does it provide a target for further therapy? It certainly is a target for further investigation at this time.

**B.J. Gersh, M.B., Ch.B., D.Phil., F.R.C.P.**

### Effect of Smoking Status on the Long-term Outcome After Successful Percutaneous Coronary Revascularization

Hasdai D, Garratt KN, Grill DE, et al (Mayo Clinic and Mayo Found, Rochester, Minn)

*N Engl J Med* 336:755–761, 1997                                     2–30

*Introduction.*—For the development and progression of coronary heart disease, cigarette smoking is a well-established risk factor. After the cessation of smoking, the excess risk of cardiovascular events gradually declines. Little is known, however, of the long-term effect of smoking status before and after percutaneous coronary revascularization. The effect of smoking status on the long-term outcome after successful percutaneous coronary revascularization was examined, and whether the cessation of smoking before or after the index intervention affected event-free survival, was also determined.

*Methods.*—The retrospective analysis included 2,009 nonsmokers who had successful percutaneous coronary revascularization, 2,259 former smokers who had stopped smoking before the procedure, 435 quitters who stopped smoking after the procedure, and 734 persistent smokers who smoked before and after the procedure. They were studied for up to 16 years.

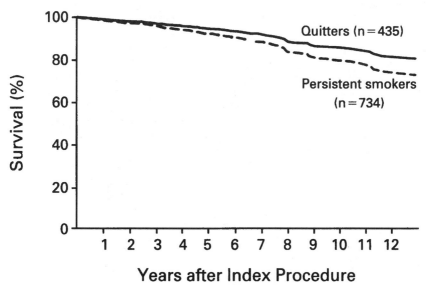

## Years after Index Procedure

FIGURE 1.—Estimated survival curves for smokers undergoing percutaneous coronary revascularization, according to subsequent smoking status. Persistent smokers were defined as patients who smoked before and after the index procedure, and quitters as those who quit smoking immediately after the procedure. (Reprinted by permission of *The New England Journal of Medicine*, from Hasdai D, Garratt KN, Grill DE, et al: Effect of smoking status on the long-term outcome after successful percutaneous coronary revascularization. *N Engl J Med* 336:755–761, 1997. Copyright 1997, Massachusetts Medical Society. All rights reserved.)

*Results.*—Similar baseline characteristics and outcomes were seen among nonsmokers and former smokers. Nonsmokers were older than the quitters and persistent smokers. More favorable clinical and angiographic characteristics were seen in the former smokers. A greater relative risk of death and O-wave infarction was seen in the persistent smokers than in the nonsmokers (Fig 1). The nonsmokers were more likely than the quitters and persistent smokers to have additional percutaneous coronary procedures or coronary bypass surgery. The quitters had a lesser risk of death than the persistent smokers. Persistent smokers had a 44% greater risk of death from any cause than those who stopped smoking.

*Summary.*—A greater risk for Q-wave infarction and death was seen among patients who continued to smoke after successful percutaneous coronary revascularization than nonsmokers. Benefits were seen among patients who stopped smoking either before or after percutaneous revascularization. Patients having percutaneous revascularization should be encouraged to quit smoking. The smaller number of referrals for repeated revascularization procedures in the smokers is still an enigma.

▶ It has previously been shown that after coronary bypass surgery, stopping smoking has an important beneficial impact upon long-term outcome after percutaneous transluminal coronary angioplasty (PTCA). This study is quite complex in that the univariate analysis demonstrated a lower risk of death from all causes and severe angina among quitters and persistent smokers, as opposed to nonsmokers. This is another example of the so-called "smoker's paradox." This apparent paradox should not be interpreted as a relative benefit of cigarette smoking. It is just that patients who smoke tend to have premature atherosclerosis, and at the age of presentation are approximately 10 years younger than former smokers and nonsmokers, in addition to their having fewer co-existing conditions that predispose to coronary atherosclerosis, such as diabetes and hypertension. Once one adjusts for these more favorable baseline characteristics in a multivariate statistical analysis, the strong adverse impact of smoking upon late outcome becomes evident.

It is of interest that quitters and persistent smokers were less likely than the nonsmokers to undergo additional or repeat revascularization procedures (PTCA or coronary artery bypass graft), but the reasons for this are not clear, and are likely multifactorial, as discussed by the authors.

In summary, it is said that "you cannot teach an old dog a new trick," but after coronary revascularization, be it bypass surgery or PTCA, smoking cessation is one risk factor that has to be modified, and the benefits accrue to all age groups.

**B.J. Gersh, M.B., Ch.B., D.Phil., F.R.C.P.**

*References*

1. Cavender JB, Rogers WJ, Fisher LD, et al: The effects of smoking on survival and morbidity in patients randomized to medical or surgical therapy in the Coronary Artery Surgery Study (CASS): Ten-year follow-up. *J Am Coll Cardiol* 20:287–294, 1992.

2. Barbash GI, Reiner J, White HD, et al: Evaluation of paradoxical beneficial effects of smoking in patients receiving thrombolytic therapy for acute myocardial infarction; Mechanism of the "smoker's paradox" from the GUSTO-I trial with angiographic insight. *J Am Coll Cardiol* 26:1222–1229, 1995.

---

### Stent Placement Compared With Balloon Angioplasty for Obstructed Coronary Bypass Grafts

Savage MP, for the Saphenous Vein De Novo Trial Investigators (Jefferson Med College, Philadelphia; Emory Univ, Atlanta, Ga; Univ of Florida, Gainesville; et al)
*N Engl J Med* 337:740–747, 1997                                    2–31

---

*Introduction.*—Severe atherosclerotic disease is found in half of all saphenous vein bypass grafts within a decade after surgery. Repeated surgery involves substantial risks and results of angioplasty have been disappointing, making management of graft disease problematic. Previous studies have suggested that stent implantation has shown superior outcomes in native vessels when compared to balloon angioplasty. For the

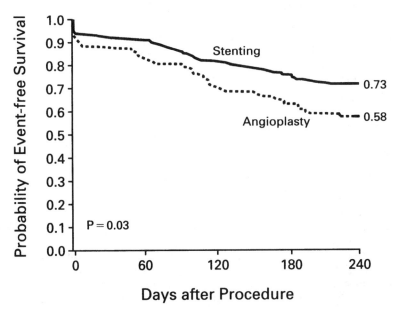

**FIGURE 2.**—Kaplan-Meier survival curves for freedom from major cardiac events. The rate of event-free survival was significantly higher among patients assigned to stenting than among those assigned to angioplasty. The relative risk of a major cardiac event after stenting was 0.82 (95% confidence interval, 0.68–0.98); after adjustment for diabetes, the relative risk was 0.82 (95% confidence interval, 0.68–0.99). (Reprinted by permission of *The New England Journal* of Medicine, from Savage MP, for the Saphenous Vein De Novo Trial Investigators: Stent placement compared with balloon angioplasty for obstructive coronary bypass grafts. *N Engl J Med* 337:740–747. Copyright 1997, Massachusetts Medical Society. All rights reserved.)

treatment of obstructive disease of various bypass grafts, stent implantation was compared to balloon angioplasty.

*Methods.*—Placement of Palmaz-Schatz stents or standard balloon angioplasty was randomly performed on 220 patients with new lesions in aortocoronary-venous bypass grafts. During the index procedure and 6 months later, coronary angiography was performed.

*Results.*—A higher rate of procedural efficacy, defined as a reduction in stenosis to less than 50% of the vessel diameter without a major cardiac complication, was seen in those patients assigned to stenting when compared to patients assigned to angioplasty (stenting 92% vs. angioplasty 69%). More frequent hemorrhagic complications were found in the stenting group than in the angioplasty group (16% vs. 5%). A larger increase in luminal diameter was seen in the stenting group (1.92±0.30 mm) than in the angioplasty group (1.21±0.37 mm). At 6 months, the stenting group had a greater gain in luminal diameter (0.85±0.96 mm) than the angioplasty group (0.54±0.91 mm). In 37% of the patients in the stent group, restenosis occurred, compared to 46% in the angioplasty group. In the stent group, the outcome in terms of freedom from death, myocardial infarction, repeated bypass surgery, or revascularization of the target lesions was significantly better (73%) than in the angioplasty group (58%) (Fig 2).

*Conclusion.*—Superior procedural outcomes, a larger gain in luminal diameter, and a reduction in major cardiac events occurred with stenting of selected venous bypass-graft lesions as compared to balloon angioplasty. In regard to the rate of angiographic restenosis, the primary end point of the study, however, there was no significant benefit.

▶ Although coronary bypass surgery and percutaneous transluminal coronary angioplasty (PTCA) are usually viewed as competitive therapeutic strategies, one should appreciate the extent to which they are complementary forms of treatment. In several studies, PTCA was utilized as opposed to reoperation in the majority of patients with prior bypass surgery who underwent revascularization.

The management of vein graft disease is difficult, particularly because the patient population is older, with a greater increase in co-morbidity, in addition to the risk of operation upon patent grafts and the difficulty of achieving complete revascularization as a result of the progression of disease in many patients. Unfortunately, the results of PTCA in vein grafts are suboptimal,[1] with a higher rate of periprocedural complications and a poorer long-term outcome. This randomized trial of stents vs. conventional angioplasty is encouraging, although the lack of any difference in the primary end point of restenosis is surprising, given the overall reduction in clinical events.

One should realize that many patients with graft disease are not suitable for either PTCA or stents. Exclusion criteria in this study included an acute myocardial infarction within 7 days, diffuse disease requiring 2 or more stents, an ejection fraction of less than 25%, and evidence of thrombosis and outflow obstruction of the graft because of distal anastomotic problems or poor run off in the native vessel. Many of the patients we see in our clinical practices, however, fall into this category, and unfortunately among these, a significant number are not candidates for either bypass surgery or a transcatheter technique. Perhaps it is in this population that translaser myocardial revascularization may have a place.

**B.J. Gersh, M.B., Ch.B., D.Phil., F.R.C.P.**

*Reference*

1. deFeyter PJ, VanSuylen R-J, deJaegere PPT, et al: Balloon angioplasty for the treatment of lesions in saphenous vein bypass graft. *J Am Coll Cardiol* 21:1539–1549, 1993.

---

**Probucol and Multivitamins in the Prevention of Restenosis After Coronary Angioplasty**
Tardif J-C, for the Multivitamins and Probucol Study Group (Univ of Montreal)
*N Engl J Med* 337:365–372, 1997                                           2–32

---

*Background.*—Oxidizing metabolites produced at the site of coronary angioplasty can cause chain reactions that may result in restenosis. Previous studies have suggested that antioxidants may prevent restenosis after angioplasty. Whether drugs with antioxidant properties reduce the incidence and severity of restenosis after angioplasty was studied.

*Methods.*—Three hundred seventeen patients were enrolled in the double-blind, randomized study. One month before angioplasty, the patients were assigned to placebo, 500 mg of probucol, multivitamins (30,000 IU of beta carotene, 500 mg of vitamin C, and 700 IU of vitamin E), or probucol plus multivitamins. Treatments were taken twice a day for 4 weeks before and for 6 months after angioplasty. Twelve hours before angioplasty, the groups received additional doses of the treatments to which they had been assigned.

*Findings.*—Six months after angioplasty, the mean decrease in luminal diameter was 0.12 mm in the probucol group, 0.22 mm in the combined treatment group, 0.33 mm in the multivitamin group, and 0.38 mm in the placebo group. Restenosis rates per segment were 20.7%, 28.9%, 40.3%, and 38.9%, respectively. The respective rates of repeated angioplasty were 11.2%, 16.2%, 24.4%, and 26.6% (Fig 1).

*Conclusions.*—The antioxidant probucol effectively decreases the rate of restenosis after balloon coronary angioplasty. It is unclear why multivitamins do not prevent restenosis, as they are also antioxidants.

▶ At last we have a trial that has shown a pharmacologic intervention may be effective in reducing restenosis. It would appear that probucol, which was initially used for lowering serum cholesterol, possesses potent antioxidant properties. This may be beneficial because oxidized lipoproteins probably result in a number of changes in cell function that promote atherogenesis.[1, 2] The accompanying editorial postulates that macrophages and smooth

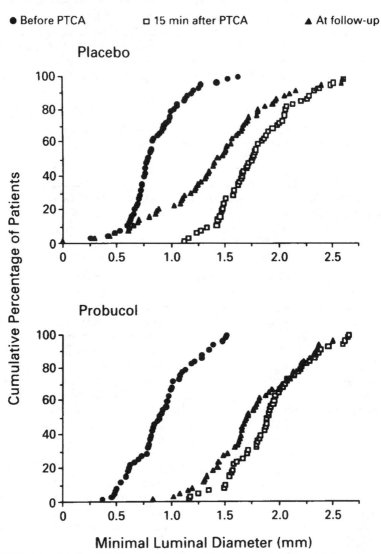

● Before PTCA     □ 15 min after PTCA     ▲ At follow-up

Placebo

Probucol

Cumulative Percentage of Patients

Minimal Luminal Diameter (mm)

FIGURE 1.—Cumulative distribution of the minimal luminal diameter before angioplasty, 15 minutes after angioplasty, and at follow-up among patients in the 4 study groups who completed the study without protocol violations. The curves clearly favor probucol at follow-up. *Abbreviation*: PTCA, percutaneous transluminal coronary angioplasty. (Reprinted by permission of *The New England Journal of Medicine*, from Tardif J-C, for the Multivitamins and Probucol Study Group: Probucol and multivitamins in the prevention of restenosis after coronary angioplasty. *N Engl J Med* 337:365–372. Copyright 1997, Massachusetts Medical Society. All rights reserved.)

muscle cells, which can produce large amounts of superoxide anions, may perhaps accumulate in the injured intima after angioplasty, but also in the adventitial layer, and that these oxygen species might signal changes in cellular behavior which initiate the cascade of atherosclerosis and resteno-

● Before PTCA         □ 15 min after PTCA         ▲ At follow-up

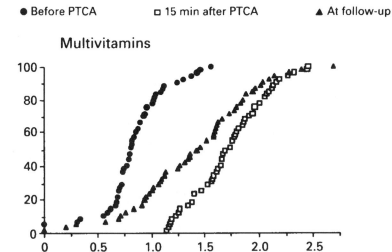

Multivitamins

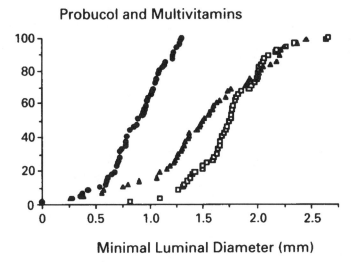

Probucol and Multivitamins

**Minimal Luminal Diameter (mm)**

sis. Perhaps probucol might reduce the severity of the inflammation after angioplasty, which in turn may reduce restenosis.[3]

This study does raise a number of clinical questions, because one of the disadvantages of probucol is that it reduces high-density lipoprotein choles-terol and, although the drug might be effective in preventing restenosis, it could, at least theoretically, adversely affect atherosclerosis in other coro-nary arteries or the peripheral vessels.[4] In any event, probucol is no longer marketed in the United States, and we will probably require a trial of an alternative antioxidant agent before adopting any widespread recommenda-tions. What is also not clear is whether the drug should be given for a short period of time and if, after withdrawal, we will see an increased incidence of late restenosis. In any event, this well-conducted clinical trial does offer a ray of hope in what has been to date a somewhat discouraging area of investigation.

**B.J. Gersh, M.B., Ch.B., D.Phil., F.R.C.P.**

*References*

1. Libby P, Ganz P: Restenosis revisited—new targets, new therapies (editorial). *N Engl J Med* 337:418–419, 1997.
2. Steinberg D, Parthasarathy S, Carew TE, et al: Beyond cholesterol. Modifications of low-density lipoprotein that increase its atherogenicity. *N Engl J Med* 312:915–924, 1989.
3. Tanaka H, Sukhova GK, Swanson SJ, et al: Sustained activation of vascular cells and leukocytes in the rabbit aorta after balloon injury. *Circulation* 88:1788–1803, 1993.
4. Walldius G, Erikson U, Olsson AG, et al: The effect of probucol on femoral atherosclerosis: The Probucol Quantitative Regression Swedish Trial (PQRST). *Am J Cardiol* 74:875–883, 1994.

## Coronary Artery Bypass Grafting

### Five-Year Clinical and Functional Outcome Comparing Bypass Surgery and Angioplasty in Patients With Multivessel Coronary Disease: A Multicenter Randomized Trial

Frye RL, and The Writing Group for the Bypass Angioplasty Revascularization Investigation (BARI) Investigators (Univ of Pittsburgh, Pa)
*JAMA* 277:715–721, 1997                                                      2–33

*Background.*—Patients with multivessel coronary artery disease may be treated by coronary artery bypass grafting (CABG) or percutaneous transluminal coronary angioplasty (PTCA). The Bypass Angioplasty Revascularization Investigation (BARI) indicated that, for most patient groups, the 2 techniques gave equivalent results in terms of 5-year survival. Their effects on symptoms and quality of life were then compared.

*Background.*—The randomized trial included 1,829 patients from BARI with multivessel coronary artery disease suitable for both CABG and PTCA. The patients were followed for an average of 5 years. The 2 treatment groups were compared by intention-to-treat analysis of symptoms, exercise test results, medications, and quality-of-life indicators. Assessments were performed at 4 to 14 weeks after treatment and repeated at 1, 3, and 5 years. Five hundred fifteen patients in the CABG group and 513 in the PTCA group were available for 5-year follow-up.

*Results.*—At 4 to 14 weeks, freedom from angina was 73% in the PTCA group vs. 95% in the CABG group, a significant difference. However, by 5 years, freedom from angina was 79% in the PTCA group and 85% in the CABG group. Similarly, CABG offered advantages in terms of exercise-induced angina and ischemia at early follow-up, compared with no significant difference at 5-year follow-up. By 1 year, there were no differences between groups in quality-of-life measures, return to work, modification of smoking and exercise behaviors, or cholesterol levels. Patients in the CABG group were more likely to be using anti-ischemic medication at follow-up. They were also more likely to be using other medications, although the difference was not as great. Of patients who were free of angina at 5 years, 52% of those in the PTCA group had required repeat revascularization, compared with 6% of those in the CABG group.

*Conclusion.*—The immediate clinical and functional results of CABG are better than those of PTCA in patients with multivessel coronary artery disease. However, the gap narrows over time, largely because of recurrent symptoms in patients treated with CABG and the need for repeat revascularization in patients with PTCA. The residual ischemia after PTCA is, apparently, well tolerated, as patients have similar quality of life and 5-year survival compared with those treated by CABG. The 2 approaches are similar in the impact on long-term employment, limitations on habits and relationships, and overall patient satisfaction.

▶ These data are similar to those reported from other clinical trials demonstrating that patients assigned to CABG were more likely to be free of angina, although the differences diminish with time, as increasing numbers of PTCA patients undergo repeat revascularization procedures. Nonetheless, it is important to mention that among patients free of angina at 5 years, 52% of patients who had PTCA underwent revascularization; on the other hand, 70% of patients who were angina-free at 5 years achieved without the need for coronary bypass surgery.

As was the case in the Randomized Intervention Treatment of Aging (RITA) Trial in the United Kingdom, there was no significant difference between the 2 treatments in regard to quality-of-life issues, return to work, modification of smoking, or exercise behavior. Serum cholesterol levels were similar between the 2 groups; however, what is quite striking is the minimal change in serum cholesterol from baseline to 5 years. In this respect, the mean low-density lipoprotein (LDL) cholesterol at baseline was 145 mg/dL in patients undergoing CABG, and at 5 years this had fallen to only 142 mg/dL. For PTCA patients, LDL cholesterol levels were 142 mg/dL at the start and 139 mg/dL at 5 years.

The use of lipid-lowering agents, at least during the first 3 years, was also relatively low given the striking results of the trials of lipid-lowering therapy in patients with coronary heart disease,[1] and taking into account the encouraging results in a recent trial of aggressive lowering of LDL cholesterol in patients with saphenous vein bypass grafts.[2]

**B.J. Gersh, M.B., Ch.B., D.Phil., F.R.C.P.**

*References*

1. Sacks FM, Pfeffer MA, Moye LA, et al: The effect of pravastatin on coronary events after myocardial infarction in patients with average cholesterol levels. *N Eng J Med* 335:1001–1009, 1996.

2. The Post Coronary Artery Bypass Graft Trial Investigators: The effect of aggressive lowering of low-density lipoprotein cholesterol levels and low-dose anticoagulation on obstructive changes in saphenous-vein coronary-artery bypass grafts. *N Eng J Med* 336:153–162, 1997.

### Effects of Acadesine on Myocardial Infarction, Stroke, and Death Following Surgery

Mangano DT, for The Multicenter Study of Perioperative Ischemia (McSPI) Research Group (Veterans Affairs Med Ctr, San Francisco)
*JAMA* 277:325–332, 1997                                              2–34

*Background.*—Morbidity and mortality associated with coronary artery bypass graft (CABG) surgery continue to increase, despite advances in technique. These increases are thought to be the result of changes in patient demographics. Patients are now older and sicker, and many have had prior CABG surgery or failed angioplasty. Of the pharmacologic interventions that have been attempted, acadesine is the only agent that has been studied in large-scale trials. This paper reports a meta-analysis of the results of 5 such trials.

*Methods.*—The 5 trials, conducted in the United States, Canada, and Europe, involved 81 institutions and 4,311 patients who underwent CABG surgery. The meta-analysis excluded 265 patients, most of whom had received an atypically low or high dose of acadesine. Therefore, the results are based on 2,031 patients who received placebo and 2,012 patients who received acadesine (0.01 mg/kg$^{-1}$/min$^{-1}$ given intravenously before and during surgery, along with 5 µg/mL in cardioplegia solution). The primary outcome was defined as MI, and the secondary outcomes were defined as cardiac death, stroke or cerebrovascular accident (CVA), or a combination of these.

*Results.*—Compared with the placebo, acadesine decreased the incidence of MI by 27%, the incidence of combined outcomes by 26%, and the incidence of cardiac death by 50%. It did not significantly affect the incidence of stroke or CVA, however. In the placebo group, the number of deaths following MI (through postoperative day 4) was 13 of 98 (13.3%). In the acadesine group, it was 1 of 71 (1.4%). The only difference in adverse events between the two groups was that acadesine caused a transient increase in serum uric acid during infusion. This resolved without clinical sequelae during hospital stay. Acadesine reduced the postoperative use of ventricular–assistance-devices by about one third.

*Conclusions.*—The meta-analysis of these trials shows that acadesine reduces the incidence of myocardial injury associated with CABG surgery. Acadesine, as well as the entire class of agents that preserve adenosine in ischemic tissue, deserve further study.

▶ Despite the limitations of meta-analysis, which are vigorously defended by the authors in the discussion section of this article, the results of acadesine use in more than 4,000 patients undergoing CABG surgery from

5 multicenter trials are quite impressive. Acadesine is a purine nucleoside analogue, which selectively raises tissue adenosine levels during ischemic conditions.[1] In the experimental situation, adenosine and adenosine-regulating agents have a favorable effect on ischemia, and they have an effect against both ischemia and reperfusion-induced injury, resulting in improved myocardial protection.[2] Despite the excellent results currently obtainable with CABG surgery, an increasingly older and higher risk population is undergoing the procedure, and it would appear, at least from the preliminary data, that this agent warrants further evaluation, particularly among these high-risk patients.

**B.J. Gersh, M.B., Ch.B., D.Phil., F.R.C.P.**

*References*

1. Mullane K: The prototype adenosine regulating agent for reducing myocardial ischemic injury. *Cardiovasc Res* 27:43–47, 1993.
2. Vinten-Johansen J, Nakanishi K, Zhao ZQ, et al: Acadesine improves surgical myocardial protection with blood cardioplegia in ischemically injured canine hearts. *Circulation* 88:350–358, 1993.

**A Comparison of Coronary-Artery Stenting With Angioplasty for Isolated Stenosis of the Proximal Left Anterior Descending Coronary Artery**
Versaci F, Gaspardone A, Tomai F, et al (Università di Roma Tor Vergata, Rome; Università Cattolica del Sacro Cuore, Rome)
*N Engl J Med* 336:817–822, 1997                                                2–35

*Background.*—Recent clinical trials have suggested that primary stent implantation in large coronary arteries results in a lower rate of restenosis and less need for repeat interventions than percutaneous transluminal coronary angioplasty (PTCA) as a treatment for coronary artery disease. The effectiveness of primary stent implantation was compared with that of PTCA in the treatment of patients with symptomatic isolated stenosis of the proximal left anterior descending coronary artery in a prospective, randomized study.

*Methods.*—The study population consisted of 120 patients with typical angina pectoris and/or confirmed myocardial ischemia; a newly diagnosed, isolated stenosis of the proximal portion of the left anterior descending coronary artery; and a left ventricular ejection fraction of at least 40%. Patients were randomly assigned to either primary stent implantation or PTCA. After discharge, patients were treated with warfarin for 3 months, and with aspirin and diltiazem indefinitely. The primary clinical end points were the rate of procedural success and the rate of event-free survival, defined as freedom from death, myocardial infarction, and angina at 12 months. The amount of restenosis was assessed 12 months after the procedure.

TABLE 2.—Clinical Outcomes in the Hospital and During Follow-up, According to Treatment Group

| EVENT | PTCA (N=60) | STENTING (N=60) | P VALUE |
|---|---|---|---|
| In hospital | | | |
| Revascularization procedure — no. (%) | 58 (97) | 58 (97) | |
| Procedural success | 54 (93) | 55 (95) | 0.98 |
| Procedural failure | 4 (7) | 3 (5) | 0.88 |
| Vascular complication | 0 | 4 (7) | 0.12 |
| Median hospital stay — days | 5.0 | 6.5 | 0.04 |
| At 12 months — no. (%) | | | |
| Event-free survival | 42 (70) | 52 (87) | 0.04 |
| Death from cardiac causes | 1 (2) | 1 (2) | 0.30 |
| Nonfatal infarction | 2 (3) | 1 (2) | 0.30 |
| Recurrence of angina | 15 (25) | 6 (10) | 0.05 |

Note: Percentages may not sum to 100 because of rounding.
Abbreviation: PTCA, percutaneous transluminal coronary angioplasty.
(Reprinted by permission of *The New England Journal of Medicine*, from Versaci F, Gaspardone A, Tomai F, et al: A comparison of coronary-artery stenting with angioplasty for isolated stenosis of the proximal left anterior descending coronary artery. *N Engl J Med* 336:817–822, 1997. Copyright 1997, Massachusetts Medical Society. All rights reserved.)

*Results.*—Between March 1992 and July 1995, 105 men and 15 women were referred for isolated, symptomatic stenosis of the proximal left anterior descending coronary artery. Sixty patients were randomly assigned to primary stent implantation and 60 to PTCA. There were no significant differences between these 2 groups in demographic, clinical, or angiographic characteristics. The rate of procedural success was similar for the 2 treatment groups (Table 2). The 12-month rate of event-free survival was 87% in the stent group and 70% in the PTCA group. The rate of restenosis was 19% in the stent group and 40% in the PTCA group.

*Conclusions.*—These results demonstrate that in symptomatic patients with isolated stenosis of the proximal left anterior descending coronary artery, primary stent implantation is associated with both a significantly lower rate of restenosis and a better clinical outcome than percutaneous transluminal coronary angioplasty.

▶ These results are not surprising and will probably form the basis of a subsequent trial comparing coronary-artery stenting with medical therapy. The key to such a trial is the use of aggressive lipid-lowering therapy in both arms. Previous trials of standard angioplasty and medical therapy did not demonstrate any difference in death or myocardial infarction, but patients undergoing PTCA had greater exercise tolerance and fewer symptoms than medically treated counterparts. All trials were confined to patients with proximal single-vessel disease.[1-3] No one would dispute that probably the most effective method of revascularization for proximal left anterior descending coronary artery disease is an internal mammary artery bypass, but it is an invasive procedure and we need more data on the results of the minimally invasive approaches.[4] This trial by Versaci et al. is encouraging, although it involves only 120 patients and is somewhat obsolete in that warfarin was continued for 3 months, followed by aspirin and diltiazem, whereas the current standard of care would include aspirin and ticlopidine after stent placement.[5]

**B.J. Gersh, M.B., Ch.B., D.Phil., F.R.C.P.**

*References*

1. Parisi AF, Folland ED, Hartigan PA: Comparison of angioplasty with medical therapy in the treatment of single vessel coronary artery disease. *N Engl J Med* 326:10–16, 1992.
2. Strauss WE, Fortin T, Hartigan P, et al: The comparison of quality of life scores in patients with angina pectoris after angioplasty compared with medical therapy; Outcomes of a randomized clinical trial. *Circulation* 92:1710–1719, 1995.
3. Hueb WA, Bellotti G, deOliveria SA, et al: The Medicine, Angioplasty or Surgery Study [MASS]; A prospective randomized trial of medical therapy, balloon angioplasty or bypass surgery for single proximal left anterior descending artery stenoses. *J Am Coll Cardiol* 26:1600–1605, 1995.
4. Lytle BW: Minimally invasive cardiac surgery. *J Thorac Cardiovasc Surg* 111:554–555, 1996.
5. Colombo A, Hall P, Nakamura S, et al: Intracoronary stenting without anticoagulation accomplished with intravascular ultravascular guidance. *Circulation* 91:1676–1688, 1995.

---

**The Effect of Aggressive Lowering of Low-density Lipoprotein Cholesterol Levels and Low-dose Anticoagulation on Obstructive Changes in Saphenous-Vein Coronary-Artery Bypass Grafts**
Campeau L, and the Post Coronary Artery Bypass Graft Trial Investigators (Maryland Med Research Inst, Baltimore, Md)
*N Engl J Med* 336:153–162, 1997                                    2–36

---

*Background.*—Patients who undergo saphenous vein coronary bypass grafts often develop obstruction caused by atherosclerosis or thrombosis. It has been proposed that lipid-lowering and low-dose anticoagulation treatments can reduce the likelihood of graft obstruction. This study used a 2-by-2 factorial design to test the following hypotheses: (1) aggressive lowering of the low-density lipoprotein (LDL) cholesterol level would be more effective than moderate lowering in delaying the progression of atherosclerosis in bypass grafts; (2) low-dose anticoagulation would be more effective than placebo in reducing graft obstruction.

*Methods.*—At 7 clinical centers, 1,351 patients were enrolled (92% male, 94% white, mean age 61.5 years, age range 21 to 74 years). The following eligibility criteria were used: a LDL cholesterol level of 130–175 mg/dL, a triglyceride level below 300 mg/dL, 2 patent saphenous vein grafts with stenosis of less than 75% (only 1 such graft for women), and an ejection fraction of at least 30%. Patients received either aggressive lovastatin treatment to lower LDL cholesterol levels (target level, 60–85 mg/dL) or moderate treatment (target level, 130–140 mg/dL). Cholestyramine was added in both groups as needed. Patients also were randomized either to low-dose anticoagulation treatment with warfarin

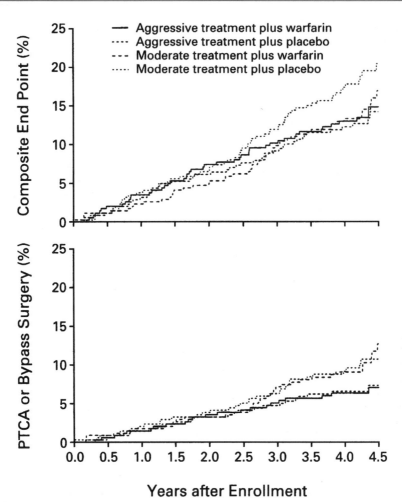

**Years after Enrollment**

FIGURE 2.—Cumulative life-table rates of events according to study group. The composite end point was death from cardiovascular or unknown causes, nonfatal myocardial infarction, stroke, bypass surgery, or angioplasty. *Abbreviation: PTCA*, percutaneous transluminal coronary angioplasty. (Courtesy of The Post Coronary Artery Bypass Graft Trial Investigators: The effect of aggressive lowering of low-density lipoprotein cholesterol levels and low-dose anticoagulation on obstructive changes in saphenous-vein coronary-artery bypass grafts. *N Engl J Med* 336:153–162, 1997. Reprinted by permission of *The New England Journal of Medicine*. Copyright 1997, Massachusetts Medical Society. All rights reserved.)

(the target was an international normalized ratio below 2) or to placebo. Angiography was performed at baseline 4 to 5 years after enrollment.

*Results.*—In the patients who received moderate lipid-lowering therapy, the target LDL cholesterol level was achieved; the mean level ranged from 132–136 mg/dL. In the patients who received aggressive therapy, the mean level ranged from 93–97 mg/dL, which was above the target. Nevertheless, atherosclerosis of the grafts progressed in only 27% of those who received aggressive therapy, compared with 39% of patients who received moderate lipid-lowering therapy. This difference was significant. Warfarin did not have a more beneficial effect on graft obstruction than placebo, even though the mean international normalized ratio (INR) in patients who received warfarin was 1.4. Differences in treatment were not associated with any differences in clinical outcome (Fig 2).

*Conclusions.*—In this group of patients, aggressive lowering of the LDL cholesterol level to below 100 mg/dL was associated with decreased progression of atherosclerosis in bypass grafts. Warfarin therapy did not influence the progression of graft disease.

▶ Vein graft disease can be divided into the following 3 distinct phases: (1) an early postoperative phase in which technical factors can lead to thrombotic occlusion; (2) an intermediate phase characterized by intimal hyperplasia and possible thrombosis within the first postoperative year; (3) a late phase characterized by lipid-rich atherosclerosis of the graft and superimposed thrombosis.[1] The third phase is associated with increased levels of LDL cholesterol and decreased levels of HDL cholesterol. This trial emphasizes the importance of aggressive risk factor reduction in preventing the progression of disease in saphenous vein grafts. Although the trial did not address clinical events, there was certainly an encouraging trend toward a reduction in the rate of revascularization procedures in the more aggressively treated patients. It would appear that in this respect, the benefits of lipid lowering apply to vein grafts as well as to native coronary arteries.

At first glance it is somewhat surprising that anticoagulation appeared to demonstrate no benefit over placebo in this trial, despite the fact that thrombosis appears to be a major factor both in early and late vein graft occlusion. In addition, we have evidence from other studies that aspirin is beneficial in the prevention of graft occlusion within the first postoperative year.[2] It should be emphasized that the anticoagulation dose was low, with a mean INR of 1.4, and the accompanying editorial discusses other mechanistic explanations for why late vein graft disease may not respond to conventional or low-dose anticoagulants.[3]

For the present, the role of aggressive lipid lowering and aspirin therapy after coronary bypass surgery is well established. It remains to be seen whether higher doses of warfarin (target INR of 2 to 3) or other antiplatelet agents, for example, ticlopidine and the platelet glycoprotein IIb/IIIa receptor inhibitors, will be more effective.

**B.J. Gersh, M.B., Ch.B., D.Phil., F.R.C.P.**

*References*

1. Pearson T, Rapport E, Criqui M, et al: Optimal risk factor management in the patient after coronary revascularization. *Circulation* 90:3125–3133, 1994.
2. Goldman S, Copeland J, Moritz T, et al: Long-term graft patency (in 3 years) after coronary artery surgery: Effects of aspirin—results of a VA cooperative study. *Circulation* 89:1138–1143, 1994.
3. Fuster V, Vorcheimer DA: Intervention of atherosclerosis in coronary-artery bypass grafts. *N Engl J Med* 336:212–213, 1997.

### Influence of Diabetes on 5-Year Mortality and Morbidity in a Randomized Trial Comparing CABG and PTCA in Patients With Multivessel Disease: The Bypass Angioplasty Revascularization Investigation (BARI)

Frye RL, for the BARI Investigators (Univ of Pittsburgh, Pa; Natl Heart, Lung, and Blood Inst, Bethesda, Md; Univ of Alabama; et al)
*Circulation* 96:1761–1769, 1997                                              2–37

*Introduction.*—The incidence of atherosclerotic cardiovascular disease is increased in patients with diabetes mellitus, and they have greater morbidity and mortality after coronary revascularization compared with patients without diabetes. Results of the Bypass Angioplasty Revascularization Investigation (BARI) suggest that the 5-year survival rate is improved after coronary artery bypass grafting (CABG) vs. percutaneous transluminal coronary angioplasty (PTCA) in patients with treated diabetes mellitus (TDM). Details of this study are reported.

*Methods.*—The multicenter study randomized 1,829 patients with multivessel coronary artery disease to undergo initial CABG or PTCA. At study entry, 353 patients (19%) met the criteria for TDM. Participants were followed up for an average of 5.4 years for all-cause mortality at 5 years (the primary end point) and for myocardial infarction and functional and symptomatic status (secondary end points). Patients with TDM differed substantially from the other patients in baseline demographic characteristics and co-morbid conditions, but, among patients with TDM, baseline characteristics were equally distributed between treatment arms.

TABLE 4.—Cause-specific Mortality Rates

| MMCC Classification Cause of Death | Treated for Diabetes | | All Others | |
|---|---|---|---|---|
| | PTCA (n=170)* | CABG (n=173)† | PTCA (n=734)‡ | CABG (n=719)§ |
| Cardiac, n (%) | 35 (20.6) | 10 (5.8) | 35 (4.8) | 34 (4.7) |
| Noncardiac, n (%) | | | | |
|   Related to atherosclerosis | 6 (3.5) | 6 (3.5) | 3 (0.4) | 6 (0.8) |
|   Medical | 13 (7.6) | 13 (7.5) | 28 (3.8) | 26 (3.6) |
| Suicide/accident/other, n (%) | 1 (0.6) | 2 (1.2) | 0 (0) | 3 (0.4) |
| Unclassifiable, n (%) | 4 (2.4) | 2 (1.2) | 4 (0.5) | 5 (0.7) |
| Total, n (%) | 59 (34.7) | 33 (19.1) | 70 (9.5) | 74 (10.3) |

*There were 2 treated patients with diabetes assigned to PTCA who received CABG. There was 1 patient who did not receive revascularization and died of a direct cardiac cause.

†There were 3 treated patients with diabetes assigned to CABG who received PTCA; 1 died of a direct cardiac cause and 1 died of a contributory cardiac cause. Four other patients assigned to CABG did not receive revascularization; 1 died of a direct cardiac cause, and 1 died of medical reasons.

‡There were 7 patients without treated diabetes assigned to PTCA who received CABG; 1 of these patients died of a direct cardiac cause. One patient never received revascularization.

§There were 12 patients without treated diabetes who were assigned to CABG but who received PTCA. There were 3 patients who never received revascularization.

*Abbreviations:* CABG, coronary artery bypass grafting; PTCA, percutaneous transluminal coronary angioplasty; MMCC, Mortality and Morbidity Classification Committee.

(Courtesy of Frye RL, for the BARI Investigators: Influence of diabetes on 5-year mortality and morbidity in a randomized trial comparing CABG and PTCA in patients with multivessel disease: The bypass angioplasty revascularization investigation (BARI). *Circulation* 96:1761–1769, 1997. Reproduced with permission from *Circulation.* Copyright 1997, American Heart Association.)

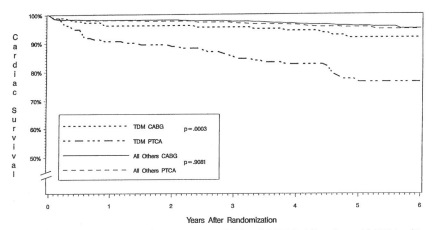

FIGURE 1.—Cardiac survival after assignment to PTCA and CABG in 353 patients with TDM and in 1,476 patients without TDM. *Abbreviations: CABG*, coronary artery bypass grafting; *PTCA*, percutaneous transluminal coronary angioplasty; *TDM*, treated diabetes mellitus. (Courtesy of Frye RL, for the BARI Investigators: Influence of diabetes on 5-year mortality and morbidity in a randomized trial comparing CABG and PTCA in patients with multivessel disease: The bypass angioplasty revascularization investigation (BARI). *Circulation* 96:1761–1769, 1997. Reproduced with permission from *Circulation.* Copyright 1997, American Heart Association.)

*Results.*—The five-year survival rate was significantly worse for patients with TDM (73.1%) than for the other patients (91.3%). Patients with TDM who underwent CABG, however, had significantly higher cumulative survival rates than those assigned to PTCA (80.6% vs. 65.5%, respectively). Cardiac mortality rates were similar after PTCA (4.8%) and CABG (4.7%) in patients without TDM. In contrast, the revascularization method was associated with a significant difference in cardiac mortality among patients with TDM: 20.6% for PTCA vs. 5.8% for CABG. Rates of noncardiac death were comparable by assigned treatment within both TDM and non-TDM groups (Table 4). Thus, among patients with TDM, a better survival rate with CABG was the result of reduced cardiac mortality (Fig 1).

*Conclusion.*—Cardiac mortality was markedly reduced in patients with TDM assigned to CABG vs. PTCA. The survival benefit of CABG is limited to the use of internal mammary artery grafts. If only saphenous vein grafts are used, cardiac mortality is similar in the 2 groups.

▶ This is one of the most important papers resulting from the BARI trial. The benefit of CABG over PTCA among the patients treated for diabetes has also been reported in a preliminary fashion in the Coronary Angioplasty vs. Bypass Revascularization Investigation (CABRI) trial, which was presented at the Annual Scientific Sessions of the American Heart Association in November 1995. In the Emory Angioplasty Surgery Trial (EAST) study, the number of diabetics was small, but their mortality was somewhat surprisingly no different from that in patients without diabetes.[1] What should be emphasized is that the significant mortality difference between PTCA and CABG in patients treated for diabetes is a result of a more than threefold reduction in cardiac mortality.

The explanation for the poorer results after PTCA in patients with diabetes is multifactorial, but the higher incidence of restenosis in patients with diabetes and the more rapid progression of disease in nondilated segments could obviously be a factor.[2]

Several basic vascular biological mechanisms might explain the more rapid progression of disease and the higher rate of restenosis in patients with diabetes, but this remains to be clarified.

There is another explanation that may account, in part, for the poorer outcomes in patients with diabetes in the BARI trials. Previous studies have shown that the mortality after PTCA in patients with multivessel disease and impaired left ventricular function may be relatively high.[3] There is additional evidence that patients with triple-vessel disease and left ventricular dysfunction require complete revascularization, which is often not possible with PTCA using current techniques because there is a high incidence of chronic total occlusions in patients with triple-vessel disease.[4] If I had to pick a subgroup of patients with multivessel disease in whom I would expect bypass surgery to be superior to PTCA, it would be the patients with the combination of triple-vessel disease and left ventricular dysfunction. In this respect, patients with diabetes comprised a "sicker" group than did patients without diabetes: there were a higher proportion with triple-vessel disease, and diffuse disease, in addition to a greater proportion of patients with histories of heart failure and ejection fractions less than 50%. The fact that such patients were randomized to PTCA, even though in clinical practice, they might well have been treated surgically, is an added explanation for the mortality difference in favor of coronary bypass surgery in this study.

From a practical standpoint, I do not believe that all patients with diabetes should be referred for coronary bypass surgery; I would rather individualize therapy according to the number of lesions, the extent and diffuseness of the disease, and the extent of ventricular function present.

**B.J. Gersh, M.B., Ch.B., D.Phil., F.R.C.P.**

*References*

1. King SB, Lembo NJ, Weintraub WS, et al: A randomized trial comparing coronary angioplasty with coronary bypass surgery. *N Engl J Med* 331:1044–1050, 1994.
2. Kip K, Faxon D, Detre K, et al: Coronary angioplasty in diabetic patients (PTCA): The NHLBI PTCA Registry. *Circulation* 94:1818–1825, 1996.
3. Ellis SG, Cowley MJ, DiSciacio G, et al: Determinants after two-year outcome after coronary angioplasty in patients with multivessel disease on the basis of comprehensive procedural evaluations: Implications for patient selection. *Circulation* 83:1905, 1991.
4. Bell MR, Gersh BJ, Chaff HV, et al: Effective completeness on revascularization on long-term outcome of patients with three-vessel disease undergoing coronary artery bypass surgery: A report from the Coronary Artery Surgery Study (CASS) Registry. *Circulation* 86:446, 1992.

## Pharmacologic Therapy

### Effect of Combination Therapy With Lipid-reducing Drugs in Patients With Coronary Heart Disease and "Normal" Cholesterol Levels

Pasternak RC, for the Harvard Atherosclerosis Reversibility Project (HARP) Study Group (Harvard Med School, Boston)
*Ann Intern Med* 125:529–540, 1996                                    2–38

*Objective.*—Although combination drug therapy has been shown to be beneficial for hyperlipidemic patients, similar efficacy studies have not been conducted for patients with coronary heart disease and normal LDL cholesterol levels. Results of a randomized, placebo-controlled, efficacy and tolerability trial of the effect of combination drug therapy on LDL and HDL cholesterol levels in patients with coronary heart disease and normal lipid levels were presented.

*Methods.*—A total of 91 patients (11 women), aged 30 to 75 years, with angiographically documented arterial stenosis $\geq 30\%$ and a total cholesterol HDL ratio > 4 was randomly allocated to receive stepped-care pharmacologic therapy ($n = 44$) (pravastatin, nicotinic acid, cholestyramine, and gemfibrozil) or placebo ($n = 47$) for an average of 125 weeks. Patients were evaluated every 6 weeks until they reached their targets and then every 3 months thereafter.

*Results.*—All lipid values decreased significantly from baseline in the treated group (214 to 159 mg/dL for mean total cholesterol, 140 to 90 mg/dL for LDL cholesterol, 159 versus 122 mg/dL for triglyceride). Throughout treatment, LDL cholesterol levels continued to decrease, whereas total cholesterol and triglyceride values stayed about the same (Fig 2). HDL cholesterol levels increased significantly in the treatment group from 42 to 46 mg/dL. Twelve of 47 patients receiving placebo required cholesterol-lowering drugs for total cholesterol levels >250 mg/dL. Adverse reactions were had by 59% of treated patients and 6% of placebo patients. Most symptoms were gastrointestinal or dermatologic and were related mainly to nicotinic acid and cholestyramine.

*Conclusion.*—The stepped-care 4-drug combination therapy approach significantly lowered LDL cholesterol and triglyceride levels and increased HDL cholesterol levels in patients with coronary heart disease and normal cholesterol levels. Gastrointestinal and dermatologic side effects were common.

▶ Effective combination therapy in patients with ostensibly "normal" cholesterol levels with pravastatin and nicotinic acid or gemfibrozil, but not with a resin, was effective in achieving optimal target levels of LDL cholesterol (160 mg/dL) in addition to lowering triglyceride and increasing HDL cholesterol levels. From a clinical standpoint, it would appear that the way to go is a "stepped care" approach with frequent and regular surveillance as necessary.[1]

**B.J. Gersh, M.B., Ch.B., D.Phil., F.R.C.P.**

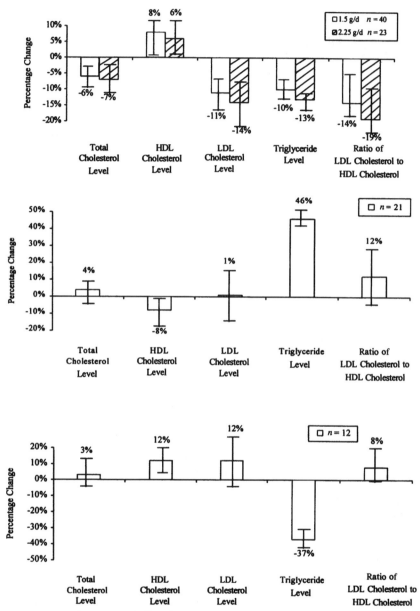

FIGURE 2.—The incremental effect of each drug added in the sequence specified by the stepped-care algorithm. *Top*, Nicotinic acid. *Middle*, Cholestyramine. *Bottom*, Gemfibrozil. Horizontal bars represent the 95% confidence intervals. Numbers given in boxes are numbers of patients who received the medication. *Abbreviations*: *HDL*, High-density lipoprotein; *LDL*, low-density lipoprotein. (Courtesy of Pasternak RC, for the Harvard Atherosclerosis Reversibility Project (HARP) Study Group: Effect of combination therapy with lipid-reducing drugs in patients with coronary heart disease and "normal" cholesterol levels. *Ann Intern Med* 125:529–540, 1996.)

*Reference*

1. Summary of the second report of the National Cholesterol Education Program (NCEP) expert panel on detection, evaluation and treatment of high blood cholesterol in adults (Adult Treatment Panel-2). *JAMA* 269:3015–3022, 1993.

---

## Effect of Long-acting and Short-acting Calcium Antagonists on Cardiovascular Outcomes in Hypertensive Patients

Alderman MH, Cohen H, Roqué R, et al (Albert Einstein College of Medicine, Bronx, NY)
*Lancet* 349:594–598, 1997                                                2–39

---

*Introduction.*—There is evidence that the use of short-acting calcium antagonists in patients with hypertension may lead to increased coronary artery morbidity, mortality, and noncardiovascular complications. Although short-acting calcium antagonists are recommended for the treatment of hypertension, the only formulations approved by the Food and Drug Administration are the long-acting ones, together with short-acting verapamil. The effects of short-acting calcium antagonists on cardiovascular risk were assessed.

*Methods.*—The case-control study was nested in a prospective cohort of 4,350 patients participating in a systematic hypertension control program. The case subjects were 189 patients with hypertension who had had an initial cardiovascular event—including cardiovascular deaths and hospitalizations for cardiovascular disease—over a 5-year period. The controls were 189 patients without such cardiovascular outcomes, matched for sex, ethnicity, age, previous antihypertensive treatment, year of entry into the study, and duration of follow-up. Information on prescription drugs taken on the day of the cardiovascular event was recorded for the case subjects, and drugs taken on the same date were noted for controls. Drug types were assessed to compare the incidence of cardiovascular events among patients taking long-acting vs. short-acting calcium antagonists.

*Results.*—One hundred thirty-six patients were taking long-acting calcium antagonists, and 27 were taking short-acting calcium antagonists. The risk of cardiovascular events was significantly increased for patients taking short-acting calcium antagonists, compared with patients taking β-blocker monotherapy (adjusted odds ratio, 3.88). No such increase in risk was noted for patients taking long-acting calcium antagonists (adjusted odds ratio, 0.76) (Table 4). On analysis of 38 matched pairs taking short-acting vs. long-acting calcium antagonists, the adjusted risk ratio for patients taking the long-acting formulations was 8.56.

*Conclusion.*—Long-acting calcium antagonists do not carry the same risk of adverse cardiovascular events as short-acting calcium antagonists. The findings support the conclusions of previous studies questioning the safety of short-acting calcium antagonists. Trials currently underway will

TABLE 4.—Adjusted Odds Ratios by Logistic Regression

| Variable* | Odds ratio (95% CI) | p |
|---|---|---|
| Long-acting calcium antagonists | 0·76 (0.41–1.43) | 0·761 |
| Short-acting calcium antagonists | 3·88 (1.25–13.11) | 0·029 |
| ACE inhibitor monotherapy | 0·52 (0.24–1.14) | 0·104 |
| Diuretic monotherapy | 1·35 (0.53–3.45) | 0·531 |
| Non-calcium antagonist combinations | 0·52 (0.22–1.19) | 0·120 |
| Withdrawn from drugs | 0·38 (0.15–0.95) | 0·039 |
| Previous history of myocardial infarction | 1·99 (0.98–4.03) | 0·057 |
| Initial cholesterol† | 1·32 (1.05–1.65) | 0·021 |
| Current smoker | 2·30 (1.38–3.83) | 0·001 |

*All variables in this table are coded yes = 1, no = 0, except cholesterol, which is continuous.
†Standard deviation change = 49 mg/dL.
*Abbreviation:* ACE, angiotensin converting enzyme.
(Courtesy of Alderman MH, Cohen H, Roqué R, et al: Effect of long-acting and short-acting calcium antagonists on cardiovascular outcomes in hypertensive patients. *Lancet* 349:594–598, copyright 1997 by The Lancet Ltd.)

provide important data on the relative cardiovascular effects of different antihypertensive drugs.

▶ The controversy continues, but the evidence against the use of short-acting calcium channel antagonists becomes increasingly persuasive.[1] The major risks of calcium channel antagonists, however, appear primarily, if not exclusively, to cluster around the adverse effects of the short-acting dihydropyridines and, in particular, short-acting or immediate-release nifedipine. Longer acting dihydropyridine compounds may be relatively safe, although further outcome data are needed. Of importance, in this case-control study by Alderman et al., there is no evidence of a harmful effect on patients treated with long-acting calcium channel antagonists, although the authors do not provide any data on the specific class of calcium channel antagonists.

Case control studies, such as this one, describe an association between exposure and an event and are subject to limitations. The ideal method of assessing the effects of drugs upon events is a randomized clinical trial. For this, we must await the results of the large Antihypertensive and Lipid Lowering Treatment to Prevent Heart Attack Trial (ALLHAT), but the results will likely not be available for another 3 to 5 years. Nonetheless, I believe that this and other studies suggest that there are significant differences between the short- and long-acting calcium channel antagonists, and the concerns understandably raised about the former—and, in particular, short-acting dihydropyridines—have not been shown to apply to the latter. In fact, preliminary data with a long-acting dihydropyridine (Amlodipine) in patients with nonischemic cardiomyopathy are favorable, and a larger trial is under way (PRAISE Study).[2]

Of interest and in need of further exploration from a therapeutic standpoint are other potentially favorable qualities of the calcium channel antagonists, including endothelial protection, relief of exercise-induced coronary vasoconstriction, antioxidant properties, antiplatelet effects[3] and inhibition of graft arteriopathy (for diltiazem).

**B.J. Gersh, M.B., Ch.B., D.Phil., F.R.C.P.**

*References*

1. Psaty BM, Heckbert SR, Koepsell TD, et al: The risk of myocardial infarction associated with antihypertensive drug therapy. *JAMA* 274:620–625, 1995.
2. Packer M, O'Connor CM, Ghali JK, et al: Effect of amlodipine on morbidity and mortality in severe chronic heart failure. Prospective Randomized Amlodipine Survival Evaluation Study Group. *N Engl J Med* 335:1107–1114, 1996.
3. Wallen NH, Heald C, Rehnquvist N, et al: Platelet aggregability in vivo as attenuated by verapamil, but not by metoprolol in patients with stable angine pectoris. *Am J Cardiol* 75:1–6, 1995.

---

**Effect of Ticlopidine on the Long-term Patency of Saphenous-vein Bypass Grafts in the Legs**
Becquemin J-P, for the Etude de la Ticlopidine après Pontage Fémoro-Poplité and the Association Universitaire de Recherche en Chirurgie (Centre Hospitalier Universitaire Henri Mondor, Créteil, France)
*N Engl J Med* 337:1726–1731, 1997                                   2–40

---

*Introduction.*—Late graft failure after infrainguinal arterial bypass surgery is often caused by progressive stenosis of the arteries on either side of the bypass. Platelet-inhibiting drugs have been evaluated as a way of improving the patency of saphenous-vein grafts, but the optimal treatment to prevent late occlusions has not been determined. A double-blind trial assessed the efficacy of ticlopidine, an inhibitor of platelet aggregation, on the long-term patency of below-knee saphenous-vein grafts.

*Methods.*—The multicenter study enrolled 243 patients with femoropopliteal or femorotibial saphenous-vein bypass grafts. Randomization was to ticlopidine (250-mg tablets) or matching placebo. Patients were instructed to take 1 tablet twice daily for 24 months. They were also given a list of anticoagulants and drugs with antiplatelet effects to avoid during the study period. Graft patency was evaluated at 1, 3, 6, 12, 18, and 24 months.

*Results.*—Study participants had a mean age of 67.4 years; 77.4% were men. Treatment and placebo groups did not differ significantly in sex, age, preoperative risk factors, site of proximal anastomosis, runoff, immediate graft patency, or mean duration of therapy. Bypass patency was assessed in 192 patients at 24 months by either duplex US (171) or angiography (21); 12 patients were assessed on the basis of clinical evaluation. The percentage of patients alive with a patent graft was greater in the ticlopidine group (66.4%) than in the placebo group (51.2%) at 2 years. The ticlopidine group also had a 2-year cumulative patency rate (Fig 1) superior to that of the placebo group (82% vs. 63%). Overall mortality (18 patients in each group) and the rate of major ischemic events did not differ significantly between the 2 groups. Nonischemic adverse events were more common in

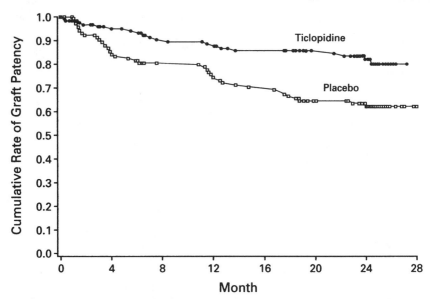

FIGURE 1.—Cumulative rates of graft patency according to the intention-to-treat analysis. There was a significant difference between groups ($P = 0.002$ by the log-rank test). (Reprinted by permission of *The New England Journal of Medicine* from Becquemin J-P, for the Etude de la Ticlopidine après Pontage Fémoro-Poplité and the Association Universitaire de Recherche en Chirurgie: Effect of ticlopidine on the long-term patency of saphenous-vein bypass grafts in the legs. *N Engl J Med* 337:1726–1731. Copyright 1997, Massachusetts Medical Society. All rights reserved.)

the ticlopidine group, which was a difference almost entirely accounted for by gastrointestinal disorders.

*Conclusion.*—Treatment with ticlopidine significantly improved the long-term patency of below-knee saphenous-vein graft¹s and reduced the need for major amputations. The drug's efficacy and lack of serious adverse effects recommend its use after femoropopliteal or femorotibial saphenous-vein bypass grafting.

▶ This is an interesting study demonstrating that ticlopidine therapy produced a significant and clinically meaningful improvement in the long-term patency or saphenous-vein grafts. Previous studies with aspirin have demonstrated varied results; there was a benefit from aspirin plus dipyridamole in 1 study of patients with infrainguinal prosthetic grafts,[1] whereas other studies have not shown any benefit.[2] Nonetheless, I still would have preferred to see this study compare ticlopidine with aspirin as opposed to placebo because antiplatelet agents such as aspirin are recommended in patients with peripheral arterial disease with the objective of preventing major cardiovascular ischemic events.[3] Unfortunately, ticlopidine is associated with a significant incidence of neutropenia, and it will be interesting to see whether its place in patients with saphenous-vein bypass grafts is taken over by a drug such as clopidogrel.

**B.J. Gersh, M.B., Ch.B., D.Phil., F.R.C.P.**

*References*

1. Sheehan SJ, Salter MCP, Donaldson DR, et al: Five year follow up of long-term aspirin/dipyridamole in femoropopliteal Dacron bypass grafts. *Br J Surg* 74:330A, 1987.
2. Edmonson RA, Cohen AT, Das SK, et al: Low-molecular weight heparin versus aspirin and dipyridamole after femoropopliteal bypass grafting. *Lancet* 344:914–918, 1994.
3. Antiplatelet Trialists' Collaboration: Collaborative overview of randomised trials of antiplatelet therapy: I. Prevention of death, myocardial infarction, and stroke by prolonged antiplatelet therapy in various categories of patients. *BMJ* 308:81–106, 1994.

**Effects of Intermittent Transdermal Nitroglycerin on Occurrence of Ischemia After Patch Removal: Results of the Second Transdermal Intermittent Dosing Evaluation Study (TIDES-II)**

Pepine CJ, Lopez LM, Bell DM, et al (Univ of Florida, Gainesville; West Virginia Univ, Morgantown)

*J Am Coll Cardiol* 30:955–961, 1997                                    2–41

*Introduction.*—Transdermal nitroglycerin (TD-NTG) patches, initially applied continuously over 24 hours, were found to be associated with partial or complete tolerance, and a 10–12-hour "patch off" period was recommended. Some patients, however, experienced more ischemia during this nitrate-free interval. In a multicenter study, the effects of intermittent TD-NTG on the occurrence of ischemia during patch-off hours were evaluated in patients with stable angina who were taking other agents to suppress angina.

*Methods.*—Period 1 of the study assessed tolerability to TD-NTG over a 3-week period during which patients were instructed to wear the patch for 14 hours a day. In period 2, 72 patients received either double-blind transdermal placebo or maximally tolerated TD-NTG for 2 weeks, then they crossed over to the alternate treatment for an additional 2 weeks in period 3. The patch was applied daily at 8 AM and removed at 10 PM; symptoms and sublingual nitroglycerin use were recorded in a diary. Ischemia during patch-on and patch-off periods was assessed by patients' perceptions of angina, a symptom-limited exercise treadmill test (ETT), and 48-hour ambulatory ECG (AECG) monitoring.

*Results.*—Compared with placebo, TD-NTG (0.2–0.4 mg/hr) significantly reduced the magnitude of ST-segment depression at angina onset during ETT. The active and placebo patch groups did not differ significantly in total angina frequency, but angina frequency increased with TD-NTG compared with placebo during patch-off hours. The AECG analyses also yielded similar trends for an increase in ischemia after TD-NTG. The frequency of ischemia tended to be higher during patch-on hours but lower during patch-off hours for placebo. The ischemia frequency decreased 58% from patch-off to patch-on periods in the placebo condition, whereas the TD-NTG condition resulted in a 14% increase in ischemia frequency. The frequency of ischemic episodes during TD-NTG therapy did not vary during 6-hour periods, but with placebo, there was a highly significant difference in the 6-hour period after midnight compared with the morning and afternoon periods.

*Conclusion.*—The normal diurnal pattern of ischemia appears to be disrupted with intermittent TD-NTG. Patients using intermittent TD-NTG experience an increase in ischemia during patch-off hours, which is a subjective finding supported by a similar trend for increased AECG ischemia during this period.

▶ This is an important study that provides new information, although I am not sure of the clinical implications. I was somewhat surprised by the lack of nitroglycerin efficacy compared with placebo, but the doses used were very low. The rebound effect, however, appears to be real, and the potential clinical implications of this are obvious, although only 46% of patients were receiving a β-blocker. Would β-blockers attenuate the rebound effect, and, in any event, does the latter result in an increase in adverse events (e.g., myocardial infarction)? We simply do not know the answers to either of these questions.

What is also somewhat disturbing in this and other studies is the large placebo effect on the frequency of both angina and asymptomatic ischemia.[1] Perhaps the actual wearing of a placebo patch does have a therapeutic effect. In any event, in my own clinical practice, the initial therapy consists of using sublingual nitroglycerin during episodes of angina and prophylactically, and, if I were to advise a long-acting nitrate, this would invariably be used in conjunction with a β-blocker, providing there were no contraindications.

**B.J. Gersh, M.B., Ch.B., D.Phil., F.R.C.P.**

*Reference*

1. Benson H, McCallie DP: Angina pectoris and the placebo effect. *N Engl J Med* 300:1424–1429, 1979.

## Socioeconomic

### Medical Care Costs and Quality of Life After Randomization to Coronary Angioplasty or Coronary Bypass Surgery

Hlatky MA, for the Bypass Angioplasty Revascularization Investigation (BARI) Investigators (Stanford Univ, Calif; Univ of Alabama, Birmingham; Univ of Pittsburgh, Pa; et al)
*N Engl J Med* 336:92–99, 1997                                                    2–42

*Background.*—Mortality and myocardial infarction rates are similar for patients with multivessel coronary artery disease undergoing coronary angioplasty vs. bypass surgery. Thus considerations of cost and quality of life play an important role in deciding between these 2 revascularization options. Long-term functional status, quality of life, employment, and

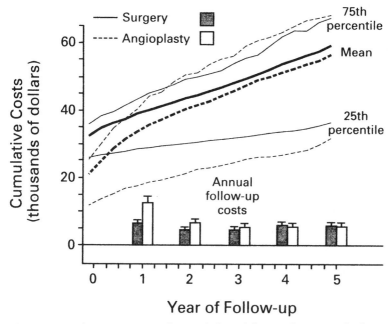

**Year of Follow-up**

FIGURE 2.—Cumulative costs at quarterly intervals during follow-up of patients randomly assigned to bypass surgery or angioplasty. The *thick curves* indicate mean cumulative costs calculated by a modification of the life-table method. The *lighter curves* at the top indicate the 75th percentile of the cumulative cost, and the lighter curves at the bottom the 25th percentile, among the patients remaining in the follow-up cohort. The *bars* at the bottom of the figure indicate the mean (+2 SE) follow-up costs accrued in the previous year among patients followed up throughout that year. (Reprinted by permission of *The New England Journal of Medicine,* from Hlatky MA, for the Bypass Angioplasty Revascularization Investigation [BARI] Investigators: Medical care costs and quality of life after randomization to coronary angioplasty or coronary bypass surgery. *N Engl J Med* 336:92–99, 1997. Copyright 1997, Massachusetts Medical Society. All rights reserved.)

costs were compared for patients undergoing angioplasty and bypass surgery.

*Methods.*—The study included 934 of 1,829 patients randomly allocated to coronary angioplasty or coronary bypass surgery for the treatment of multivessel coronary disease in the Bypass Angioplasty Revascularization Investigation. Each year, the patients were assessed on the Duke Activity Status Index, which evaluates functional status in terms of the ability to perform common activities of daily living. Emotional health and employment status were assessed as well. Utilization of medical services was evaluated quarterly.

*Results.*—All patients showed a significant improvement in the Duke Activity Status Index 1 year after treatment. On a scale of 0–58.2, the mean improvement was 5.7 units overall, 7.0 units for patients undergoing bypass surgery, and 4.4 units for those undergoing angioplasty. The difference remained significant at 2 and 3 years, but not at 4 years. The proportion of patients who continued working declined to 45% by 5

TABLE 4.—Cost and Life Expectancy Over the Five Years of Follow-up, According to Clinical Characteristics

| CHARACTERISTIC | PATIENTS | | COST ($) | | YEARS OF LIFE ADDED | |
|---|---|---|---|---|---|---|
| | SURGERY | ANGIOPLASTY | SURGERY | ANGIOPLASTY | SURGERY | ANGIOPLASTY |
| All patients | 469 | 465 | 58,889 | 56,225* | 4.4 | 4.3 |
| No of diseased vessels | | | | | | |
| 2 | 274 | 273 | 58,498 | 52,930* | 4.4 | 4.3 |
| 3 | 195 | 192 | 59,430 | 60,918 | 4.4 | 4.3 |
| Diabetes mellitus | | | | | | |
| No | 355 | 373 | 54,777 | 51,709 | 4.4 | 4.4 |
| Yes | 114 | 92 | 71,776 | 74,427 | 4.3 | 3.8† |
| Nondiabetics | | | | | | |
| 2-Vessel disease | 215 | 218 | 55,129 | 51,039 | 4.4 | 4.4 |
| 3-Vessel disease | 140 | 155 | 54,166 | 52,659 | 4.4 | 4.4 |
| Diabetics | | | | | | |
| 2-Vessel disease | 59 | 55 | 70,830 | 60,445 | 4.4 | 4.0† |
| 3-Vessel disease | 55 | 37 | 72,837 | 95,376 | 4.3 | 3.5† |

*$P < 0.05$ for the comparison with surgery by the Wilcoxon rank-sum test (for cumulative cost) and by the log-rank test (for survival), each through June 5, 1995.
†$P < 0.01$ for the comparison with surgery.
(Reprinted by permission of *The New England Journal of Medicine*, from Hlatky MA, for the Bypass Angioplasty Revascularization Investigation [ARI] Investigators: Medical care costs and quality of life after randomization to coronary angioplasty or coronary bypass surgery. *N Engl J Med* 336:92–99, 1997. Copyright 1997, Massachusetts Medical Society. All rights reserved.)

years, with no significant difference between groups. Total costs at 5 years were $58,889 in the bypass group and $56,225 in the angioplasty group, a difference of 5% (Fig 2). The costs of angioplasty were lower for patients with 2-vessel disease, but not for those with 3-vessel disease. For patients with 2-vessel disease, the cost-effectiveness ratio of bypass surgery was $60,057 per year of life added (Table 4).

*Conclusion.*—For the first 3 years after treatment for multivessel coronary disease, quality of life is better with coronary artery bypass surgery than with coronary angioplasty. Although angioplasty is initially less expensive, subsequent costs for hospitalization and medication may reduce the savings. By 5 years, the costs of angioplasty are lower only in patients with 2-vessel disease.

▶ This is one of the most important papers emanating from the BARI Trial and demonstrates that in most respects the quality of life is equivalent with the 2 forms of revascularization. Functional status, assessed by the Duke Activity Status Index, which evaluates the ability to perform common activities of daily living,[1] was higher in the bypass surgery group at 1 and 3 years, but there was no significant difference at 5 years. The findings about the costs of angioplasty and bypass surgery are similar to those noted in previous randomized trials and this is not surprising. The initial costs are much higher with bypass surgery, but the differences narrow over a period of time because of the need for repeat hospitalization and repeat revascularization in the percutaneous transluminal coronary angioplasty group. Nonetheless, there was still an overall 5% reduction in costs in patients treated with angioplasty, but this was confined to patients with 2 diseased vessels, whereas total costs were almost identical in patients with 3 diseased vessels. Among diabetic patients with triple-vessel disease, in whom the BARI Trial did demonstrate a mortality difference, cost of treatment was considerably higher with angioplasty, whereas in diabetic patients with 2-vessel disease it was less.[2] Further follow-up and cost data will be interesting to see the impact of saphenous vein graft failure and progression of disease in unbypassed or nondilated vessels upon the costs of both procedures. I suspect that we will see additional analysis that would speculate upon the impact of stents upon the cost data in this study, because BARI antedated widespread stent replacement.

There does appear to be some evidence that bypass surgery was more "cost-effective" as a result of the very small mortality difference in favor of bypass surgery. Nonetheless, the authors address the limitations of this analysis and the methodology of cost-effective analysis is still evolving.

What is of interest and less explicable is that the relatively poor rate of employment did not differ between the 2 groups. Only 57% of patients who were initially employed continued to work either full-time or part-time after 3 years and this fell to 45% after 5 years. Because the median age was approximately 63 years at the time of entry, this could reflect attrition from the work force as a result of retirement. Other studies in the past have shown a relatively high rate of failure to return to full-time employment.

**B.J. Gersh, M.B., Ch.B., D.Phil., F.R.C.P.**

*References*

1. Hlatky MA, Boineau RE, Higginbotham MB, et al: A brief self-administered questionnaire to determine functional capacity (The Duke Activity Status Index.) *Am J Cardiol* 64:651–654, 1989.
2. The Bypass Angioplasty Revascularization Investigation (BARI) Investigators: Comparison of coronary bypass surgery with angioplasty in patients with multivessel disease. *N Engl J Med* 335:217–225, 1996.

---

**Racial Variation in the Use of Coronary-Revascularization Procedures: Are the Differences Real? Do They Matter?**

Peterson ED, Shaw LK, DeLong ER, et al (Duke Univ, Durham, NC)

*N Engl J Med* 336:480–486, 1997                                                  2–43

---

*Background.*—Through multiple studies, researchers have confirmed that blacks in the United States undergo fewer revascularization procedures than whites. However, these studies often have been based on medical claims data, which do not necessarily allow researchers to accurately identify patients with coronary artery disease, adjust for differences in disease severity, or determine the effect of differences in treatment. This study was designed to correct those deficiencies by investigating whether there are racial differences in the use of coronary angioplasty and bypass surgery.

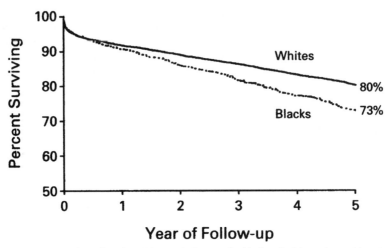

FIGURE 4.—Unadjusted Kaplan-Meier survival curves for black and white patients with coronary disease. (Courtesy of Peterson ED, Shaw LK, DeLong ER, et al: Racial variation in the use of coronary-revascularization procedures: Are the differences real? Do they matter? *New Engl J Med* 336:480–486, 1997. Reprinted by permission of *The New England Journal of Medicine.* Copyright 1997, Massachusetts Medical Society. All rights reserved.)

*Methods.*—Of 21,989 patients who underwent a first cardiac catheterization at a single institution from March 1984 to December 1992, 12,402 were enrolled in this study. The study population comprised 11,127 white patients (89.7%) and 1,275 black patients (10.3%) who had obstructive coronary artery disease. After catheterization, the patients were contacted yearly (mean duration of follow-up, 5.6 years) and were asked about their clinical status and whether they had undergone a revascularization procedure. The data were adjusted for differences in clinical history, disease severity, anginal symptoms, coexisting illness, and access to subspecialty care.

*Results.*—Even after adjustment for disease severity and other characteristics, blacks were 32% less likely than whites to undergo bypass surgery. The difference for angioplasty was not statistically significant. The 5-year survival rate was significantly lower for blacks than for whites (Fig 4). This was true even after the investigators controlled for the fact that blacks have a higher baseline risk of coronary disease, higher rates of diabetes and hypertension, and worse ventricular function.

*Conclusion.*—In this patient population, revascularization seems to have been underused in treating blacks.

▶ This is a disturbing paper, particularly since an adjustment was made to account for disease severity, angina status, and the estimated survival benefit from revascularization. What is of particular concern is the poorer 5-year survival rate of blacks. Even after adjusting for baseline prognostic factors, blacks remained 18% more likely to die than whites during the 5 years of follow-up. After further adjustment for both baseline risk factors and stratification according to the initial treatment received, blacks were only at marginally higher risk for death than whites, and this suggests that the higher mortality rate in blacks was partly the result of *treatment received* as well as differences in baseline risk, such as the prevalence of hypertension and diabetes.

These concerns are similar to those raised by gender differences in the use of invasive procedures.[1, 2] Are these differences the result of bias or clinical judgment, and if the answer is the latter, is this appropriate or inappropriate? These are tremendously important and complex issues with profound implications, both medical and societal. This and other studies pose new questions that need to be answered. First, can the results of this study reflecting practice patterns at a single institution be generalized to the rest of the country? Second, race may be a marker of other socioeconomic factors such educational level, employment status, and family structure, all of which can have an impact on the use of procedures. Third, as the authors point out, they did not have access to information about the patients' preferences regarding therapy, and there are data to suggest racial differences in the acceptance of a recommendation to undergo bypass surgery or cardiac catheterization.[3, 4] Whatever the mechanisms, these issues must be resolved because no one feels comfortable with the thought that patients are unable to obtain equal access to procedures on the basis of race, gender, or any other nonmedical factor.

**B.J. Gersh, M.B., Ch.B., D.Phil., F.R.C.P.**

*References*

1. Ayanin JZ, Epstein AM: Differences in the use of procedures between women and men hospitalized for coronary heart disease. *N Engl J Med* 325:221–225, 1991.
2. Steingart RM, Packer M, Hamm P, et al: Sex differences in the management of coronary artery disease. *N Engl J Med* 3256:226–230, 1991.
3. Maynot C, Fisher LD, Passamani ER, et al: Blacks and the Coronary Artery Surgery Study [CASS]: Race and clinical decision making. *Am J Public Health* 76:1446–1448, 1986.
4. Schecter AD, Goldschmidt-Clermont PJ, McKee G, et al: Influence of gender, race and education on patient preferences and receipt of cardiac catheterizations amongst coronary care unit patients. *Am J Cardiol* 78:996–1001, 1996.

---

**Functional Recovery After Myocardial Infarction in Men: The Independent Effects of Social Class**
Ickovics JR, Viscoli CM, Horwitz RI (Yale Univ, New Haven, Conn)
*Ann Intern Med* 127:518–525, 1997                                                    2–44

---

*Introduction.*—Although left ventricular function is the most important single clinical determinant of death after myocardial infarction, other clinical indicators, life style factors, and social and psychological characteristics also significantly influence outcome. The effect of social class on functional recovery from myocardial infarction was determined using prospective data from a multicenter trial.

TABLE 2.—Association of Social Class With Baseline Functional Status and Change in Functional Status From Baseline to Follow-up

| Social Class Category | Baseline Functional Limitation: New York Heart Association Classes II–IV | Improvement in Functional Status from Baseline to Follow-up |
|---|---|---|
| | % (n) | |
| High (n = 750) | 40.4 (303) | 72.1 (541) |
| Middle (n = 949) | 44.8 (425) | 64.1 (608) |
| Low (n = 446) | 54.7 (244) | 57.4 (256) |

(Courtesy of Ickovics JR, Viscoli CM, Horwitz RI: Functional recovery after myocardial infarction in men: The independent effects of social class. *Ann Intern Med* 127:518–525, 1997.)

*Methods.*—Data were drawn from the Beta-Blocker Heart Attack Trial, a randomized, placebo-controlled trial conducted to assess the efficacy of propranolol administered after myocardial infarction. Patients had been treated at 25 hospitals or clinical sites in the United States and Canada. The 2,145 patients recruited for the trial were men who ranged in age from 29 to 69 years (mean, 54 years). The trial's primary outcome was change in New York Heart Association functional class between baseline assessment and 12-month follow-up. Social class was defined by a composite of education and occupation.

*Results.*—Most patients were white, and 37.6% had a history of hypertension. Social class was defined as high in 35.0% of patients, middle in 44.2%, and low in 20.8%. Baseline cardiovascular risk factors were most

TABLE 3.—Bivariate Logistic Regression Analysis Predicting No Functional Improvement From Baseline to 1 Year After Infarction

| Risk Factor | Bivariate Odds Ratio (95% CI) |
|---|---|
| Demographic features | |
| Social class (change in 1 category) | 1.39 (1.23–1.57) |
| Age (10-year categories) | 1.28 (1.15–1.43) |
| Black race (black compared with nonblack) | 1.85 (1.31–2.60) |
| Clinical features | |
| Medical history* | |
| History of myocardial infarction | 2.31 (1.83–2.92) |
| History of stroke | 1.58 (0.85–2.92) |
| History of diabetes | 1.42 (1.07–1.88) |
| History of hypertension | 1.38 (1.15–1.65) |
| Current smoking | 1.47 (1.19–1.82) |
| Use of β-blockers | 1.03 (0.86–1.23) |
| Severity of myocardial infarction† | |
| Congestive heart failure | 1.53 (1.23–1.92) |
| Electrical events | 1.06 (0.88–1.28) |
| Psychosocial features‡ | |
| Life stress | 1.40 (1.16–1.68) |
| Social isolation | 1.19 (0.99–1.45) |
| Depression | 1.99 (1.41–2.81) |

(Courtesy of Ickovics JR, Viscoli CM, Horwitz RI: Functional recovery after myocardial infarction in men: The independent effects of social class. *Ann Intern Med* 127:518–525, 1997.)

likely to be reported in the low social class group and least likely to be reported in the high social class group. There was a clear inverse relationship between social class and baseline functional status. Even after controlling for relevant prognostic factors, patients of high social class were significantly more likely than those of low or middle social class to have improved functional status 1 year after infarction (Table 2). Bivariate logistic regression analyses identified baseline demographic, clinical, and psychosocial factors associated with a change in functional status (Table 3). Factors adversely affecting functional status included a history of myocardial infarction, the presence of congestive heart failure, smoking at baseline, and high levels of stress and depression.

*Conclusion.*—Patients of high social class had more improvement in functional status 1 year after myocardial infarction than patients in the middle or low social classes. This difference was not explained by clinical risk at baseline, nor was it strongly influenced by access to health care. Clinicians need to be aware that lower social class confers an independent risk for a poorer outcome.

▶ The study confirms and extends previous data that have linked social class to cardiovascular outcomes.[1] What is particularly important about this study is that the results were probably not influenced by access to health care or differences in the quality of care, because all the patients were enrolled in a clinical trial in which health status was evaluated regularly. Although the relationship between social class and cardiovascular health is well established, the mechanisms need clarification. In some studies, occupation has been identified as a key factor, but in others, education has been the strongest and most powerful predictor.[2] In this study, variables such as smoking and previous infarctions were measured, but others, such as exercise and alcohol use, which were not taken into account, may well be important mechanisms that underlie the impact that social class has on outcome. The important message of this study is that it is not enough just to treat the patient and the disease, but the broader socioeconomic implications of data such as these point to the need to address the primary causes of poverty and poor education as a means of improving the health of all our citizens.

**B.J. Gersh, M.B., Ch.B., D.Phil., F.R.C.P.**

*References*

1. Blane D, Hart CL, Smith GD, et al: Association of cardiovascular disease risk factors with socioeconomic position during childhood and during adulthood. *BMJ* 313:1434–1438, 1996.
2. Winkleby MA, Jatulis DE, Frank E, et al: Socioeconomic status and health: How education, income, and occupation contribute to risk factors for cardiovascular disease. *Am J Public Health* 82:816–820, 1992.

## The Association Between Birthplace and Mortality From Cardiovascular Causes Among Black and White Residents of New York City

Fang J, Madhavan S, Alderman MH (Albert Einstein College of Medicine, Bronx, NY)

*N Engl J Med* 335:1545–1551, 1996                                          2–45

*Objective.*—Black Americans have a higher mortality rate from cardiovascular disease and a shorter life expectancy than do white Americans. Because country of origin adds to the genetic and environmental risk factors for mortality, the association between birthplace and mortality from cardiovascular disease in New York City between 1988 and 1993 was examined in blacks born in the southern United States, blacks born in the Caribbean, and blacks and whites born in the northeastern United States.

*Methods.*—Death records and census data were obtained and information on age, sex, race, ethnic group, birthplace, and education was statistically compared with death rates from cardiovascular disease for residents of New York City and the United States as a whole.

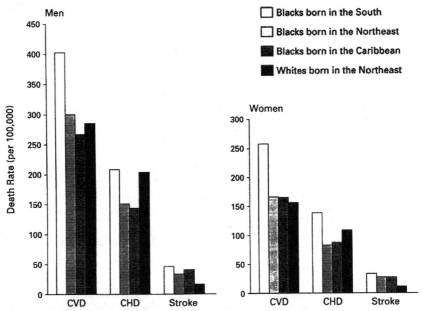

FIGURE 1.—Age-adjusted annual rates of death from selected cardiovascular diseases in non-Hispanic blacks and whites in New York City from 1988 through 1992, according to birthplace. Mortality rates were adjusted for age in 10-year age categories, with the U.S. population in 1940 used as the standard. *Abbreviations*: CVD, Cardiovascular disease; CHD, coronary heart disease. (Courtesy of Fang J, Madhavan S, Alderman MH: The association between birthplace and mortality from cardiovascular causes among black and white residents of New York City. *N Engl J Med* 335:1545–1551, 1996. Reprinted by permission of *The New England Journal of Medicine*. Copyright 1997 by the Massachusetts Medical Society. All rights reserved.)

*Results.*—Birthplace was the northeastern United States for 73.1% of whites and 54.1% of blacks, the South for 20% of blacks, and the Caribbean for 17% of blacks. The average ages of blacks in the Northeast, South, and Caribbean were 23.2, 51.1, and 37.7 years, respectively. Cardiovascular mortality rates for blacks born in the Northeast were higher than for whites born in the Northeast (299 per 100,000 vs. 285 for men and 165 vs. 155 for women). Death rates from cardiovascular disease for city blacks and whites were 34.1% and 51.8%, respectively, with age-adjusted cardiovascular death rates per 100,000 population of 264.9 for blacks and 209.9 for whites. This rate was higher for both male and female blacks (Fig 1). Blacks born in the South had substantially higher death rates from cardiovascular disease than did blacks born in the Northeast or the Caribbean. Blacks born in the Caribbean had the lowest death rates among the black populations studied and had significantly lower mortality rates than whites. Young black men born in the South had a cardiovascular death rate 30% higher than young black men born in the Northeast and 4 times higher than young black men born in the Caribbean.

*Conclusion.*—The heterogeneous mortality rates among blacks depending on birthplace is significant. Most of the differences between black and white cardiovascular mortality rates are from the high mortality rate among blacks born in the South. Although death rates from hypertension and stroke are high among all blacks, mortality rates for cardiovascular deaths vary by birthplace and may be the result of genetic or environmental factors.

▶ This study is limited by reliance on death certificates and census data. Nonetheless, the findings are of great interest. The coronary mortality difference between black and white in the United States is well documented, but it would appear, at least in New York City, that this is almost completely accounted for by blacks born in the South. Studies like this raise questions and the answers will come from several different avenues of investigation. Are the differences due to genetic or environmental influences or both?[1] Genetic heterogeneity may explain the lower risk of coronary artery disease in Caribbean-born blacks and, if so, the next question is to identify those genetic factors that are "protective." Obviously, other explanations lie in the realm of socioeconomic and sociocultural differences which may relate to lifestyle, diet, risk factor modification, and access to medical care, etc. All of this remains to be teased out, but it would appear from this study that the findings cannot be accounted for purely on the basis of the well-documented higher incidence of hypertension in blacks. An accompanying editorial by Gillum develops a fascinating hypothesis on the stages and the epidemiologic evolution of patterns of cardiovascular disease among persons of sub-Saharan African origin. It does draw attention to the methodologic problems of this study but also highlights the complex and fascinating issue of studies on "migrant" populations. It would appear that there are multiple factors including selection, origin, and destination which may determine the incidence of disease in migrant populations with a similar genetic background.[2]

**B.J. Gersh, M.B., Ch.B., D.Phil., F.R.C.P.**

*References*

1. Miller GJ, Kotecha S, Wilkenson WH, et al: Dietary and other characteristics relevant for coronary heart disease in men of Indian, West Indian and European descent in London. *Atherosclerosis*, 70:6372, 1988.
2. Gillum RF: The epidemiology of cardiovascular disease in black Americans. *N Engl J Med* 335:1597–1599, 1996.

---

**Excess Mortality Among Blacks and Whites in the United States**
Geronimus AT, Bound J, Waidmann TA, et al (Univ of Michigan, Ann Arbor; Natl Bureau for Economic Research, Cambridge, Mass; Urban Inst Health Policy Ctr, Washington, DC)
*N Engl J Med* 335:1552–1558, 1996                                                 2–46

---

*Objective.*—Young and middle-aged blacks have higher morbidity and mortality rates than do whites of the same age. To better understand patterns of excess mortality, the life expectancies and mortality rates of people in disadvantaged vs. more advantaged areas were compared.

*Methods.*—Age- and sex-specific overall and specific death rates for black and white groups, aged 15 to 64 years, from 16 study areas were determined and compared with standardized rates to determine annualized excess death rates (Fig 1). Life tables were calculated, and measures of mortality were compared statistically.

*Results.*—The death rates for poor black men and women in every area were excessively high. The mortality ratios for black men and women from Harlem were 4.11 and 3.38 compared with ratios of 1.18 and 1.08 for black men and women from Queens-Bronx, which was similar to the rate for white men and women nationally. Poor white men and women had higher mortality rates than white men and women nationally. Mortality ratios for white men and women in Detroit were 2.01 and 1.90 compared with ratios of 0.41 and 0.54 for white men and women in Sterling Heights, Mich. The average number of years of life lost varied significantly among groups (Table 1). Causes of excess mortality rates were diseases of the circulatory system in every group; HIV among men and women from Harlem and the Lower East Side; accidents among Appalachian men and men in Black Belt Alabama; homicide among men from Watts, Calif., and Harlem and all men in Detroit; cancer among men and women in Harlem, Watts, and poor white and poor black areas of Detroit; and infections in men and women from Harlem.

*Conclusion.*—Although all disadvantaged groups had excess mortality rates, the patterns of excess mortality differed among communities.

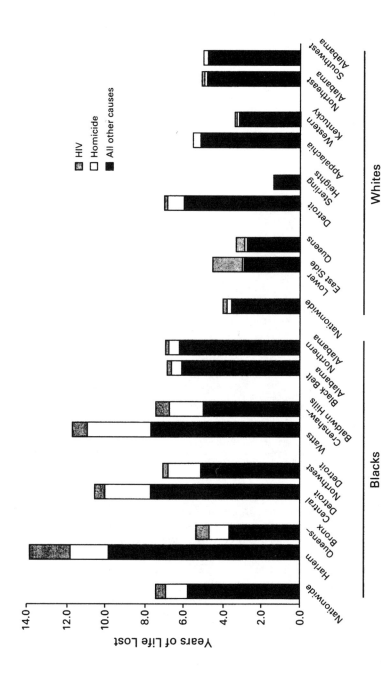

**FIGURE 1.**—Average years of life lost between the ages of 15 and 65 in men and boys, according to study area and for selected causes of death. (Courtesy of Geronimus AT, Bound J, Waidmann TA, et al: Excess mortality among blacks and whites in the United States. *N Engl J Med* 335:1552–1558, 1996. Reproduced by permission of *The New England Journal of Medicine.* Copyright 1997, Massachusetts Medical Society. All rights reserved.)

TABLE 1.—Summary Data on the Study Areas, 1990*

| AREA | NO. OF INHABITANTS† | MEAN FAMILY INCOME ($) | FAMILIES BELOW THE POVERTY LEVEL‡ (%) |
|---|---|---|---|
| U.S. population | | | |
| Total | 248,709,873 | 43,803 | 10.0 |
| Whites | 199,827,064 | 49,248 | 6.4 |
| Blacks | 29,930,524 | 29,337 | 25.7 |
| **Blacks** | | | |
| New York City | | | |
| Harlem | 101,697 | 24,174 | 33.1 |
| Queens–Bronx | 170,380 | 51,606 | 5.7 |
| Detroit | | | |
| Central | 98,833 | 19,841 | 44.3 |
| Northwest | 132,668 | 41,127 | 15.1 |
| Los Angeles | | | |
| Watts | 98,488 | 23,743 | 35.4 |
| Crenshaw–Baldwin Hills | 100,744 | 40,419 | 15.7 |
| Alabama | | | |
| Black Belt | 93,695 | 17,222 | 48.7 |
| Northern | 116,490 | 23,935 | 28.6 |
| **Whites** | | | |
| New York City | | | |
| Lower East Side | 158,452 | 34,208 | 21.3 |
| Queens | 144,216 | 54,836 | 5.7 |
| Detroit metropolitan area | | | |
| Detroit | 126,752 | 29,334 | 22.0 |
| Sterling Heights | 113,452 | 54,424 | 2.7 |
| Kentucky | | | |
| Appalachia | 109,794 | 18,925 | 34.6 |
| Western | 113,163 | 31,002 | 14.1 |
| Alabama | | | |
| Northeast | 167,037 | 30,480 | 13.6 |
| Southwest | 102,527 | 36,500 | 8.6 |

*Data are from the 1990 U.S. Census. The makeup of the study groups is described in the Methods section, and the 16 regions are described in the Appendix. In each pair of areas, the one listed first is the lower-income area, and the one listed second is the comparison area of higher socioeconomic status.
†Numbers shown refer to only black residents or only white residents, depending on the area studied.
‡The poverty levels were those defined by the Bureau of the Census.
(Courtesy of Geronimus AT, Bound J, Waidmann TA, et al: Excess mortality among blacks and whites in the United States. *N Engl J Med* 335:1552–1558, 1996. Reproduced by permission of *The New England Journal of Medicine.* Copyright 1997, Massachusetts Medical Society. All rights reserved.)

▶ It is well established that rates of death from cardiovascular causes amongst black Americans are among the highest in the industrialized world, and the decline in mortality from coronary heart disease has been less in black Americans than in other population groups in the United States. This case study by Geronimus et al. really draws attention to the vulnerability of inner-city populations to death from coronary heart disease, but also emphasizes the heterogeneity of mortality rates from cardiovasular disease among different black American populations. An interesting editorial by Gillum[1] points out not only the limitations of this study but also suggests new directions of research that will define the socioeconomic, cultural, behavioral, and ethnic factors that account for these differences between blacks and whites and within the black population. He develops a fascinating hypothesis on the stages and epidemiologic evolution of cardiovascular disease among persons of sub-Saharan African origin and points out that in precolonial Africa, hypertensive cardiovascular disease and atherosclerotic cardiovascular disease were virtually nonexistent. He closes on an encouraging note in which he states that perhaps in the next century "American blacks will return to their ancestral low rates of cardiovascular disease while retaining the positive aspects of a western lifestyle."

**B.J. Gersh, M.B., Ch.B., D.Phil., F.R.C.P.**

*Reference*

1. Gillum RF: The epidemiology of cardiovascular disease in black Americans. *N Engl J Med* 335:1597–1598, 1996.

## Pathophysiology of Coronary Artery Disease

### Association Between Prior Cytomegalovirus Infection and the Risk of Restenosis After Coronary Atherectomy

Zhou YF, Leon MB, Waclawiw MA, et al (Natl Heart, Lung and Blood Inst, Bethesda, Md; Washington Hosp Ctr, Washington, DC)
*N Engl J Med* 335:624–630, 1996                                    2–47

*Purpose.*—Up to 50% of patients undergoing coronary angioplasty have restenosis. The mechanisms by which restenosis develops are unclear. A recent study found cytomegalovirus (CMV) DNA in restenotic lesions from atherectomy specimens, suggesting that CMV might play a role in the development of restenosis. Latent CMV may be locally reactivated in response to vascular injury in some patients undergoing coronary angioplasty. The possible link between CMV and restenosis was assessed in a prospective study.

*Methods.*—Seventy-five consecutive patients with symptomatic coronary artery disease who were scheduled for direction coronary atherectomy were studied. Anti-CMV IgG antibodies were measured before atherectomy in all patients. Six months later, coronary angiography was performed to see if restenosis had occurred.

*Results.*—The results of CMV antibody testing were positive in 49 patients and negative in 26. The mean minimal luminal diameter in the treated vessel was 3.18 mm in seropositive patients vs. 2.89 mm in seronegative patients. Six months later, the reduction in luminal diameter was 1.24 mm in the seropositive group and 0.68 mm in the seronegative group. The restenosis rates were 43% and 8%, respectively (Fig 1). Multivariate analysis showed that CMV seropositivity and CMV titer were independently associated with restenosis, with odds ratios of 12.9 and 8.1, respectively. Neither group of patients had evidence of acute CMV infection.

*Conclusions.*—Previous exposure to CMV is a major risk factor for the development of restenosis after coronary atherectomy. If the results are confirmed by further studies, CMV antibody testing may become a useful method of predicting patients' risk of restenosis. This knowledge may be useful in deciding whether to perform atherectomy or coronary artery

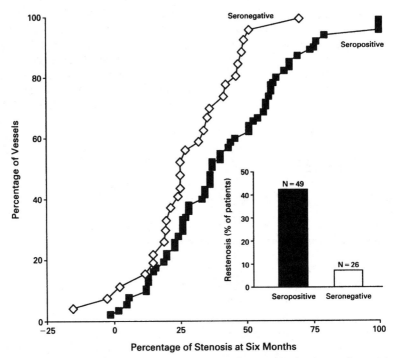

**FIGURE 1.**—Influence of prior cytomegalovirus (CMV) infection on the distribution of stenosis in 85 target vessels in 75 patients, as determined by angiography six months after directional coronary atherectomy. The patients were divided into two groups on the basis of whether they were seropositive or seronegative for anti-CMV IgG antibodies at baseline. A seropositive status was defined prospectively as an assay value of 0.25 unit or higher. At six months, vessels in the seropositive patients had a higher percentage of stenosis than vessels in the seropositive patients ($P=0.01$). The inset shows the incidence of restenosis (> 50% narrowing of the vessel diameter), which was also higher in the seropositive patients. (Courtesy of Zhou YF, Leon MB, Waclawiw MA, et al: Association between prior cytomegalovirus infection and the risk of restenosis after coronary atherectomy. *N Engl J Med* 335:624–630, 1996. Reprinted by permission of *The New England Journal of Medicine*. Copyright 1996, Massachusetts Medical Society. All rights reserved.)

bypass grafting. If CMV proves to be a cause of restenosis, then preventive antiviral treatment strategies could be developed.

▶ This study reports further fascinating data on the association between inflammation and various manifestations of atherosclerosis. The hypothesis is that latent CMV infection may be reactivated locally by vascular injury (e.g., balloon inflation) and that proteins expressed by the virus in turn initiate a series of actions that enhance the accumulation of smooth muscle cells and cause restenosis.[1]

The next question is whether antiviral agents will be successful in inhibiting the process and preventing restenosis.

**B.J. Gersh, M.B., Ch.B., D.Phil., F.R.C.P.**

*Reference*

1. Speir E, Modali R, Huang ES, et al: Potential role of human cytomegalovirus and p53 interaction in coronary restenosis. *Science* 265:391–394, 1994.

## Vulnerable Plaque: Relation of Characteristics to Degree of Stenosis in Human Coronary Arteries

Mann JM, Davies MJ (St George's Hosp Med School, London)
*Circulation* 94:928–931, 1996                                                2–48

*Background.*—An individual coronary artery will usually contain a spectrum of plaques, ranging from the lipid-rich type implicated in thrombosis to the solid, fibrous type that has no risk of disruption. In addition to a large lipid core, plaques at risk for disruption have a thin cap and a high macrophage content. Atherosclerotic plaques obtained from 31 individuals who died suddenly of ischemic heart disease were examined for plaque size, size of the lipid core, cap thickness, and the relations among these variables.

*Methods.*—Twenty-seven men and 4 women with a mean age of 59 years died in the hospital receiving room after attempts at resuscitation. Twenty-five (81%) had chest pain in the 6 hours before death. Coronary arteries were fixed by perfusion with 10% formaldehyde at a pressure of 120 mm Hg, then dissected intact from the heart and decalcified. The arteries were divided into 2-mm transverse slices and processed for histology. Stenosis was measured by comparison of the minimal lumen size at the site of a plaque with that of the lumen in the adjacent normal segment of artery. Forty-nine entire arteries containing 160 types IV and V plaques were studied.

*Results.*—The plaques were quite varied, exhibiting every permutation of plaque size, stenosis, core size, and cap thickness (Table 1). Lipid core size ranged from 0% to 82% of overall plaque size. In 17% of plaques the core size was >50%. There was no correlation between core size and degree of stenosis or between absolute plaque size and lipid core size (Fig 3). Minimal cap thickness (mean 0.25 mm) had no relation to core size.

TABLE 1.—Lipid Core Size as a Proportion of Overall Plaque Size in 160 Plaques

| Totally Fibrous | Core Size | | |
| --- | --- | --- | --- |
| | 5%–20% | 21%–50% | >50% |
| Type Vc | | Type IV Va | |
| 12 (7%) | 45 (28%) | 76 (48%) | 27 (17%) |

(Courtesy of Mann JM, Davies MJ: Vulnerable plaque: Relation of characteristics to degree of stenosis in human coronary arteries. *Circulation* 94:928–931, 1996. Copyright 1996, American Heart Association.)

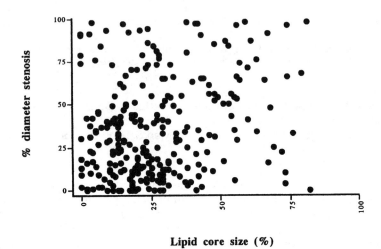

**Lipid core size (%)**

FIGURE 3.—Lipid core size as a percentage of overall plaque size plotted against percentage of diameter stenosis. There is no significant correlation ($r = 0.21$). Plaques with a very large lipid core can cause stenosis ranging from negligible to high grade. (Courtesy of Mann JM, Davies MJ: Vulnerable plaque: Relation of characteristics to degree of stenosis in human coronary arteries. *Circulation* 94:928–931, 1996. Copyright 1996, American Heart Association.)

Cores >50% were present in 10% of plaques predicted to be angiographically invisible.

*Discussion.*—The concordance of a large lipid core and a thin cap is the major determinant of plaque vulnerability, but these characteristics cannot be identified at angiography. A lack of correlation among absolute plaque size, core size, and plaque thickness suggests that these variables are independent. Patients with all fibrous plaques may have slowly progressive angina, whereas those with all lipid-rich plaques have a very high risk of repeated acute ischemic episodes. It is more common, however, for patients to have mixtures of all types of plaques.

▶ This is a most important paper that illustrates that angiography, which can determine the severity of a stenosis, cannot identify which plaques are vulnerable to subsequent rupture or fissuring, leading to the development of an acute ischemic syndrome.[1] The impact of this finding on the selection of patients for revascularization, and in particular percutaneous transluminal coronary angioplasty, is far reaching. In the absence of symptoms or objective evidence of ischemia, percutaneous transluminal coronary angioplasty is not indicated as a method of preventing the development of a future culprit because angiography alone does not tell us which plaques are likely to be the cause of acute ischemic syndromes in the future. On the other hand, particularly in patients with single-vessel disease, the presence of symptoms or ischemia would suggest that the most severe lesion is the culprit and, as such, dilatation is likely to be of value.

**B.J. Gersh, M.B., Ch.B., D.Phil., F.R.C.P.**

*Reference*

1. Ambrose J, Tannenbaum M, Alexopoulos D, et al: Angiographic progression of coronary artery disease in the development of myocardial infarction. *JACC* 12:56–62, 1988.

## Prevalence and Associations of Abdominal Aortic Aneurysm Detected Through Screening
Lederle FA, for the Aneurysm Detection and Management (ADAM) Veterans Affairs Cooperative Study Group (Veterans Affairs Med Ctr, Minneapolis)
*Ann Intern Med* 126:441–449, 1997                                        2–49

*Objective.*—Although abdominal aortic aneurysm (AAA) is a leading cause of death, key questions remain about its cause and epidemiology. Most epidemiologic data on this condition have come from screening studies. No multivariate analyses have been conducted in large patient populations to determine the independent risk factors for AAA. Risk factors for AAA and the prevalence of previously unrecognized AAA were studied as part of a large cross-sectional screening study.

*Methods.*—The study included 73,451 subjects undergoing ultrasonographic screening at 15 VA medical centers. The veterans, aged 50 to 79 years at the time of the screening, had no history of AAA (Table 3). The screening findings, along with the responses to a prescreening questionnaire, were used to determine the prevalence of AAA in various demographic and risk groups. Factors independently associated with AAA were evaluated as well.

*Results.*—The prevalence of previously unrecognized AAA was 1.4%. The main risk factor was smoking (odds ratio [OR] for AAA measuring 4 cm or larger was 5.57), compared with normal aortas with an infrarenal aortic diameter of less than 3.0 cm. The greater the number of years the

TABLE 3.—Prevalence of Abdominal Aortic Aneurysm 4.0 cm or Larger Detected by Screening in Men

| Age | Patients Who Never Smoked | Prevalence of AAA | Patients Who Smoked* | Prevalence of AAA |
|-----|---------------------------|-------------------|----------------------|-------------------|
| y | n | % | n | % |
| 50–54 | 1152 | 0 | 4359 | 0.3 |
| 55–59 | 1481 | 0 | 5819 | 0.9 |
| 60–64 | 2985 | 0.2 | 11 119 | 1.5 |
| 65–69 | 4198 | 0.2 | 14 129 | 1.9 |
| 70–74 | 4679 | 0.5 | 13 008 | 2.5 |
| 75–79 | 2544 | 0.8 | 5669 | 2.7 |

*Abbreviation: AAA,* abdominal aortic aneurysm.
*More than 100 cigarettes over lifetime.
(Courtesy of Lederle FA, for the Aneurysm Detection and Management (ADAM) Veterans Affairs Cooperative Study Group: Prevalence and associations of abdominal aortic aneurysm detected through screening. *Ann Intern Med* 126:441–449, 1997.)

subject smoked, the greater the risk of AAA. This risk decreased progressively as the number of years since quitting smoking increased. Smoking-related risk explained 78% of all AAAs measuring 4 cm or larger. Other risk factors associated with AAA were female sex (OR 0.22), African-American race (OR 0.49), and diabetes (OR 0.54). Subjects with a family history of AAA were at double the risk (OR 1.95). However, just 5% of the veterans studied reported such a history. Age, height, coronary artery disease, atherosclerosis, high cholesterol, and high blood pressure also were independently associated with AAA.

*Conclusions.*—Many different factors are related to risk of AAA. However, smoking is the major risk factor and may account for most clinically significant instances of previously undiagnosed AAA. The prevalence of previously undiagnosed AAA in this large screening population was about 1%.

▶ This is the largest study of screening for AAA to date, and the first that describes a detailed multivariate analysis of potential risk factors in all previously undetected cases in a population. The most powerful association was with smoking, and these data strongly suggest that AAA is a smoking-related illness, although the mechanisms for it are not clear.[1] Other independently associated risk factors included elevated cholesterol levels, coronary artery disease, atherosclerosis elsewhere, older age and a family history of AAA, although a family history of AAA was reported by only 5.1% of participants. The negative association with diabetes is of interest, and at first glance puzzling, but other studies have pointed in the same direction.

There are several limitations to this study, including its generalizability to individuals other than U.S. Veterans age 50 to 79 years, the low response rate (30%) to the invitation to participate in the study (which raises the question of selection bias, and the self-reporting of risk factors. Nonetheless, this study provides important new evidence for use in planning future screening programs, although other studies will be required to address whether such programs are justified and whether surgery for small AAAs will reduce mortality.[2, 3]

**B.J. Gersh, M.B., Ch.B., D.Phil., F.R.C.P.**

*References*

1. MacSweeney ST, Ellis M, Worrell PC, et al: Smoking and growth rate of small abdominal aortic aneurysms. *Lancet* 344:651–652, 1994.
2. Lederle FA, Wilson SE, Johnson GR, et al: Design of the abdominal aortic aneurysm detection and management study. *J Vasc Surg* 20:296–303, 1994.
3. UK Small Aneurysm Trial, Design, Methods and Progress: The UK small aneurysm trial participants. *Eur J Vasc Endovasc Surg* 9:42–48, 1995.

## Investigation of the Mechanism of Chest Pain in Patients With Angiographically Normal Coronary Arteries Using Transesophageal Dobutamine Stress Echocardiography

Panza JA, Laurienzo JM, Curiel RV, et al (NIH, Bethesda, Md)
*J Am Coll Cardiol* 29:293–301, 1997                    2–50

*Background.*—Approximately 20% of patients with angina-like chest pain, or persistent chest pain after successful angioplasty, have normal cardiac arteriograms. It has been suggested that such patients have a coronary microvascular abnormality that leads to myocardial ischemia and chest pain. However, the research has been inconclusive. This study used stress echocardiography to study whether patients with chest pain and normal coronary arteriograms have myocardial ischemia.

*Methods.*—The subjects were 70 patients (44 women and 26 men; mean age, 49 years) who had normal or near-normal results on cardiac catherization (epicardial coronary stenoses less than 30%) for angina-like chest pain. The mean duration of pain had been 4 years (range 0.5 to 28 years). The patients underwent conventional symptom-limited treadmill exercise testing and transesophageal stress echocardiography with dobutamine infusion. In addition, 62 patients underwent exercise radionuclide angiography and exercise thallium scintigraphy. Their results were compared with those of 26 control subjects.

*Results.*—Infusion of dobutamine provoked angina-like chest pain, similar to that experienced during daily activities, in 59 (84%) patients and none of the control subjects. A similar percentage (80%) of patients developed chest pain during exercise testing. However, even though 31% of patients developed ischemic appearing repolarization changes during exercise testing, no patient developed regional wall motion abnormalities (Fig 2). Radionuclide test results did not correlate with each other or with the presence of repolarization changes during exercise testing.

*Conclusions.*—It is reasonable to assume a cardiac origin of the chest pain in these patients, because chest pain was induced by both exercise and dobutamine infusion. However, it is unlikely that myocardial ischemia was a common cause of the pain, even in patients who developed repolarization abnormalities, because no regional wall motion abnormalities were induced. The absence of left ventricular functional evidence of ischemia supports the theory that abnormal cardiac pain perception is a potential source of chest pain. Dobutamine stress echocardiography may be useful in distinguishing between patients who will benefit from anti-ischemic therapy and those who need treatment for abnormal cardiac nociception.

▶ The occurrence of angina-like chest pain in patients without evidence of constructive CAD, which is often called *syndrome X*, is a puzzling and frequently troublesome clinical entity, although not uncommon. It has been suggested by some that this is because microvascular dysfunction leads to myocardial ischemia as a consequence of an inappropriate vasodilator response to increases in myocardial oxygen demand.[1] This study certainly

# Coronary Artery Disease

**Basal**            **Dobutamine**

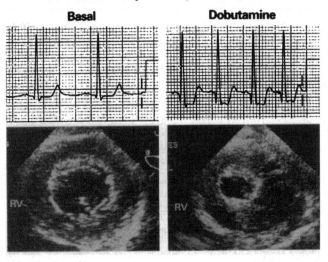

# Chest Pain With Normal Coronary Arteries

**Basal**            **Dobutamine**

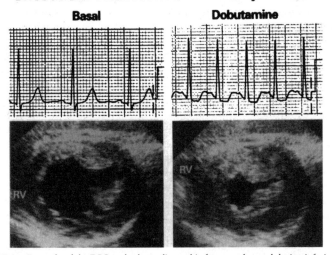

FIGURE 2.—Example of the ECG and echocardiographic features observed during infusion of dobutamine in a patient with CAD (**top**) and a patient with chest pain and normal coronary arteries (**bottom**). For each patient, 1 ECG lead obtained before and during the peak dose of dobutamine is shown in the **top panels**. The **bottom panels** show the end-systolic frames obtained from the short-axis view at baseline and during the infusion of the peak dose of dobutamine. The patient with CAD had significant ST-segment depression with the infusion of dobutamine, which was accompanied by the development of hypokinesia in the interventricular septum. Coronary angiography demonstrated significant stenosis of the left anterior descending coronary artery. The patient with chest pain and normal coronary arteries also developed repolarization abnormalities with dobutamine infusion. However, no regional wall motion abnormalities developed. Instead, there was a homogeneous increase in systolic thickening of all segments (*RV*, Right ventricle). (Courtesy of Panza JA, Laurienzo JM, Curiel RV, et al: Investigation of the mechanism of chest pain in patients with angiographically normal coronary arteries using transesophageal dobutamine stress echocardiography. *J Am Coll Cardiol* 29:293–301, 1997. Reprinted with permission from the American College of Cardiology.)

points in the opposite direction. The provocation of chest pain by dobutamine in the absence of left ventricular functional evidence of myocardial ischemia suggests an alternative hypothesis, which is that syndrome X is a disorder of pain perception, or the so-called sensitive heart syndrome.[2] Clearly, syndrome X is a sobriquet for a number of clinical entities with different pathophysiologic mechanisms resulting in angina-like chest pain with exercise, in the absence of angiographically documented obstructive epicardial CAD. However, documentation of an absence of overt ischemia during dobutamine stress echocardiography may be helpful in identifying patients who probably will not benefit from anti-ischemic therapy but might respond to other drugs such as imipramine, which may alter pain threshold at a central level.[3]

**B.J. Gersh, M.B., Ch.B., D.Phil., F.R.C.P.**

*References*

1. Cannon RO, Camici PG, Epstein SE: Pathophysiological dilemma of Syndrome X. *Circulation* 85:583–592, 1992.
2. Cannon RO, Quyumi AA, Schenke WH, et al: Abnormal cardiac sensitivity in patients with chest pain and normal coronary arteries. *J Am Coll Cardiol* 16:1359–1366, 1990.
3. Cannon RG, Quyumi AA, Mincemoyer R, et al: Imipramine in patients with chest pain and normal coronary angiogram. *N Engl J Med* 330:1411–1417, 1994.

## Inflammation, Aspirin, and the Risk of Cardiovascular Disease in Apparently Healthy Men

Ridker PM, Cushman M, Stampfer MJ, et al (Brigham and Women's Hosp, Boston; Harvard Med School, Boston; Harvard School of Public Health, Boston )
*N Engl J Med* 336:973–979, 1997                              2–51

*Background.*—Both laboratory and pathologic data have suggested that inflammation plays a role in the initiation and progression of atherosclerosis, but little information is available on the role of inflammation in first myocardial infarction, stroke, or venous thrombosis. C-reactive protein is a marker of systemic inflammation. Baseline plasma C-reactive protein concentration was assessed in 1,086 healthy men who participated in the Physicians' Health Study to examine the association between inflammation and the risk of a first cardiovascular event.

*Methods.*—The Physicians' Health Study was a randomized, double-blind, placebo-controlled 2-×-2 factorial trial of aspirin and beta carotene in the primary prevention of cardiovascular disease and cancer. Before randomization, participants were asked to provide baseline blood samples. Each participant who provided an adequate baseline blood sample and had a confirmed myocardial infarction, stroke, or venous thrombosis during at least 8 years of follow-up was matched with 1 control who provided an adequate blood sample and reported no cardiovascular dis-

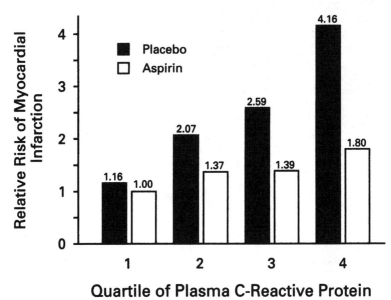

**Quartile of Plasma C-Reactive Protein**

FIGURE 2.—Relative risk of a first myocardial infarction associated with baseline plasma concentrations of C-reactive protein, stratified according to randomized assignment to aspirin or placebo therapy. Analyses are limited to events occurring before the unblinding of the aspirin component of the Physicians' Health Study. The reduction in the risk of myocardial infarction associated with the use of aspirin was 13.9% in the first (lowest) quartile of C-reactive protein values, 33.4% in the second quartile, 46.3% in the third quartile, and 55.7% in the fourth (highest) quartile. (Reprinted by permission of *The New England Journal of Medicine*, from Ridker PM, Cushman M, Stampfer MJ, et al: Inflammation, aspirin, and the risk of cardiovascular disease in apparently healthy men. *N Engl J Med* 336:973–979, 1997. Copyright 1997, Massachusetts Medical Society. All rights reserved.)

ease. Patients and controls were matched for age, smoking status, and length of time since randomization.

*Results.*—Cardiovascular disease developed in 543 participants during the course of the study and these participants were matched with 543 controls. Baseline plasma C-reactive protein levels were higher among men who had a myocardial infarction or ischemic stroke than among men without cardiovascular events or men who had venous thrombosis. The men in the highest C-reactive protein quartile had 3 times the risk of myocardial infarction and 2 times the risk of ischemic stroke as the men in the lowest quartile. This risk was stable over long periods of time, and was independent of smoking, body mass index, blood pressure, and plasma levels of total or high-density lipoprotein cholesterol, triglyceride, lipoprotein(a), tissue plasminogen activator antigen, D-dimer, fibrinogen, or homocysteine. Aspirin intake was associated with significant reductions in the risk of myocardial infarction among men in the highest quartile, but not with significant risk reductions among men in the lowest quartile (Fig 2).

*Conclusions.*—The baseline plasma concentration of C-reactive protein (a marker for inflammation) in healthy men can be used to predict the risk of first myocardial infarction and ischemic stroke, but not of venous thromboembolism, suggesting that the effect of inflammation on vascular risk may be limited to the arterial circulation. The benefits of aspirin ingestion in reducing the risk of a first cardiovascular event were directly related to the level of C-reactive protein. This result not only implicates aspirin's anti-inflammatory activity, as well as its antiplatelet activity, in its beneficial effects on cardiovascular health, but also suggests that other anti-inflammatory agents could play a role in the prevention of cardiovascular disease.

▶ An accumulating mass of experimental evidence supports the concept that inflammation plays a role in both the initiation and progression of atherosclerosis. C-reactive protein is an acute-phase reactant in response to infectious agents, immunologic stimuli, and tissue damage, which is a marker for systemic inflammation, and in this study was independently associated with the risk of myocardial infarction and stroke, but not venous thrombosis. This study on apparently healthy men with favorable risk factor profiles for coronary disease extends prior observations, demonstrating an association between an elevated C-reactive protein level in the serum in patients with acute ischemic syndromes or patients at high risk as a result of cigarette smoking.[1, 2] What is also of interest in this study is that the association was present in both smokers and nonsmokers.

Another fascinating aspect of this study is the association between the use of aspirin and significant reductions in the risk of myocardial infarction among men in the highest quartile of C-reactive protein levels, with only small reductions among those in the lowest quartile. It is traditionally and logically accepted that the powerful effects of aspirin in patients with coronary artery disease are related to its effect on platelet inhibition. These data also suggest the possibility that, in fact, part of the benefit of aspirin may be through its anti-inflammatory action. This also raises the question of whether other anti-inflammatory agents may have a role in preventing cardiovascular disease.[3] In fact, the apparent efficacy of aspirin in acute ischemic syndromes is somewhat surprising, given the fact that there are other pathways of platelet aggregation that are not affected by aspirin. One would not expect aspirin, therefore, to be as powerful as an agent that interferes with the platelet glycoprotein IIb/IIIa receptors. Nonetheless, aspirin is effective, even if from the theoretical standpoint, it is not the "complete antiplatelet agent." Perhaps the explanation lies in the additional anti-inflammatory effect.

In any event, the association between inflammation and atherosclerosis appears to be strengthening, and this study suggests that the effects are stable over long periods, as opposed to a short-term action on clotting factors alone. Whether the inflammation will be found to be caused by an infectious agent such as *Chlamydia, Helicobacter,* or cytomegalovirus, or whether C-reactive protein is a surrogate for other cytokines that can cause inflammation, remains to be seen. Should C-reactive protein levels be measured in high-risk patients, based upon the results of this study? Certainly not—this remains an area of investigation and not clinical practice at this stage.

B.J. Gersh, M.B., Ch.B., D.Phil., F.R.C.P.

References

1. Liuzzo G, Biasucci LM, Gallimore JR, et al: Prognostic value of C-reactive protein in serum amyloid A-protein in severe unstable angina. N Engl J Med 331:417–424, 1994.
2. Kuller LH, Tracy RP, Shaten J, et al: Relation of C-reactive protein in coronary heart disease in the MRSIT Case-Control Study. Am J Epidemiol 144:537–547, 1996.
3. Vane J: The evolution of non-steroidal anti-inflammatory drugs and their mechanisms of action. Drugs 33:185–275, 1997.

## Propafenone During Acute Myocardial Ischemia in Patients: A Double-blind, Randomized, Placebo-controlled Study

Faber TS, Zehender M, Krahnefeld O, et al (Universitätsklinik Freiburg, Germany; Universitätsklinik Hamburg, Germany)
J Am Coll Cardiol 29:561–567, 1997                                     2–52

*Introduction.*—When used in patients with coronary artery disease, class I antiarrhythmic agents have been recognized as increasing the risk of sudden cardiac death. The effect of class Ic antiarrhythmic activity in association with myocardial ischemia is still unknown. QT interval dispersion may be a noninvasive marker of inhomogeneous ventricular repolarization and susceptibility to ventricular arrhythmias. Little is known, however, about the effects of the combination of antiarrhythmic agents and myocardial ischemia. The effect of acute myocardial ischemia on ventricular repolarization dispersion (QT dispersion) on the surface ECG was assessed in patients pretreated with either propafenone or placebo before percutaneous transluminal coronary angioplasty.

*Methods.*—There were 98 patients undergoing percutaneous transluminal coronary angioplasty who were treated with placebo or propafenone in a randomized, double-blind study. The definition of QT dispersion was maximal minus minimal QT interval on the 12-lead ECG before and after percutaneous transluminal coronary angioplasty.

*Results.*—During occlusion of the left anterior descending coronary artery, the QT interval increased by 9% and the corrected QT interval increased by 11%. There was no effect with occlusion of the circumflex and right coronary arteries. In the propafenone group during ischemia, corrected QT dispersion increased by a significant 52% (Fig 2). During left anterior descending coronary artery occlusion and ischemia of the anterior wall, the most considerable effect on QT dispersion was seen, with an increase of 74%. The results were not influenced by plasma levels of propafenone which were 522 ±165 µg/L.

*Conclusion.*—A significant increase in QT dispersion resulted with propafenone during myocardial ischemia, particularly during left anterior

QTc duration in msec

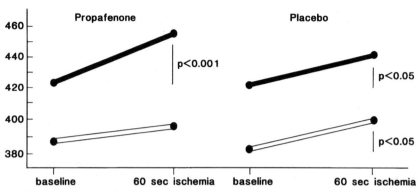

FIGURE 2.—Maximal (*solid lines*) and minimal (*open lines*) corrected QT duration in patients treated with either propafenone or placebo at baseline and after 60 seconds of myocardial ischemia. There was no difference in minimal corrected QT duration, but a significant increase in corrected QT maximal duration, in patients pretreated with propafenone. (Reprinted by permission of the American College of Cardiology from Faber TS, Zehender M, Krahnefeld O, et al: Propafenone during acute myocardial ischemia in patients: A double-blind, randomized, placebo-controlled study. *J Am Coll Cardiol* 29:561–567, 1997.)

descending coronary artery occlusion. Inhomogeneous ventricular repolarization generated by the ischemic anterior wall of the myocardium is reflected by QT interval prolongation and enhanced QT dispersion. Myocardial ischemia, repolarization variables, and propafenone may have clinically important interactions.

▶ The link between class I antiarrhythmic agents, proarrhythmia, and sudden cardiac death is well-established.[1, 2] It has been suggested that the proarrhythmic effects of the drug may be enhanced in the setting of ischemia, which by increasing the degree of conduction delay may increase the heterogeneity of the repolarization process, leading to reentrant ventricular arrhythmias.[3]

QT interval dispersion has been suggested as a noninvasive marker of inhomogeneous ventricular repolarization.[4] This randomized study quite convincingly demonstrates that ischemia in the distribution of the left anterior descending coronary artery increases QT dispersion, and this is enhanced by propafenone. This is the first study to provide clinical data on the effects of class Ic antiarrhythmic agents in patients with ischemic episodes, and strongly suggests that the antiarrhythmic drug in the setting of ischemia enhances the heterogeneity of ventricular repolarization. These observations certainly support a clinically significant interaction between myocardial ischemia, repolarization, and antiarrhythmic agents.

**B.J. Gersh, M.B., Ch.B., D.Phil., F.R.C.P.**

*References*

1. Cardiac Arrhythmia Suppression Trial (CAST) Investigators: Preliminary Report: Effect of encainide and flecainide on mortality in a randomized trial of arrhythmias suppression after myocardial infarction. *N Engl J Med* 321:406–412, 1989.
2. Belbit B, Podrid P, Lowen B, et al: Aggravation and provocation of ventricular arrhythmias by antiarrhythmic drugs. *Circulation* 65:886–894, 1982.
3. Nattel S, Pedersen DH, Zipes DP: Alterations in regional myocardial distribution and arrhythmogenic effects of aprindine produced by coronary artery occlusion in the dog. *Cardiovasc Res* 15:80–85, 1989.
4. Higham PD, Furniss SS, Campbell, RWF: QT dispersion and components of the QT interval on ischemia and infarction. *Br Heart J* 73:32–36, 1995.

**Population-based Analysis of the Effect of the Northridge Earthquake on Cardiac Death in Los Angeles County, California**

Kloner RA, Leor J, Poole WK, et al (Univ of Southern California, Los Angeles; Ben-Gurion Univ of the Neger, Beer-Sheva, Israel; Research Triangle Inst, Research Triangle Park, NC)

*J Am Coll Cardiol* 30:1174–1180, 1997                                                        2–53

*Introduction.*—Reports from the Los Angeles Coroner's Office and coronary care units suggest that the Northridge earthquake (NEQ) of January 17, 1994 increased the number of myocardial infarctions and cases of sudden cardiac death in the area. The effect of the NEQ on the number of deaths caused by cardiovascular disease, both on the day of the earthquake and during the weeks after the event, was determined by analyzing all deaths in the entire population of Los Angeles County.

*Methods.*—Daily death certificate data for January 1994 were analyzed, together with similar data for the control periods of January 1992 and January 1993. Cases of ischemic heart disease (IHD) and atherosclerotic cardiovascular disease (ASCVD), as well as other causes of death, were sought using the International Classification of Diseases, 9th Revision, codes.

*Results.*—During the 3 January periods (1992, 1993, and 1994), the total number of deaths reported in Los Angeles County were 6,689, 5,995, and 6,933, respectively. The total number of deaths caused by IHD and ASCVD during these periods were 2,089 for January 1992, 1,886 for January 1993, and 2,094 for January 1994. From January 1 to January 16, 1974, an average of 73 deaths per day were caused by IHD and ASCVD. On the day of the NEQ, however, 125 deaths were attributed to these causes (Fig 2). The average number of cardiac deaths per day decreased to 57 for the remainder of January 1994. A geographic analysis of data showed a redistribution of IHD–ASCVD-related deaths toward the epicenter on the day of the NEQ. The age and sex trends in IHD–ASCVD-related deaths on the earthquake day did not differ from those reported during the weeks before and after the earthquake.

*Conclusion.*—The major stress of the NEQ increased the number of deaths caused by IHD and ASCVD throughout Los Angeles County. This

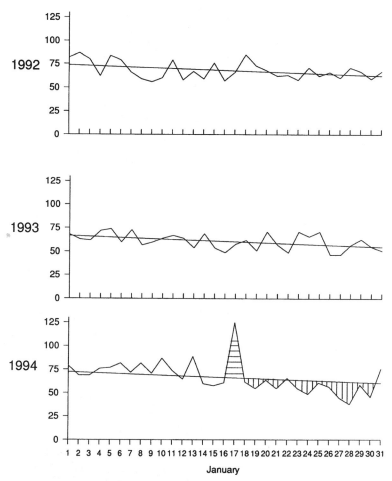

**FIGURE 2.**—Daily deaths in Los Angeles County caused by IHD and ASCVD during January of 1992, 1993 (control periods), and 1994. There was an increase in these deaths on the day of the NEQ (January 17, 1994), followed by a decrease during a 2-week period and eventual recovery. During the 2 weeks after the NEQ, there was a decrease in deaths caused by IHD and ASCVD, which overcompensated for the increase on the day of the NEQ. The *horizontal bars* represent the excess number of deaths on the day of the NEQ. The *vertical bars* represent the decrease in deaths during the 14 days after the NEQ. *Abbreviations: NEQ,* Northridge earthquake; *IHD,* ischemic heart disease; *ASCVD,* atherosclerotic cardiovascular disease. (Reprinted with permission from the American College of Cardiology from Kloner RA, Leor J, Poole WK, et al: Population-based analysis of the effect of the Northridge earthquake on cardiac death in Los Angeles County, California. *J Am Coll Cardiol* 30:1174–1180, 1997.)

increase was followed by a significant decrease in the last 2 weeks of January 1994, which is an effect that may represent a possible preconditioning effect of stress or a population that is more resistant to stress or both.

▶ This fascinating paper complements a prior study that documented an increase in death caused by ASCVD and sudden cardiac death on the day of the NEQ in Los Angeles.[1] In this population based study, the decrease in deaths during the subsequent 2 weeks, which overcompensated for the increase on the day of the earthquake, is intriguing. The authors speculate on the mechanisms, including the possibility that stress may have preconditioned the population. Preconditioning because of periods of brief ischemia, catecholamines, or other illnesses has been shown in experimental and clinical studies to be cardioprotective.[2] This and other studies from Greece and Japan suggest that emotional and physical stress in response to natural disasters and other events can precipitate acute myocardial infarction and sudden cardiac death.[3]

**B.J. Gersh, M.B., Ch.B., D.Phil., F.R.C.P.**

*References*

1. Leor J, Poole WK, Kloner RA: Sudden cardiac death triggered by an earthquake. *N Engl J Med* 34:413–419, 1996.
2. Kloner RA, Shook T, Przyklenk K, for TIMI 4 Investigators: Previous angina alters in-hospital outcome in TIMI 4: A clinical correlate to preconditioning? *Circulation* 91:37–45, 1995.
3. Muller JE, Abela GS, Nesto GH, et al: Triggers, acute risk factors and vulnerable plaques: The lexicon of a new frontier. *J Am Coll Cardiol* 23:809–813, 1994.

---

**Hormonal Therapy Increases Arterial Compliance in Postmenopausal Women**
Rajkumar C, Kingwell BA, Cameron JD, et al (Baker Med Research Inst, Prahran, Australia; Latrobe Univ, Melbourne, Australia)
*J Am Coll Cardiol* 30:350–356, 1997                                      2–54

---

*Introduction.*—In reducing the incidence of coronary heart disease and possibly stroke, postmenopausal use of estrogen-containing hormonal therapy appears to be beneficial. Significantly lower death rates are also found among postmenopausal women taking estrogens when compared to age-matched controls who did not take hormonal therapy. In both men and women, arterial stiffness, determined by pulse wave velocity, increases with age. The increase in arterial stiffness may be partially reversed with long-term treatment with estrogen-containing hormonal therapy. The capacity of long-term treatment with estrogen-containing therapy to influence the age-related decrease in arterial compliance in postmenopausal women was investigated.

*Methods.*—In 26 premenopausal women and in 52 postmenopausal women, 26 of whom were taking hormonal therapy, total systemic arterial compliance and pulse wave velocity were determined.

*Results.*—In the premenopausal group, arterial compliance was greater (0.57 ± 0.04 arbitrary compliance units) than in the postmenopausal group not taking hormonal therapy (0.26 ± 0.02 arbitrary compliance units). A significantly increased systemic arterial compliance was found in postmenopausal women taking hormonal therapy (0.43 ± 0.02 arbitrary

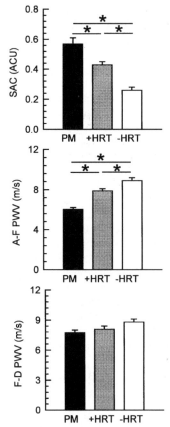

**FIGURE 1.**—Systemic arterial compliance and pulse wave velocity in premenopausal women (PM) and postmenopausal women with (+HRT) and without hormonal therapy (−HRT). *Abbreviations: A-F PNV,* pulse wave velocity over the aortofemoral region; *F-D PWV,* pulse wave velocity over the femorodorsalis pedis region; *SAC,* systemic arterial compliance. Data shown are mean value ± SEM. *Significant differences (*P* < 0.05). (Reprinted with permission from the American College of Cardiology, from Rajkumar C, Kingwell BA, Cameron JD, et al: Hormonal therapy increases arterial compliance in postmenopausal women. *J Am Coll Cardiol* 30:350–356, 1997.)

compliance units) compared to women not taking hormonal therapy (0.26 ± 0.02 arbitrary compliance units) (Fig 1). In the premenopausal women, the pulse wave velocity in the aortofemoral region was 6.0 ± 0.2 m/sec compared to untreated postmenopausal women, who had a pulse velocity of 8.9 ± 0.3 m/sec. A significantly lower pulse wave velocity was seen in postmenopausal women taking hormonal therapy (7.9 ± 0.2 m/sec) compared to women not taking hormonal therapy (8.9 ± 0.3 m/sec). For 4 weeks, 11 postmenopausal women had their hormone replacement therapy withdrawn, which resulted in a significant increase in aortofemoral pulse wave velocity and a significant decrease in systemic arterial compliance.

*Conclusion.*—Stiffness of the aorta and large arteries may be decreased in postmenopausal women receiving hormonal therapy, as evidenced by the increased systemic arterial compliance and decreased pulse wave velocity, with potential benefit for age-related cardiovascular disorder. Hormonal therapy appears to alter the reduction of arterial compliance with age.

▶ There is increasing evidence that the postmenopausal use of estrogen-containing hormonal therapy is beneficial in reducing the incidence of coronary heart disease and possibly stroke, and that estrogens have beneficial effects upon lipoprotein profiles.[1-3] It has been suggested, however, that the changes in the lipoprotein levels account for only 25% to 50% of the observed risk reduction in cardiovascular mortality[4] and that additional factors may be involved. The data from this study support others suggesting that estrogens exert a direct effect on the vasculature, and it has been previously established that pulse pressure, which is a surrogate measure of arterial stiffness and compliance, is an independent predictor of future events.[5] The mechanisms for the beneficial effects of sex hormones on the properties of the arterial wall are not well understood, but one explanation may be that estrogen causes vasodilation, mediated through endothelium-dependent nitric oxide and that dilation in turn may affect arterial compliance, both acutely and through long-term structural adaptative mechanisms.

As we await the results of large placebo-controlled trials that will take into account not only the benefits, but also the risks of estrogen therapy, it is appropriate to continue to evaluate the mechanisms, and this particular effect of estrogens on arterial compliance should be easily validated by a small, controlled, randomized trial.

**B.J. Gersh, M.B., Ch.B., D.Phil., F.R.C.P.**

*References*

1. Martin KA, Freeman MW: Post menopausal hormone replacement therapy. *N Engl J Med* 328:1115–1117, 1993.
2. Paganini-Hill A, Ross RA, Henderson BE: Post menopausal oestrogen treatment and stroke: A prospective study. *BMJ* 297:519–522, 1988.
3. Wahl P, Walden C, Knopp R, et al: Effects of estrogen/progestin potency on lipid/ lipoprotein cholesterol. *N Engl J Med* 308:862–867, 1983.
4. Bush TR, Barrett-Connor E, Cowen LD, et al: Cardiovascular mortality in non-contraceptive use of estrogen in women: Results from the Lipid Research Clinic's Program Follow-up Study. *Circulation* 75:1102–1109, 1987.
5. Madhavan S, Ooi WL, Cohen H, et al: Relation of pulse pressure and blood pressure reduction to the incidence of myocardial infarction. *Hypertension* 3:395–401, 1994.

**Attenuation of Severity of Myocardial Ischemia During Repeated Daily Ischemic Episodes**
Tzivoni D, Maybaum S (Shaare Zedek Med Ctr, Jerusalem, Israel)
*J Am Coll Cardiol* 30:119–124, 1997                                    2–55

*Introduction.*—A worse prognosis is found in patients with coronary artery disease who have frequent ischemic episodes than those without such episodes. Some have suggested that repeated ischemia adversely affects prognosis, whereas others have suggested that repeated ischemia may confer myocardial protection from further ischemia, which was termed "preconditioning" in previous animal studies. Few studies in humans have been conducted on the outcomes of preconditioning. Whether severity of myocardial ischemia would be attenuated in patients with repeated and adjacent ischemic episodes was investigated.

*Methods.*—On 3 consecutive occasions, 21 patients with known coronary artery disease and ischemia on exercise testing and ambulatory ECG monitoring walked a distance known to have previously caused myocardial ischemia. The patients walked for about 15 minutes and then had 5 minutes of rest.

*Results.*—During the 3 walks, the mean maximal heart rate was similar. There was a decrease in mean maximal ST-segment depression from the first walk at 2.21 mm to the second walk at 1.61 mm and the third walk at 1.43 mm. There was also a decrease in ischemia duration from the first

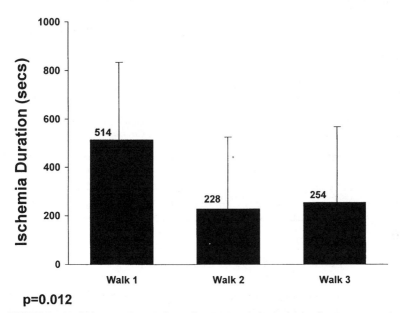

p=0.012

FIGURE 2.—Marked attenuation in ischemia duration is seen during the 3 walks. Data are presented as mean value ± 1 SD. (Reprinted with permission from the American College of Cardiology, from Tzivoni D, Maybaum S: Attenuation of severity of myocardial ischemia during repeated daily ischemic episodes. *J Am Coll Cardiol* 30:119–124, 1997.)

walk by 514 seconds to 228 seconds during the second walk and 254 seconds during the third walk, representing a 56% decrease (Fig 2). On the first walk, the heart rate at onset of ischemia (ischemic threshold) increased from 99 beats/min to 101 beats/min at the second walk and to 106 beats/minute on the third walk.

*Conclusion.*—In patients with repeated and adjacent ischemic episodes, there was attenuation of myocardial ischemia with an associated increase in ischemic threshold. During ordinary activity, this form of myocardial protection is likely to be found and may represent the clinical counterpart of myocardial preconditioning.

▶ The phenomenon of ischemic preconditioning, both early and late, is well documented in animals and to a lesser extent in humans.[1, 2] There is some evidence to suggest that this mechanism may reduce infarct size after coronary occlusion and reperfusion, protect against ischemia-induced arrhythmias, and enhance the recovery of contractile functioning after ischemia. Whatever the mechanism, several studies have suggested that antecedent angina may result in an improved outcome after myocardial infarction.[3] The current study, using ambulatory ECG monitoring, implies that ischemic preconditioning may be the pathophysiologic basis for the clinical phenomena of "walk-through or warm-up" angina. This particular study cannot exclude that the recruitment of collaterals or a local vascular adaptation was the explanation, although the experimental data suggest that local metabolic protective mechanisms provide the most plausible explanation.

**B.J. Gersh, M.B., Ch.B., D.Phil., F.R.C.P.**

*References*

1. Murry CE, Richard BJ, Jennings RV, et al: Myocardial protection is lost before contractile function recovers from ischemic preconditioning. *Am J Physiol* 260:H796–804, 1991.
2. Deutch E, Berger M, Kussman WG, et al: Adaptation to ischemia during PTCA: Clinical, hemodynamic and metabolic features. *Circulation* 82:2044–2051, 1990.
3. Kloner RA, Shook T, Prizyklenk K, et al: Previous angina alters in-hospital outcome in TIMI-IV. A clinical correlate to preconditioning? *Circulation* 91:37–45, 1995.

---

**Age-specific Incidence Rates of Myocardial Infarction and Angina in Women With Systemic Lupus Erythematosus: Comparison With the Framingham Study**
Manzi S, Meilahn EN, Rairie JE, et al (Univ of Pittsburgh, Pa; Boston Univ)
*Am J Epidemiol* 145:408–415, 1997                                    2–56

*Background.*—Several conditions appear to increase the risk of cardiovascular events in premenopausal women. The age-specific incidence rates of myocardial infarction and angina pectoris in a large number of women with systemic lupus erythematosus (SLE) were determined.

TABLE 2.—Incidence Rates of Cardiovascular Events per 1,000 Person-years in the 498 Women With Systemic Lupus Erythematosus, University of Pittsburgh, and 2,208 Women, Framingham Offspring Heart Study, 1980–1993

| Age (years) | SLE Rate | SLE 95% CI | Framingham Rate | Framingham 95% CI | Rate ratio | 95% CI |
|---|---|---|---|---|---|---|
| | | | *Myocardial infarction* | | | |
| 15–24 | 6.33 | 0.2–35.3 | 0.00 | 0.0–11.8 | ∞ | |
| 25–34 | 3.66 | 0.8–10.7 | 0.00 | 0.0–1.2 | ∞ | |
| 35–44 | 8.39 | 4.2–15.0 | 0.16 | 0.0–0.9 | 52.43 | 21.6–98.5 |
| 45–54 | 4.82 | 1.0–14.1 | 1.95 | 0.9–3.6 | 2.47 | 0.8–6.0 |
| 55–64 | 8.38 | 1.7–24.5 | 1.99 | 0.6–4.6 | 4.21 | 1.7–7.9 |
| 65–74 | 7.94 | 1.0–28.7 | 0.00 | 0.0–17.1 | ∞ | |
| | | | *Angina* | | | |
| 15–24 | 0.00 | 0.0–23.4 | 0.00 | 0.0–11.8 | ∞ | |
| 25–34 | 1.22 | 0.0–6.8 | 0.62 | 0.1–2.3 | 1.96 | 0.0–9.0 |
| 35–44 | 1.53 | 0.2–5.5 | 0.65 | 0.2–1.7 | 2.35 | 0.4–11.1 |
| 45–54 | 1.61 | 0.0–8.9 | 1.56 | 0.7–3.1 | 1.03 | 0.2–4.6 |
| 55–64 | 5.59 | 0.7–20.2 | 2.39 | 0.9–5.2 | 2.33 | 0.9–5.5 |
| 65–74 | 15.87 | 4.3–40.6 | 0.00 | 0.0–17.1 | ∞ | |

*Abbreviations: SLE, systemic lupus erythematosus; CI, confidence interval.*
(Courtesy of Manzi S, Meilahn EN, Rairie JE, et al: Age-specific incidence rates of myocardial infarction and angina in women with systemic lupus erythematosus: Comparison with the Framingham Study. *Am J Epidemiol* 145:408–415, 1997.)

*Methods.*—Four hundred ninety-eight women with SLE seen at 1 center between 1980 and 1993 were included in the study. Cardiovascular event rates in this group were compared with those occurring among 2,208 women without SLE of similar age during the same period.

*Findings.*—Thirty-three first events occurred among the women with SLE after the diagnosis of lupus. There were 11 cases of myocardial infarction, 10 of angina pectoris, and 12 of both. Two thirds of the women were younger than 55 years at the time of these events. Women with SLE aged 35–44 years were more than 50 times more likely to have a myocardial infarction than women in that age group but without SLE. Compared to women with SLE who did not have an event, those with SLE who did have such an event were older at the time of their lupus diagnosis, had a longer duration of disease and of corticosteroid use, and were more likely to have hypercholesterolemia and to be postmenopausal (Table 2).

*Conclusions.*—Premature cardiovascular disease is much more common in premenopausal women with SLE than in unaffected women of similar age. Because improved treatment has increased the life expectancy of patients with SLE, cardiovascular disease has become a significant threat to the health of these patients.

▶ The frequency of cardiovascular disease among women with systemic lupus erythematosus is well documented,[1] but what is quite striking in this case-control study, is the high event rate among women younger than 55 years, the majority of whom were younger than 45 years.

The pathophysiology of coronary artery disease in lupus is likely multifactorial. Inflammation in the development of atherosclerosis in the general population is a highly topical subject at present and, although an inflammatory, coronary vasculitis occurs in lupus, it is not common. Nonetheless, an interaction between inflammatory mediators and thrombosis by antiphospholipid antibodies, causing vascular injury and thrombosis in patients with lupus, is certainly plausible. Other factors include concomitant hypertension and renal disease and the effects of steroids, either directly upon the atherosclerotic disease process or via risk factors such as hyperlipidemia, hyperglycemia, hypertension or obesity.[2]

As the improved therapy of lupus increases life expectancy from this disease, the impact of premature cardiac disease and the need for vigorous control of risk factors warrant careful attention.

**B.J. Gersh, M.B., Ch.B., D.Phil., F.R.C.P.**

*References*

1. Petri M, Perez-Gutthann S, Spence D, et al: Risk factors for coronary artery disease in patients with systemic lupus erythematosus. *Am J Med* 93:513–519, 1992.
2. Barkely HB, Roberts WC: The heart in systemic lupus erythematosus and the changes induced in it by corticosteroid therapy. *Am J Med* 58:243–264, 1975.

## Miscellaneous

### Endoluminal Stent-Grafts for Infrarenal Abdominal Aortic Aneurysms
Blum U, Voshage G, Lammer J, et al (Univ Hosp, Freiburg, Germany; Henriettenstiftung, Hannover, Germany; Univ Hosp, Vienna)
*N Engl J Med* 336:13–20, 1997                                    2–57

*Introduction.*—Mortality rate is high with surgical management of aortic aneurysms. One promising alternative is the use of endovascular stents or stent-graft prostheses. The short- and mid-term results of stent-grafting for infrarenal abdominal aortic aneurysms using stents made of nitinol and covered with polyester fabric are reported.

*Methods.*—The study included 154 patients with infrarenal abdominal aortic aneurysms who were referred to 1 of 3 hospitals. There were 150 men and 4 women, mean age 68 years. One hundred thirty-three patients had aortic aneurysms involving the bifurcation and common iliac arteries; they received bifurcated stent grafts. The other 21 patients did not have aneurysmal involvement of the aortic bifurcation, and they received straight stent-grafts. The polyester-covered nitinol endoprostheses were placed through a unilateral surgical arteriotomy of the femoral artery under fluoroscopic guidance. Each patient underwent follow-up computed tomography and intraarterial angiography at an average of 12.5 months after the procedure. Primary success was defined as complete exclusion of the abdominal aortic aneurysm.

*Results.*—Primary success rates were 87% in the patients receiving bifurcated grafts and 86% in those receiving straight grafts. Conversion to open surgery was necessary in 3 patients. The complication rate was 10%; there were 3 major procedure-related complications, including 1 death. A postimplantation syndrome was noted in all patients, including leukocytosis and increased C-reactive protein levels.

*Conclusions.*—Endovascular stent-graft placement can achieve a high success rate in patients with infrarenal abdominal aortic aneurysms, preliminary results suggest. This approach may offer an effective and safe alternative to conventional surgical repair, particularly for patients at high surgical risk. The authors call for a prospective, randomized trial of endoluminal vs. surgical repair.

► What a way to start the year! This study of 154 patients is the largest reported to date, and only one trial of endovascular stenting has been initiated in the United States.[1] The potential for the noninvasive treatment of aortic aneurysms is of course extraordinarily exciting and opens up a multitude of options, particularly among the elderly. Nonetheless, this remains an experimental technique at present, with a significant morbidity rate, primarily from emboli reported in this and other series. The follow-up on all reports to date has been relatively short at 13–17 months.[2] As pointed out in an editorial, the long-term integrity of the endovascular stent and its site of attachment is crucial to the success of this approach.[3] What would also be emphasized is that late mortality rate in patients with peripheral vascular disease is from cardiac causes in the majority, and in such patients the presence of peripheral vascular disease should be considered a marker for high-risk coronary artery disease, which is either already present or likely to develop in the future.[4] Whatever the caveats, the future is promising indeed.

**B.J. Gersh, M.B., Ch.B., D.Phil., F.R.C.P.**

*References*

1. Moore SS, Rutherford RB: Transfemoral endovascular repair of abdominal aortic aneurysm: results of the north American NAEVT phase I trial. *J Vasc Surg* 23:543–553, 1996.
2. Parodi JC: Endovascular repair of abdominal aortic aneurysms and other arterial lesions. *J Vasc Surg* 21:549–557, 1995.
3. Ernst CB: Current therapy for infrarenal aortic aneurysms [editorial]. *N Engl J Med* 336:59–60, 1996.
4. Gersh BJ, Rihal CS, Rooke TW, et al. Evaluation and management of patients with both peripheral vascular and coronary artery disease. *JACC* 18:203–214, 1991.

---

**Acute Ischaemia: A Dynamic Influence on QT Dispersion**
Sporton SC, Taggart P, Sutton PM, et al (UCL Hosps, London)
*Lancet* 349:306–309, 1997                                        2–58

---

*Objective.*—The term QT dispersion refers to the range of QT intervals across the 12-lead electrocardiogram. It has been suggested that increased dispersion of electrical activity after activation is a major contributor to the development of ischemia-related arrhythmias. The effects of acute myocardial ischemia on QT dispersion were evaluated.

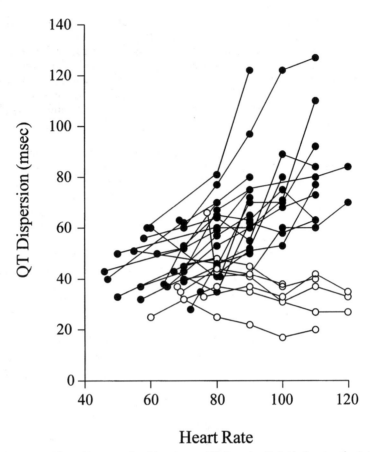

**FIGURE 1.**—Effect of incremental atrial pacing on QT dispersion (individual patient data). *Closed circles,* coronary artery disease; *open circles,* normal coronary arteries. (Courtesy of Sporton SC, Taggart P, Sutton PM, et al: Acute ischaemia: a dynamic influence on QT dispersion. *Lancet* 349:306–309, 1997. Copyright by The Lancet Ltd.)

*Methods.*—The study included 18 patients with coronary artery disease and 6 normal controls. Each subject underwent coronary catheterization, during which mild myocardial ischemia was induced by incremental atrial pacing. The ischemia was intended to be similar to that encountered by patients with coronary artery disease during their everyday activities. Its effects on QT dispersion were measured.

*Results.*—In the patients with coronary artery disease, induced ischemia was accompanied by angina or ST depression. They also had a marked increase in QT dispersion, with a mean of 38 msec. The alteration in QT dispersion was correlated with the patients' extent of coronary artery disease. The controls had no symptoms, no ST changes, and no significant change in QT dispersion (Fig 1). Baseline QT dispersion was similar in the 2 groups: 44 msec in patients with coronary artery disease and 40 msec in controls.

*Conclusions.*—In patients with coronary artery disease, inducing mild myocardial ischemia by incremental atrial pacing produces an acute increase in QT dispersion. No such effect is noted in controls with normal coronary arteries. For diagnostic purposes, "inducible" QT dispersion may be a better indicator of arrhythmia risk than resting QT dispersion.

▶ Experimental work has demonstrated that the increased dispersion of electrical recovery after activation is a key factor in the genesis of arrhthymias in response to ischemia.[1] There are also extensive epidemiologic, morphologic, and clinical data that suggest that a substantial proportion of sudden cardiac deaths is ischemic in nature, even in the absence of acute myocardial infarction. A study using QT dispersion as a marker of homogeneity or inhomogeneity of electrical recovery suggests that ischemia does indeed result in a dynamic increase in QT dispersion in patients with otherwise stable coronary artery disease and no prior myocardial infarction.

Although there is little doubt that ischemia causes serious or fatal ventricular arrhythmias in a substantial proportion of patients, it is a case of the "glass being half empty or half full." It would appear that in another equally sizable proportion of patients with sudden cardiac death (perhaps the majority), there is no evidence of an acute ischemic event as the causal mechanism. The postulate is that ventricular fibrillation was the result of a sustained ventricular tachycardia degenerating into ventricular fibrillation, but that the original ventricular tachycardia emanates from a fixed substrate (a mixture of scar and viable tissue).

Clinically, the issue is important in that among some survivors of a cardiac arrest or sudden cardiac death from an acute ischemic cause, revascularization alone should suffice without the need for additional antiarrhthymic therapy or the implantation of a device. Unfortunately, such patients are a minority, perhaps only 10% to 15% of all survivors of sudden cardiac death. In my practice, revascularization alone is confined to patients with single-vessel disease, a clear culprit lesion, normal left ventricular function without any regional wall motion abnormalities, and an unequivocal history of an acute ischemic event preceding the cardiac arrest. For the remainder who require revascularization, implantation of an implantable cardioverter defibrillator is the norm.

**B.J. Gersh, M.B., Ch.B., D.Phil., F.R.C.P.**

*Reference*

1. Janse MJ, Wit AL: Electrophysiological mechanisms of ventricular arrhythmias resulting from myocardial ischemia and infarction. *Physiol Rev* 69:1049–1069, 1989.

### Sex and Test Verification Bias: Impact on the Diagnostic Value of Exercise Echocardiography

Roger VL, Pellikka PA, Bell MR, et al (Mayo Clinic, Rochester, Minn)
Circulation 95:405–410, 1997                    2–59

*Introduction.*—Exercise echocardiography has been validated as a diagnostic test for coronary artery disease (CAD). However, its use in clinical practice has not been documented, including its use in women vs. men. The effects of sex and test verification bias on the diagnostic value of exercise echocardiography were investigated.

*Methods.*—The analysis included 3,679 consecutive patients undergoing exercise echocardiography, all entered into a prospective database. The patients included 1,965 men and 1,714 women. Angiography was performed in 340 of these patients—244 men and 96 women—permitting calculation of the sensitivity, specificity, and correct classification rate of exercise echocardiography. Data on the entire group were used to estimate the effects of test verification bias, sensitivity, and specificity.

*Results.*—Angiography revealed an 80% prevalence of CAD in men and a 60% prevalence in women. Exercise echocardiography had a 78% sensitivity in men and a 79% sensitivity in women. Specificity values were 44% and 37%, respectively. The correct classification rate was 71% in men and 63% in women (Table 4). Sensitivity dropped to 42% in men vs. 32% in women after adjustment for test verification bias. This difference was significant, although there was no difference in "debiased" specificity. Positive predictive value was 84% in men vs. 66% in women. The main source of test verification bias was the tendency to refer patients with a positive echocardiogram result to angiography. The rate of referral to angiography after a positive exercise echocardiogram result was 27% in men vs. 19% in women.

*Conclusions.*—In clinical use of exercise echocardiography, specificity decreases and sensitivity increases as a result of test verification bias. This test has lower positive predictive value and adjusted sensitivity in women than in men. Referral to angiography differs between the sexes, although

TABLE 4.—Results of Exercise Echocardiography in Relation to the Results of Coronary Angiography

| Coronary Angiography | Exercise Echocardiography | |
| --- | --- | --- |
| | − | + |
| Women (n=96) | | |
| − | 14 | 24 |
| + | 12 | 46 |
| Men (n=96) | | |
| − | 22 | 28 |
| + | 43 | 151 |

no assessment of appropriateness of care can be made with the current data. The results are consistent with previous studies showing a reduced sensitivity of stress test modalities in women.

▶ This is one of the best of many papers comparing the predictive accuracy of noninvasive stress testing for coronary artery disease between men and women. The unique aspect of this study is the attempt to take into account the phenomenon of "verification bias," which in this situation leads to a higher proportion of patients with a positive stress test result being referred to angiography (the verification test). Although this is clinically appropriate, it does introduce a statistical bias that markedly increases the sensitivity and reduces the specificity of any given test.[1] In this study, the lower yield and lower positive predictive value of exercise echocardiography in women compared with men is not surprising. This finding is consistent with a lower prevalence and a lesser severity of coronary artery disease compared with men in addition to intrinsic test performance.[2]

What is more disturbing and less explicable is the lower sensitivity in women, although this has been noted in other studies of different stress testing modalities.[3] Potential explanations include differences in the severity and presence of multivessel disease between men and women, different levels of maximum exercise capacity, and perhaps differences in the physiologic consequences of coronary artery disease.

**B.J. Gersh, M.B., Ch.B., D.Phil., F.R.C.P.**

*References*

1. Diamond GA: Reverend Bayes' silent majority: an alternative factor affecting sensitivity and specificity of exercise electrocardiography. *Am J Cardiol* 57:1175–1180, 1986.
2. Weiner DA, Ryan TJ, McCabe CH, et al: Exercise stress testing: correlations among history of angina, ST segment response and prevalence of coronary artery disease and the Coronary Artery Surgery Study (CASS). *N Engl J Med* 301:230–235, 1979.
3. Kong BA, Shore L, Miller DD, et al: Comparison of accuracy for detecting coronary artery disease and side-effect profile of dipyridmole-thallium-201 myocardial perfusion imaging in women versus men. *Am J Cardiol* 70:168–173, 1992.

## Ischemia During Ambulatory Monitoring as a Prognostic Indicator in Patients With Stable Coronary Artery Disease

Mulcahy D, Husain S, Zalos G, et al (NIH, Bethesda, Md)
*JAMA* 277:318–324, 1997                                                   2–60

*Background.*—Previous research has shown that in patients with stable coronary artery disease (CAD), transient ischemia rarely occurs in those patients with a negative exercise test; whereas it occurs in more than half of patients with a positive exercise test and is more likely to occur in patients with more severe CAD or normal left ventricular function. This study was designed to assess the prognostic significance of transient ischemia in patients with stable angina and the relationship between coronary lesions that cause ischemia and those that are responsible for acute cardiac events.

*Methods.*—Of 450 patients who underwent ambulatory ST segment monitoring over a 7-year period, 221 with documented CAD were entered in the study. All underwent exercise testing and ventriculography. Of these, 32 were classified as high risk, and 189 were classified as low risk. Patients were classified as low risk if they were asymptomatic or mildly symptomatic and had (1) single-vessel disease; (2) 2-vessel disease with a negative exercise test, left ventricular ejection fraction (LVEF) ≥40%, or both; or (3) 3-vessel disease with negative exercise test and LVEF ≥40%. All patients (or their families or physicians) were contacted after 6 to 84 months (mean, 52 months) and questioned about present symptoms, medications, and history of hospital admissions and coronary angiography.

*Results.*—When all 221 patients were considered, the only significant predictor of outcome was the number of diseased vessels. Apart from that, the best predictor was the conventional classification into high risk or low risk. No clinical measure or noninvasive test of ischemia had prognostic significance in either the overall group or the low-risk group. Angiography was reported by 27 of 30 patients who had acute, nonfatal cardiac events during follow-up. In 74% of these, significant stenoses had developed at previously unobstructed sites. The stenosis that had been responsible for the initial ischemia was rarely the site of new acute cardiac events.

*Conclusions.*—These results suggest that in low-risk patients with stable angina, ischemia is not associated with significantly worse long-term results. The data do not support the hypothesis that ambulatory ischemia reflects plaque instability that might precipitate an acute cardiac event. Efforts to reduce or abolish ambulatory ischemia seem unlikely to improve prognosis.

▶ This careful study on a selected group of relatively low-risk patients with stable CAD reinforces the following increasingly accepted concept: in many patients, we can identify "culprit" lesions, which are responsible for symptoms, but we are notoriously ineffective at identifying "future culprits." This is because the lesions that have *subsequently* been shown to be responsible for an acute ischemic syndrome are usually not the site of a significant stenosis at the time of the *initial* angiogram.[1] In fact, plaques that are less stenotic but more lipid rich appear to be those most likely to rupture in the future and to be the underlying cause of a subsequent myocardial infarction, episode of unstable angina, or sudden cardiac death.[2]

Of note is that the only significant, independent predictor of outcome for all events, including the "soft" end point of revascularization, was the number of diseased vessels. This may be the result of a direct correlation between the severity of the disease and the number of diseased vessels and the amount of minor, but nonetheless vulnerable, plaques in other vessels, which may be the sites for future acute coronary events.[3, 4]

Irrespective of our ability to predict the prognosis of patients with stable CAD, there are measures we can take to stabilize the endothelium and plaques, preventing future rupture. These measures include aspirin and above all, aggressive lipid lowering.[5] The role of the newer platelet inhibitors in estrogen therapy remains to be determined.

**B.J. Gersh, M.B., Ch.B., D.Phil., F.R.C.P.**

*References*

1. Little WC, Constantinescu MS, Applegate RJ, et al: Can coronary angiography predict the site of a subsequent myocardial infarction in patients with mild to moderate coronary artery disease. *Circulation* 78:1157–1166, 1988.
2. Mann JM, Davies MJ: Vulnerable plaque: Relation of characteristics to degree of stenosis in human coronary arteries. *Circulation* 94:928–931, 1996.
3. Nakagomi A, Celermager DS, Lumley T, et al: Angiographic severity of coronary narrowing is a surrogate marker for the extent of coronary atherosclerosis. *Am J Cardiol* 78:516–519, 1996.
4. Ambrose JA, Fuster V: Can we predict future acute coronary events in patients with stable coronary artery disease (editorial)? *JAMA* 277:343–344, 1997.
5. Scandinavian Simvastatin Survival Study Group. Randomized trials of cholesterol lowering in 4,444 patients with coronary heart disease: The Scandinavian Survival Study (IVS). *Lancet* 344:1383–1389, 1994.

---

**Cardiac Risk of Noncardiac Surgery: Influence of Coronary Disease and Type of Surgery in 3368 Operations**
Eagle KA, for the CASS Investigators and University of Michigan Heart Care Program (Univ of Michigan, Ann Arbor)
*Circulation* 96:1882–1887, 1997                                                    2–61

---

*Objective.*—The most common cause of death after surgery is a cardiac complication. There is little information about surgery-specific risks of noncardiac procedures. The interaction between the extent of coronary disease and procedure-related stresses on the heart can be assessed by using the Coronary Artery Surgery Study (CASS) registry.

*Methods.*—Of the 24,959 patients enrolled at 15 clinical sites between 1974 and 1979, 3,368 patients had undergone at least 1 noncardiac surgery. Patients were stratified into those who had coronary artery disease (CAD), those who did not, and those who had undergone coronary bypass surgery (CABG) before noncardiac operations (abdominal 36%, urologic 21%, orthopedic 15%, vascular 9%, head and neck 7%, thoracic 5%, and breast 2%). The end point was operative mortality, myocardial infarction, or perioperative death. Univariate analysis was used to compare patients with and without myocardial infarction and/or perioperative death and risk factors.

*Results.*—Patients with known coronary disease, described as "high-risk" for noncardiac surgery, had a lower preoperative risk if they had undergone CABG (Figure). Multivariate predictors of 30-day death or myocardial infarction after noncardiac surgery, in addition to coronary disease not treated by CABG in patients with CAD, included congestive heart failure, advanced age, and hypertension. Multivariate predictors of 30-day death or myocardial infarction after higher risk noncardiac surgery in patients with known CAD included coronary disease not treated by

Type of Non Cardiac Surgery and Postop MI+ or Death

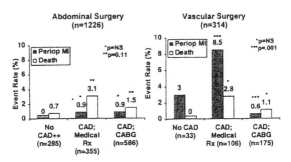

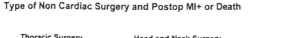

Type of Non Cardiac Surgery and Postop MI+ or Death

Total Event Rates in High Risk Surgery (n=1961)

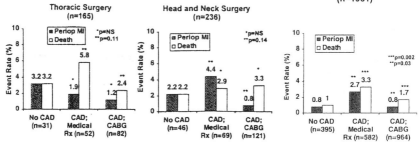

**FIGURE.**—Type of noncardiac surgery and postoperative myocardial infarction (*MI*) or death among higher risk procedures (combined MI and death rate of 4% or higher in medically treated patients). Rates of MI or death among patients undergoing abdominal, vascular, thoracic, and head and neck surgeries are stratified by the presence or absence of coronary artery disease (*CAD*) and whether it was previously treated medically or with coronary artery bypass surgery (*CABG*). (Reproduced with permission, from Eagle KA, for the CASS Investigators and University of Michigan Heart Care Program: Cardiac risk of noncardiac surgery: Influence of coronary disease and type of surgery in 3368 operations. *Circulation* 96:1882–1887, Copyright 1997, American Heart Association.)

CABG, congestive heart failure, hypertension, and smoking. Patients having urologic, orthopedic, breast, and skin surgery were at no increased risk regardless of whether pre-existing CAD was treated medically or surgically. Coronary bypass surgery protected noncardiac surgical patients for at least 6 years.

*Conclusion.*—Patients undergoing low-risk surgical procedures such as urologic, orthopedic, breast, and skin operations, and patients who have undergone CABG will probably not benefit from extensive coronary evaluations. Mortality and risks of myocardial infarction are reduced in patients with coronary disease having noncardiac surgery if they have undergone CABG.

▶ The protective shield of CABG in patients undergoing noncardiac surgery is highlighted by this study from the CASS Registry (Coronary Artery Surgery Study), but it comes at a price.[1] There is a morbidity and mortality associated with CABG, and among patients with peripheral vascular disease and the elderly, this is substantial. In the modern era of perioperative care in the ICU setting, I do not see a role for "prophylactic" coronary revascularization as a method of reducing the morbidity and mortality of noncardiac surgery. In recent years, there have been significant improvements in the outcomes of noncardiac and in particular peripheral vascular surgery.[2, 3]

The objectives of CABG among patients undergoing noncardiac surgery should be the same as in the population at large, namely, the improvement in symptoms and prolongation of *late* survival as opposed to lessening the morbidity and mortality of the noncardiac surgical procedure. Among subsets of patients in whom CABG or percutaneous transluminal coronary angioplasty is indicated to either relieve symptoms or prolong late survival, the need to perform additional noncardiac surgery influences the *timing* of the coronary revascularization procedure. In many patients, and in particular those undergoing major noncardiac surgery, it may be preferable to perform the coronary revascularization first, whereas in other patients with stable coronary disease, the clinical situation may dictate performing the noncardiac procedure initially, followed by coronary revascularization at a later date. In this setting, meticulous perioperative care is essential.

**B.J. Gersh, M.B., Ch.B., D.Phil, F.R.C.P.**

*References*

1. Gersh BJ, Rihal CS, Rooke TW, et al: Evaluation of management of patients with both peripheral vascular and coronary artery disease. *J Am Coll Cardiol* 18:203–214, 1991.
2. Ashton CM, Petersen NJ, Wrapy NP, et al: The incidence of perioperative myocardial infarction in men undergoing noncardiac surgery. *Ann Intern Med* 118:504–510, 1993.
3. Mangano DT, Goldman L: Current concepts: Preoperative assessment of patients with known or suspected coronary disease. *N Engl J Med* 333:1750–1756, 1995.

---

**Cardiac Troponin T Is Elevated in Asymptomatic Patients With Chronic Renal Failure**

Frankel WL, Herold DA, Ziegler TW, et al (VA Med Ctr, San Diego, Calif; Univ of California-San Diego, La Jolla, Calif)
*Am J Clin Pathol* 106:118–123, 1996                                          2–62

---

*Background.*—Patients with chronic renal failure (CRF) are at high risk for coronary artery disease and need to be examined for potential myocardial infarcts. Their underlying diseases, however, can mask typical symptoms, and protein markers of cardiac damage may be elevated on a long-term basis in some patients. Investigators assessed the value of cardiac troponin T (cTnT), a sensitive marker of cardiac injury, in patients with CRF and no symptoms of myocardial infarction.

*Methods.*—The cTnT assay was performed on blood samples obtained from 38 randomly selected patients with CRF immediately before hemodialysis. Also analyzed were samples from 16 of these patients postdialysis

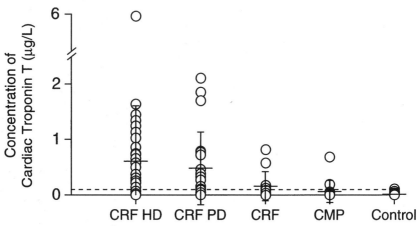

**FIGURE 1.**—Distribution of cTnT concentrations in various adult patient groups. *Side bars* represent mean and standard deviation cTnT concentrations. The *dotted line* indicates the cutoff for normal values (0.1 µg/L). *Abbreviations: cTnT,* cardiac troponin T; *CRF,* chronic renal failure; *HD,* hemodialysis, *PD,* peritoneal dialysis, *CMP,* cardiomyopathy. (Courtesy of Frankel WL, Herold DA, Ziegler TW, et al: Cardiac troponin T is elevated in asymptomatic patients with chronic renal failure. *Am J Clin Pathol* 106:118–123, 1996.)

and from 4 other groups: 21 patients undergoing peritoneal dialysis, 10 patients with CRF but not undergoing dialysis, 11 patients with cardio-myopathy, and 10 adolescent patients with CRF undergoing hemodialysis. Thirty healthy controls were included for comparison. Blood samples were analyzed for cTnT, myoglobin, creatine kinase, creatine kinase isoen-zyme-MB (CK-MB), lactate dehydrogenase, and lactate dehydrogenase isoenzyme-1 (LD-1).

*Results.*—Patients in the CRF hemodialysis group had a mean age of 60 years. None had specific symptoms of myocardial infarction at the time of evaluation, but 32% had known severe CAD and more than half had hypertension and/or diabetes mellitus. Twenty-seven patients (71%) had elevated cTnT levels and all but 1 had elevated myoglobin concentrations. Cardiac TnT concentrations were significantly correlated with concentra-tions of CK-MB and myoglobin. Values of cTnT before and after dialysis did not differ significantly in this group. Elevated cTnT was also present in 57% of patients with CRF undergoing peritoneal dialysis, 30% with CRF not undergoing dialysis, 18% with cardiomyopathy (Fig 1), and 20% of adolescent patients with CRF undergoing hemodialysis. Almost all pa-tients with CRF, regardless of whether they were undergoing dialysis, had elevated myoglobin levels; few had elevated CK-MB or LD-1 levels.

*Conclusion.*—Patients with CRF often exhibit elevated levels of cTnT, but the relationship of this finding to cardiac damage is uncertain. There may be a decreased clearance of cTnT because of renal failure, and most patients with elevated cTnT levels are not known to have had cardiac events.

▶ The prevalence of coronary artery disease in patients with CRF is increased for a number of reasons, including pre-existing hypertension, diabetes, and hyperlipidemia. Moreover, among patients with CRF who are undergoing dialysis, the hemodynamic derangements caused by fluid overload and marked volume shifts in conjunction with hypertension, tachycardia, and anemia may precipitate ischemic events in patients with underlying coronary artery disease. Furthermore, the diagnosis of myocardial infarction is often masked by nonspecific symptoms of chest pain and/or the presence of pericarditis, in addition to markedly abnormal repolarization changes on the ECG. A reliable marker of myocardial infarction would therefore be helpful, given that creatine phosphokinase (CPK) and CPK-MB isoenzymes may be elevated in CRF despite the absence of cardiac symptoms or other evidence of myocardial infarction.[1]

Unfortunately, cTnT will not be helpful despite its initial promise. This study demonstrates elevated levels in the majority of patients with CRF, both in patients undergoing hemodialysis and ambulatory peritoneal dialysis and also among patients with CRF who are not undergoing dialysis. The authors discuss in detail the potential mechanisms for troponin T elevation, and it would appear that reduced troponin T clearance is the most likely, although other factors may be operative in some patients. Irrespective of the cause, a different biochemical marker of cardiac injury is needed in patients with CRF.

**B.J. Gersh, M.B., Ch.B., D.Phil., F.R.C.P.**

*Reference*

1. Jaffe AS, Ritter C, Meltzer V, et al: Unmasking artifactual increases in creatine kinase isoenzymes in patients with renal failure. *J Lab Clin Med* 104:193–202, 1984.

---

**Sleep-related Myocardial Ischemia and Sleep Structure in Patients With Obstructive Sleep Apnea and Coronary Heart Disease**
Schäfer H, Koehler U, Ploch T, et al (Univ of Bonn, Germany; Univ of Marburg, Germany)
*Chest* 111:387–393, 1997                                                         2–63

---

*Background.*—Obstructive sleep apnea is a condition in which frequent arousals occur during nighttime sleep. It is common in middle-aged men and is associated with cardiovascular mortality. Patients with a combination of coronary heart disease (CHD) and obstructive sleep apnea may be at increased cardiac risk as a result of apnea-induced hypoxemia. Their sleep quality may be compromised by both apnea-associated arousals and ischemia-associated arousals. The association between nocturnal myocardial ischemia and sleep apnea was examined in patients with CHD.

*Methods.*—Fourteen male patients with both obstructive sleep apnea and CHD and 7 male patients with obstructive sleep apnea alone were analyzed for 6 consecutive nights in the sleep laboratory, with standard sleep and cardiorespiratory measurements, plus 6-lead ECG monitoring. Cardiac patients did not take any cardiovascular medication for 48 hours before sleep testing. All patients received a single dose of a sustained-release, high-dose nitrate or placebo on nights 3, 4, 5, and 6, in a double-blind crossover, placebo-controlled design, to test the effect of nitrate therapy on nocturnal ischemia.

*Results.*—During 3 nights of recordings, 144 episodes of nocturnal myocardial ischemia were detected in 6 participants. Of these 6 study participants, 5 had underlying CHD and 1 had diffuse coronary artery wall defects. During 85.4% of the ischemic episodes, there were concomitant apneas with greater than 3% oxygen desaturation. Although REM sleep accounted for only 18% of total sleeptime, 77.8% of ischemic episodes occurred during REM sleep (Fig 1). The mean oxygen saturation was significantly lower during apnea-associated ischemic periods than during ischemic periods without associated apnea. Nitrate administration had no effect on ischemia. Sleep periods with myocardial ischemia were associated with significantly more frequent and severe arousals than those without ischemia. The microstructure of sleep was also disturbed by myocardial ischemia in the absence of apnea.

*Conclusions.*—Patients with both CHD and obstructive sleep apnea should be considered to be at cardiovascular risk, as apnea-associated oxygen desaturation can lead to nocturnal myocardial ischemia. Nocturnal myocardial ischemia can cause arousal, which may result in increased daytime sleepiness. Patients with nocturnal ischemia should be screened for underlying sleep apnea, even if they fail to respond to nitrate therapy.

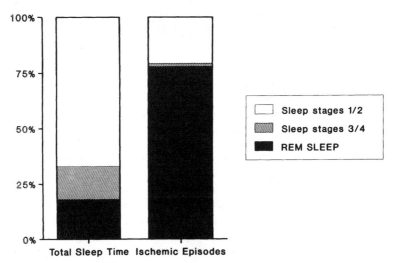

FIGURE 1.—Distribution of ischemic episodes and total sleep time in relation to sleep stages. (Courtesy of Schäfer H, Koehler U, Ploch T, et al: Sleep-related myocardial ischemia and sleep structure in patients with obstructive sleep apnea and coronary heart disease. *Chest* 111:387–393, 1997.)

▶ This is an interesting clinical study, which suggests that the combination of obstructive coronary artery disease and sleep apnea identifies a group with a particularly high incidence of nocturnal ischemia. Apnea-associated oxygen desaturation reduces myocardial oxygen supply, but another component of this imbalance between supply and demand is provided by the hemodynamic changes that occur in sleep apnea, which may alter left ventricular preload and afterload so as to increase oxygen demands. What is also of interest is that the "silent" myocardial ischemic episodes lead to an activation of the CNS, which causes additional sleep disturbances and increased daytime sleepiness. Whether the activation of the autonomic nervous system is responsible for an increased incidence of cardiovascular events such as sudden death, myocardial infarction, etc. is unproved, but it is at least theoretically possible.[1]

Sleep apnea needs to be treated for its own sake, but studies such as this strengthen the case further in patients with coronary artery disease. Interestingly, sustained-release nitrates were no better than placebo in ameliorating these episodes, but one wonders what the effect would be of beta-blockers, calcium-channel blockers, or their combination.

**B.J. Gersh, M.B., Ch.B., D.Phil., F.R.C.P.**

*Reference*

1. Schwartz PJ, LaRobert MC, Vanoli V: Autonomic nervous system and sudden cardiac death. *Circulation* 85:775–915, 1992.

# 3 Hypertension

## Introduction

Despite increasing recognition and treatment, hypertension remains largely uncontrolled in the United States and elsewhere. As noted in the 1997 Sixth Joint National Committee Report (JNC-6), only 27% of U.S. hypertensives have their condition under adequate control. The striking falls in stroke and coronary disease mortality observed in the United States since the early 1970s seem to have slowed, and the incidence of congestive heart failure and end-stage renal disease—two conditions closely allied to hypertension—are rising progressively.

These stark findings call attention, not to the continued unknowns but to the overriding need to focus on what is known: Hypertension must be more effectively treated; if it is, morbidity and mortality will fall.

The first abstract to be reviewed is perhaps the most important, since the JNC-6 report is a concise yet complete portrayal of where we are and what we can do.

Norman M. Kaplan, M.D.

---

**The Sixth Report of the Joint National Committee on Prevention, Detection, Evaluation, and Treatment of High Blood Pressure**
Sheps SG, for the Joint National Commitee on Prevention, Detection, Evaluation and Treatment of High Blood Pressure and the National High Blood Pressure Education Program Coordinating Committee (Mayo Clinic and Found, Rochester, Minn; Rush-Presbyterian-St. Luke's Med Ctr, Chicago; St. Louis Univ; et al)
*Arch Intern Med* 24:2413–2446, 1997                                    3–1

---

*Objective.*—Since the last Joint National Committee report on prevention, detection, evaluations, and treatment of high blood pressure in 1993, the trend toward improved awareness, treatment, and control of hypertension has slowed. Mortality from strokes and coronary heart disease have leveled off during this time, while the incidence of end-stage renal disease and the prevalence of heart failure have increased. Although randomized, controlled trials are the best source of information for directing clinical policy, they cannot answer all questions. The prevention and treatment of hypertension and the resultant target organ damage still pose considerable public health challenges. The Sixth Report of the Joint National Committee (JNC VI) is presented.

*Measurement and Clinical Evaluation.*—The JNC VI presents a revised classification of blood pressure stages in adult patients, combining stage 3 and 4 hypertension. However, recommendations for detection, confirmation, and evaluation of high blood pressure are little changed. For self-measurement or ambulatory blood pressure measurement, readings of 135/85 mmHg may be considered elevated. Current knowledge of the genetics of hypertension is discussed, along with clinical clues for identifying causes of hypertension. The report also includes new information on cardiovascular risk factors and risk stratification.

*Prevention and Treatment.*—The report notes the importance of lifestyle modifications in protecting against high blood pressure and cardiovascular disease. Benefits of reducing blood pressure include decreased deaths from strokes, coronary events, and heart failure. Reducing hypertension can also slow the progression of renal failure, prevent progression to more severe hypertension, and decrease all-cause mortality. When drug therapy is necessary, the drug of first choice is a diuretic and/or a β-blocker, unless another form of treatment is specifically indicated. A multidisciplinary team approach can improve patient compliance with treatment. Randomized, controlled trials have proved that treating high blood pressure can reduce cardiovascular events; this finding has important implications in the current era of managed health care. The JNC VI report includes new information on the management of hypertensive emergencies.

*Special Populations and Situations.*—Different racial and ethnic groups vary in their prevalence and control rates of hypertension. The treating clinician should always bear these social and cultural factors in mind. The new report includes guidelines for the treatment of high blood pressure in women and children. Elderly patients with hypertension should be managed with diuretics, if possible; long-acting dihydropyridine calcium antagonists may be considered as well. The report includes specific recommendations for the management of patients with left ventricular hypertrophy, coronary artery disease, and heart failure. Blood pressure goals for patients with renal insufficiency vary, from 125/75 mmHg for patients with proteinuria levels of more than 1 g/day to 130/85 mmHg for those with a lesser degree of proteinuria. Treatment with angiotensin-converting enzyme inhibitors can enhance renal protection. For patients with diabetes mellitus, the goal of treatment should be a blood pressure of less than 130/85 mmHg. The report also discusses some of the other conditions and pressor agents that can induce hypertension.

*Summary.*—The JNC VI provides guidelines for primary care physicians in the prevention and treatment of hypertension. Compared with previous reports, the JNC VI emphasizes absolute risks and benefits and incorporates risk stratification into the treatment approach. For uncomplicated cases, drug therapy should start with diuretics and β-blockers; other agents are indicated in specific clinical situations.

▶ This report should be carefully read by every health care provider who sees patients with hypertension, and that obviously includes every reader of the YEAR BOOK OF CARDIOLOGY. Because I am 1 of the 4 coeditors under the chairman, Dr. Sheldon Sheps, my views may be biased, but I believe that the report is succinct, up-to-date, comprehensive, and as unbiased as it possibly can be. Critics will find faults: for instance, the "compelling" indication (after diuretics) for use of long-acting dihydropyridine calcium channel blockers for elderly patients with systolic hypertension, as shown in Figure 8 of the original article. As with the other major recommendations, this one is evidence based, mainly from the SYST-EUR trial[1] but also from other controlled trials showing the capability of such agents to reduce morbidity and mortality.

One of the main differences in JNC-VI from the 1993 JNC-V is the recognition that drug therapy need not be the initial treatment for all patients. Lifestyle modifications are recommended for 6–12 months for those with stage 1 hypertension (blood pressure, 140/90–160/100) who are free of target organ damage, major other risk factors, and overt cardiovascular disease. Although such paragons may be relatively rare, they have not been shown to benefit from drug therapy in the 3–6 year clinical trials,[2] so the aggressive pursuit of lifestyle changes is certainly appropriate.

There are multiple other changes, in keeping with the many advances made in our understanding of the mechanisms and treatment of hypertension during the past few years. The report certainly deserves a careful reading.

**N.M. Kaplan, M.D.**

*References*

1. Staessen JA, Fagard R, Thijs L, et al: Randomised double-blind comparison of placebo and active treatment for older patients with isolated systolic hypertension. *Lancet* 350:757–764, 1997.
2. Gueyffier F, Boutitie F, Boissel J-P, et al: Effect of antihypertensive drug treatment on cardiovascular outcomes in women and men. *Ann Intern Med* 126:761–767, 1997.

## Diagnosis and Monitoring

### INTRODUCTION

Home and ambulatory blood pressure measurements are increasingly being recognized as lower than clinic readings and closer to long-term therapeutic needs and prognosis as well.

**Norman M. Kaplan, M.D.**

## Ambulatory and Home Blood Pressure Normality in the Elderly: Data From the PAMELA Population

Sega R, Cesana G, Milesi C, et al (Università di Milano, Italy; IRCCS Centro Auxologico Italiano, Milano, Italy; ISTRA, Milano, Italy)
*Hypertension* 30:1–6, 1997                                        3–2

*Introduction.*—Population studies of men and women aged 25 to 64 have found the upper limit of normality of ambulatory blood pressure (BP) to be lower (120-130/75-81 mmHg) than the accepted upper limit of normality of clinic BP (140/90 mmHg). To provide data on ambulatory BP normality in the elderly, 24-hour recordings were made in a random sample of individuals 65 or older.

*Methods.*—The study location was the city of Monza, Italy. A sample of 800 men and women was selected from residents between the ages of 65 and 74. At outpatient clinic visits, the participants had a medical history taken, a physical examination, and 3 sitting BP measurements. An ambulatory BP-monitoring device was provided for use during normal activities, and 2 sitting home BPs were also obtained.

*Results.*—Clinic, home, and ambulatory BP measurements were obtained in only half of the selected participants, but the final sample was representative of the original sample. Twenty-four hour average BP (Table 3) was much lower than clinic BP, and daytime average BP, though greater than 24-hour average BP, was still significantly and markedly less than clinic BP. Men and women differed only slightly or not at all in BP and heart rate values. Compared with younger individuals, clinic BP was steeply and progressively increased in the elderly group. The 24-average BP showed a much flatter age-dependent change. Clinic, home, and 24-hour average heart rates did not differ substantially between younger and older groups. And as reported for younger individuals, clinic BP in older study participants showed a positive correlation with home and ambulatory BPs, which were also correlated with each other. In contrast to younger subjects, home BP in the elderly was higher than 24-hour average BP. All

TABLE 3.—Home and Ambulatory Blood Pressure Values
Corresponding to a Clinic Blood Pressure of 140/90 mmHg in
Normotensive and Untreated Hypertensive Subjects of the
PAMELA Study Aged 65 to 74 Years

| Blood Pressure | SBP (mmHg) | DBP (mmHg) |
|---|---|---|
| Home | 133 (131–135) | 82 (80–83) |
| 24-Hour mean | 120 (118–121) | 76 (75–77) |
| Daytime mean | 124 (123–126) | 80 (79–81) |
| Nighttime mean | 109 (106–111) | 67 (66–68) |

SBP indicates systolic blood pressure; DBP, diastolic blood pressure.
Values are mean (95% confidence interval).
(Courtesy of Sega R, Cesana G, Milesi C, et al: Ambulatory and home blood pressure normality in the elderly: Data from the PAMELA population. *Hypertension* 30:1–6, 1997. Reproduced with permission. *Hypertension* Copyright 1997, American Heart Association.)

readings were higher in treated hypertensive than normotensive elderly subjects.

*Conclusion.*—Individuals aged 65 to 74 were found to have 24-hour average, daytime average, and home systolic and diastolic BPs that were significantly less than clinic BPs. Because the upper limit of normality in ambulatory and home BPs is well below 140/90 mmHg (about 120/76 mmHg), elevations may be missed in a large number of the elderly. It was also apparent that antihypertensive therapy may not achieve full BP control in older patients.

▶ The main attraction of these data is that they were obtained in a random sample of presumably ambulatory, free-living people, so they should be applicable to the majority of outpatients. The main objection to these data is the repeated comparisons between 24-hour average BP to the clinic and home readings. As shown in the Table, the inclusion of the typically much lower nighttime (sleeping) readings makes the mean 24-hour level much less comparable to the home and clinic readings, which are obviously taken during the day.

The 9 mmHg difference between the 2 home BPs and the multiple ambulatory readings likely reflects some "white-coat" effect when people initially take their own readings. Most find little difference between multiple home readings and daytime ambulatory readings. Moreover, home readings are much more reproducible over prolonged intervals than are occasional office readings.[1]

As shown in the Table, the lower home and ambulatory readings likely will translate into different criteria for hypertension based on those readings than the 140/90 used for office readings. Home BP of 135/85 is probably about right, although a home level of 140/90 or higher is probably appropriate to start therapy. Regardless, home readings should be used both for diagnosis and for follow-up management, providing much better data than a few office readings.

**N.M. Kaplan, M.D.**

*Reference*

1. Sakuma M, Imai Y, Nagai K, et al: Reproducibility of home blood pressure measurements over a 1-year period. *Am J Hypertens* 10:798–803, 1997.

---

**Prognostic Significance of the White Coat Effect**
Verdecchia P, Schillaci G, Borgioni C, et al (Ospedale Generale Regionale Raffaello Silvestrini, Italy; Area Omogenea di Cardiologia e Medicina, Perugia, Italy; Ospedale Beato G Villa, Città della Pieve, Italy)
*Hypertension* 29:1218–1224, 1997                                    3–3

---

*Introduction.*—A transient pressor rise in the patient may be triggered by the physician in the clinic environment who is measuring blood pressure. On the assumption that average daytime ambulatory blood pressure reflects the blood pressure immediately before the visit, the "white coat effect" has been estimated by the difference between clinic blood pressure and the average daytime ambulatory blood pressure. It has been suggested that white coat hypertension may be a condition of low cardiovascular morbidity. Subjects were measured for baseline off-therapy clinic blood pressure and 24-hour noninvasive ambulatory blood pressure to assess cardiovascular morbidity and mortality.

*Methods.*—Baseline off-therapy clinic blood pressure measurements were obtained and 24-hour noninvasive ambulatory blood pressure monitoring was performed in 1,522 patients who were followed up for 9 years. Echocardiography and electrocardiography were also performed.

*Results.*—With increasing clinic blood pressure, the predicted values of ambulatory blood pressure progressively diverged from the identity line, but the predicted values of clinic blood pressure tended toward the identity line with increasing ambulatory blood pressure. During the 9-year follow-up, there were 157 major cardiovascular morbid events. According to the log-rank test, the rate of total cardiovascular morbid events or the rate of fatal cardiovascular events did not differ among the distribution of the clinic-ambulatory blood pressure difference. In hypertensive subjects, cigarette smoking evoked a persistent rise in ambulatory blood pressure, and women had a higher blood pressure reactivity to clinic visits.

*Conclusion.*—In patients with essential hypertension, the clinic-ambulatory blood pressure difference, or white coat effect, did not predict cardiovascular morbidity and mortality.

▶ The recognition over the past 10 years of white-coat hypertension in ≥20% of patients with persistent office hypertension (but, by definition, normotension out of the office) has given rise to considerable uncertainty as to the course and prognosis in these patients. These data are the best currently available, following the largest group of patients more carefully for a longer duration than any other study. They obviously support the view that the white-coat (alerting) effect that occurs in most people when their pressures are taken in the office setting and which may be so large as to induce office (white-coat) hypertension in ≥20% is not a serious problem—at least for 5 years or so.

Even more, longer term data are clearly needed, since some have noted more cardiovascular risk factors and a fairly high rate of progression from white-coat to persistent hypertension in such patients.[1] Nonetheless, I believe out-of-office readings should always be obtained so that white-coat hypertension can be identified and that patients so identified should be advised to follow appropriate lifestyle changes and to monitor their blood pressure more closely but not be diagnosed as hypertensive or treated with antihypertensive agents.

Home blood pressure measurements with inexpensive arm devices are usually reliable; those obtained by more expensive finger devices are not.[2]

**N.M. Kaplan, M.D.**

*References*

1. Cerasola G, Cottone S, Nardi E, et al: White-coat hypertension and cardiovascular risk. *J Cardiovasc Risk* 2:545–549, 1995.
2. Ristuccia HL, Grossman P, Watkins LL, et al: Incremental bias in Finapres estimation of baseline blood pressure levels over time. *Hypertension* 29:1039–1043, 1997.

---

**Antihypertensive Treatment Based on Conventional or Ambulatory Blood Pressure Measurement: A Randomized Controlled Trial**
Staessen JA, for the Ambulatory Blood Pressure Monitoring and Treatment of Hypertension Investigators (Katholieke Universiteit Leuven, Belgium; et al)
*JAMA* 278:1065–1072, 1997                                              3–4

---

*Introduction.*—Blood pressure can be recorded throughout the day with ambulatory monitoring while patients engage in their normal daily activities. It would take several weeks to acquire this same information with conventional recording methods. Conventional blood pressure (CBP) and ambulatory blood pressure (ABP) were compared during the Ambulatory Blood Pressure Monitoring and Treatment of Hypertension Trial, a multicentered randomized investigation.

*Methods.*—A total of 419 patients with untreated average diastolic blood pressure (DBP) of 95 mmHg or higher were randomized to the CBP or ABP arms. Antihypertensive treatment was adjusted in a stepwise fashion, based on the average daytime ambulatory DBP from 10 AM to 8 PM in the ABP group or the average of 3 sitting DBP readings in the CBP group. A blinded physician intensified, left unchanged, or decreased antihypertensive treatment, based on DBP readings.

*Results.*—At a median follow-up of 182 days, significantly more patients in the ABP than CBP group had stopped antihypertensive treatment (26.3% vs. 7.3%) and significantly fewer progressed to sustained multiple-drug treatment (27.2% vs. 42.7%). The final average differences between treatment groups for systolic blood pressure ranged between 2.6 and 3.5 mmHg. For DBP, the range was 1.4 to 1.9 mmHg. The 2 groups were similar in measurements of left ventricular mass and symptoms reported by questionnaire. The possible savings from less intensive drug treatment and fewer physician visits in the ABP group were offset by costs of ABP monitoring.

*Conclusion.*—Adjusting antihypertensive treatment based on ABP monitoring vs. CBP resulted in less intensive drug treatment. This cost savings was offset by the cost of ABP monitoring. General well-being and inhibition of ventricular enlargement were similar for both groups.

▶ These data confirm the presence of "white-coat" hypertension in about 20% of all patients with office blood pressures above 140/90. The new and important information from this study is the recognition that removal or reduction of antihypertensive drug therapy in patients with white-coat hypertension did not lead to any obvious target organ damage, specifically left ventricular enlargement, in a 6 month follow-up. Obviously more patients need to be followed for much longer to ensure the benignity of white-coat hypertension. Others have observed no increase in cardiovascular morbidity or mortality in such patients without treatment over as long as 7 years.[1] On the other hand, subtle cardiovascular dysfunction may be found,[2] so such patients should at the very least be closely followed while they are encouraged to modify unhealthy lifestyle habits.

**N.M. Kaplan, M.D.**

*References*

1. Verdecchia P, Schillaci G, Borgioni C, et al: Prognostic significance of the white coat effect. *Hypertension* 29:1218–1224, 1997.
2. Ferrara LA, Guida L, Pasanisi F, et al: Isolated office hypertension and end-organ damage. *J Hypertens* 15:979–985, 1997.

---

**Ambulatory Blood Pressure Is Superior to Clinic Blood Pressure in Predicting Treatment-induced Regression of Left Ventricular Hypertrophy**
Mancia G, for the SAMPLE Study Group (Università di Milano, Italy)
*Circulation* 95:1464–1470, 1997                                              3–5

---

*Introduction.*—To improve the diagnosis of hypertension and estimation of the efficacy of antihypertensive treatment, ambulatory blood pressure monitoring has become more common. Previous studies have shown that ambulatory blood pressure is clinically superior to clinical blood pressure by suggesting a closer association of cardiovascular morbidity or target-organ deterioration, but these studies have not provided a definitive conclusion. Patients with echocardiographic evidence of left ventricular hypertrophy (LVH) were prospectively examined with clinic or 24-hour average blood pressure to determine which blood pressure measurement more accurately predicts reduction of left ventricular mass induced by long-term antihypertensive treatment.

*Methods.*—Clinic supine blood pressure, 24-hour ambulatory blood pressure, and left ventricular mass index (LVMI were measured in 206 patients with essential hypertension, before and after 12 months of treatment. Treatment consisted of lisinopril at 20 mg UID with or without hydrochlorothiazide at 12.5 or 25 mg UID.

*Results.*—Clinic supine blood pressure was 165 ± 15/105 ± 5 mmHg before treatment. The 24-hour average blood pressure was 149 ± 16/95 ± 11 mmHg, and LVMI was 158 ± 32 g/m². The clinical supine blood pressure was 139 ± 12/87 ± 7 mmHg after treatment; 24-hour average blood pressure was 131 ± 12/83 ± 10 mmHg; and LVMI was 133 ± 26 g/m². Clinic blood pressure did not correlate with LVMI before treatment, but there was a correlation between systolic and diastolic 24-hour average

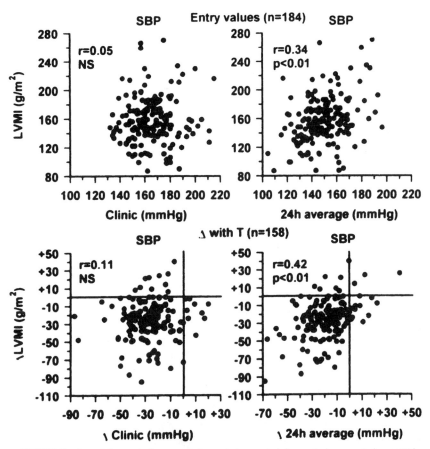

FIGURE 2.—Entry left ventricular mass index and changes in left ventricular mass index at 12th-month treatment vs. corresponding supine clinical and 24-hour average systolic blood pressure values in individual patients. (Courtesy of Mancia G, for the SAMPLE Study Group: Ambulatory blood pressure is superior to clinic blood pressure in predicting treatment-induced regression of left ventricular hypertrophy. *Circulation* 95:1464–1470, 1997.)

blood pressure and LVMI (Fig 2). A reduction in the 24-hour average blood pressure was related to LVMI reduction, but not to clinic blood pressure reduction. In average daytime and nighttime blood pressure measurements, treatment-induced changes correlated with LVMI changes as strongly as 24-hour blood pressure changes. Clinic orthostatic, random-zero, and home blood pressure did not show any substantial advantage over clinic supine blood pressure.

*Conclusion.*—Regression of LVH was predicted much more closely by treatment-induced changes in ambulatory blood pressure than in clinic blood pressure. Ambulatory blood pressure may be clinically superior to traditional blood pressure measurements according to the results of this first longitudinally controlled study.

▶ These data add to the already overwhelming evidence that 24-hour ambulatory blood pressure measurements obtained by automatic monitors are better than office measurements for estimating the risks for hypertension, and in particular, LVH and, as shown in this paper, the ability of treatment to regress LVH.

A particular aspect of the 24-hour pattern of blood pressure may be most closely correlated to the degree of LVH, the abrupt rise in blood pressure on arising from overnight sleep. Gosse et al.[1] found a closer correlation between left ventricular mass and the blood pressure after arising than with other portions of the 24-hour pattern or with office measurements. These findings fit well with the well-documented increase in heart attacks, strokes, and sudden death in the early morning, post-arising hours.[2]

Further evidence that it is the effect of arising from sleep and not the time of day that gives the abrupt rise in blood pressure has come from measurements of blood pressure in subjects undergoing long transmeridian air travel.[3]

Despite the advantages of 24-hour ambulatory monitoring and the availability of efficient, relatively inexpensive (around $5,000) equipment, U.S. third-party payers usually will not pay for the procedure, so it is being very rarely performed in clinical practice. Considering the demands to reduce the cost of health care and the overuse of every technology ever introduced into cardiology and all other areas of medicine, we shouldn't expect the situation to change.

Fortunately, almost all of the useful information provided by ambulatory monitoring can be provided by less expensive and easily available home blood pressure devices. As they are being more widely used, the criteria for hypertension by home measurements is being set at around 135/85 mmHg.[4]

**N.M. Kaplan, M.D.**

*References*

1. Gosse P, Ansoborlo P, Lemetayer P, et al: Left ventricular mass is better correlated with arising blood pressure than with office or occasional blood pressure. *Am J Hypertens* 10:505–510, 1997.
2. Muller J, Stone P, Turi ZG, et al., and the MILIS Study Group: Circadian variation in the frequency of onset of acute myocardial infarction. *N Engl J Med* 313:1315–1322, 1985.
3. Fogari R, Lusardi P, Zoppi A, et al: Effect of a westward transmeridian flight on ambulatory blood pressure monitoring in normotensive subjects. *J Hypertens* 15:143–146, 1997.
4. Tsuji I, Imai U, Nagai K, et al: Proposal of reference values for home blood pressure measurement. *Am J Hypertens* 10:409–418, 1997.

# Mechanisms

## INTRODUCTION

Evidence for the contribution of previously known factors, including age, obesity, intrauterine growth retardation, insulin resistance, and stress, continues to expand along with the role of anxiety both in causing hypertension and, in an even more obvious manner, contributing to its symptoms. Meanwhile, the possible role of neurovascular compression of the ventral medulla has received more support, but I remain highly skeptical.

**Norman M. Kaplan, M.D.**

---

**Hemodynamic Patterns of Age-related Changes in Blood Pressure: The Framingham Heart Study**

Franklin SS, Gustin W IV, Wong ND, et al (Univ of California, Irvine; Framingham Heart Study, Mass; Natl Heart, Lung and Blood Inst, Bethesda, Md; et al)

*Circulation* 96:308–315, 1997                                        3–6

---

*Introduction.*—Age-related changes in blood pressure are well documented, but the hemodynamic factors responsible for these changes are uncertain. Data from the Framingham Heart Study were used to identify, in both normotensive and untreated hypertensive individuals, age-related changes in systolic blood pressure (SBP), diastolic blood pressure (DBP), pulse pressure (PP), and mean arterial pressure (MAP). An attempt was made to infer underlying hemodynamic mechanisms from longitudinal changes in blood pressure components.

*Methods.*—The sample analyzed for this study included individuals with no clinical evidence of coronary heart disease and who had measurements of high density lipoprotein cholesterol available. All were aged 50 to 79 at the index examination, had not received antihypertensives at or before baseline and had 4 or more examinations at which untreated blood pressure levels were measured. The 2,036 eligible participants were divided into 4 groups according to SBP at the index examination: optimal SBP (less than 120 mmHg), normal and high normal SBP, stage 1 systolic hypertension (140 to 159 mmHg), and stages 2 to 4 systolic hypertension (up to 160 mmHg). One-way ANOVA was used to compare means of blood pressure slopes and curvatures among groups.

*Results.*—Optimal blood pressure was recorded in 22% of study participants; 41% had normal or high normal readings and 37% had hypertension. Systolic blood pressure exhibited a linear rise from age 30 through 84, with concurrent increases in DBP and MAP. After age 50 to 60 there were declines in DBP, a steep rise in PP, and MAP reached an asymptote. Women made up 47% of those with combined systolic-diastolic hypertension, but 62% of those with isolated systolic hypertension. Both normotensives and hypertensives showed an early rise and late fall in DBP, and all 4 groups had a consistent linear rise with aging. These patterns were unchanged when subsequent deaths and individuals with nonfatal myocardial infarction or heart failure were excluded. Individuals with the highest baseline SBP exhibited the greatest age-related linear increases in SBP, PP, and MAP, and as the early rise and late fall in DBP.

*Conclusion.*—Increases in MAP, SBP, and DBP age 50 are consistent with increasing peripheral vascular resistance, and the late fall in DBP with increased large artery stiffness. Untreated hypertension may accelerate the rate of development of large artery stiffness, thereby perpetuating a vicious cycle of accelerated hypertension.

▶ These data were obtained from the largest numbers of people followed as long as 30 years. They confirm what has been noted in smaller populations followed longitudinally and in cross-sectional observations from larger populations.

Obviously, systolic pressures typically continue to rise with age, even more in those who start with already higher pressure. Isolated systolic hypertension (ISH) was noted in more than 60% of the Framingham population older than age 65 who had an elevated blood pressure above 140 systolic or 90 diastolic.

For the past 5 years, strong proof of the value of treating those with ISH has become available, first from the SHEP study in the U.S.[1] and most recently from the SYST-EUR study from Europe.[2] In those studies, drugs were the primary treatment, a low-dose diuretic in SHEP, a long-acting dihydropyridine calcium antagonist in SYST-EUR. Fortunately, the elderly respond very well to a lower-sodium diet[3] and that, along with other lifestyle changes, should often be the initial therapy.

**N.M. Kaplan, M.D.**

*References*

1. SHEP Cooperative Research Group: Prevention of stroke by antihypertensive drug treatment in older persons with isolated systolic hypertension. *JAMA* 265:3255–3264, 1991.
2. Staessen JA, for the Systolic Hypertension in Europe (Syst-Eur) Trial Investigators: Randomised double-blind comparison of placebo and active treatment for older patients with isolated systolic hypertension. *Lancet* 350:757–764, 1997.
3. Fotherby MD, Potter JF: Metabolic and orthostatic blood pressure responses to a low-sodium diet in elderly hypertensives. *J Hum Hypertens* 11:361–366, 1997.

---

**Are Symptoms of Anxiety and Depression Risk Factors for Hypertension? Longitudinal Evidence From the National Health and Nutrition Examination Survey I Epidemiologic Follow-up Study**

Jonas BS, Franks P, Ingram DD (Natl Ctr for Health Statistics, Hyattsville, Md; Univ of Rochester, NY)
*Arch Fam Med* 6:43–49, 1997

3–7

---

*Background.*—Some studies have suggested that anxiety and depression may have a pressor effect on the cardiovascular system that could lead to hypertension. To examine the role of anxiety and depression in the subsequent development of hypertension, data from the National Health and Nutrition Examination I (NHANES I) Epidemiologic Follow-Up Study were used.

*Study Design.*—The NHANES I study was conducted from 1971 to 1975 with a nationwide probability sample of the civilian noninstitutionalized population of the United States. The Epidemiologic Follow-Up Study is a longitudinal study of 14,407 of the original NHANES I participants. The subjects of this study included 2,992 white and black participants from NHANES I who were 25 to 64 years old at baseline and normotensive at the beginning of the study period. These participants were followed for 7 to 16 years. The association between anxiety and depression at baseline and hypertension at follow-up was analyzed.

*Results.*—Multivariate analysis indicated that for whites and blacks aged 45 to 64 years, high anxiety and depression at baseline assessment were independent predictors of subsequent hypertension and treatment for hypertension. For whites aged 25 to 44 years, intermediate anxiety and depression were independent predictors of treated hypertension.

*Conclusion.*—This prospective study suggests that among both whites and blacks aged 25 to 64 years, there was an association between self-perceived anxiety and depression and subsequent hypertension. Further studies are required to understand the mechanism by which anxiety and depression exert their effects on blood pressure to increase the incidence of subsequent hypertension.

▶ Starting with a genetic predisposition (perhaps involving capillary rarefaction as noted in Abstract 3–11), at least 3 environmental factors seem most likely to be involved in the pathogenesis of hypertension: obesity (involving insulin resistance as noted in Abstract 3–9), sodium (as noted in Abstract 3–22) and stress, as described in this abstract. The progress can be accelerated by the lasting effects of low birth weight, as described in Abstract 3–10.

Of the 3 environmental factors, stress has been the hardest to document, largely because it is so hard to quantitate but also because long-term associations between increased stress and the subsequent incidence of hypertension have rarely been examined. These data involve a 7- to 16-year follow-up of a random sample of a large number of normotensives who had an assessment of anxiety and depression. Both were significantly predictive of the subsequent development of hypertension.

Other data show an association between the cardiovascular reactivity to psychological stress and the progression of carotid artery plaque formation over a 2 year period.[1] Moreover, Palatini and Julius[2] have reviewed the considerable evidence for increased hypertension and cardiovascular disease the faster the heart rate, presumably reflecting heightened sympathetic nervous system activity which could be medicated by stress.

The problem with all of this evidence is, how to get rid of stress, particularly when relaxation therapies seem to do so little.[3] With the accelerating turmoil in health care organization and delivery, physicians seem unlikely to be any less stressed for the immediate future.

**N.M. Kaplan, M.D.**

*References*

1. Barnett PA, Spence JD, Manuck SB, et al: Psychological stress and the progression of carotid artery disease. *J Hypertens* 15:49–55, 1997.
2. Palatini P, Julius S. Heart rate and the cardiovascular risk. *J Hypertens* 15:3–17, 1997.
3. Hunyor SN, Henderson RJ, Lal SKL, et al. Placebo-controlled biofeedback blood pressure effect in hypertensive humans. *Hypertension* 29:1225–1231, 1997.

## Anxiety-induced Hyperventilation: A Common Cause of Symptoms in Patients With Hypertension

Kaplan NM (Univ of Texas, Dallas)
*Arch Intern Med* 157:945–948, 1997                                              3–8

*Introduction.*—Anxiety-induced hyperventilation occurs often in patients with difficult-to-control hypertension. Treatment of the hypertension often becomes more difficult in such patients, and unnecessary diagnostic tests may be performed. A prospective study examined the prevalence of anxiety-induced hyperventilation and the mechanisms by which hyperventilation induces symptoms and a transient rise in blood pressure.

*Methods.*—The study population included 300 patients with primary hypertension who were referred for difficulty in controlling the condition (254 cases) or for various symptoms attributed to antihypertensive agents (46 cases). Uncontrolled hypertension was defined as office blood pressure readings greater than 140/90 mmHg despite treatment with at least 2 antihypertensive medications. Once a thorough history was taken, patients were asked to breathe rapidly and deeply for up to 3 minutes or as long as needed to relate their symptoms to hyperventilation.

*Results.*—The average age of the patients was 54; 278 were white and 163 were women. Their average office-seated blood pressure was 168/108 mmHg. On the basis of preexisting symptoms, anxiety-induced hypertension was considered likely in 104 patients. The typical symptoms complex (paresthesias, dizziness, palpitations) was reproduced in 86 patients by a brief period of voluntary hyperventilation. Hyperventilation was diagnosed in 16% of the men and 45% of the women in the study group. The process of overbreathing was explained to patients recognized as hyperventilators, and the technique of rebreathing into a No. 6 paper sack for prevention and relief of symptoms was demonstrated. Four patients with more severe anxiety were referred for psychotherapy.

*Conclusion.*—There was a high prevalence of hyperventilation in this group of patients referred for uncontrolled hypertension or symptoms ascribed to antihypertensive agents. Only 8 of 88 patients, however, had been previously diagnosed as having hyperventilation. This condition should be more frequently considered in cases of difficult-to-control hypertension. Once patients recognize the cause of their symptoms and learn the paper sack technique, hypertension can be better treated and unnecessary procedures minimized.

▶ I seldom include a review of my own papers in the YEAR BOOK, but this one deserves wide recognition because the problem is commonly found in patients seen by cardiologists (and all doctors), but it is often undiagnosed.

A recent patient portrays the problem: a 46-year-old man who was admitted to the Dallas VA hospital for the *tenth* time to rule out myocardial infarction because of "atypical chest pain." He was increasingly anxious about his heart, despite having been ruled out each time and having multiple normal stress tests and even 2 clean coronary angiograms. His anxiety began after a younger brother had a massive myocardial infarction, after which the patient was warned about his vulnerability and advised to "take an aspirin and rush to the ER" if any chest pain appeared.

His chest pain was related to a fast and forceful heartbeat against the chest wall, usually starting after a period of worry about his potential for a heart attack. The pain was associated with tingling of his fingers, band-like headache, dizziness, and a "smothering" sensation. The entire constellation was easily reproduced by voluntary overbreathing and relieved by rebreathing into a No. 6 paper sack.

Despite the overwhelming certainty that this "chest pain" was secondary to hyperventilation, the patient was unconvinced saying, "I know I have heart trouble, but the doctors haven't been able to find it yet." Obviously, each admission and each procedure further accentuated the likelihood of organic disease in his mind. He had become a virtual cardiac cripple because the psychosomatic nature of his problem had not been recognized and emphasized.

Atypical chest pain (more chest wall discomfort), palpitations, and dyspnea are some of the frequent manifestations of hyperventilation that will be noted in many patients seen by cardiologists. When taken to its extreme, overt panic attacks can occur[1] so it should always be considered in patients with anxiety and symptoms suggestive of hyperventilation. I've come across it rather frequently in the cardiac care unit. Certainly a patient who has just had a potentially lethal myocardial infarction and is being managed with all sorts of high-tech procedures is entitled to lots of anxiety. This anxiety can be manifested by acute hyperventilation.

**N.M. Kaplan, M.D.**

*Reference*

1. Hegel MT, Ferguson RJ: Psychophysiological assessment of respiratory function in panic disorder: evidence for a hyperventilation subtype. *Psychosom Med* 59:224–230, 1997.

### Hyperinsulinemia and Clustering of Cardiovascular Risk Factors in Middle-aged Hypertensive Finnish Men and Women

Vanhala MJ, Kumpusalo EA, Pitkäjärvi TK, et al (Pieksämäki District Health Centre, Naarajärvi, Finland; Kuopio Univ, Finland; Community Health Centre of the City of Tampere, Finland)
J Hypertens 15:475–481, 1997                                     3–9

*Introduction.*—Obesity, abdominal adiposity, and metabolic disorders are often associated with essential hypertension. Hyperinsulinemia–insulin resistance are linked to these abnormalities and are independent risk factors for cardiovascular disease. Little is known, however, about the association between cardiovascular risk factor cluster status and the level of fasting plasma insulin for hypertension. The prevalence of obesity, abdominal adiposity, hypertriglyceridemia, a low level of high-density lipoprotein cholesterol, and abnormal glucose metabolism was compared among hypertensive and normotensive subjects according to fasting levels of plasma insulin.

*Methods.*—One hundred sixty-one hypertensive men and women, ages 36 to 51 years, were compared with 177 normotensive patients. Measurements were taken according to the statistical quartiles of the fasting plasma insulin concentration of clusters of obesity, measured as body mass index >30.0 $kg/m^2$; abdominal adiposity, measured as waist-hip ratio >1.00 for men and >0.88 for women; a low level of high-density lipoprotein cholesterol, measured as <1.0 mmol/L in men and <1.20 mmol/L in women; hypertriglyceridemia, measured as >1.70 mmol/L; and abnormal glucose metabolism.

*Results.*—Compared with normotensive subjects, patients with hypertension were at 2.0- to 3.6-fold higher risk for clustering of the insulin resistance–associated cardiovascular risk factors. There was a 6- to 12-fold increase in risk associated with having 2 or more insulin resistance–associated cardiovascular risk factors among the hypertensive patients in the highest quartile of fasting plasma insulin, compared with those in the lowest quartile. There was a positive correlation between high levels of fasting plasma insulin and a high number of certain risk factors.

*Conclusion.*—These data confirm the association between hyperinsulinemia in middle-aged hypertensive patients and the presence of a cluster of risk factors for premature cadiovascular diseases.

▶ These data add to the large body of evidence incriminating hyperinsulinemia arising from insulin resistance as a precursor for hypertension, dyslipidemia, and diabetes—a combination noted most frequently in patients with upper body (abdominal or visceral) obesity but also in about a third of nonobese hypertensive patients.[1] This study both benefits and suffers from the use of fasting plasma insulin levels as the index for insulin resistance: the benefit derives from the relative ease of measuring plasma insulin levels; the downside comes from the rather weak association between a single fasting insulin measurement and insulin resistance as measured by more complicated techniques.

Regardless, the study is useful in that it examines a relatively representative sample of middle-aged normotensive and hypertensive subjects and documents further a significant association between major cardiovascular risk factors and fasting insulin levels.

Should a fasting plasma insulin measurement be added to the battery of cardiovascular risk factor markers? Probably not, despite these and other indicators of an association with diverse indices of target organ damage, such as left ventricular hypertrophy and microalbuminuria[2] and carotid artery intima-media thickness.[3] The reason is that traditional and widely used measures—blood pressure, lipid and glucose levels—seem adequate to document cardiovascular risk. However, like my mother's chicken soup, a fasting insulin level certainly wouldn't hurt, and might help.

**N.M. Kaplan, M.D.**

*References*

1. Masuo K, Mikami H, Ogihara T, et al: Prevalence of hyperinsulinemia in young, nonobese Japanese men. *J Hypertens* 15:157–165, 1997.
2. Tomiyama H, Doba N, Kushiro T, et al: The relationship of hyperinsulinemic state to left ventricular hypertrophy, microalbuminuria, and physical fitness in borderline and mild hypertension. *J Hypertens* 10:587–591, 1997.
3. Fujii K, Abe I, Ohya Y, et al: Association between hyperinsulinemia and intima-media thickness of the carotid artery in normotensive men. *J Hypertens* 15:167–172, 1997.

---

**Fetal Nutrition and Cardiovascular Disease in Later Life**
Barker DJP (Southampton Gen Hosp, England)
*Br Med Bull* 53:96–108, 1997                                               3–10

---

*Introduction.*—Studies have shown that many fetuses have had to adapt to a limited amount of nutrients, which can change their metabolism and physiology. Fetal growth is usually limited by the supply of nutrients and oxygen in the intrauterine environment. At particular stages of gestation, markers of lack of nutrients are low birth weight, and disproportion in head circumference, length, weight, and placental weight. The origin of a number of diseases in later life, such as coronary heart disease, hypertension, and diabetes, may be a result of these changes.

*Coronary heart disease.*—Variations in the death rate from coronary heart disease according to geographic region have correlated to the same variations in death caused by low birth weight in newborn babies. The development of coronary heart disease in adult life may be linked to low rates of growth before birth. One study compared death rates from coronary heart disease according to birth weight and found a correlation between low birth weight and coronary heart disease.

*Other diseases.*—Persons who were small at birth but are obese as adults are at risk of non-insulin-dependent diabetes and impaired glucose tolerance. A study showed that low birth weight is associated with resistance to insulin and its associated disorders in later life. Disturbances of cholesterol metabolism and blood coagulation have been linked to being born with a short body in relation to the size of its head although within the normal range of weight. There has been extensive demonstration of the association between low birth weight and elevated blood pressure in childhood and adult life.

*Conclusion.*—The growth of the fetus is influenced not only by its genes but also by the nutrient and oxygen supply it receives. The mother's dietary intake and nutrient stores, together with nutrient delivery to the placenta and the placenta's transfer capabilities, determine fetal nutrition. The true effects of maternal nutrition on fetal development are still not fully understood. The long-term sequelae of fetal adaptations to undernutrition should be studied.

▶ Barker has been the leading proponent of the low-birth-weight hypothesis for the origins of hypertension, diabetes, stroke, and coronary disease, as summarized in this review of the evidence.

The evidence is strong and makes a compelling argument, in part because it opens the way to a major preventive approach: the ability to prevent adult cardiovascular diseases by preventing intrauterine growth retardation through delay of adolescent pregnancies and improved maternal nutrition. Now, if only the pseudo-religious ultraconservatives will allow sex education, contraceptive availability, and federal support for prenatal care, we might be able to make a significant impact on the heavy cost in life and money that accrue to those not blessed with affluence and position.

My liberal leanings make me want to believe this hypothesis. Support continues to grow for its validity. For instance, a strong inverse association has been found between birth weight and blood pressure that cannot be explained by confounding socioeconomic circumstances.[1] On the other hand, some data do not support this hypothesis: no effect on later survival has been found among cohorts subjected to prolonged and extreme nutritional deprivation in utero during a major famine in Finland.[2]

If the hypothesis holds, as I believe it will, the mechanisms likely include in utero stunting of vital organ development, particularly the kidneys, in relation to later blood pressure. Other possible mechanisms include an effect of low maternal protein intake to lowering placental 11-β-hydroxysteroid dehydrogenase activity so that more cortisol floods the fetal circulation, programming the fetus for subsequent hypertension and diabetes.

**N.M. Kaplan, M.D.**

*References*

1. Koupilová I, Leon DA, Vägerö D: Can confounding by sociodemographic and behavioral factors explain the association between size at birth and blood pressure at age 50 in Sweden? *J Epidemiol Community Health* 51:14–18, 1997.
2. Kannisto V, Christensen K, Vaupel JW: No increased mortality in later life for cohorts born during famine. *Am J Epidemiol* 145:987–994, 1997.

3. Langley-Evans SC: Hypertension induced by foetal exposure to a maternal low-protein diet, in the rat, is prevented by pharmacological blockade of maternal glucocorticoid synthesis. *J Hypertens* 15:537–544, 1997.

**Impaired Microvascular Dilatation and Capillary Rarefaction in Young Adults With a Predisposition to High Blood Pressure**
Noon JP, Walker BR, Webb DJ, et al (Univ of Edinburgh, Scotland; Univ of Exeter, England; Ladywell Med Centre, Edinburgh, Scotland; et al)
*J Clin Invest* 99:1873–1879, 1997                                  3–11

*Introduction.*—Resistance across vessels less than 100 μm in luminal diameter is a sign of peripheral vascular resistance. In essential hypertension, capillary pressures are elevated and venous pressure is normal. Hypertensive patients tend to have decreased luminal diameter, predominantly in larger arterioles, and a reduction in the density of vessels per volume of tissue. It is still unknown whether microvascular abnormalities are a cause or a consequence of a rise in blood pressure. Patients identified as either having high or low blood pressure in early adulthood and who were further classified on the basis of their parents' blood pressure were studied to distinguish microvascular abnormalities that could cause high blood pressure from those that are a consequence of high blood pressure.

*Methods.*—Recordings of blood pressure and cardiac function were made. Maximum vasodilation of skin microvessels was measured by laser Doppler fluximetry in the right arm in response to local heating to 42°C, followed by the addition of a period of ischemia. Intravital videomicroscopy was used to measure nailfold capillary blood velocity and red cell column width, and capillary numbers on the dorsum of the ring finger. Strain gauge plethysmography was used to measure blood flow before and after ischemia in the right arm.

*Results.*—Following ischemia and heating, offspring with high blood pressure whose parents also have high blood pressure had more impaired dermal vasodilation in the forearm and fewer capillaries on the dorsum of the finger, compared with the other groups. In young adult men, impaired microvascular vasodilation and capillary rarefaction are associated with the expression of familial predisposition to essential hypertension. At this stage in the development of high blood pressure, capillary luminal diameter and blood flow are not reduced and are more likely to be consequences rather than causes of elevated blood pressure.

*Conclusion.*—Increased minimum resistance and capillary rarefaction are exhibited in the dermal vessels of men with a familial predisposition to high blood pressure. In the inheritance of high blood pressure, defective angiogenesis may be an etiologic component.

▶ The experimental approach used by these investigators, looking at a variety of possible contributors to the pathogenesis of hypertension in those most likely to become hypertensive (higher personal and parenteral blood pressure) in comparison with those least likely to become hypertensive (lower personal and parental blood pressure), continues to deliver interesting data.

The significant differences in microvascular dilatation and the number of capillaries suggest that one of the ways that heredity is involved is the transmission of defective blood vessel formation (angiogenesis). Presumably, over time these changes would translate into increased peripheral vascular resistance, the hemodynamic hallmark of established hypertension.

Hopefully, these investigators will still be around when these subjects develop hypertension, so that their hypothesis can be documented.

**N.M. Kaplan, M.D.**

---

**The Prevalence of Hypertension in Seven Populations of West African Origin**
Cooper R, Rotimi C, Ataman S, et al (Loyola Univ, Maywood, Ill; Univ of Ibadan, Nigeria; Univ Ctr for Health Science, Yaounde, Cameroon; et al)
*Am J Public Health* 87:160–168, 1997                                    3–12

---

*Background.*—Hypertension is more prevalent among American blacks than it is among American whites. Although the reasons for this discrepancy have been sought, the influence of genetic differences and environmental factors have yet to be understood. The role of environmental factors in the risk for hypertension was explored by comparing the prevalence of hypertension and its association with known risk factors among 7 populations of West African descent.

*Methods.*—Study populations were chosen in Nigeria; rural Cameroon; urban Cameroon; Jamaica; St. Lucia, Barbados; and Maywood, Illinois. A total of 10,014 subjects from these populations were recruited to participate in the study. Interviews, measurements of anthropometric characteristics, and blood pressure measurements were performed for each participant. As an estimate of dietary sodium and potassium intake, 24-hour urinary sodium and potassium excretion was measured on a subset of the participants.

*Results.*—Hypertension prevalence was lowest in West Africa (16%), midrange in the Caribbean (26%), and highest in the United States (33%). Although the prevalence of hypertension was similar among participants ages 25–34 years across all populations, it increased with age twice as rapidly in the United States as it did in West Africa. There was a strong correlation between body mass, standardized for sex and age, and hypertension prevalence across all study populations (Fig 5). A similar, but less consistent, gradient was detected for the sodium–potassium ratio. In a regression analysis, mean body mass indices and sodium–potassium ratios accounted for 70% of the geographic differences in age- and sex-adjusted hypertension prevalence.

*Conclusions.*—The participants shared common ancestry, minimizing any potential role of genetic factors in the outcome of the project. These findings demonstrate the influence of sociocultural factors on hypertension

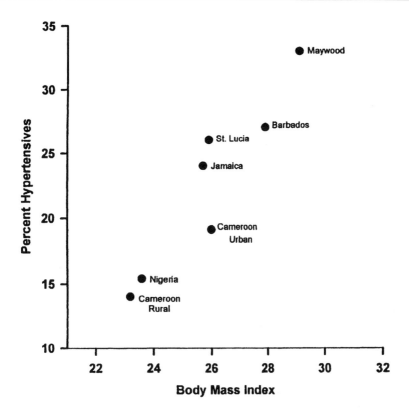

*Note.* ICSHIB = International Collaborative Study of Hypertension in Blacks.

FIGURE 5.—Prevalence of hypertension among seven populations of West African origin, by mean body mass index: the ICSHIB Study, 1995. *Abbreviation: ICSHIB*, International Collaborative Study of Hypertension in Blacks. (Courtesy of Cooper R, Rotimi C, Ataman S, et al: The prevalence of hypertension in seven populations of West African origin. *Am J Public Health* 87:160–168, 1997. Copyright 1997 by the American Public Health Association.)

prevalence among peoples of African descent and are supportive of the hypothesis that the greater prevalence of hypertension among black, compared with white, Americans is the result of external environmental factors rather than of differing genetic predispositions to the disease. Further research is needed to identify more precisely the risk factors for hypertension among black Americans and to explore potential preventive strategies.

▶ Hypertension is more prevalent and more deadly in U.S. blacks than it is in U.S. Hispanics or Whites.[1] This could reflect a genetic predisposition or a selective migration of people more susceptible to hypertension. Such selective migration has been attributed to the survival of those Africans transported in slave ships, who were able to conserve sodium, protecting them from the exigencies of trans-Atlantic travel but exposing them to additional sodium retention when they reached the United States, with its salt-rich diet.

These data display a progressive increase in the prevalence of hypertension in blacks in Africa, the Caribbean, and the United States. Thus, genetics likely plays a secondary role, whereas environmental exposures must be primary. Because more obesity and higher sodium–lower potassium intakes were observed, along with gradient of hypertension, these 2 environmental factors likely are involved. The salt-conservation hypothesis could be part of the association with sodium. Greater psychosocial stress obviously could be added to these other factors.

**N.M. Kaplan, M.D.**

*Reference*

1. Klag MJ, Whelton PK, Randall BL, et al: End-stage renal disease in African-American and white men. *JAMA* 277:1293–1298, 1997.

---

**Neurovascular Compression of the Rostral Ventrolateral Medulla Related to Essential Hypertension**
Morimoto S, Sasaki S, Miki S, et al (Kyoto Prefectural Univ, Japan)
*Hypertension* 30:77–82, 1997                                                     3–13

---

*Introduction.*—The rostral ventrolateral medulla (RVLM) is a major center of the sympathetic nervous system and is involved in regulating the cardiovascular system. An association between essential hypertension and neurovascular compression of the ventrolateral medulla at the root-entry zone of glossopharyngeal and vagus nerves has been observed clinically and experimentally. Magnetic resonance imaging was performed using a high-resolution $512 \times 512$ matrix, a new magnetic device, and MR angiography to determine more precise information about the relationship between essential hypertension and neurovascular compression of the RVLM.

*Methods.*—Twenty-one patients with essential hypertension, 10 patients with secondary hypertension, and 18 normotensive research subjects underwent MRI and MR angiography assessments. Significance of the differences in the distances between the center of the RVLM and nearest arteries and between the surface of the medulla oblongata and the nearest arteries among the 3 groups was analyzed.

*Results.*—Neurovascular compression of the RVLM was detected in 15 of 20 (75%) patients with essential hypertension, 1 of 10 (10%) patients with secondary hypertension, and 2 of 18 (11%) normotensive research subjects. The rate of neurovascular compression detected in the essential hypertension group was significantly higher, in contrast to the secondary hypertension group and the normotensive group. In the essential hypertension group, the distances between the RVLM and the nearest arteries were significantly shorter than that of the secondary hypertension and normotensive groups.

*Conclusion.*—Using a new MR device (proton density weighted images with a high-resolution 512 × 512 matrix), the distances between the surface of the RVLM, but not other regions of the medulla oblongata and neighboring arteries, were significantly shorter in patients with essential hypertension than in patients who were normotensive and those with secondary hypertension. Neurovascular compression in the RVLM and essential hypertension might be related.

▶ I continue to doubt the causal association between neurovascular compression of the RVLM and hypertension espoused first and repeatedly by Jannetta et al. in Pittsburgh.[1] The anatomical finding in some hypertensive patients cannot be denied and is further documented in this study from Japan. Investigators from Germany have also found such compression in 15 patients with a syndrome of autosomal dominant hypertension and brachydactyly.[2]

Since blood vessels in patients with long-standing hypertension are often more tortuous, the anatomical finding is not, in itself, surprising. No specific pathophysiological role that could arise from neurovascular compression has been noted in these patients. The proof must come from a properly controlled trial of decompression providing long-term relief of hypertension. Such evidence has not been provided.

**N.M. Kaplan, M.D.**

*References*

1. Jannetta PJ, Segal R, Wolfson SK: Neurogenic hypertension: Etiology and surgical treatment. I: Observations in 53 patients. *Ann Surg* 201:391–398, 1985.
2. Naraghi R, Schuster H, Toka HR, et al: Neurovascular compression at the ventrolateral medulla in autosomal dominant hypertension and brachydactyly. *Stroke* 28:1749–1754, 1997.

## Complications

### INTRODUCTION

There are obvious cardiovascular sequelae of untreated hypertension, in particular on the myocardium. These cardiac effects, increasingly recognized by echocardiography, are being found to be closely correlated to subsequent morbidity and mortality. Other factors than blood pressure—including clotting components and lipoprotein levels—play a role, and the brain obviously may suffer as well.

**Norman M. Kaplan, M.D.**

### The Role of Blood Pressure in Cognitive Impairment in an Elderly Population

Rengo F for the 'Osservatorio Geriatrico Campano Group' (Università delgi Studi di Napoli 'Federico II', Napoli, Italy)
J Hypertens 15:135–142, 1997                                                3–14

*Introduction.*—There is continuing debate over how cognitive function is affected by blood pressure. Studies of this issue have given inconsistent results; however, many have found a high prevalence of cognitive impairment among elderly patients with hypertension. A cross-sectional study of a Mediterranean population was performed to assess the relationships among aging, blood pressure, and cognitive performance.

*Methods.*—Interviews were conducted with a random sample of 1,339 elderly subjects (mean age, 74 years) in southern Italy. Variables assessed included sociodemographic factors, Mini-Mental State Examination (MMSE) score, Geriatric Depression Scale (GDS) score, blood pressure, and whether the patient was receiving antihypertensive medication. After exclusion of patients who had neurologic diseases or were receiving psychotropic medication, the analysis included 1,106 subjects.

*Results.*—Twenty-eight percent of subjects had an MMSE score of less than 24. The sample population had a mean blood pressure of 145/82 and a mean GDS score of 10.8. Significant predictive factors for cognitive impairment on logistic regression analysis were female sex, GDS score, and diastolic blood pressure. Systolic blood pressure was not a significant predictor. Subjects who had higher educational attainment and who were taking antihypertensive medication had lower rates of cognitive impairment. The link between diastolic blood pressure and cognitive impairment held for subjects aged 75 years and for those older than 75 years (odds ratios, 1.62 and 5.16, respectively) but not for subjects aged 65 to 74 years.

*Conclusion.*—Diastolic blood pressure is an independent predictor of cognitive impairment in subjects aged 75 years and older who are free of neurologic disorders. This relationship is unaffected by potential confounders such as age, education, depression, and antihypertensive therapy. Systolic blood pressure is not a significant predictor, however.

▶ Next to the heart, the brain is the most commonly afflicted target organ of hypertension. Strokes are the usual manifestation of cerebrovascular disease and are the third leading cause of death in the United States. Even more common as a cause of morbidity is dementia. Most previously published studies have shown an association between hypertension and cognitive impairment varying from minimal loss of cognitive performance by psychometric test all the way to overt dementia. However, some studies have not shown a clear association, so this study was performed on a sizable elderly population, 1,106 subjects aged 65 to 95 years.

The results are somewhat surprising in that only elevated diastolic, but not systolic, pressure was associated with cognitive impairment in those over age 75. Systolic blood pressure is more predictive of the risk of stroke (and heart attack) in the elderly, presumably reflecting the contribution of atherosclerotic thickening to the rising systolic blood pressure of aging. The data underscore the importance of effective therapy for both systolic and diastolic hypertension in the elderly—the former perhaps more to prevent stroke, the latter perhaps more to prevent cognitive impairment.

**N.M. Kaplan, M.D.**

---

**Antecedent Hypertension Confers Increased Risk for Adverse Outcomes After Initial Myocardial Infarction**
Haider AW, Chen L, Larson MG, et al (Natl Heart, Lung, and Blood Inst's Framingham Heart Study, Mass; Natl Heart, Lung, and Blood Inst, Bethesda, Md; Boston Univ; et al)
*Hypertension* 30:1020–1024, 1997                3–15

---

*Introduction.*—The association between blood pressure (BP) after myocardial infarction (MI) has been extensively assessed regarding risk for adverse outcome. Few trials have evaluated prognosis after MI as a function of BP before MI. The relation of antecedent hypertension to risk of adverse outcomes after initial MI was evaluated in research subjects from the Framingham Heart Study.

*Methods.*—From 1967 to 1990, 404 of 5,209 male and female research subjects from the Framingham Heart Study had an initial MI. Research subjects with initial MI were classified according to BP before MI: 118 normotensive (BP less than 140/90 mmHg and not receiving antihypertension treatment), 89 stage I—untreated hypertension (BP 140 to 159/90 to 99 mmHg), 197 stage II–IV or treated hypertension (BP ≥160/100 mmHg or treated hypertension).

*Results.*—The post-MI median survival was 12.19, 8.88, and 4.18 years, respectively, for patients with normotensive, stage I, and stage II–IV hypertension (Fig 2) before MI. Research subjects with stage I hypertension before MI were at marginally increased risk for reinfarction, and those with stage II–IV hypertension were at significantly increased risk for reinfarction, compared to research subjects who were normotensive. Research subjects with stage II–IV hypertension before MI were at increased risk for all-cause mortality, compared to those who were normotensive. Research subjects in stage I and stage II–IV hypertension before MI were at similar risk for coronary heart disease death, compared to those who were normotensive.

*Conclusion.*—Antecedent hypertension is a risk factor for adverse outcome after initial MI, particularly for recurrent MI. The risk increases with increasing hypertension stage and is higher after excluding early events. More effective blood pressure control may decrease the risk of initial MI and improve outcome if an MI occurs.

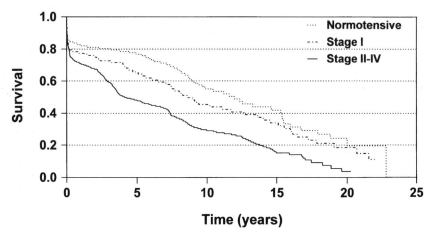

**FIGURE 2.**—Survival after myocardial infarction according to blood pressure status before infarction. Kaplan-Meier curves for survival after initial myocardial infarction for normotensive individuals (systolic blood pressure less than 140 mmHg and diastolic blood pressure less than 90 mmHg and not receiving antihypertensive therapy), stage I hypertensive individuals (systolic blood pressure 140 to 159 mmHg or diastolic blood pressure 90 to 99 mmHg and not receiving antihypertension treatment), and stage II to IV hypertensive individuals (systolic blood pressure ≥160 mmHg or diastolic blood pressure ≥100 mmHg or current use of antihypertensive therapy). Median survival times were 12.19 years, 8.88 years, and 4.18 years, respectively. (Courtesy of Haider AW, Chen L, Larson MG et al: Antecedent hypertension confers increased risk for adverse outcomes after initial myocardial infarction. *Hypertension* 30:1020–1024, 1997.)

▶ As the authors note in their introduction, many papers have documented an increased mortality after an acute MI among patients with antecedent hypertension, particularly if the post-MI blood pressure is significantly lower suggesting poor pump function.

The beauty of this paper from Framingham is the long-term follow up of a carefully observed cohort, as perhaps can come from this ongoing study better than from any other. As the authors note, however, these data don't address the issue in groups other than Caucasians and don't adequately answer the question as to whether effective antihypertensive therapy will minimize the post-MI troubles.

**N.M. Kaplan, M.D.**

---

**Left Atrial Size in Hypertensive Men: Influence of Obesity, Race and Age**
Gottdiener JS, for the Department of Veterans Affairs Cooperative Study Group on Antihypertensive Agents (Georgetown Univ, Washington, DC)
*J Am Coll Cardiol* 29:651–658, 1997                                               3–16

---

*Purpose.*—Patients with hypertension have increased left ventricular (LV) mass and left atrial (LA) size. In the population, blood pressure has less of an effect on LA size than age and body mass index do. However, these interrelationships in patients with established hypertension are unknown. The effects of blood pressure, obesity, race, age, and LV mass in LA size in hypertensive patients were studied.

*Methods.*—The study sample comprised 690 men with mild-to-moderate hypertension and a high prevalence of LV hypertrophy. Fifty-eight percent of the subjects were African-American; the mean blood pressure was 152/98 mmHg. Univariate and multivariate analyses were performed to assess the effects of LV mass, adiposity, race, age, physical activity, height, weight, sodium excretion, plasma renin activity, and heart rate.

*Results.*—The mean LA size was 44 mm in obese patients, 42 mm in overweight patients, and 39 mm in normal-weight patients. At a cutoff point of 43 mm, 56% of obese patients, 42% of overweight patients, and 25% of normal-weight patients had LA enlargement. Left atrial size increased with age to a greater extent in Caucasian men than in African-American men. In obese patients, LV mass was significantly and positive related to LA size, whereas in normal-weight men, there was no relationship between these 2 factors. Obesity was the main independent predictor of increased LA size on multiple regression analysis, followed by race, an interaction between LV mass and body mass, an interaction between age and race, and LV mass.

*Conclusion.*—In hypertensive patients, the main factor affecting LA size is obesity. Obesity also amplifies the relationship between LA size and LV mass, whereas race alters the effects of age and hypertension on LA size. Left atrial size and LV mass are both influenced by obesity and associated with adverse outcomes; obesity, race, and age all have an important influence on the cardiac effects of hypertension.

▶ The left ventricle is usually the cardiac chamber that is measured and analyzed when the effects of hypertension on the heart are considered. However, the left atrium is also affected by hypertension, with the subsequent possibility of alteration of LV filling and induction of atrial arrhythmias.

This study involved almost 700 of the 1,292 men with diastolic BP of 95 to 109 mmHg enrolled in a Department of Veterans Affairs cooperative trial of various antihypertensive drugs, using 2-dimensional M-mode echocardiography. The greater importance of obesity compared with levels of systolic or diastolic BP as the strongest predictor of LA size may reflect the relative mildness of these patients' hypertension and the confounding effects of prior antihypertensive therapy, which was discontinued for only 6 to 12 weeks before entry into the study. Regardless, LA enlargement is frequently seen in hypertensives and may contribute to the cardiac sequelae of the condition.

**N.M. Kaplan, M.D.**

### Usefulness of Subnormal Midwall Fractional Shortening in Predicting Left Ventricular Exercise Dysfunction in Asymptomatic Patients With Systemic Hypertension

Schussheim AE, Devereux RB, de Simone G, et al (New York Hosp-Cornell Med Ctr)

Am J Cardiol 79:1070–1074, 1997                                    3–17

*Background.*—In a recent study, the authors found that some asymptomatic patients with hypertension have below-normal left ventricular (LV) midwall fiber shortening at rest. This characteristic is an independent predictor of morbidity and mortality, independent of age, blood pressure, or LV hypertrophy. This study sought to determine whether abnormal midwall fractional shortening in asymptomatic hypertensive patients is associated with subnormal LV functional reserve or extracardiac damage.

*Methods.*—Two groups of patients with an average diastolic blood pressure of 90 mmHg or greater were studied. Echocardiography showed subnormal midwall fractional shortening in 16 patients, whereas this finding was normal in 89 patients. The radionuclide cineangiographic LV ejection fraction was assessed at rest and at maximal exercise in all patients. The results, as well as the clinical findings, were compared between groups.

*Results.*—The 2 groups were comparable in sex, age, and systolic blood pressure. However, mean diastolic blood pressure and body mass index were higher in the group with normal shortening. The resting ejection fraction was 56% in the group with normal shortening and 55% in the group with subnormal midwall fractional shortening. However, LV mass was greater in the patients with subnormal shortening. Urinary protein excretion and serum creatinine levels tended to be higher in this group, as well. A subnormal exercise LV ejection fraction—i.e., less than 54%—was present in 15% of patients with normal midwall fractional shortening vs. 44% of patients with subnormal shortening. Midwall fractional shortening was an independent predictor of exercise performance on multiple linear regression analysis.

*Conclusion.*—In patients with asymptomatic hypertension, subnormal LV midwall fractional shortening is associated with reduced LV functional reserve. Subnormal shortening may be a useful indicator of extracardiac target-organ damage and, thus, useful for identifying high-risk hypertensive patients who need particularly intensive treatment.

▶ These investigators had previously shown that the assessment of LV function in hypertensives with an increased myocardial afterload as assessed by radionuclide cineangiography using the "conventional practice of relating LV minor axis shortening at the endocardium to the mean level of wall stress across the LV wall represents a conceptual mismatch that may introduce potential errors in assessment of LV contractile state." Therefore, they introduced fractional shortening at the midwall level as a more physiologically appropriate measure of LV systolic function and found it to be an independent predictor of cardiovascular risk in hypertensive patients.[1]

The study abstracted here was performed to determine whether subnormal midwall fractional shortening could be used to predict impaired LV functional reserve during exercise. The results show that midwall fractional shortening independently predicts exercise performance in asymptomatic hypertensives. However, the separation between patients with normal vs. subnormal LV ejection fraction during exercise was not complete: A subnormal LV ejection fraction during exercise was seen in 15% of patients with normal midwall fractional shortening and in 44% of those with subnormal shortening. It seems doubtful whether the procedure will find much clinical utility because easier-to-obtain indicators of risk seem adequate to identify high risk hypertensives.

**N.M. Kaplan, M.D.**

*Reference*

1. de Simone G, Devereux RB, Koren MJ, et al: Midwall left ventricular mechanics: An independent predictor of cardiovascular risk in arterial hypertension. *Circulation* 93:259–265, 1996.

---

**Left Ventricular Mass Is Better Correlated With Arising Blood Pressure Than With Office or Occasional Blood Pressure**
Gosse P, Ansoborlo P, Lemetayer P, et al (Hôpital Saint André, Bordeaux, France)
*Am J Hypertens* 10:505–510, 1997                                        3–18

---

*Introduction.*—The elevation in blood pressure that occurs on morning waking and arising appears to increase the risk of cardiovascular events. Although the peak incidence of myocardial infarction, stroke, and sudden death is between 6 AM and 12 PM, there is no firm evidence linking the extent of blood pressure elevation and risk of cardiovascular complications. The significance of arising blood pressure was examined in a retrospective study of previously untreated patients with hypertension.

*Methods.*—Eligible patients had good-quality echocardiograms enabling measurement of left ventricular mass and records of 24-hour ambulatory blood pressure monitoring during which a measurement was triggered on arising in the morning. The product of the arising systolic blood pressure and heart rate and the difference between the arising blood pressure and mean nighttime blood pressure were calculated.

*Results.*—The study group included 128 men and 53 women with a mean age of 50. Their mean office blood pressure was 162/101 mmHg and their mean blood pressure at the time when the monitoring device was fitted was 156/102 mmHg. During the monitoring period, mean arising blood pressure was 141/96 mmHg and mean arising heart rate was 82 beats/min. Mean left ventricular mass, indexed for height, height$^{2.7}$, and body surface area, was 132 g/m, 54.5, and 122 g/m$^2$, respectively. Mean posterior wall thickness was 9.2 mm. Elevation in blood pressure on rising averaged 18 mmHg for systolic and 16 mmHg for diastolic blood pressure. Systolic blood pressure on arising was significantly better correlated than office blood pressure with left ventricular mass index and wall thickness. Multivariate analysis revealed that the values of systolic blood pressure on arising and mean 24-hour systolic blood pressure contributed significantly and independently to the correlation with left ventricular mass and wall thickness.

*Conclusion.*—In this group of patients who were previously untreated for hypertension, there was a highly significant correlation between blood pressure measured immediately after arising in the morning and left ventricular mass. This steep elevation in blood pressure can persist for several hours and may contribute to the triggering of cardiac complications.

▶ These data add to the considerable evidence that getting out of bed is a dangerous thing to do. The abrupt rise in blood pressure that accompanies standing and ambulating is clearly involved in the markedly increased propensity for sudden death, myocardial infarction, arrhythmias, and strokes to occur in the early morning hours.[1] From these data, it appears that an increased left ventricular mass could be an intermediary to these vascular catastrophes.

All of this calls attention to the need for 24-hour control of hypertension by use of long-acting, once-a-day formulations of whatever drug is used to treat the condition.

**N.M. Kaplan, M.D.**

*Reference*

1. Muller J, and the MILIS study group: Circadian variation in the frequency of onset of acute myocardial infarction. *N Engl J Med* 313:1315–1322, 1985.

---

**Relation of Left Ventricular Mass and QT Dispersion in Patients With Systematic Hypertension**
Ichkhan K, Molnar J, Somberg J (Finch Univ of Health Sciences/Chicago Med School, North Chicago, Ill)
*Am J Cardiol* 79:508–512, 1997                    3–19

---

*Purpose.*—QT dispersion refers to the difference between the minimum and maximum QT measured in any of the 12 ECG leads. It is a measure of regional variation in ventricular repolarization and is thought to be useful in predicting the risk of ventricular arrhythmia. This study sought to determine whether QT dispersion is increased in patients with left ventricular (LV) hypertension.

*Methods.*—Electrocardiograms and echocardiograms from 2 groups of patients with hypertension were studied. There were 25 patients with LV hypertrophy and 24 without. QT dispersion, corrected QT dispersion,

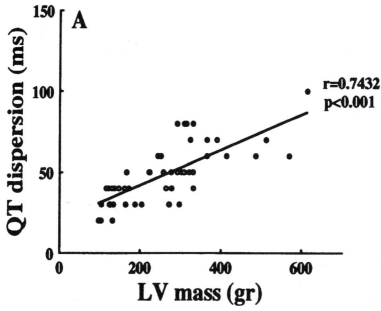

FIGURE 1.—A, correlation between QT dispersion and left ventricular (*LV*) mass. (Reprinted by permission of the publisher from Ichkhan K, Molnar J, Somberg J: Relation of left ventricular mass and QT dispersion in patients with systematic hypertension. *American Journal Of Cardiology* 79:508–512, copyright 1997 by Excerpta Medica, Inc.)

percent normalized QT dispersion, and percent normalized corrected QT dispersion were calculated and compared with LV mass.

*Results.*—QT dispersion was significantly correlated with LV mass, ($r = -0.74$ (Fig 1A). Left ventricular mass was correlated with the other measures of QT dispersion as well. The mean QT dispersion was 58 msec in patients with hypertension and LV hypertrophy vs. 39 msec in those with hypertension but without LV hypertrophy.

*Conclusion.*—In patients with hypertension, a larger LV mass is associated with greater QT dispersion. Hypertensive patients with LV hypertrophy have significantly increased QT dispersion, whereas hypertensive patients without LV do not. Thus, increased QT dispersion results not from hypertension as such but from LV hypertrophy. Long-term studies are needed to see whether changes in QT dispersion, as an index of electric instability, are correlated with regression of left ventricular hypertrophy.

▶ These data add to the large body of evidence that LV hypertrophy is both common in patients with hypertension and an indicator of increased risk for arrhythmias, coronary disease, sudden death, and congestive heart failure. The data connect the presence of a known marker for malignant arrhythmias and sudden death—prolongation of the rate-corrected QT interval—to the presence of LV hypertrophy, a connection that is stronger than just the mere presence of hypertension.

The authors question whether regression of LV hypertrophy will reduce the risk for arrythmia, a logical question which has not yet been addressed in an adequately large and long study. Meanwhile, evidence continues to define the increased risks of LV hypertrophy, with little difference in predictive value among the various methods used to assess it. Additional comparisons between the relative abilities of various classes of antihypertensive agents to regress LV hypertrophy have been published.[2] In the Gottdiener study, better effects were noted with an angiotensin converting enzyme inhibitor, β-blocker, or diuretic than with a calcium blocker, α-blocker, or central α-agonist. However, as noted by Devereux,[3] this study included too few patients and used questionable methods to assess changes in LV hypertrophy, so the issue remains unsettled.

As Devereux concludes: "The ultimate question with regard to hypertensive LVH is not whether one agent or another is somewhat more effective in reversing it but rather whether regression of hypertensive LVH confers a prognostic benefit over and above the degree of induced lowering of blood pressure."

Studies to answer this, the "ultimate question," are in progress. Meanwhile, small studies measuring surrogate end points suggest that regression may not be all that beneficial. For instance, regression of LV hypertension over 6 months by various antihypertensives did not improve exercise performance in hypertensive patients.[4]

**N.M. Kaplan, M.D.**

*References*

1. Roman MJ: How best to identify prognostically important left ventricular hypertrophy: A cut to the chase. *J Am Coll Cardiol,* 29:648–650, 1997.
2. Gottdiener JS, Reda DJ, Massie BM, et al: Effect of single-drug therapy on reduction of left ventricular mass in mild to moderate hypertension. *Circulation* 95:2007–2014, 1997.
3. Devereux RB: Do antihypertensive drugs differ in their ability to regress left ventricular hypertrophy? *Circulation* 95:1983–1985, 1997.
4. Fagard RH, Lijnen PJ: Reduction of left ventricular mass by antihypertensive treatment does not improve exercise performance in essential hypertension. *J Hypertens* 15:309–317, 1997.

**Production of Plasminogen Activator Inhibitor 1 by Human Adipose Tissue: Possible Link Between Visceral Fat Accumulation and Vascular Disease**

Alessi MC, Peiretti F, Morange P, et al (Laboratoire d'Hématologie, Marseille, France)
*Diabetes* 46:860–867, 1997        3–20

*Introduction.*—The pathogenesis of atherothrombosis may be affected by plasminogen activator inhibitor type 1 (PAI-1), because elevated concentrations decrease endogenous and therapeutic fibrinolysis and increase extension of thrombosis. Patients with cardiovascular diseases have demonstrated increased levels of PAI-1. Insulin resistance syndrome may be a regulator of PAI-1 expression, and the participation of adipose tissue in its increase in insulin-resistant patients has attracted much attention. Plasminogen activator inhibitor type 1 expression by human adipose tissue and its different cellular fraction was investigated.

*Methods.*—Subcutaneous adipose tissue was removed during elective abdominoplasty in 15 healthy female patients with body mass index 25–29 kg/m². Tissue explants and adipocytes were incubated, and immunocytochemical staining, PAI-1 and leptin antigen determination, RNA and DNA extraction, riboprobe preparation, ribonuclease protection, and statistical analysis were performed.

*Results.*—At the stromal and adipocyte levels, PAI-1 protein was present. In stromal vascular cells freshly isolated and under culture conditions, PAI-1 mRNA was detected. In whole adipose tissue and adipocyte fraction under culture conditions, PAI-1 was also detected. Within 2 hours of incubation, the mRNA signal from the adipocyte fraction was detected. In the conditioned medium that was suppressed by treatment with cycloheximide, the increase in PAI-1 mRNA was followed by an increase in PAI-1 antigen. Plasminogen activator inhibitory-1 antigen production by the adipocyte fraction was significantly increased by transforming growth factor-β1. No effect was seen with tumor necrosis factor-α. Omental tissue explants produced significantly more PAI-1 antigen than did subcutaneous tissue from the same individual after 5 hours of incubation. The two territories, however, demonstrated similar production of leptin.

*Conclusion.*—An important contributor to the elevated PAI-1 levels observed in central obesity is human adipose tissue, particularly visceral tissue.

▶ These data provide another possible explanation for the common association between upper body (abdominal or visceral) obesity and cardiovascular disease, beyond the contribution of insulin resistance–hyperinsulinemia described in Abstract 3–9.

As Alessi et al. note, PAI-1 seems to be involved in atherothrombosis. Their new recognition of a greater production of PAI-1 from human visceral fat cells compared with subcutaneous fat cells adds to the evidence that PAI-1 derived from visceral fat cells could be involved in the pathogenesis of the cardiovascular consequences of visceral obesity.

Now, if we could only prevent the development of visceral obesity.

**N.M. Kaplan, M.D.**

### Association of Serum Lipoprotein(a) Levels and Apolipoprotein(a) Size Polymorphism With Target-Organ Damage in Arterial Hypertension

Sechi LA, Kronenberg F, De Carli S, et al (Univ of Udine, Italy; Univ of Innsbruck, Austria)
*JAMA* 277:1689–1695, 1997                                                      3–21

*Background.*—In patients with hypertension, many different factors affect the risk of target-organ damage (TOD). One of these factors is lipoproteins, which have a major influence on cardiovascular morbidity and mortality. Previous studies have suggested that high plasma levels of lipoprotein (a) (Lp[a])—a heterogeneous lipoprotein consisting of a low-density lipoprotein particle and the highly polymorphic apolipoprotein(a) (apo[a])—are an independent risk factor for atherosclerosis and athero-sclerotic complications. This study examined Lp(a) as a possible risk factor for TOD in hypertensive patients.

*Methods.*—Two hundred seventy-seven patients with untreated, mild-to-moderate essential hypertension and 102 healthy controls underwent measurement of Lp(a) and apolipoproteins. An independent sample of 106 patients with hypertension and 105 controls underwent apo(a) phenotype analysis. Each patient was evaluated by World Health Organization guidelines for the staging of TOD, including clinical evaluation, laboratory measurements of creatinine clearance and proteinuria, ophthalmoscopy, ECG, echocardiography, and ultrasound examination of the major arteries.

*Results.*—Univariate analysis found that the presence and severity of TOD were significantly related to blood pressure; duration of hypertension; and low-density lipoprotein cholesterol, apolipoprotein B, Lp(a), and fibrinogen levels. On multivariate analysis, the best indicator of TOD was Lp(a) level, followed by systolic blood pressure, duration of hypertension, and low-density lipoprotein cholesterol. The relationship between Lp(a) and TOD was unaffected by the severity of blood pressure. Studies of the independent sample confirmed the link between Lp(a) and TOD. As the severity of TOD increased, so did the frequency of low–molecular-weight apo(a) isoforms.

*Conclusion.*—In patients with essential hypertension, the Lp(a) and apo(a) phenotype are both related to the severity of TOD. These may function as sensitive indicators for identification of patients prone to the development of hypertensive TOD. Patients with TOD show an increased frequency of low–molecular-weight apo(a) isoforms, suggesting that they are genetically predisposed to the development of hypertensive TOD.

▶ It appears from these very strong associations between Lp(a) levels and the extent of multiple target damages that the measurement of LP(a) should be added to the traditional lipid profile of total, low-density lipoprotein, and high-density lipoprotein cholesterol. The LP(a) assay is widely available and quite reproducible. Whether it adds enough to the other measurements will require longitudinal observations beyond such cross-sectional data as these.

As Sechi et al. note, LP(a) levels are genetically determined, so they may be able to identify patients susceptible to cardiovascular disease even earlier. Moreover, these data add to the evidence that hypertension and dyslipidemia often go together, much more often than would be likely by chance alone. As a deadly duo, they must be diagnosed in every adult and aggressively treated. Fortunately, antihypertensive agents need not worsen lipid levels, and lowering lipid levels will help correct the endothelial dysfunction seen in hypertensives.[1]

**N.M. Kaplan, M.D.**

*Reference*

1. Lithell H, Andersson P-E: Metabolic effects of carvedilol in hypertensive patients. *Eur J Clin Pharmacol* 52:13–17, 1997.

## Non-Drug Therapies

### INTRODUCTION

The value of various lifestyle modifications has been further confirmed. These modifications not only reduce blood pressure but ameliorate other cardiovascular and cancer risk factors. The search for factors that may be involved in the very beginnings of hypertension has been extended to young children, but the data remain sketchy.

**Norman M. Kaplan, M.D.**

---

**Diet and Blood Pressure in Children and Adolescents**
Simons-Morton DG, Obarzanek E (Natl Heart, Lung, and Blood Inst, Bethesda, Md)
*Pediatr Nephrol* 11:244–249, 1997                                    3–22

---

*Introduction.*—Pediatric patients with upper-range blood pressure (BP) measurements are at increased risk of hypertension in adulthood. Associations between diet and BP are well demonstrated in adults but little studied in children. Forty-six different studies—many of them examining more than 1 nutrient—were reviewed to assess what is known about the relationships between dietary nutrient intake and BP in children and adolescents.

*Sodium.*—The nutrient that has been best studied in this regard is sodium, with 25 observational and 12 intervention studies identified. Interpretation of the results was hindered by methodologic flaws in many studies. However, the better-quality observational studies and the several randomized, controlled trials reported suggested that children and adolescents with a higher sodium intake have higher BP. However, in the intervention trials, it was sometimes difficult to achieve a significant difference in sodium intake between the intervention and control groups. When a large reduction in sodium intake was achieved, BP was not always lower than in studies with a lesser reduction in sodium intake.

*Potassium.*—Thirteen observational and 2 intervention studies of potassium were identified. The results did not provide a consistent depiction of the association between potassium and BP in pediatric patients. Higher potassium intake was linked to lower BP in about half of the observational studies; however, 1 such study found the opposite relationship. In the intervention trials, potassium supplementation did not significantly reduce BP.

*Calcium.*—There were 8 observational and 1 intervention study of calcium. Again, the relationship between the nutrient and blood pressure in children and adolescents was unclear. One fourth of the observational studies suggested that calcium intake was negatively associated with BP. Calcium supplementation had no significant effect on BP.

*Magnesium.*—Five observational studies of magnesium suggested that higher levels of magnesium intake may be associated with lower BP. There were no intervention studies.

*Macronutrients and Dietary Patterns.*—Nine studies assessed the BP effects of macronutrients and food groups or dietary patterns in children and adolescents. There is some evidence that macronutrients and fiber can affect BP. No conclusions could be drawn regarding the effects of dietary patterns or food groups.

*Discussion.*—Relatively little is known about the effects of nutrient intake on BP in children and adolescents. More study is needed to identify dietary factors that can affect BP in pediatric patients and to test dietary approaches to modify BP. The authors suggest some important methodologic considerations for future studies.

▶ The roots of hypertension likely are nourished in the responses of children's BP to various stresses of early life. This review of the relationship between various dietary factors and blood pressure in children and adolescents largely confirms what has also been noted in adults: sodium seems most closely connected to higher BP, potassium may be connected, calcium and other minerals probably are not. Whether the association between the typically high sodium intake in the United States (and most of the developed world) and hypertension is strong enough to mandate universal moderation of sodium intake continues to be debated. I am convinced by the evidence of the role of sodium, as recently reviewed by Law.[1] Moreover, even if high sodium intake does not cause hypertension, it can cause lots of other mischief, including osteoporosis and kidney stones.[2]

There is no doubt that modest sodium restriction will lower high blood pressure.[3] It is, however, very difficult to maintain a moderately restricted sodium diet when almost all processed, packaged, and fast foods have so much salt added for taste enhancement and other purposes. If only we could get Campbell's, McDonald's, et al. to slowly but steadily reduce the sodium they add to what most of us eat, we might be able to accomplish populationwide what is very difficult to accomplish individually—a moderate sodium intake that could significantly reduce the incidence of hypertension.

**N.M. Kaplan, M.D.**

*References*

1. Law MR: Epidemiologic evidence on salt and blood pressure. *Am J Hypertens* 10:42S–45S, 1997.
2. MacGregor GA: Salt: More adverse effects. *Am J Hypertens* 10:37S–41S, 1997.
3. Cutler JA, Follmann D, Allender PS: Randomized trials of sodium reduction: An overview. *Am J Clin Nutr* 65:643S–651S, 1997.

---

**Randomized Trials of Sodium Reduction: An Overview**
Cutler JA, Follmann D, Allender PS (Natl Heart, Lung, and Blood Inst, Bethesda, Md)
*Am J Clin Nutr* 65(suppl):643S-651S, 1997                                    3–23

---

*Purpose.*—Randomized trials provide the best evidence for answering questions about reducing dietary sodium intake and its effects on risk of cardiovascular disease. Previously, the authors reported an overview of published studies regarding sodium reduction in adults, including a descriptive summary and pooled analyses of unconfounded randomized trials. They have updated that review through 1994.

*Methods.*—The meta-analysis included 32 trials with outcome data on 2,635 subjects. Twenty-two trials included hypertensive subjects and 12 included normotensive subjects. Studies that had confounded designs included pre-adolescent subjects, tested sodium intakes outside the usual range for the United States population, or did not report on systolic or diastolic blood pressure were excluded. All information was abstracted by 2 independent reviewers, with differences reconciled by consensus. Data from the studies were pooled for analysis.

*Results.*—The pooled data on blood pressure differences between treated and control groups showed highly significant differences for all trials combined and on separate analyses of data from trials in hypertensive and normotensive subjects pooled separately. With trials weighted according to sample size, the effect of reducing sodium intake was a 4.8-mmHg systolic and a 2.5-mmHg diastolic reduction in hypertensive subjects and a 1.9/1.1-mmHg reduction in normotensive subjects. The median difference in sodium excretion between sodium-reduction and control arms was 77 mmol/24 hr for hypertensive subjects and 76 mmol/24 hr for normotensive subjects. The blood pressure reduction per each 100 mmol/24 hr–reduction in sodium was 5.8/2.5 mmHg in hypertensive subjects and 2.3/1.4 mmHg in normotensive subjects (Fig 2). There were no apparent safety concerns related to sodium reduction.

*Conclusion.*—This meta-analysis suggests that significant reductions in blood pressure can be achieved by moderately reducing dietary sodium. The effect is greater in hypertensive subjects but is seen in normotensive

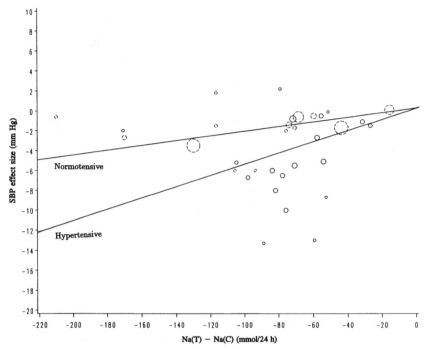

**FIGURE 2.**—Dose-response analysis: weighted linear regression of systolic blood pressure (*SBP*) as a function of mean net change in sodium excretion. Lines are forced through the origin. Trials involving hypertensive and normotensive subjects are analyzed separately. *Abbreviations*: *T*, treatment group; *C*, control group. (Courtesy of Cutler JA, Follmann D, Allender PS: Randomized trials of sodium reduction: An overview 65(suppl):643S–651S, 1997. Copyright *Am J Clin Nutr*. American Society for Clinical Nutrition.)

subjects as well. The pooled data probably underestimate the magnitude of the blood pressure reductions possible through reduction of dietary sodium, which could lead to significant reductions in stroke, coronary artery disease, and overall mortality.

▶ This most recent and most thorough analysis of the effects of dietary sodium restriction on blood pressure confirm what has been noted for over 20 years: moderate, attainable sodium restriction will lower blood pressure, not massively but enough to have a significant benefit. The larger effect in hypertensives could enable many to remain free of medications. The smaller effect in normotensives is still enough to keep as many as 20% of the population in the normotensive range rather than having them progress into hypertension.

All agree that moderate sodium restriction will lower blood pressure in most hypertensives, the effect being greater the older the patients and the higher the pressure.[1] Some argue that caution is needed because very low sodium intake may induce numerous aberrations, including sympathetic nervous activation.[2] As true as that may be, in practice, patients simply will not, cannot, and should not reduce sodium intakes to the absurdly low levels that have been shown to have various adverse effects (mostly short-term).

The truth is that even when strenuous efforts are made to help patients follow a moderately restricted diet, one down to 100 mmol per day (2.4 g sodium or 6 g sodium chloride), most of them do not sustain the reduced intake. The problem largely reflects the almost ubiquitous presence of the large amounts of sodium that are added to processed, packaged, and fast foods—originally as a preservative but now as a taste enhancer, filler, and, some argue, a device to encourage consumption of more bottled drinks. (Ever wonder why salted nuts and popcorn are free in bars?) Achieving meaningful and sustained reductions in sodium intake will require the cooperation of food processors in slowly and continually reducing the amount of salt they add to their products. Unfortunately, the food processors, through their lobby, the Salt Institute, have taken a strong adversarial posture, refusing to acknowledge any benefit but loudly proclaiming the putative dangers of sodium restriction.

As strong as I feel about the benefits of moderate sodium restriction, I recognize that it has not, by itself, been proved to prevent hypertension.[3] Nonetheless, few other preventive options are available, so I believe we should continue to cut down on salt.

**N.M. Kaplan, M.D.**

*References*

1. Law MR, Frost CD, Wald NJ: Analysis of data from trials of salt reduction. *BMJ* 302:819–824, 1991.
2. Grassi G, Cattaneo M, Seravalle G, et al: Baroreflex impairment by low sodium diet in mild or moderate essential hypertension. *Hypertension* 29:802–807, 1997.
3. Anonymous: Effects of weight loss and sodium reduction intervention on blood pressure and hypertension incidence in overweight people with high-normal blood pressure. The Trials of Hypertension Prevention, phase II. The trials of Hypertension Prevention Collaborative Research Group. *Arch Intern Med* 157:657–667, 1997.

## A Clinical Trial of the Effects of Dietary Patterns on Blood Pressure

Appel LJ, for the DASH Collaborative Research Group (Johns Hopkins Univ, Baltimore, Md; et al)
*N Engl J Med* 336:1117–1124, 1997                                                 3–24

*Introduction.*—Numerous dietary changes have been recommended for the prevention and treatment of hypertension, including weight control, reduced salt intake, reduced alcohol consumption, and increased potassium consumption. Trials of vegetarian diets have resulted in reduced blood pressure in normotensive and hypertensive subjects. However, trials testing individual nutrients, often in the form of dietary supplements, have shown little effect. A multicenter, randomized dietary study was performed to assess the effects of diet on blood pressure.

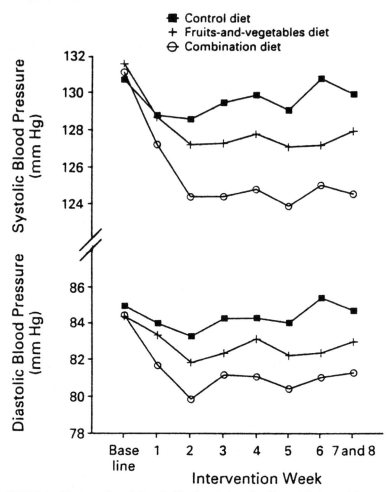

FIGURE 1.—Mean systolic and diastolic blood pressures at baseline and during each intervention week, according to diet, for 379 subjects with complete sets of weekly blood-pressure measurements. (Reprinted by permission of *The New England Journal of Medicine*, courtesy of Appel LJ, for the DASH Collaborative Research Group. *N Engl J Med* 336:1117–1124, copyright 1997, Massachusetts Medical Society. All rights reserved.)

*Methods.*—The study included 459 adult subjects with a systolic blood pressure of less than 160 mmHg and a diastolic blood pressure of 80 to 95 mmHg. For the first 3 weeks of the study, all patients received a control diet with a fat content typical of the average United States diet; the control diet contained few fruits, vegetables, and dairy products. The subjects were then randomized to continuation of the control diet; a diet high in fruits and vegetables; or a combination diet that was high in fruits, vegetables, and low-fat dairy products and had reduced levels of saturated and total fat. The subjects' sodium levels and body weight were held steady at all times.

*Results.*—The mean blood pressure at baseline was 131/85 mmHg. Compared with subjects assigned to the control diet, subjects assigned to the combination diet had a 5.5 mmHg–reduction in systolic blood pressure and a 3.0 mmHg–reduction in diastolic blood pressure. Those receiving the high–fruit-and-vegetable diet had a 2.8 mmHg–reduction in systolic blood pressure and a 1.1 mmHg–reduction in diastolic blood pressure (Fig 1). One hundred thirty-three patients had hypertension, defined as a blood pressure of 140/90 mmHg or greater. In this group, the combination diet yielded a 11.4/5.5 mmHg reduction in blood pressure. For subjects without high blood pressure, the reduction was 3.5/2.1 mmHg.

*Conclusion.*—Blood pressure can be lowered by following a diet high in fruits, vegetables, and low-fat dairy foods and low in saturated and total fat. This "combination" diet provides an effective nutritional alternative in the prevention of hypertension. It achieves significant reductions in blood pressure with no change in body weight, a sodium intake of about 3 g/day, and an alcohol intake of no more than 2 drinks/day.

▶ Some of the lowering of blood pressure by the higher fruit and vegetable intake may reflect the increased intake of potassium from an average of 1,700 mg per day in the control diet to over 4,000 mg per day in the fruit and vegetable diet. Increased amounts of fiber and antioxidants plus lots of other ingredients of fruits, vegetables, and low-fat dairy products obviously could be involved. For instance, an oral antioxidant supplement has been shown to lower blood pressure in a placebo-controlled, crossover study.[1]

This study is particularly important because it shows what can be accomplished by relatively simple and readily attainable changes in the usual American diet. A Pritikin-type diet may work even better, but only a gifted few can follow such a restricted program. Everyone can eat more fresh fruits and vegetables and low-fat dairy products, so the benefits should be applicable to the larger population. Moreover, the effects were seen without weight reduction or sodium restriction. If those had been added, even greater decreases in blood pressure might have occurred.

**N.M. Kaplan, M.D.**

*Reference*

1. Galley JF, Thornton J, Howdle PD, et al: Combination oral antioxidant supplementation reduces blood pressure. *Clin Sci (Colch)* 92:361–365, 1997.

### Effects of Oral Potassium on Blood Pressure: Meta-analysis of Randomized Controlled Clinical Trials

Whelton PK, He J, Cutler JA, et al (Johns Hopkins Univ, Baltimore, Md; Natl Heart, Lung, and Blood Inst, Bethesda, Md )
*JAMA* 277:1624–1632, 1997                                   3–25

*Background.*—Previous studies have shown that blood pressure is inversely related to potassium. However, blood pressure is also related to other nutritional variables, some of which are highly correlated with one another. Although there have been many trials of potassium supplementation in hypertensive patients, most studies have been too small to yield definitive results. Data from randomized, controlled trials were pooled to examine the effects of oral potassium supplementation on blood pressure.

*Methods.*—The analysis included 33 randomized, controlled trials comparing potassium supplementation for patients vs. none for controls. Potassium supplementation was the only difference between groups. The studies included information on 2,609 subjects. Information on sample size, study duration, design, potassium dose, subject characteristics, and treatment results was abstracted according to a standardized protocol by 2 independent reviewers. A random-effects model was used to pool the data, with the results of each trial weighted by the inverse of its variance.

*Results.*—One trial found an extreme blood pressure–lowering effect of potassium; this trial was excluded as an outlier. The remaining data suggested that potassium supplementation significantly reduced blood pressure. The size of the effect was −3.11 mmHg for systolic blood pressure, with a 95% confidence interval of −1.91 to −4.31 mmHg. For diastolic blood pressure, the effect was −1.97 mmHg, with a 95% confidence interval of −0.52 to −3.42 mmHg. The results suggested that a 53 mmol/day increase in urinary potassium excretion would yield a 2.4/1.5 mmHg reduction in blood pressure. Studies in which the participants had a high sodium intake seemed to derive the greatest blood pressure–reducing effect from potassium supplementation.

*Conclusion.*—This meta-analysis suggests that oral potassium supplementation is associated with a reduction in blood pressure. Low potassium intake may be a major causative factor in high blood pressure. An increased intake of oral potassium may be recommended for the prevention and treatment of high blood pressure, particularly for patients who cannot reduce their sodium intake.

▶ The overall impact of these trials on blood pressure is fairly impressive. With exclusion of the 1 outlier trial that reported a rather unbelievable reduction in blood pressure, an overall 3/2 mmHg reduction in BP was noted in these 31 trials. As is true for every nondrug and drug therapy, the effect is greater in hypertensives who averaged a 4.4/2.5 mmHg decrease in blood pressure compared with normotensives, who average a 1.8/1.0 mmHg fall.

The greater impact of potassium supplements the higher the level of sodium intake may reflect a natriuretic effect of potassium or a special effect of the sodium-potassium ratio beyond the actual levels of their intake. Potassium supplements may be useful, but they are too expensive and may cause some gastrointestinal discomfort. Extra potassium can be ingested by substitution of natural foods (all high in potassium and low in sodium) for processed foods (most are high in sodium and lower in potassium). Nature knows best.

**N.M. Kaplan, M.D.**

---

**Effect of Regular Aerobic Exercise on Elevated Blood Pressure in Post-menopausal Women**
Seals DR, Silverman HG, Reiling MJ, et al (Univ of Colorado, Boulder; Univ of Colorado, Denver)
*Am J Cardiol* 80:49–55, 1997                                               3–26

---

*Introduction.*—A study of postmenopausal women with elevated blood pressure (BP) was conducted to determine whether regular aerobic exercise, apart from the influences of dietary intake or body weight, would lower arterial BP. The efficacy of aerobic exercise in this setting has not been determined.

*Methods.*—Nine of 16 women enrolled in the study completed the 12 weeks of aerobic exercise training and all measurements. Inclusion criteria were postmenopausal status, age 50 and over, BP at rest in the high normal or stage I hypertensive ranges, no other chronic degenerative diseases, and no regular exercise during the previous 2 years. Three women were taking hormone supplements and 3 were being treated for hypertension; these drugs were maintained at baseline levels throughout the exercise period. Five women took part in a 12-week lead-in period during which BP measurements were obtained. Exercise consisted of regular walking, which was increased in duration and intensity during the 12 weeks.

*Results.*—The women had a mean age of 55 and a mean BP at rest of 138/89 mmHg in the sitting position and 142/95 mmHg in the standing position. They exercised an average of 3.2 days per week with a mean duration of exercise sessions of 44 minutes. Mean intensity of exercise was equivalent to 69% of maximal heart rate or 62% of baseline maximal oxygen consumption. Maximal aerobic capacity was unchanged in the group after 12 weeks of exercise, but exercise tolerance as measured by treadmill walking increased by approximately 10%. Although heart rate at rest was unchanged, there was a reduction in heart rate during submaximal treadmill walking compared with baseline. Resting BP was lowered by an average of 10/7 and 12/5 mmHg in the sitting and standing positions, respectively. There was a trend for greater mean reductions in systolic BP in the 5 women with stage I essential hypertension than in the 4 with high normal systolic BP. Training significantly reduced levels of systolic and diastolic BP (Fig 3) during standardized submaximal exercise.

*Discussion.*—Postmenopausal women with modestly elevated BP at baseline benefited from regular aerobic exercise. During the 12-week train

## Systolic Blood Pressure

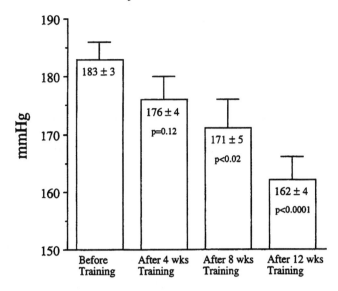

## Diastolic Blood Pressure

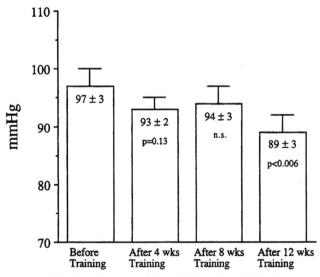

**FIGURE 3.**—Mean level of systolic (*top*) and diastolic (*bottom*) arterial blood pressure during standardized exercise* before and after 4, 8, and 12 weeks of aerobic exercise training. *Workload = 80% of maximal heart rate at baseline. (Reprinted by permission of the publisher from Seals DR, Silverman HG, Reiling MJ, et al: Effect of regular aerobic exercise on elevated blood pressure in postmenopausal women, *Am J Cardiol* 80:49–55, Copyright 1997 by Excerpta Medica, Inc.)

ing period, reductions in resting BP were clinically important, and if sustained could reduce the risk of cardiovascular disease. The effects of exercise occurred without changes in body weight, dietary intake, or maximal aerobic capacity.

▶ This relatively small but very well conducted and intense study of aerobic exercise documents further a fall in BP with repeated exercise over time. These women walked; swimming will likely do as well.[1]

One nagging doubt arises from these and previous data from the same authors[2]: the routinely recorded BP fell but the 24-hour ambulatory BP did not. Could it be that what is seen is removal of the "white-coat" or "alerting" reaction that is frequently noted when BP is measured repeatedly over time by routine manometry with no intervention of any kind? This seems unlikely since all of these women were monitored until their BPs were stable before starting the exercise program, and 5 women were simply watched over 12 weeks and they had no significant change in BP. Nonetheless, it would make me feel more positive about the antihypertensive potency of exercise if the ambulatory readings had also fallen. Regardless, aerobic exercise is good for lots of other reasons, perhaps most importantly to prevent obesity.

**N.M. Kaplan, M.D.**

*References*

1. Tanaka H, Bassett DR, Howley ET, et al: Swimming training lowers the resting blood pressure in individuals with hypertension. *J Hypertens* 15:651–657, 1997.
2. Seals DR, Reiling MJ: Effect of regular exercise on 24-hour arterial pressure in older hypertensive humans. *Hypertension* 18:583–592, 1991.

---

**Smoking Is Associated With Higher Cardiovascular Risk in Young Women Than in Men: The Tecumseh Blood Pressure Study**
Vriz O, Nesbitt S, Krause L, et al (Univ of Michigan, Ann Arbor)
*J Hypertens* 15:127–134, 1997                                           3–27

---

*Objective.*—Smoking is a major risk factor for coronary heart disease and predisposes to myocardial infarction and sudden death. Women who smoke have a strikingly high incidence of coronary heart disease; the metabolic effects of smoking may be greater in women than in men. Possible sex differences in the effects of smoking on hemodynamic and biochemical variables were evaluated.

*Methods.*—The study included 851 subjects from the Tecumseh Blood Pressure Study, all healthy men and women between 18 and 42 years of age. Group 1 consisted of nonsmokers (258 men and 234 women); group 2 consisted of smokers (185 men and 174 women). Home- and clinic-measured blood pressures, clinical examination and laboratory testing results, and echocardiographic findings were compared between groups.

*Results.*—Especially for female smokers, home systolic blood pressure measurements were nonsignificantly higher than clinic blood pressure measurements. The only variable that was significantly different between smokers and nonsmokers in both sexes was hematocrit: 43.9 in male smokers vs. 44.6 in male nonsmokers, and 39.2 in female nonsmokers vs. 40.3 in female smokers. Compared with nonsmokers, female smokers had significant elevations in triglycerides (80.6 vs. 99.6 mg/dL), left ventricular mass index (95.4 vs. 100.0 g/m$^2$), and posterior wall thickness (9.5 vs. 9.71 mm). Female smokers also had a significant reduction in high-density lipoproteins (48.7 vs. 44.5 mg/dL). The difference in posterior wall thickness was no longer significant after adjustment for home systolic blood pressure measurements; all of the other differences remained significant.

*Conclusion.*—Smoking appears to be even more harmful in women than in men. By smoking, women seem to lose their lower risk of ischemic heart disease relative to men. Women—who are targeted by tobacco company advertisements—should be made aware of the sex-specific deleterious effects of smoking.

▶ The evils of smoking, then, may be even worse for women than for men. Not measured in this study are other adverse effects of smoking that are peculiar to women (and their children): the higher likelihood of giving birth to growth-retarded infants and the transmission of respiratory illness to their infants from their second-hand smoke.

The authors observed even higher blood pressures in smokers when they were measured at home vs. measurements taken in the office. This reflects the often significant but usually short-term pressor effect of cigarettes, likely to be captured at home but hardly ever recognized in smoke-free doctors' offices and clinics.

Americans seem increasingly alerted to the evils of cigarettes, as witnessed by the multiple lawsuits that have brought tobacco companies to the bargaining table. However, more young girls are taking up smoking, presumably to make themselves look older (even though the extra wrinkles don't show up for some years) and keep thin (a specious argument for a benefit of smoking by avoiding obesity). Data such as these need to be widely disseminated to emphasize further the extra dangers of smoking for women.

As I travel overseas, I am repeatedly struck by the continued widespread prevalence of smoking by doctors and nurses in much of the rest of the world. Some people can claim ignorance and others the difficulty of breaking the most tenacious addiction known, but doctors and nurses have no excuse.

**N.M. Kaplan, M.D.**

### Comparison of Single Versus Multiple Lifestyle Interventions: Are the Antihypertensive Effects of Exercise Training and Diet-Induced Weight Loss Additive?

Gordon NF, Scott CB, Levine BD (Presbyterian Hosp of Dallas; Univ of Texas, Dallas; Candler Hosp, Savannah, Ga)
*Am J Cardiol* 79:763–767, 1997                                                                3–28

*Background.*—Lifestyle modifications are used widely as definitive or adjunctive therapy for high blood pressure. Separately, aerobic exercise training and diet-induced weight loss have been shown to reduce blood pressure (BP). However, the possible additive effect of their combined use is unknown. This issue was addressed in a 3-way randomized trial.

*Methods.*—Fifty-five sedentary, overweight adults with high-normal BP or stage 1 or 2 hypertension participated in the study. The patients were assigned into 3 intervention groups, and each intervention lasted 12 weeks. One group was assigned aerobic exercise only; patients exercised for 30 to 45 minutes 3 to 5 days per week at 60% to 85% of maximal heart rate. Another group was assigned to dietary modification only, with reduction of energy intake and dietary fat for the purpose of weight loss. The third group was assigned to both exercise training and dietary modification. Outcome measures included BP, body weight, and maximal graded treadmill testing.

*Results.*—Seven patients dropped out of the study for various reasons, leaving 48 patients for analysis. The mean reduction in body weight was 7 kg with exercise plus diet, compared with 6 kg with diet only and 1 kg with exercise only. Patients assigned to both diet and exercise also had a greater improvement in maximal oxygen uptake: 4.3 mL/kg/min, compared with 1.9 mL/kg/min with diet only and 2.5 mL/kg/min with exercise only. However, there was no significant difference between groups in the mean BP reduction achieved: 12.5/8 mmHg with exercise and diet, 11/7.5 mmHg with diet only, and 10/6 mmHg with exercise only.

*Conclusion.*—Although each is effective in reducing hypertension, aerobic exercise training and diet-induced weight loss do not have additive effects on BP. In terms of BP only, no greater effect is to be expected when both diet and exercise are prescribed for patients with high-normal BP or stage 1 or 2 hypertension. However, both interventions have important benefits other than their antihypertensive effect.

▶ Although this was a well-designed and conducted study, I'm not willing to concede the main conclusion: various lifestyle interventions are not additive in their effects. My reasons for doubt include the following:

1.  Each intervention provided some really marked falls in blood pressure, almost 10/6 mmHg for the exercise group, over 11/7 mmHg for the diet group. There may be a floor beyond which no further falls from individual or combined therapies can occur. After all, human physiology provides many defenses against marked falls in BP.

2. With more severely hypertensive patients, a greater possible effect of the combination might have been noted.

3. The numbers of subjects were small, so that a β-type error could have occurred that would be overcome by larger numbers of subjects.

4. With a larger number of subjects, the little bit of additive effect that was seen could have grown to become highly significant.

Nonetheless, different lifestyle changes, including exercise and weight loss, may produce their antihypertensive effects through similar mechanisms, including a decrease in insulin resistance and a modulation of sympathetic nervous activity. Therefore, the lack of additive effects may be a reflection of each modality working through similar mechanisms.

Regardless, in the real world, patients should be asked to do all that they can as it is unlikely that they will be as assiduous in following any one modality enough to accomplish its full benefit. Certainly it's hard to lose weight and keep it off unless physical activity is increased. When one cuts calories, it's likely going to involve the reduction of sodium and maybe alcohol as well. So, combining lifestyle changes should be helpful even if one alone, carried to its maximum, would be enough.

In this regard, the evidence for a cardioprotective effect of moderate daily consumption of alcohol continues to grow, now even including we physicians who were enrolled in the Physicians Health Study.[1] So when we advise cutting back on alcohol, remember that most people who drink do so in (healthful) moderation. Only the boozers need to really cut back.

Two other lifestyle modifications that have been widely touted, calcium supplements and relaxation therapies, continue to receive little support. Calcium supplements not only don't lower BP, they may increase the risk for kidney stones.[2] Relaxation doesn't seem to keep BP down,[3] though some find it helps when used with medications.[4]

**N.M. Kaplan, M.D.**

*References*

1. Camargo CA, Hennekens CH, Gaziano JM, et al: Prospective study of moderate alcohol consumption and mortality in US male physicians. *Arch Intern Med* 157:79–85, 1997.

2. Curhan GC, Willett WC, Speizer FE, et al: Comparison of dietary calcium with supplemental calcium and other nutrients as factors affecting the risk for kidney stones in women. *Ann Intern Med* 126:497–504, 1997.

3. Hunyor SN, Henderson RJ, Lal SKL, et al: Placebo-controlled biofeedback blood pressure effect in hypertensive humans. *Hypertension* 29:1225–1231, 1997.

4. Shapiro D, Hui KK, Oakley ME, et al: Reduction in drug requirements for hypertension by means of a cognitive-behavioral intervention. *Am J Hypertens* 109:9–17, 1997.

# Drug Therapy

## INTRODUCTION

While the controversy over possible dangers from the use of calcium antagonists continues to fester, the overwhelming problem remains that of keeping patients on enough of whatever it takes to control their blood pressure. The problems of noncompliance are compounded among the indigent and, as managed care threatens to restrict further the uninsured from obtaining adequate health care, we may witness even worse.

**Norman M. Kaplan, M.D.**

---

**Blood-Pressure Control in the Hypertensive Population**
Mancia G, Sega R, Milesi C, et al (Centro Studi di Patologica Cronico-Degenerativa, Milano, Italy; Centro di Fisiologia Clinica e Ipertensione, Milano, Italy; Università di Milano, Italy; et al)
*Lancet* 349:454–457, 1997                                    3–29

---

*Background.*—Adequate control of hypertension is achieved infrequently in the United States and Europe. Although generally blamed on poor therapeutic compliance, this finding may be artifactual, secondary to stress normally experienced by patients in a medical environment, or the "white coat effect," rather than to poor control of hypertension. The blood pressure of 1,651 study participants was measured both in a clinic setting and in the home, to test for and to quantify stress-related blood pressure elevation in a clinical situation.

*Methods.*—Blood pressure was measured in a cohort of 1,651 study participants by a physician in a clinic and again outside the clinic, using both an automatic device to generate a 24-hour ambulatory blood pressure profile and a semiautomatic device, which allowed participants to measure their own blood pressure while sitting. Participants with systolic and diastolic clinic blood pressures greater than 140 mmHg or greater than 90 mmHg, respectively, were considered hypertensive. Hypertensive participants who had received hypertensive drugs for 15 days or less were considered untreated.

*Results.*—Mean systolic and diastolic pressures measured in the clinic were significantly greater in hypertensive participants than they were in normotensive ones (Fig 1) and were insignificantly or only slightly lower in treated patients than they were in untreated ones. Blood pressure means generated by the 24-hour profiles, or measured in the home, were only several mmHg lower than pressures determined in the clinic for all 3 groups of participants. When blood pressure was measured outside the clinic, treated hypertensive participants had pressures similar to, or only slightly less than, those of untreated hypertensive participants. Adequate control of hypertension was achieved in only 28% of treated hypertensive subjects, based on pressure measurements in the clinic, and 36%, based on 24-hour blood pressure profiles.

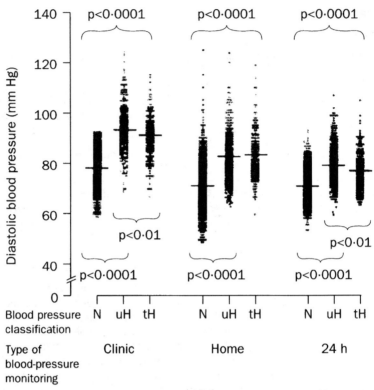

**FIGURE 1.**—Individual diastolic blood pressure values in normotensive, untreated hypertensive, and treated hypertensive participants. *Abbreviations: N,* normotensive participants; *uH,* untreated hypertensive participants; *tH,* treated hypertensive participants. Horizontal bars = mean values. (Courtesy of Mancia G, Sega R, Milesi C, et al: Blood-pressure control in the hypertensive population. *Lancet* 349:454–457, 1997. Copyright by the Lancet Ltd., 1997.)

*Conclusions.*—Blood pressure measured in a clinic setting is typically elevated in treated hypertensive patients to a level comparable to that in patients with untreated hypertension. Therefore, adequate control of hypertension in patients receiving treatment for the disease appears to be relatively rare, which is likely the result of poor compliance with treatment. Although pressures measured outside a clinic are slightly lower, a high clinic pressure is truly indicative of the high pressure of daily life and is not simply a "white coat effect."

▶ Only about 1 in 4 Americans with hypertension have their condition under adequate control, that is, blood pressure below 140/90 mmHg.[1] Many reasons have been offered for this poor record—one that the higher readings obtained in the presence of a physician or the "white-coat effect," is largely discounted by these data. As expected, readings taken outside the office were usually lower than those obtained in the office. However, most cases of hypertensives were poorly controlled both in-office and out-of-office.

The problem of poor control is inherent in hypertension, which is a lifelong condition that is asymptomatic and for which no obvious benefit is provided by therapy. In addition, treatment may be expensive and may cause side effects. I have often thought that patients would be better managed if their hypertension hurt just a little, with their discomfort relieved by lowering their blood pressure.

Despite the short-fall in control, the overall impact of the more widespread treatment of hypertension has clearly played a role in the recent decline in mortality from coronary heart disease noted in the United States.[2] Reduction in the risk factors for coronary heart disease, including hypertension, account for approximately half the decrease in mortality.

**N.M. Kaplan, M.D.**

*References*

1. Kaplan NM: Hypertension in the population at large, in Kaplan NM (ed): *Clinical Hypertension*, ed 7. Baltimore, Williams & Wilkins, 1998.
2. Hunink MGM, Goldman L, Tosteson ANA, et al: The recent decline in mortality from coronary heart disease, 1980–1990: The effect of secular trends in risk factors and treatment. *JAMA* 277:535–542, 1997.

**Correlates of Controlled Hypertension in Indigent, Inner-City Hypertensive Patients**

Ahluwalia JS, McNagny SE, Rask KJ (Emory Univ, Altanta, Ga; Rollins School of Public Health, Atlanta, Ga)

*J Gen Intern Med* 12:7–14, 1997                                        3–30

*Introduction.*—The most common medically treatable chronic disease is hypertension, which affects 50 million Americans. Nevertheless, the level of blood pressure control in known hypertensive patients currently under treatment is poor, despite the availability of 5 classes of effective antihypertensive agents. In minority and disadvantaged populations, uncontrolled hypertension is even more prevalent. Hypertension is controlled in only 25% of African-Americans who are aware of their diagnosis. Correlates of controlled hypertension were identified in a largely minority population of patients with treated hypertension.

*Methods.*—Eighty-eight patients with hypertension who had a mean blood pressure of 193/106 mmHg were compared with 133 control subjects with a mean blood pressure of 130/80 mmHg. The study was conducted over 12 weeks. An interview and patient self-report were conducted to determine age, gender, ethnicity, mode of transportation, home ownership, educational level, household income, marital status, use of health services, and employment. Hospital administration records were examined for insurance status. Patients were also evaluated for having a regular source of care, their general health status, and compliance with medications.

*Results.*—Having a regular source of care and having been to a physician in the previous 6 months, reporting that cost was not a deterrent to buying antihypertensive medication, and having insurance were factors associated with blood pressure control, according to a logistic regression model after adjustments were made for age, gender, race, education, owning a telephone, and family income. There was borderline significance with being compliant with antihypertensive medication. Cost was reported as a barrier to purchasing antihypertensive medications and seeing a physician more often by uninsured patients than by those with Medicaid coverage.

*Conclusion.*—Blood pressure control may be affected significantly by out-of-pocket expenses under Medicaid for medications and physician care. In an indigent, inner-city population, improved blood pressure control may result from improved access to a regular source of care and increased sensitivity to medication costs for all patients.

▶ As bad as is our record of the control of hypertension in the United States, with fewer than 1 in 4 patients having their condition under good control,[1] we continue to make it even more difficult for those who are the most vulnerable to the cardiovascular damages induced by high blood pressure.[2]

The data by Ahluwalia et al. are somewhat surprising in finding the overriding role of a lack of a regular source of health care to be more important than the cost of medications or the availability of insurance. As we continue to remove the net of support for relatively inexpensive preventive care for indigent, inner-city patients, we will pay far more eventually in providing expensive terminal care for their end-stage renal disease, strokes, and heart attacks.[2] The evidence continues to document the value of lowering blood pressure for both primary and secondary prevention of heart attacks and strokes.[3]

**N.M. Kaplan, M.D.**

*References*

1. Burt VL, Cutler JA, Higgins M, et al. Trends in the prevalence, treatment, and control of hypertension in the adult U.S. population. *Hypertension* 26:60–69, 1995.
2. Klag MJ, Whelton PK, Randall BL, et al. End-stage renal disease in African-American and white men. *JAMA* 277:1293–1298, 1997.
3. MacMahon S, Rodgers A, Neal B, et al: Blood pressure lowering for the secondary prevention of myocardial infarction and stroke. *Hypertension* 29:537–538, 1997.

**The Effects of Initial Drug Choice and Comorbidity on Antihypertensive Therapy Compliance: Results From a Population-based Study in the Elderly**

Monane M, Bohn RL, Gurwitz JH, et al (Harvard Med School, Boston)
*Am J Hypertens* 10:697–704, 1997                                    3–31

*Introduction.*—The treatment of elevated blood pressure is a major concern in the elderly. Despite the widespread use of antihypertensive agents, normotension is often not achieved in patients 65 and older. To address the problem of noncompliance in elderly populations, researchers examined the effect of initial drug choice and comorbidity on antihypertensive therapy (AHT) compliance.

*Methods.*—The study population was identified by reviewing files of New Jersey's Medicaid and Medicare programs from 1982 to 1988. The initial screen identified 9,468 new users of at least 1 antihypertensive drug; 8,643 of these patients made up the final cohort. Compliance was calculated in terms of the number of days in which AHT was available to the patients during the 12 months after therapy was started. Various factors that might influence compliance were examined, including demographic data, number of antihypertensive and other medications, class of antihypertensive, and the presence of comorbid cardiac disease.

**ADJUSTED ODDS RATIO**

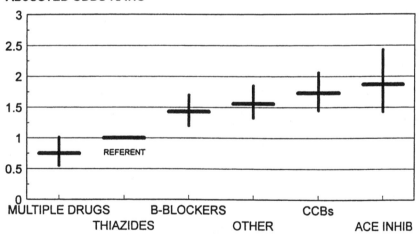

FIGURE 1.—Initial drug choice as a factor related to antihypertensive therapy (AHT) compliance, adjusted for age, gender, race, and year of therapy. The y axis depicts the odds ratio for good compliance (≥80% of days covered) for patients beginning antihypertensive therapy. MULTIPLE, initiation of therapy with two or more drugs; THIAZIDES, thiazide or related diuretics; B-BLOCKERS, β-adrenergic blockers; OTHER, central adrenergic agonists, peripheral adrenergic antagonists, or vasodilators; CCBs, calcium channel blockers; and ACE INHIB, angiotensin converting enzyme inhibitors. For each variable, the odds ratio is indicated by the horizontal line and the 95% confidence interval is indicated by the vertical line. (Courtesy of Monane M, Bohn RL, Gurwitz JH, et al: The effects of initial drug choice and comorbidity on antihypertensive therapy compliance: results from a population-based study in the elderly. *Am J Hypertens* 10:697–704, 1997. Reprinted by permission of Elsevier Science Inc. Copyright 1997 by American Journal of Hypertension, Inc.)

*Results.*—The study population had a mean age of 76.5 and was predominantly female (77%) and white (67%). Diuretics accounted for 50% of first prescriptions; calcium channel blockers (CCBs) and β-adrenergic blockers each accounted for 12%. Only 20% of patients who started AHT achieved good levels of compliance, defined as greater than or equal to 80% based on physicians' instructions for use. Compliance was highest (Fig 1) among users of angiotensin converting enzyme (ACE) inhibitors, CCBs, and β-blockers. Other factors that had a positive effect on compliance were multiple physician visits and the presence of heart disease in the 120 days before the initial antihypertensive prescription. There was an inverse association between good compliance and the use of multiple pharmacies and number of medications prescribed overall.

*Conclusion.*—Among newly treated elderly hypertensives, good compliance with AHT was strongly related to drug choice, comorbidity, and health services utilization. Patients with multiple physician visits and comorbid cardiovascular disease were likely to achieve good compliance, and those on ACE inhibitors and CCBs were almost twice as likely as thiazide users to be compliant.

▶ Although there are lots of unknown possible confounders, these data suggest that elderly patients take some antihypertensive drugs more regularly than others. As the authors state, one reason why they took ACE inhibitors or calcium channel blockers more regularly than diuretics may be that "patients with more severe hypertension or greater comorbidity may have been more likely to be started on ACE inhibitors and CCB, whereas those with milder hypertension were started on diuretic therapy . . . . Sicker patients are more likely to take medications because of the perceived need to treat their condition effectively."

The better compliance to the newer agents seen here was not seen in England, where only 40% to 50% of patients continued on any of the 4 major classes of drugs.[1] Perhaps the major point is that so many patients do not adhere to their antihypertensive therapy, not so much from side effects as from the inherent difficulty of keeping asymptomatic people on any therapy that doesn't provide immediate and obvious benefit.

**N.M. Kaplan, M.D.**

*Reference*

1. Jones JK, Gorkin L, Lian JF, et al: Discontinuation of and changes in treatment after start of new courses of antihypertensive drugs: a study of a United Kingdom population. *BMJ* 311:293–295, 1995.

### Health Outcomes Associated With Antihypertensive Therapies Used as First-line Agents: A Systematic Review and Meta-analysis

Psaty BM, Smith NL, Siscovick DS, et al (Univ of Washington, Seattle; Bowman Gray School of Medicine, Winston-Salem, NC)

*JAMA* 277:739–745, 1997          3–32

*Introduction.*—Despite guidelines in 1993 and 1997 by the Joint National Committee on the Detection, Evaluation, and Treatment of High Blood Pressure (JNC-V) and JNC-V1 recommending low-dose diuretics and β-blockers as first-line agents, angiotensin-converting enzyme (ACE) inhibitors and calcium channel blockers continue to be widely used in the first-line treatment of hypertension. Scientific evidence concerning the safety and efficacy of various antihypertensive agents used as first-line agents was reviewed and evaluated for major disease end points.

*Methods.*—MEDLINE searches were conducted (1980–1995) and previous meta-analyses were used to identify long-term trials that evaluated major disease end points as an outcome. Placebo-controlled randomized trials were used for the meta-analysis. In random trials that used surrogate end points, such as blood pressure, the largest investigations that assessed multiple drugs were used. Observational trials were used when clinical trial evidence was lacking.

*Results.*—Eighteen randomized long-term trials (48,220 patients) from the United States, Europe, Scandinavia, Australia, and Japan evaluated diuretics and β-blockers. Congestive heart failure and stroke were effectively prevented by β-blockers, compared with placebo. High-dose diuretic therapy was similarly effective in preventing stroke and congestive heart failure. Low-dose diuretic therapy was effective in preventing these illnesses and coronary disease and total mortality. Calcium channel blockers and ACE inhibitors decreased blood pressure in patients with hypertension, but their influence on health outcomes was slight. In fact, available evidence suggested the possibility of harm for some short-acting dihydropyridine calcium channel blockers. It is not known whether the long-acting formulations or the dihydropyridine calcium channel blockers are safe or prevent major cardiovascular events in patients with hypertension.

*Conclusion.*—The available scientific evidence supports the current national guidelines for treating hypertension with diuretics and β-blockers. Long-term clinical trials are needed before it can be determined whether calcium channel blockers and ACE inhibitors are good treatment options for hypertension.

▶ This meta-analysis takes everything available through 1995 to make an obvious point: the only modalities used in multiple randomized controlled trials (RCTs) for the treatment of hypertension were diuretics and adrenergic inhibitors, mainly β-blockers. Since the results from RCTs are the strongest evidence on which clinical decisions should be made, they are certainly correct in their conclusion that diuretics (in low doses) and β-blockers be given preference.

There are, however, two problems with their conclusions—one that they should have recognized, the other that has become obvious only after they completed their analysis. The first problem relates to the use of β-blockers in the elderly. As noted by others,[1] β-blockers have shown absolutely no benefit in reducing morbidity or mortality in the elderly when used alone. Therefore, the JNC-VI report[2] will recommend either diuretics alone or diuretics with β-blockers for the elderly.

The second problem has come from the publication of the first RCT involving long-acting calcium channel blockers. In a large study[3] of almost 5,000 elderly patients with predominately systolic hypertension who were given either a placebo or the dihydropyridine CCB nitrendipine, the benefits were as good as those seen with diuretics given in the previously published RCTs (see Abstract). Therefore, JNC-VI adds a dihydropyridine CCB to the alternative choices for elderly patients with systolic hypertension.

That's the problem with meta-analyses: by the time they're published, more data become available.

**N.M. Kaplan, M.D.**

*References*

1. Michalewicz L, Chambers R, Grodzicki T: Primary prevention of cardiovascular disease endpoints using β-blockers. *JAMA* 277:1759, 1997.
2. Joint National Committee on Detection, Evaluation, and Treatment of High Blood Pressure: The Sixth Report of the Joint National Committee on *Detection, Evaluation*, and Treatment of High Blood Pressure (JNCVI). *Arch Intern Med* 157:2413–2446, 1997.
3. Staessen JA, Fagard R, Thijs L. Morbidity and mortality in the placebo-controlled European trial on isolated systolic hypertension in the elderly. *Lancet* 350:757–764, 1997.

---

**Cardiovascular Morbidity and Mortality Among Hypertensive Patients in General Practice: The Evaluation of Long-term Systematic Management**
Harms LM, Schellevis FG, van Eijk JTM, et al (Vrije Universiteit, Amsterdam)
*J Clin Epidemiol* 50:779–786, 1997                                            3–33

---

*Introduction.*—In 1978, 4 general practitioners in Einhoven, The Netherlands, began a systematic hypertension management program in a large series of patients who were employed by an electronic company—the largest employer in the region. A comparison was made between patients with hypertension under systematic management and those under general practice care.

*Methods.*—The index group was composed of 120 employees in the systematic management program who were hypertensive. The reference group was 120 patients under general practice care. The groups were matched for age, gender, fasting blood glucose, and frequency of occupational health examination. Age range of the mostly male (78%) cohort was

50–65 years. Morbidity and mortality were evaluated for a period of 12 successive years (1978–1989).

*Results.*—The total follow-up duration was 2,628 patient-years. Mean follow-up duration for the index and reference groups was 10.8 and 11.1 years, respectively. In contrast to the reference group, the index group had less left ventricular hypertrophy, less angina pectoris, and less peripheral artery disease. The index group had a difference in blood pressure that was a mean of 11.3 mmHg systolic and 5.9 mmHg diastolic lower than that of the reference group. There were no between-group differences regarding changes in other cardiovascular risk factors.

*Conclusion.*—Patients aged 50–65 years with hypertension who were in the systematic management group had significantly lower cardiovascular morbidity and blood pressure, compared with patients under general practice care. These findings should be subjected to randomized, controlled settings.

▶ It's nice to see such documentation that antihypertensive therapy carefully administered by general practitioners can provide such significant benefit in the "real world." We've known for 30 years that patients enrolled in large-scale clinical trials benefit from therapy. But the ability to transfer these benefits from controlled clinical trials to ordinary clinical practice has not been adequately addressed. These results, then, are most welcome, giving further support for our efforts to improve the management of hypertension.

**N.M. Kaplan, M.D.**

---

**Long-term Effects on Sexual Function of Five Antihypertensive Drugs and Nutritional Hygienic Treatment in Hypertensive Men and Women: Treatment of Mild Hypertension Study (TOMHS)**
Grimm RH Jr, Grandits GA, Prineas RJ, et al (Hennepin County Med Ctr, Minneapolis, Minn; Univ of Minnesota, Minneapolis; Univ of Pittsburgh, Pa; et al)
*Hypertension* 29:8–14, 1997                                                    3–34

---

*Introduction.*—The relationship between hypertensive drugs and sexual dysfunction has been addressed in only a few placebo-controlled trials. Some have questioned whether the sexual dysfunction is caused by drug treatment for hypertension or by hypertension itself. Data from the Treatment of Mild Hypertension Study (TOMHS) were used to explore the relation between 5 antihypertensive drugs and placebo on sexual function in men and women aged 45–69 years with stage I diastolic hypertension.

*Methods.*—The TOMHS was a double-blind, placebo-controlled, randomized trial with 902 patients with hypertension. The effects of placebo and 5 active drugs (acebutolol, amlodipine maleate, chlorthalidone, doxazosin maleate, and enalapril maleate) on sexual function were evaluated at baseline and at annual follow-up visits by means of physician interview.

*Results.*—Baseline interviews revealed that 14.4% of men and 4.9% of women had problems with sexual function. Problems maintaining or obtaining an erection were reported by 12.2% of men at baseline; 2% of women reported problems with achieving orgasm. For men, problems with erection were positively associated with age, systolic pressure, and previous antihypertensive drug use. At 24- and 48-month follow-up, 9.5% and 14.7% of men experienced erection dysfunction that was related to type of antihypertensive therapy. Compared with placebo, patients randomized to receive chlorthalidone reported significantly higher incidence of erection dysfunction through 24 months (8.1% vs. 17.1%). At 48 months, the incidence rates of erection dysfunction were similar among treatment groups. The lowest rate for drugs was observed in the doxazosin group, but it was not significantly different from the placebo group. The incidence rate was similar for placebo, acebutolol, amlodipine, and enalapril. Erection dysfunction did not require medication withdrawal for most patients.

*Conclusion.*—The incidence of erection dysfunction in men treated for hypertension was low in all treatment groups, but higher for men in the chlorthalidone group. The rate of sexual problems was even lower for women, and did not seem to differ by type of drug. The similar dysfunction rates for drug and placebo groups indicate that problems should not automatically be attributed to antihypertensive medications.

▶ Diuretics may be the class of drugs that have been used in most of the large randomized controlled trials (RCTs) of the treatment of hypertension, and thereby found to reduce cardiovascular morbidity and mortality. Thus they have been recommended for initial therapy in most patients with hypertension. However, there is more to life than cardiovascular disease, and these findings suggest that, for one important aspect of living, diuretics may not be so preferable.

This study is the only one currently available that has carefully assessed the effects representative of all of the major classes of antihypertensive drugs on sexual function. The fact that diuretics came out worst is not that surprising since they also caused twice more impotence than β-blockers in the Medical Research Council[1] trial published in 1985.

Fortunately, the other drugs didn't impair sexual function, whereas only one, the α-adrenergic blocker doxazosin, was accompanied by less impotence than seen with placebo.

The lessons include: Watch out for diuretics, even in low doses; consider an α-adrenergic blocker for those with some sexual dysfunction already present; if impotence appears, try a low dose of another type of drug, slowly increased to achieve adequate blood pressure control.

The same patients in the TOMHS study had no overall worsening of their quality of life with any of the various agents or the combined lifestyle regimen that they all followed.[2]

**N.M. Kaplan, M.D.**

*References*

1. Anonymous: MRC trial of treatment of mild hypertension: Principal results. *Br Med J* (*Clin Res Ed*). 291:97–104, 1985.
2. Grimm RH, Grandits GA, Cutler JA: Relationships of quality-of-life measures to long-term lifestyle and drug treatment in the Treatment of Mild Hypertension Study. *Arch Intern Med* 157:638–648, 1997.

---

**Prevention of Heart Failure by Antihypertensive Drug Treatment in Older Persons With Isolated Systolic Hypertension**
Kostis JB, for the SHEP Cooperative Research Group (UMDNJ, New Brunswick, NJ; et al)
*JAMA* 278:212–216, 1997

3–35

---

*Introduction.*—More than 2 million persons are affected by heart failure in the United States. A common antecedent is hypertension and isolated systolic hypertension. The incidence of total stroke was reduced by 36% and of major cardiovascular events by 32% in the Systolic Hypertension in the Elderly Program (SHEP), in which participants aged 60 years and older had antihypertensive stepped-care drug treatment with low-dose chlorthalidone. The occurrence of heart failure in active and placebo groups in SHEP was studied among patients with a history of ECG evidence of prior myocardial infarction and compared with the other patients.

*Methods.*—There were 4,736 persons aged 60 years and older with diastolic blood pressure below 90 mmHg and systolic blood pressure between 160 and 219 mmHg who received stepped-care antihypertensive drug therapy with the step 1 drug as chlorthalidone at 12.5 to 25 mg or matching placebo, and the step 2 drug as atenolol at 25 to 50 mg or matching placebo.

*Results.*—In the active therapy group 55 of 2,365 patients had heart failure compared with 105 of 2,371 patients in the placebo group. A predictor of risk of fatal or hospitalized nonfatal heart failure was a history of ECG evidence of myocardial infarction at baseline. For the different heart failure end points examined, the risk reduction in the group with a history of ECG evidence of myocardial infarction at baseline ranged from 59% to 85%. A higher risk of heart failure occurred among older patients, men, and those with higher systolic blood pressure or a history of ECG evidence of myocardial infarction.

*Conclusion.*—A strong protective effect was exerted in preventing heart failure among older persons with isolated systolic hypertension who received stepped-care treatment based on low-dose chlorthalidone. An 80% risk reduction was seen among patients with prior myocardial infarction.

▶ These results are truly remarkable: a 50% reduction in the incidence of heart failure in older patients with isolated systolic hypertension by therapy based on 12.5 mg of the diuretic chlorthalidone. Even more remarkable is the 80% reduction in congestive heart failure (CHF) in those with a prior acute myocardial infarction.

Two obvious questions should be addressed: First, can these results apply to all older hypertensive patients? Second, can other drugs, in particular angiotensin-converting enzyme (ACE) inhibitors, do as well or better?

The answer to the first question is certainly and unfortunately, no. The SHEP patients were "healthy" in most other ways, free of known coronary, cerebrovascular, renal disease, and arrhythmias, and had to be ambulatory. Most older hypertensive patients likely have one or more of these concomitant conditions that will make them more vulnerable to CHF. Nonetheless, reduction of their systolic hypertension will surely help, as the SHEP data show, since uncontrolled hypertension is a major contributor to the hospitalization of patients for CHF.[1]

As to the second question, there are no definitive data comparing various antihypertensive drugs in a large enough number of patients to document a difference between them. Of course, ACE inhibitors have been shown to be effective in improving survival of patients with reduced left ventricular systolic function, as in the SAVE trial[2] and with clinical signs of heart failure, as in the AIRE study.[3] Moreover, the benefits of ACE inhibitors in patients after myocardial infarction are even greater in the background of coexisting hypertension.[4] Therefore, it may be that ACE inhibitors will be as good or even better than diuretics in primary prevention of CHF in hypertensive patients without a prior myocardial infarction, but such evidence simply is not yet available.

**N.M. Kaplan, M.D.**

*References*

1. Chin MH, Goldman L: Factors contributing to the hospitalization of patients with congestive heart failure. *Am J Public Health* 87:643–648, 1997.
2. Pfeffer MA, Braunwald E, Moye LA, et al: Effect of captopril on mortality and morbidity in patients with left ventricular dysfunction after myocardial infarction: Results of the Survival and Ventricular Enlargement Trial. *N Engl J Med* 327:669–677, 1992.
3. The Acute Infarction Ramipril Efficacy (AIRE) Study Investigators: Effect of ramipril on mortality and morbidity of survivors of acute myocardial infarction with clinical evidence of heart failure. *Lancet* 342:821–828, 1993.
4. Gustafsson F, Pedersen-Torp C, Kober L, et al: Effect of angiotensin-converting enzyme inhibition after acute myocardial infarction in patients with arterial hypertension. *J Hypertens* 15:793–798, 1997.

**Different Concepts in First-line Treatment of Essential Hypertension: Comparison of a Low-dose Reserpine-Thiazide Combination With Nitrendipine Monotherapy**
Krönig B, for the German Reserpine in Hypertension Study Group (Technical Univ of Dresden, Germany; Univ of Regensburg, Germany)
*Hypertension* 29:651–658, 1997                                        3–36

*Introduction.*—For patients who do not respond adequately to monotherapy, fixed-dose combinations have been given that usually contained the full conventional doses of each drug. An entirely different approach is to use low doses of two agents with documented additive antihypertensive effects. Few studies have compared low-dose combinations and monotherapy in usual doses.

*Methods.*—In a randomized, double-blind, parallel study of 273 patients with hypertension with diastolic blood pressure 100–114 mmHg, the efficacy and tolerability of the fixed combination of reserpine at 0.1 mg plus the thiazide clopamid at 5 mg was compared with those of its single components and the calcium antagonist nitrendipine at 20 mg. The patients had a mean age of 58 years, and 51% were men. After a 2-week placebo period, their blood pressure was 158–160/103–104 mmHg.

*Results.*—The mean reduction in sitting blood pressure (systolic [SBP] and diastolic [DBP], respectively) from baseline at 24 hours after 6 weeks of treatment with 1 capsule daily for the reserpine-clopamid combination was −23.0 and −17.1; for reserpine alone, −14.0 and −11.7; for clopamid alone, −13.6 and −11.9; and for nitrendipine, −11.6 and −12.3. The normalization rate (SBP and DBP) for combination treatment was 63% and 55%; for reserpine alone, 46% and 40%; for clopamid alone, 41% and 36%; and for nitrendipine, 30% and 33%. Two capsules of medication were given during weeks 7–12 for patients whose blood pressure had not been normalized in the first 6 weeks. At week 12, the mean blood pressure reduction for the combination treatment was −25.7 and −18.1; for reserpine alone, −14.6 and −12.2; for clopamid alone, −17.7 and −13.4; for nitrendipine, −14.9 and −15.3 mmHg. The normalization rate at week 12 for the combination treatment was 76% and 66%; for reserpine alone, 44% and 35%; for clopamid alone, 46% and 39%; and for nitrendipine, 39% and 45%. Reserpine and clopamid combined acted more than additively, according to linear regression modeling. The adverse reaction rate for the reserpine-clopamid combinations was 27%; for reserpine, 28%; for clopamid, 29%; and for nitrendipine, 48%.

*Conclusion.*—Blood pressure was lowered significantly more by the combination of reserpine and clopamid than by either of the components alone or by nitrendipine. The combination was tolerated as well as the individual components and significantly better than nitrendipine. In the first-line treatment of hypertension, the use of a low-dose reserpine-thiazide combination appears to be a rational alternative to conventional monotherapy.

▶ Despite all of our enthusiasm for the newer drugs, the old-timers still have a place. Reserpine, in particular, remains an inexpensive, once-a-day, effective, and usually well-tolerated agent when used, as in this study, in a low dose in combination with a low dose of a diuretic. When given in larger doses, reserpine does cause sedation and depression. Although these may still occur with low doses, they are not common; depressed patients shouldn't be given the drug. Others have found that an even lower dose than used in this study, 0.05 mg/day, in combination with a diuretic may give good antihypertensive efficacy.

We shouldn't forget old friends as new drugs continue to become available. On the other hand, some old-timers may need to be used more appropriately; a good example is the β-blockers. They may worsen lipid levels and impair the ability to achieve cardiovascular fitness by exercise,[1] but they provide important secondary protection after an acute myocardial infarction, additive to the effects seen with angiotensin converting enzyme inhibitors.[2] Therefore, therapy should be individualized: young, physically active people shouldn't be burdened with a β-blocker, and elderly hypertensive patients have not been shown to be protected by β-blockers, but those with coronary disease may find them life-saving.

**N.M. Kaplan, M.D.**

*References*

1. Gordon NF, Scott CB, Duncan JJ: Effects of atenolol versus enalapril on cardiovascular fitness and serum lipids in physically active hypertensive men. *Am J Cardiol* 79:1065–1069, 1997.
2. Vantrimpont P, Rouleau JL, Wun CC, et al: Additive beneficial effects of betablockers to angiotensin-converting enzyme inhibitors in the Survival and Ventricular Enlargement (SAVE) study. *J Am Coll Cardiol* 29:229–236, 1997.

**Doxazosin for Benign Prostatic Hyperplasia: Long-term Efficacy and Safety in Hypertensive and Normotensive Patients**
Lepor H, Kaplan SA, Klimberg I, et al (New York Univ; New York; Columbia Univ, New York; Pfizer Central Research, NY; et al)
*J Urol* 157:525–530, 1997                                                          3–37

*Objective.*—The prevalence of benign prostatic hyperplasia (BPH) increases with age and is almost 50% in men 60 to 80 years old. A recent study demonstrated that the antihypertensive drug doxazosin also increased urinary flow in normotensive and hypertensive men. Results of a study and sustained efficacy of doxazosin for long–term treatment of normotensive and hypertensive men with BPH are presented.

*Methods.*—Two hundred seventy-two normotensive and 178 mildly to moderately hypertensive men were enrolled in a 4-year, open-label, dose titration extension treatment of BPH with 1 mg/d doubling at 2-week intervals to 8 mg/d for normotensive and to as high as 16 mg/d for hypertensive patients, if warranted. Efficacy and safety data were evaluated and compared statistically with baseline values.

*Results.*—Mean daily doses were 4 mg for normotensive and 6.4 mg for hypertensive patients. Maximum and average urinary flow rates and symptoms improved significantly in the intent-to-treat group. Blood pressure and heart rate decreased significantly in both groups with blood pressure readings decreasing more in the hypertensive group. The incidence of adverse reactions for the long-term study were similar to those for the shorter-term studies and included dizziness, fatigue, hypotension, edema, and dyspnea. Most adverse reactions were mild or moderate, and only 75 patients were withdrawn because of adverse events.

*Conclusion.*—Doxazosin, as treatment for BPH, was safe, effective, and well tolerated in normotensive or hypertensive men for up to 48 months. The drug also significantly lowered heart rate and blood pressure in hypertensive patients.

▶ The use of an α-blocker for an elderly hypertensive with prostatism is an excellent application of the concept of individualized therapy for hypertension. In a very short time, α-blockers have become the most widely recommended initial therapy for relief of the obstructive symptoms from an enlarged prostate. Although their antihypertensive efficacy and other attractive ancillary properties (lowering of plasma lipids, improving insulin sensitivity) have been long recognized, they have not been used widely just for the treatment of hypertension. For the man with both hypertension and prostatism, they are a natural.

**N.M. Kaplan, M.D.**

---

**The Antihypertensive Efficacy of the Novel Calcium Antagonist Mibefradil in Comparison With Nifedipine GITS in Moderate to Severe Hypertensives With Ambulatory Hypertension**
Lacourcière Y, Poirier L, Lefebvre J, et al (le Centre Hospitalier de l'Université Laval, Sainte-Foy, Quebec, Canada; Hoffmann-LaRoche, Ont, Canada; Hoffmann-LaRoche, Mississauga LaRoche, Basel, Switzerland)
*J Hypertens* 10:189–196, 1997                                    3–38

---

*Introduction.*—In the treatment of moderate to severe essential hypertension, calcium antagonists are increasingly used in single and combination therapies. A new benzimidazalyl-substituted tetraline derivative, mibefradil, is of a new class of calcium channel blockers. It has a unique receptor site and selectively blocks the T-type channels. Previous studies have shown it has a high oral bioavailability of about 90% and a half-life of 17–25 hours, decreases blood pressure by decreasing peripheral vascular resistance, and has no negative inotropic effects, compared with verapimil and diltiazem. Mibefradil was compared with nifedipine GITS, a once daily dihydropyridine calcium antagonist used to treat moderate to severe hypertension.

*Methods.*—In 71 patients with moderate to severe hypertension, a comparison was made between the effects of mibefradil at 50, 100, and 150 mg, and nifedipine GITS at 30, 60, and 90 mg monotherapies or combined with lisinopril at 20 mg.

*Results.*—During treatment with mibefradil and nifedipine GITS alone and combined with lisinopril, an incremental dose-response effect was seen in clinic and ambulatory blood pressure. A greater reduction in clinic and ambulatory diastolic blood pressures, as well as a greater response rate, was seen at maximal dosage with mibefradil. At each dose level, trough/peak ratios for systolic and diastolic blood pressures were more than 90%. With mibefradil 150 mg alone or combined with lisinopril, a significant decrease was seen in baseline heart rate, but no patients had clinically significant atrioventricular conduction abnormalities. In the nifedipine GITS group, adverse events related to vasodilation were more prevalent.

*Conclusion.*—In reducing clinic and 24-hour blood pressures while decreasing heart rate, the new calcium channel blocker mibefradil, either alone or in combination with lisinopril, is effective and well tolerated in patients with moderate or severe hypertension.

▶ If we thought we had enough calcium channel blockers, here comes another that has some different properties from those now available by having a preferentially greater effect on the T-type calcium channel rather than on the L-type channel, which is blocked primarily by the other calcium channel blockers. Mibefradil seems to combine some of the best features of both rate-slowing verapamil-diltiazem and the dihydropyridines.

As shown in this study, mibefradil is an effective antihypertensive, either alone or in combination with an angiotensin converting enzyme inhibitor, and seems to be better tolerated than the dihydropyridines. Greater clinical experience and large-scale trials will put it in its place.

**N.M. Kaplan, M.D.**

---

### Association of Calcium Channel Blocker Use With Increased Rate of Acute Myocardial Infarction in Patients With Left Ventricular Dysfunction

Kostis JB, Lacy CR, Cosgrove NM, et al (Robert Wood Johnson Med School, New Brunswick, NJ)
*Am Heart J* 133:550–557, 1997                                    3–39

---

*Introduction.*—Increased risk for acute myocardial infarction and death may be associated with calcium channel blockers (CCBs). Previous studies have highlighted the increased risk for myocardial infarction in hypertensive patients taking CCBs. The effects of enalapril were assessed in patients

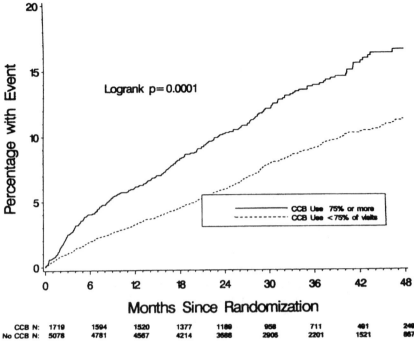

FIGURE 1.—Effect of reported use of calcium channel blockers (CCBs) during follow-up on cumulative incidence of myocardial infarction (fatal or nonfatal) in the participants of the combined trials of Studies of Left Ventricular Dysfunction. Events occurring in participants reporting calcium channel blocker (CCB) use at ≥75% of follow-up visits are denoted by CCB. Significant at $P < 0.0001$ by log-rank test. (Courtesy of Kostis JB, Lacy CR, Cosgrove NM, et al: Association of calcium channel blocker use with increased rate of acute myocardial infarction in patients with left ventricular dysfunction. *Am Heart J* 133:550–557, 1997.)

with systolic left ventricular dysfunction in the Studies of Left Ventricular Dysfunction, which included 2 placebo-controlled, randomized clinical trials.

*Methods.*—In these patients, a retrospective analysis was conducted to determine the association between CCB use and fatal and nonfatal myocardial infarction. There was a treatment trial for patients with clinical heart failure requiring treatment with diuretics or digitalis, and a prevention trial for patients with low ejection fraction but without overt heart failure. Average follow-up was 40 months.

*Results.*—In the enalapril group, myocardial infarction in 11.5% of 845 patients receiving CCBs, compared with 7.5% of 2,551 patients not receiving CCBs. In the placebo group, myocardial infarction occurred in 14.4% of 874 patients receiving CCBs, compared with 9.3% of 2,527 patients not receiving CCBs. Calcium channel blocker was an independent predictor of myocardial infarction according to multivariate Cox regression analysis, adjusting for comorbidity, cause and severity of left ventricular dysfunction, concomitant drug use, and heart failure. Patients with a higher heart rate and lower blood pressure were at greater risk for myocardial infarction (Fig 1). For all-cause mortality associated with CCBs, the adjusted risk ratio was 1.14.

*Conclusion.*—A significant increased risk for fatal or nonfatal myocardial infarction was seen with CCBs in this analysis of patients with left ventricular dysfunction. Calcium channel blockers should be avoided in patients with left ventricular dysfunction until randomized trials prove their safety. This conclusion, however, is not applicable in patients without left ventricular dysfunction.

▶ As has been abundantly clear since 1989,[1] large doses of short-acting CCBs are bad when given to hemodynamically vulnerable patients right after an acute myocardial infarction. These data show the bad effects to extend to short-acting diltiazem when given to patients with left ventricular dysfunction, as reflected by an ejection fraction below 35%.

These deleterious effects of short-acting CCBs almost certainly reflect their inherent vasodilatory effects, which translate into a fast and marked fall in systemic blood pressure, setting off compensatory sympathetic activity and putting an additional strain on a sick left ventricle.[2] As a result, these agents are contraindicated in the post–myocardial infarction and congestive heart failure settings, where they have never been recommended.

However, the sins of short-acting CCBs in certain conditions have been assumed by some to carry over to long-acting CCBs in circumstances where they are indicated and recommended. Increasingly strong evidence shows this is not true: Whereas the risk for myocardial infarction was almost 4-fold greater for short-acting CCBs than for β-blockers, the risk was less than that for β-blockers with long-acting CCBs.[3] In the placebo-controlled SYST-EUR trial, the long-acting CCB nitrendipine reduced coronary events.[4] Therefore, I am even more certain now than a year ago that long-acting CCBs are not responsible for increased coronary ischemic events.

**N.M. Kaplan, M.D.**

*References*

1. Held PH, Yusuf S, Furberg CD: Calcium channel blockers in acute myocardial infarction and unstable angina: An overview. *Br Med J* 299:1187–1192, 1989.
2. Pepi M, Maltagliati A, Berti M, et al: Relation between exercise-induced left ventricular wall motion abnormalities and coronary artery disease in hypertensive patients. *Am J Hypertens* 10:297–305, 1997.
3. Alderman MH, Cohen H, Roqué R, et al: Effect of long-acting and short-acting calcium antagonists on cardiovascular outcomes in hypertensive patients. *Lancet* 349:594–598, 1997.
4. Staessen JA, Fagard R, Thijs L: Morbidity and mortality in the placebo-controlled European trial on isolated systolic hypertension in the elderly. *Lancet* 350:757–764, 1997.

### Calcium-Channel Blockers and Risk of Cancer

Jick H, Jick S, Derby LE, et al (Boston Univ)
*Lancet* 349:525–528, 1997                                        3–40

*Introduction.*—Findings of an earlier report suggest that patients receiving calcium channel blockers (CCBs) are at increased risk for cancer (61 of 750 patients), compared with patients taking β-blockers. A large group of patients with hypertension were evaluated to determine the relation of CCBs and cancer.

*Methods.*—Data were gathered from the General Practice Research Database regarding use and dose of CCBs, angiotensin converting enzyme (ACE) inhibitors, and β-blockers. A nested case-control analysis was performed to determine the risk for cancer among users of CCBs and ACE inhibitors; patients receiving β-blockers acted as a reference group. The cohort was limited to patients with at least 4 years of medical history recorded on computer. For each patient with cancer, up to 4 controls with hypertension were matched for age, sex, and the general practice they attended.

*Results.*—There were 446 patients with cancer and 1,750 controls. The relative risk estimates for all cancers combined were 1.27 for patients receiving CCBs and 0.79 for patients taking ACE inhibitors, relative to patients taking β-blockers. There was a slight difference in risk estimates with duration of use of CCBs of <1.0 years (relative risk 1.46), 1.0–3.9 years (1.26), and ≥4.0 years (1.23).

*Conclusion.*—The small positive association between CCBs and risk for cancer (relative to use of β-blockers) was small, and was not likely causal because there was no increase in cancer risk with increasing use of CCBs.

▶ These data are only a small part of the rapidly growing evidence that CCBs do not cause cancer, as was claimed by Pahor et al.[1] on the basis of a case-control study of older hypertensives. The case-control study by Jick et al. is of much greater statistical strength, and now data of a large prospective randomized placebo-controlled study show a decrease in the incidence of cancer in those who took the CCB nitrendipine compared with those who took a placebo.[2]

The problem with such claims as Pahor et al's., based on weak data that received prominent press coverage, is that they scare both physicians and patients and make it even more difficult to use effective drugs for appropriate indications. It is unfortunate that proper large prospective studies of CCBs (or ACE inhibitors or angiotensin-II receptor blockers) were not performed *before* they were widely used. But the nature of drug approval and the patterns of drug use will likely leave us vulnerable to such unsubstantiated claims.

**N.M. Kaplan, M.D.**

*References*

1. Pahor M, Guralnik JM, Salive ME, et al: Do calcium channel blockers increase the risk of cancer? *Am J Hypertens* 9:695–699, 1996.
2. Staessen JA, Fagard R, Thijs L: Morbidity and mortality in the placebo-controlled European trial on isolated systolic hypertension in the elderly. *Lancet* 350:757–764, 1997.

---

**Randomised Double-blind Comparison of Placebo and Active Treatment for Older Patients With Isolated Systolic Hypertension**

Staessen JA, for the Systolic Hypertension in Europe (Syst-Eur) Trial Investigators (Univ of Leuven, Belgium)

*Lancet* 350:757–764, 1997                                    3–41

---

*Introduction.*—The prevalence of isolated systolic hypertension is 8% and over 25%, respectively, among persons aged 70 and 80 or older. The Systolic Hypertension in Europe trial was begun in 1989 to evaluate whether active treatment could decrease cardiovascular complications of isolated systolic hypertension; fatal and non-fatal stroke combined was the primary end point. The trial was stopped on February 14, 1997. Morbidity and mortality results are reported.

*Methods.*—Patients were recruited from 198 centers in 23 European countries. Eligible patients were age 60 or older and were started on masked placebo. Three run-in visits were held 1 month apart. The average sitting systolic blood pressure ranged from 160–219 mmHg and the average diastolic pressure was below 95 mmHg. Patients (4,695) were stratified for center, sex, and previous cardiovascular complications, then randomized to nitrendipine 10–40 mg daily, with the possible addition of enalapril 5–20 mg daily and hydrochlorothiazide 12.5–25.0 mg daily or to matching placebo. The occurrence of major end points were compared by intention to treat.

*Results.*—At a median 2 year follow-up, sitting systolic blood pressure dropped 13 mmHg and diastolic blood pressure dropped 2 mg Hg in the placebo group. These numbers were 23 and 7 mmHg in the active treatment group. The between-group differences in systolic and diastolic blood pressures were 10.1 mmHg and 4.5 mmHg, respectively. The total rate of stroke in the active treatment group dropped significantly from 13.7 to 7.9 end points per 1,000 patient-years (42% decrease). In the active treatment group: non-fatal stroke was reduced by 44%; all fatal and non-fatal cardiac end points, including sudden death, decreased by 26%; non-fatal cardiac end points were reduced by 33%, and all fatal and non-fatal cardiovascular end points decreased by 31%. There was a slight decrease in cardiovascular mortality with active treatment. There was no change in all-cause mortality.

*Conclusions.*—Initial active antihypertensive treatment with nitrendipine decreases the rate of cardiovascular complications in elderly people with isolated systolic hypertension. If 1,000 patients were treated using this regimen for 5 years, 29 strokes and 53 major cardiovascular end points could be prevented.

▶ This is the first large-scale, randomized, controlled trial of any antihypertensive drug beyond diuretics and adrenergic inhibitors to be published. Therefore, it is a true breakthrough of the barrier that previously held against all of the antihypertensive agents marketed in the past 10 years.

The SYST-EUR trial is remarkable for having achieved a highly significant reduction in strokes (the primary end point) and overall cardiovascular morbidity and mortality in an average of only 2 years of therapy—half the time required to achieve similar effects in a similar population with a diuretic-based regimen in the Systolic Hypertension in the Elderly Program (SHEP) done in the United States.

With this evidence, the use of a long-acting dihydropyridine calcium-channel blocker (CCB) has been added to the choices of initial therapy for elderly patients with systolic hypertension in the Sixth Joint National Committee report (1997).[1] Meanwhile, many more randomized controlled trials of other CCBs, angiotensin-converting enzyme inhibitors, A-II receptor blockers, and alpha-blockers are in progress so their place in the antihypertensive armamentarium will soon be solidified.

**N.M. Kaplan, M.D.**

*Reference*

1. Joint National Committee, 1997. The Sixth Report of the Joint National Committee on Detection, Evaluation, and Treatment of High Blood Pressure (JNCVI). *Arch Intern Med* 157:2413–2446, 1997.

---

**Effects of Controlled-onset Extended-release Verapamil on Nocturnal Blood Pressure (Dippers Versus Nondippers)**
White WB, and the COER-Verapamil Study Group (Univ of Connecticut, Farmington; et al)
*Am J Cardiol* 80:469–474, 1997                                          3–42

---

*Introduction.*—The usual circadian pattern of blood pressure (BP) is altered in approximately 1 in 4 patients with systemic hypertension, who exhibit an absent or blunted nocturnal decline in BP. Such patients (nondippers) may be at increased risk for cardiovascular events. A prospective clinical trial evaluated the effects of a chronotherapeutic delivery system of controlled-onset extended-release (COER) verapamil hydrochloride in patients with and without a greater than 10% decline in nocturnal BP.

*Methods.*—The multicenter, double-blind trial randomized 193 dippers and 64 nondippers to COER verapamil or placebo. The 8-week treatment period followed a 1-week washout and a 2-week single-blind placebo period to establish baseline ambulatory BP values. Medication was taken once nightly at 10 PM; COER verapamil doses ranged from 120 to 540 mg.

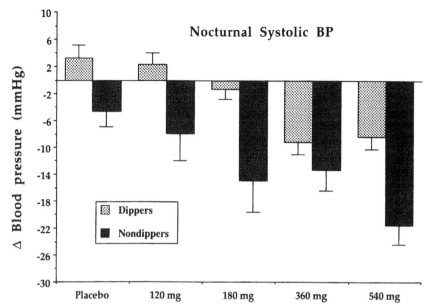

FIGURE 1.—Changes (Δ) in nocturnal (10 P.M. to 5 A.M.) BP from baseline measured by ambulatory BP monitoring in dippers (decline in mean BP from daytime period to the nocturnal period was >10%) contrasted with changes in nocturnal BP in nondippers (<10% decline in nocturnal BP) on placebo and 4 doses of COER verapamil. *Upper panel*, changes in systolic BP. *Abbreviations: BP*, blood pressure; *COER*, controlled-onset extended-release. (Courtesy of White WB, and the COER-Verapamil Study Group: Effects of controlled-onset extended-release verapamil on nocturnal blood pressure (dippers versus nondippers). *Am J Cardiol* 80:469–474, 1997. Reprinted by permission of the publisher. Copyright 1997 by Excerpta Medica, Inc.)

Average BPs during the nighttime, daytime, and 24-hour periods were computed for each patient and summarized by subgroup and treatment.

*Results.*—The various treatment groups were similar in age, gender, and ethnicity distributions. Dippers and nondippers did not differ in daytime BPs; average nighttime BPs were 136/81 mmHg in dippers and 153/94 mmHg in nondippers. Treatment of dippers and nondippers with COER verapamil led to similar decreases in placebo-subtracted BP during daytime. During nighttime, placebo increased nocturnal BP in dippers and reduced BP in nondippers (Fig 1). The mean changes from baseline (3.3/3.2 and −4.6/−3.2 mmHg, respectively) were not significant for either systolic or diastolic BP. With adjustment for covariates and subtraction of the placebo effect, nondippers had a 5.8 mmHg greater reduction in nighttime systolic BP than dippers and a 2.4 mm greater reduction in nighttime diastolic BP. Reductions in systolic and diastolic nocturnal BP showed a significant dose relationship independent of the regression to the mean effect and demographic variables.

*Conclusion.*—Treatment with COER verapamil decreased nocturnal BP to a greater extent in nondipper hypertensives than in dipper hypertensives. Nocturnal hypertensives can thus be treated by COER verapamil, and dippers will not experience excessively low BP even at high doses.

▶ This study involved a special formulation of verapamil that doesn't release the drug for 4–6 hours. It is taken at bedtime to provide antihypertensive efficacy in the morning hours after arising, when the largest portion of cardiovascular catastrophes occur. The data are comforting in that they show a much greater fall in nighttime BP in those whose nocturnal BP does not dip normally, providing the nondippers with probable protection while not exposing the dippers to potentially too-low BP during sleep.

As the authors note, similar effects have been reported with other drugs, including other 24-hour formulations of verapamil.[1] Moreover, long-acting formulations of antianginal agents are clearly better in providing relief from ambulatory myocardial ischemia than are short-acting formulations.[2] The longer, the better.

**N.M. Kaplan, M.D.**

*References*

1. Rosito GA, Gebara OCE, McKenna CA, et al: Effect of sustained-release verapamil on the morning systemic arterial pressure surge during daily activity in patients with systemic hypertension. *Am J Cardiology* 79:1252–1255, 1997.
2. Deedwania PC, Pool PE, Thadani U, et al: Effect of morning versus evening dosing of diltiazem on myocardial ischemia detected by ambulatory electrocardiographic monitoring in chronic stable angina pectoris. *Am J Cardiol* 80:421–425, 1997.

---

**Comparative Effects of Enalapril and Verapamil on Myocardial Blood Flow in Systemic Hypertension**
Parodi O, Neglia D, Palombo C, et al (Inst of Clinical Physiology of the Natl Council of Research, Pisa, Italy; Università di Firenze, Italy)
*Circulation* 96:864–873, 1997                                     3–43

---

*Introduction.*—Very few reports have assessed the effects of antihypertensive drugs on myocardial perfusion. Some antihypertensive agents, such as ACE inhibitors or calcium channel blockers, may affect the structural and functional properties of the coronary microcirculation. The long-term comparative effects of ACE inhibitors and calcium channel blockers on myocardial blood flow (MBF) were assessed in a randomized, single-blind trial of 20 patients with hypertension.

*Methods.*—Patients were randomly assigned to receive verapamil (240–240 mg/day) or enalapril (10–40 mg/day). Dynamic positron emission tomography (PET) and $^{13}$N-ammonia were used to quantitatively assess MBF at rest, during atrial pacing tachycardia, and after IV dipyridamole infusion at baseline and 6 months after treatment (after 1 week of pharmacological washout).

*Results.*—There were no between-group differences in blood pressure and heart rate during flow measurements before or after therapy. At baseline, there was no significant difference in the 2 treatment groups in mean MBF at rest, during pacing tachycardia, and after dipyridamole infusion. Pacing and dipyridamole flows were significantly lower in the treatment groups, compared to a control group of normotensive research subjects. At completion of therapy, the MBF did not change at rest, during pacing tachycardia, or after dipyridamole infusion in enalapril-treated patients but increased significantly during pacing and after dipyridamole in the verapamil-treated group. Using the coefficient of variation, the inhomogeneity of regional MBF distribution was lower at rest after both treatment regimens and during pacing in the enalapril group. There was no association between changes in MBF and changes in left ventricular mass.

Conclusion.—Successful long-term treatment with verapamil did not change myocardial perfusion at rest, but significantly decreased coronary resistance and increased MBF during metabolic and pharmacological vasodilation. The favorable changes were unrelated to left ventricular mass, indicating that the improvement in coronary vasodilating capability after verapamil was primarily due to regression of coronary microcirculatory abnormalities. Patients in the enalapril treatment group did not have significant changes in MBF. A more homogeneous MBF distribution was observed in both treatment groups, especially the enalapril group, compared to pretreatment. This may be because of an improved matching between myocardial mass and perfusion after therapy.

▶ This study, although involving only 20 hypertensive patients who were treated for only 6 months, has important implications. First, reduced coronary flow reserve has been identified in many hypertensive patients, particularly in the presence of left ventricular hypertrophy, and such reduced reserve has been held responsible for coronary ischemia in the absence of demonstrable atherosclerotic disease, i.e., syndrome X.

Second, ACE inhibitors have been shown to be effective in preventing deleterious remodeling after myocardial infarction, and a major pathogenetic role has been ascribed to intracardiac renin-angiotensin. On the other hand, calcium antagonists have claimed to have multiple adverse effects (although a long-acting dihydropyridine reduced coronary events in the randomized, placebo-controlled SYST-EUR trial).[1]

Thus, these results showing better improvement in myocardial blood flow with the calcium antagonist verapamil than with the ACE inhibitor enalapril provides another potential difference between these agents and suggests that calcium antagonists may have additional benefits beyond their antihypertensive effect in patients with reduced coronary reserve.

**N.M. Kaplan, M.D.**

*Reference*

1. Staessen JA, Fagard R, Thijs L, et al: Randomised double-blind comparison of placebo and active treatment for older patients with isolated systolic hypertension. *Lancet* 350:757–764, 1997.

### Combined Enalapril and Felodipine Extended Release (ER) for Systemic Hypertension

Gradman AH, for the Enalapril-Felodipine ER Factorial Study Group (Western Pennsylvania Hosp, Pittsburgh; et al)

*Am J Cardiol* 79:431–435, 1997                                    3–44

*Introduction.*—A single-dose drug is generally the initial step in treating hypertension. Only if blood pressure cannot be controlled are additional drugs used. Combination therapy with low doses of multiple agents is now being advocated by many authorities as an alternative strategy for achieving control of blood pressure. An evaluation was made of combination treatment with the angiotensin-converting enzyme (ACE) inhibitor enalapril and the vascular selective dihydropyridine calcium antagonist felodipine extended release (ER).

*Methods.*—In patients with essential hypertension, the safety and efficacy of combination treatment with enalapril and felodipine ER were evaluated in this multicenter, placebo-controlled, double-blind trial. Placebo, enalapril (5 or 20 mg), felodipine ER (2.5, 5, or 10 mg), or their combinations were given for 8 weeks to 707 patients with sitting diastolic blood pressure 95–115 mmHg.

*Results.*—In reducing both systolic and diastolic blood pressure, all doses of enalapril and felodipine ER had a statistically significant additive effective. For the combinations, the trough to peak ratios ranged from 0.63 (enalapril 5 mg–felodipine ER 2.5 mg) to 0.79 (enalapril 20 mg–felodipine ER 10 mg), consistent with effective blood pressure control with 1 dose per day. A greater reduction in diastolic blood pressure was seen in patients $\geq$65 years. Compared with felodipine ER monotherapy, the combination of enalapril–felodipine ER was associated with less drug-induced peripheral edema (10.8% vs. 4.1%). During the study, no serious drug-related adverse effects were seen (Table 3).

*Conclusion.*—Blood pressure was effectively lowered by the combination of enalapril and felodipine ER. When used in the treatment of hyper-

TABLE 3.—Drug-related Adverse Events

| | | Treatment Group | | |
| Adverse Events | Placebo (79 patients) | Felodipine ER Monotherapy (176 patients) | Enalapril Monotherapy (133 patients) | Combination Therapy (319 patients) |
|---|---|---|---|---|
| Headache | 6 (7.6%) | 18 (10.2%) | 5 (3.8%) | 33 (10.3%) |
| Dizziness | 0 (0.0%) | 5 (2.8%) | 2 (1.5%) | 14 (4.4%) |
| Edema swelling | 1 (1.3%) | 19 (10.8%) | 3 (2.3%) | 13 (4.1%) |
| Cough | 0 (0.0%) | 1 (0.6%) | 3 (2.3%) | 7 (2.2%) |

*Abbreviation:* ER, extended release.
(Reprinted by permission of the publisher from Gradman AH, for the Enalapril-Felodipine ER Factorial Study Group: Combined Enalapril and Felodipine Extended Release (ER) for Systemic Hypertension. *Am J Cardiol* 79:431–435, 1997. Copyright 1997 by Excerpta Medica, Inc.)

tension, the combination therapy was generally well tolerated, with an excellent safety profile.

▶ One of the major moves occurring in the treatment of hypertension is the reapplication of an old concept with a new twist: the use of two drugs in combination. The data described in the large, double-blind trial of the ACE inhibitor trandolapril and the calcium channel blocker (CCB) felodipine, each given separately and then together, show why the idea has resurfaced: When combined in low doses, the 2 drugs provided additive effects and actually reduced the incidence of a major side effect, dihydropyridine-induced pedal edema (see Table 3).

The explanation for this lesser incidence of pedal edema likely reflects the venodilation provided by the ACE inhibitor, resolving the local sequestration of fluid induced by the intense arteriolar dilation by the CCB.

Similar good hemodynamic effects of combinations have been noted with other ACE inhibitors and CCBs,[1] and excellent antihypertensive efficacy with various other combinations as well.[2]

Perhaps the most sensible combination is a low dose of a diuretic with a drug from any of the other classes, thereby enhancing efficacy and minimizing side effects.[3] Lots of combinations are already here, and more are on their way.

**N.M. Kaplan, M.D.**

*References*

1. Aepfelbacher FC, Messerli FH, Nunez E, et al: Cardiovascular effects of a trandolapril/verapamil combination in patients with mild to moderate essential hypertension. *Am J Cardiol* 79:826–828, 1997.
2. de Leeuw PW, Notter T, Zillez P: Comparison of different fixed antihypertensive combination drugs: A double-blind, placebo-controlled parallel group study. *J Hypertens* 15:87–91, 1997.
3. Abernethy DR: Pharmacological properties of combination therapies for hypertension. *Am J Hypertens* 10:13S-16S, 1997.

---

**Effects of Long-term Antihypertensive Treatment With Lisinopril on Resistance Arteries in Hypertensive Patients With Left Ventricular Hypertrophy**
Rizzoni D, Muiesan ML, Porteri E, et al (Univ of Brescia, Italy)
*J Hypertens* 15:197–204, 1997                                   3–45

---

*Introduction.*—Common accompaniments of chronic hypertension are structural abnormalities of resistance vessels. Increased arterial wall thickness is an important factor in the increase in vascular resistance. The possible regression of changes in small artery structure in hypertension is a goal of antihypertensive treatment. Previous studies have shown an improvement with an angiotensin converting enzyme (ACE) inhibitor. In hypertensive patients with left ventricular hypertrophy, the effects of long-term antihypertensive therapy with the ACE inhibitor lisinopril on structural alterations and the endothelial function of small resistance arteries was evaluated.

*Methods.*—Lisinopril was used to treat 14 patients with left ventricular hypertrophy for 3 years. At baseline and during the first and third years of treatment, patients underwent echocardiographic evaluation of left ventricular mass index. Biopsy of the subcutaneous fat from the gluteal region was taken to dissect subcutaneous small resistance arteries at the end of treatment so that a calculation could be made of the medial lumen ratio. Results were compared with those in 14 patients with untreated essential hypertension and 14 patients with normal blood pressure.

*Results.*—In the treated hypertensive patients, there was a significantly lower media/lumen ratio than in the untreated hypertensive patients, but it was still significantly higher than in the normotensive patients. A significant reduction in clinical blood pressure was seen in the treated hypertensive patients, but was still significantly higher than in the normotensive patients. Observations were made of significant correlations between the media/lumen ratio and blood pressure, left ventricular mass index, or changes in left ventricular mass index during treatment. In untreated hypertensive patients, the response to acetylcholine administration was reduced, compared with that in normotensive patients. The vasodilation obtained was greater with the 2 higher doses of acetylcholine in patients treated with lisinopril than in those with untreated hypertension, suggesting an improvement of endothelial function.

*Conclusion.*—A smaller media/lumen ratio in the subcutaneous small resistance arteries was associated with long-term therapy based on lisinopril in hypertensive patients with left ventricular hypertrophy. Lisinopril therapy probably improved endothelial function.

▶ The hemodynamic hallmark of established hypertension is increased peripheral vascular resistance. This resistance presumably reflects both structural remodeling with an increased media/lumen ratio and impaired vasodilation from endothelial dysfunction.

These data confirm the ability of ACE inhibitors to correct both of these abnormalities, providing an experimental underpinning to their obvious antihypertensive efficacy. These agents provide additional unique effects (that may be shared by the angiotensin II receptor blockers). These include prevention of myocardial remodeling after a myocardial infarction, removal of the afterload attributed to an activated renin-angiotensin system in congestive heart failure, and relaxation of renal efferent arterioles so that introglomerular pressures are lowered and progression of glomerulosclerosis is slowed.

Obviously, ACE inhibitors will continue to be major players in the field of cardiovascular therapy.

**N.M. Kaplan, M.D.**

### Increased Left-Ventricular Mass After Losartan Treatment

Cheung B (Queen Mary Hosp, Pokfulam, Hong Kong)
*Lancet* 349:1743–1744, 1997                                                    3–46

*Introduction.*—Although angiotensin II antagonists have several advantages over angiotensin–converting-enzyme (ACE) inhibitors, the clinical effects of these 2 groups of drugs may differ. The effect of losartan, an angiotensin II antagonist, on left-ventricular mass (LVM) was assessed in 12 patients before comparative studies of ACE inhibitors and angiotensin II antagonists were undertaken.

*Methods.*—Patients were 6 men and 6 women with untreated mild hypertension. The mean age of the group was 50.4; mean baseline blood pressure was 147/94 mmHg. A 2-week placebo run-in to treatment was followed by randomization to placebo or losartan (50 mg titratable to 100 mg daily). Treatment continued for 12 weeks, during which time no concurrent antihypertensive agents were allowed. The LVM index was

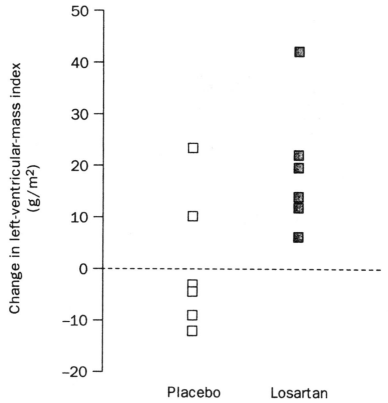

**FIGURE 1.**—(Bottom half) Changes in left-ventricular-mass index after 12 weeks of treatment with losartan or placebo. (Courtesy of Cheung B: Increased left-ventricular mass after losartan treatment. *Lancet* 349:1743–1744, 1997. Copyright by The Lancet Ltd., 1997.)

measured by echocardiography before and 12 weeks after treatment by a sonographer unaware of patient data or treatment group.

*Results.*—The losartan and placebo groups were comparable in baseline characteristics, family history of hypertension, blood pressure, renal function, LVM index, and systolic and diastolic left-ventricular function. Compliance with the once-daily regimen was more than 90%. The mean decrease in sitting diastolic blood pressure in the losartan group was 6.7 mmHg, which was not significantly different from the mean decrease that occurred with placebo. Treatment with losartan was associated with a mean increase of 19.3 $g/m^2$ in LVM index; the LVM index in the placebo group was essentially unchanged after the treatment period (Fig 1). No adverse events were reported in losartan-treated patients.

*Discussion.*—Losartan was no more effective than placebo in reducing blood pressure in patients with mild untreated hypertension, but the angiotensin II antagonist significantly increased the LVM index compared with placebo. In contrast, even low doses of ACE inhibitors may cause left-ventricular hypertrophy to regress. More long-term data are needed before losartan is used as a first-line antihypertensive agent.

▶ This small study does not prove that angiotensin II (A II) receptor blockers will not regress left ventricular hypertrophy but, as small as it is, it certainly suggests that we wait for large, long-term trials with these new agents before we make the jump to use them instead of ACE inhibitors.

One of the major differences between ACE inhibitors and the A II-receptor blockers is the rise in bradykinin and perhaps other endogenous substances that is seen with inhibition of ACE but is not seen with A II-receptor blockade. These data may reflect a major positive role for the increase in bradykinin and other substances that are also normally inactivated by the ACE enzyme. For instance, increased endogenous bradykinin has been shown to be involved in the peripheral vasodilation seen with ACE inhibitors[1] and in the potentiation of preconditioning in the human heart.[2]

Only one study comparing an ACE inhibitor (captopril) and an A II-receptor blocker (losartan) has been published.[3] In this study of more than 700 patients with class II-IV heart failure given one of these agents for 48 weeks, all-cause mortality was 46% less in those given losartan, 4.8% vs. 8.7%. A larger such comparison is in progress.

Thus, divergent results have been noted. Cough is certainly a problem with ACE inhibitors, presumably because of the increased bradykinin levels and because A II-receptor blockers do not cause cough.[4] Whether there are other benefits from the newer agents remains to be seen.

**N.M. Kaplan, M.D.**

*References*

1. Horning B, Kohler C, Drexler H: Role of bradykinin in mediating vascular effects of angiotensin-converting enzyme inhibitors in humans. *Circulation* 95:1115–1118, 1997.

2. Morris SD, Yellon DM: Angiotensin-converting enzyme inhibitors potentiate pre-conditioning through bradykinin B₂ receptor activation in human heart. *J Am Coll Cardiol* 29:1599–1606, 1997.
3. Pitt B, Segal R, Martinez FA, et al: Randomised trial of losartan versus captopril in patients over 65 with heart failure (Evaluation of Lorsartan in the Elderly Study, ELITE). *Lancet* 349:747–752, 1997.
4. Benz J, Oshrain C, Henry D, et al: Valsartan, a new angiotensin II receptor antagonist: a double-blind study comparing the incidence of cough with lisinipril and hydrochlorothiazide. *J Clin Pharmacol* 37:101–107, 1997.

## Randomised Placebo-controlled Trial of Lisinopril in Normotensive Patients With Insulin-Dependent Diabetes and Normoalbuminuria or Microalbuminuria

Chaturvedi N, and the EUCLID Study Group (Univ College, London et al)
*Lancet* 349:1787–1792, 1997                                3–47

*Background.*—People with insulin-dependent diabetes mellitus (IDDM) have higher rates of morbidity and mortality than the general population. Some of this increased risk is the result of renal and cardiovascular complications of IDDM. A prognostic factor for these complications is the appearance of protein, mostly albumin, in the urine. Elevated blood pressure is a modifiable risk factor for renal disease progression. Inhibitors of angiotensin-converting enzyme (ACE) appear to be especially effective in controlling renal disease progression in those with IDDM and macroalbuminuria. To determine its effects in IDDM patients with microalbuminuria or normoalbuminuria, a 2-year, randomized, placebo-controlled, clinical trial with the ACE inhibitor lisinopril was performed.

*Study Design.*—EUCLID, the EURODIAB controlled trial of lisinopril in IDDM, was a double-blind, randomized, parallel-design clinical trial of lisinopril and placebo conducted at 18 European centers. Men and women aged 20 to 59 years with IDDM were recruited for this study if their resting blood pressure was at least 75 and no more than 90 mmHg diastolic and no more than 155 mmHg systolic. At their initial visit, participants had blood pressure readings to determine eligibility and were issued 1 month's supply of placebo to determine compliance. One month later at the randomization visit, blood pressure was reassessed and 530 patients were stratified by center and albuminuric status. Patients reexamined at 1, 3, 6, 12, 18, and 24 months.

*Results.*—There were no significant differences in baseline characteristics of the participants by treatment group. Intention-to-treat analysis at 2 years demonstrated that albumin excretion rate (AER) was 2.2 µg/min lower in the treatment group than in the placebo group. This was equivalent to an 18.8% difference between these two groups. Among the patients with microalbuminuria, the AER difference was 34.2 µg/min. For those who completed the full 2 years of this trial, the difference was 38.5 µg/min in those with microalbuminuria and 0.23 µg/min in those with normoalbuminuria at baseline. There was no difference in hypoglycemic events or in metabolic control between the two treatment groups.

*Conclusions.*—The ACE inhibitor lisinopril was of clinical benefit to a large group of patients with IDDM with early signs of renal disease, but without hypertension. A much greater effect was observed in patients with microalbuminuria than in those with normoalbuminuria, but the exact threshold where therapy should begin could not be determined. Long-term follow-up is required to determine the full impact of lisinopril therapy on outcome. Care guidelines for those with IDDM should include treatment of early-stage renal disease with ACE inhibitors.

▶ Evidence for the value of treating hypertensive patients with IDDM with macroalbuminuria to prevent the progression of diabetic nephropathy has been available for almost a decade. Subsequently, evidence for the value of antihypertensive therapy has broadened to include hypertensive patients with diabetes with microalbuminuria and nondiabetic hypertensive patients with renal insufficiency. In earlier studies, various antihypertensive agents were used. In the more recent ones, ACE inhibitors have been the primary drug, based on the experimental evidence that they preferentially dilate renal efferent arterioles and thereby lower intraglomerular pressure and the clinical evidence that they reduce proteinuria and slow the progression of renal damage better than other agents.[1] However, the reduction in proteinuria may not always reflect a slowing of the loss of renal function; in one study of diabetic nephropathy, treatment with the ACE inhibitor lisinopril provided a greater decrease in proteinuria but a faster loss of glomerular filtration rate than did the calcium-channel blocker nisoldipine.[2]

The EUCLID data extend the evidence for renoprotection down into normotensive, patients with IDDM with microalbuminuria and suggest that even those who have no albuminuria may be protected by use of an ACE inhibitor even before the initial manifestation of nephropathy becomes obvious.

Because diabetic nephropathy is now the single most common cause of end-stage renal disease and diabetic nephropathy develops in about 40% of IDDM patients, the use of such preventive drug therapy may be appropriate. However, better control of diabetes will also slow progression of nephropathy (and other diabetic complications), so that should be the primary preventive approach. Moreover, fewer patients with non-insulin dependent diabetes develop nephropathy; thus control of their diabetes, preferable by weight reduction and newer insulin-sensitizing agents, remains the best therapy. ACE inhibitors and perhaps calcium channel blockers certainly should be used when microalbuminuria first is noted, regardless of the presence of hypertension.

In diabetic patients with hypertension, the goal of therapy must be maintenance of blood pressure well below 140/90 mmHg likely as low as 120/75 mmHg.[3] Clearly, effective lowering of blood pressure is critical to protection of the kidneys in patients with diabetes. This should be accomplished with ACE inhibitors and whatever other measures are deemed necessary.

**N.M. Kaplan, M.D.**

*References*

1. Giatras I, for the Angiotensin-Converting-Enzyme Inhibition and Progressive Renal Disease Study Group: Effect of angiotensin-converting enzyme inhibitors on the progression of nondiabetic renal disease: a meta-analysis of randomized trials. *Ann Intern Med* 127:337–345, 1997.
2. Rossing P, Tarnow L, Boelskifte S, et al: Differences between nisoldipine and lisinopril on glomerular filtration rates and albuminuria in hypertensive IDDM patients with nephropathy druing the first year of treatment. *Diabetes* 46:481–487, 1997.
3. Hasslacher C: Hypertension as a risk factor in non-insulin-dependent diabetes mellitus: How far should blood pressure be reduced? *J Diabetes Complications* 11:90–91, 1997.

## Metabolic and Cardiovascular Effects of Carvedilol and Atenolol in Non–Insulin-Dependent Diabetes Mellitus and Hypertension

Giugliano D, Acampora R, Marfella R, et al (Second Univ of Naples, Italy)
*Ann Intern Med* 126:955–959, 1997                                             3–48

*Introduction.*—Patients with diabetes are at increased risk for hypertension and its vascular consequences. Physicians have been reluctant to prescribe β-blockers for diabetics with hypertension because of the risk for worsened glucose and lipid metabolism. In a randomized, double-blind trial, investigators compared the metabolic and cardiovascular effects of atenolol with those of carvedilol, an antihypertensive drug that prevents lipid peroxidation and the depletion of endogenous antioxidants.

*Methods.*—Study participants were 45 men and women with non-insulin dependent diabetes mellitus and a supine diastolic blood pressure of 90 to 105 mmHg. After a 4- to 6-week run-in period during which placebo was given in a single-blind manner, patients were randomized to carvedilol (25 mg once daily) or atenolol (50 mg once daily) for 24 weeks of treatment. Doses were doubled for patients without decreases of at least 10 mmHg in diastolic blood pressure after 4 weeks.

*Results.*—Forty-one patients completed the study. Approximately one-third in each group required upward dose titration at week 4. Both groups exhibited decreases in average systolic and diastolic blood pressure and left ventricular mass, and the differences between groups were small. Atenolol was associated with a greater decrease in heart rate; carvedilol produced larger decreases in mean triglyceride level and greater increases in high-density lipoprotein cholesterol level. Other responses showing an advantage for carvedilol vs. atenolol included increase in total glucose disposal, decrease in plasma glucose response, decrease in insulin response to oral glucose, and decrease in lipid peroxidation.

*Conclusion.*—Both carvedilol and atenolol were equally effective in lowering blood pressure in patients with diabetes and hypertension. The metabolic effects of the 2 agents, however, are considerably different. Their effects on plasma glucose and insulin levels indicate that carvedilol improves insulin sensitivity, whereas atenolol weakens it.

▶ Diabetic hypertensives are an increasingly large segment of the overall hypertensive population, reflecting the rapidly increasing number of type II diabetics from the rapidly increasing pool of obese Americans and the longer survival of type I diabetics who are living long enough to develop nephropathy. Hypertension commonly accompanies obesity-related type II diabetes and commonly appears when nephropathy and renal insufficiency develop in either type I or type II patients.

Concerns about the use of β-blockers in diabetic patients relate to their propensity to further worsen insulin resistance and to raise triglycerides and lower high-density lipoprotein cholesterol, adding to the premature cardiovascular damages that haunt all diabetics. Many are hesitant to give diabetics a β-blocker even when they are clearly indicated, as after an acute myocardial infarction.

The new α–β-blocker carvedilol has an even greater ratio of β- to α-blocking potency than labetalol, and it has some additional antioxidant effects. Moreover, as this comparison to atenolol shows, it may improve glucose tolerance, insulin sensitivity, and lipid levels in diabetics. In a study of 56 non-diabetic hypertensives given carvedilol, Lithell and Andersson[1] found a 13% increase in triglycerides and a 17% decrease in insulin sensitivity. However, changes were much less than they had observed in previous studies with various non-selective β-blockers. Therefore, even if the metabolic effects of carvedilol are not as positive as Giugliano et al. found, they are certainly not as negative as most β-blockers.

In view of the evidence that carvedilol is effective in the treatment of heart failure,[2] this agent will likely have a wide use among diabetic hypertensives. The data in this abstract suggest that it will not have adverse metabolic effects.

**N.M. Kaplan, M.D.**

*References*

1. Lithell H, Andersson P-R: Metabolic effects of carvedilol in hypertensive patients. *Eur J Clin Pharmacol* 52:13–17, 1997.
2. Packer M, Bristow MR, Cohn JN, et al: A β-blocker improved outcomes of congestive heart failure. *N Engl J Med* 334:1349–1355, 1996.

## Secondary Hypertension

**Obstructive Sleep Apnea as a Cause of Systemic Hypertension: Evidence From a Canine Model**
Brooks D, Horner RL, Kozar LF, et al (Univ of Toronto)
*J Clin Invest* 99:106–109, 1997                                              3–49

*Introduction.*—Obstructive sleep apnea (OSA) is a serious sleep disorder characterized by repetitive episodes of upper airway collapse during sleep, resulting in interruption of airflow despite persisting respiratory efforts. Several epidemiological studies have categorized OSA as an important risk factor for stroke, systemic hypertension, myocardial infarction, and sudden death. The strongest association is between OSA and hypertension, but a direct etiological link has not been definitely determined between these 2 disorders. A canine model of OSA was used to systematically examine the effects of OSA on daytime and nighttime blood pressure (BP).

*Methods.*—Intermittent airway occlusion during nocturnal sleep was used to induce OSA in 4 dogs. During and after a 1–3 month period of OSA, daytime and nighttime BPs were taken.

*Results.*—The induced OSA resulted in acute transient increases in nighttime BP to a maximum of 13 mmHg. This eventually caused an acute transient increase in nighttime BP to a maximum of 15.7 mmHg. Recurrent arousal from sleep without airway occlusion did not result in daytime hypertension in a subsequent sleep protocol using the same 4 dogs.

*Conclusion.*—In this canine model of recurrent upper airway occlusion during sleep, OSA caused systemic nighttime and daytime hypertension. When the dogs were aroused from sleep without airway occlusion, daytime hypertension disappeared. Thus, the development of hypertension could not be attributed to recurrent arousals from sleep. These findings suggest that the high prevalence of hypertension and OSA in the general population should prompt an evaluation for possible OSA in all patients with essential hypertension.

▶ The ability to induce sustained hypertension in an experimental model by intermittent airway occlusion during sleep settles the issue as to the causal connection between obstructive sleep apnea and systemic hypertension. Our thanks to the investigators and their dogs for having proven the connection.

As for people, sleep apnea induces considerable sympathetic nervous system overactivity, and plasma norepinephrine levels are particularly high during the day in those apneics who are hypertensive.[1]

The absence of the usual nocturnal fall in blood pressure, i.e., nondipping, has been found to be usually associated with previously undiagnosed sleep apnea.[2] Thus, if ambulatory blood pressure monitoring reveals nondipping, a sleep study may be indicated.

Fortunately, antihypertensive drug therapy, including 1 kind that often induces daytime sleepiness by acting as a central α-agonist (methyldopa), does not worsen sleep apnea.[3]

**N.M. Kaplan, M.D.**

*References*

1. Ziegler MG, Nelesen R, Mills P, et al: Sleep apnea, norepinephrine-release rate, and daytime hypertension. *Sleep* 20:224–231, 1996.
2. Portaluppi F, Provini F, Cortelli P, et al: Undiagnosed sleep-disordered breathing among male nondippers with essential hypertension. *J Hypertens* 15:1227–1233, 1997.
3. Bartel PR, Loock M, Becker P, et al: Short-term antihypertensive medication does not exacerbate sleep-disordered breathing in newly diagnosed hypertensive patients. *Am J Hypertens* 10:640–645, 1997.

**Tumor Recurrence and Hypertension Persistence After Successful Pheochromocytoma Operation**
Plouin P-F, Chatellier G, Fofol I, et al (Hôpital Broussais, Paris)
Hypertension 29:1133–1139, 1997                                          3–50

*Introduction.*—Tumor resection is undertaken in patients with pheochromocytoma in order to normalize blood pressure and prevent subsequent tumor growth. Some studies indicate good long-term postoperative outcome, whereas others report persistent hypertension and recurrence rates as high as 23%. A series of 129 patients with a pheochromocytoma identified between March 1975 and March 1994 were followed-up from initial resection to death or to December 1994.

*Methods.*—Patients ranged in age from 13 to 80. Postoperative follow-up included measurement of urinary metanephrines at regular intervals. Patients with a blood pressure of 140 mmHg or greater were considered to have sustained hypertension. Recurrence was defined as the reappearance of disease after complete tumor eradication. Prognostic indicators examined included sex, age, body mass index, plasma catecholamines, tumor site and size, and the ratio of epinephrine to epinephrine plus norepinephrine (an index of tumor differentiation).

*Results.*—Pheochromocytoma caused death or persistent or recurrent disease in 28 patients. Three died within 28 days after operation and 10 died at later periods. Metastases were the cause of death in 9 patients, 7 of whom had initially malignant tumors and 2 whose initially benign tumors had malignant recurrence. Three patients with normal metanephrine excretion at follow-up died of reasons unrelated to pheochromocytoma (stroke, myocardial infarction, or colonic cancer). The 5-year survival probability was significantly higher for patients with benign tumor at first operation (96.8%) than for those with malignant tumor at first operation (22.7%). Metanephrine excretion normalized in 117 patients who survived the initial operation; 116 had benign tumors and 1 had a malignant tumor. Overall, Kaplan-Meier estimates of pheochromocytoma-free survival were 92% at 5 years and 80% at 10 years. Among the 98 living patients without recurrence, Kaplan-Meier estimates of hypertension-free survival were 74% at 5 years and 45% at 10 years. Pheochromocytoma was associated with a genetic disease in 25 patients. Variables independently associated with recurrence in the Cox model were familial pheochromocytoma and a low ratio of plasma epinephrine to total catecholamines; familial hypertension and age were independently associated with hypertension persistence.

*Discussion.*—Patients treated surgically for pheochromocytoma require periodic clinical and biochemical follow-up, particularly those with familial disease or a low epinephrine secretion. Hypertension can also persist after surgery, with an increased risk among older patients and those with familial hypertension.

▶ These findings are a bit of a wake-up call for those of us who believe that once a "curable" form of hypertension is "cured," the patient will live happily ever after. Of course, recurrences of pheos in the contralateral adrenal are well known to occur in those with familial syndromes wherein bilateral tumors or hyperplasia are likely invariable. Similarly, malignant pheos are known to recur even after many years. Therefore, the risk for recurrence is really not that great for the majority of pheo patients who have a unilateral, benign adrenal tumor.

**N.M. Kaplan, M.D.**

# 4 Pediatric Cardiovascular Disease

## Introduction

As I reflect on the trends in pediatric cardiovascular disease, the increased emphasis on treatment of the complex patient is exceedingly clear as I review the selections for this YEAR BOOK. Out of 49 selections, 15 are devoted to some aspect of the Fontan procedure or superior vena caval shunts for patients with single ventricle physiology, including surgical results, long-term follow-up, and medical therapy complications. Seventeen selections are on surgical aspects of treatment of congenital heart disease, and 6 are related to medical treatment. I have added a new category of follow-up studies. Much of what we do today or in the near future, hopefully, will become more evidence-based, and follow-up studies frequently give us some data on which to base our current decisions. There continues to be a small section related to the epidemiology of congenital or acquired heart disease, and hopefully this will become a more prominent part of the pediatric cardiovascular section in future YEAR BOOKS. We are beginning to learn more about the genetic basis for pediatric cardiovascular disease, and in the not-too-distant future, therapy related to specific genetic defects may be possible.

Thomas P. Graham, M.D.

## Arrhythmias, Pacing, and Sudden Death

### Factors That Influence the Development of Atrial Flutter After the Fontan Operation

Fishberger SB, Wernovsky G, Gentles TL, et al (Harvard Med School, Boston)

*J Thorac Cardiovasc Surg* 113:80–86, 1997                    4–1

*Background.*—Atrial flutter is a common complication of the Fontan operation and can be fatal. Atrial flutter is the most common atrial arrhythmia in patients who have this procedure, but risk factors are not well-defined. The high rate of atrial arrhythmias may result from extensive atrial surgical procedures, high atrial pressures, and atrial enlargement. Other studies have used small populations or have combined various supraventricular arrhythmias with different mechanisms.

*Methods.*—A review was conducted of the records of 334 of 500 patients who had the Fontan operation between 1973 and 1991. Medical records, ECGs, and Holter monitor recordings were examined. The modified Fontan operations included an extracardiac conduit, an atriopulmonary anastomosis, and a total cavopulmonary anastomosis. Risk factors for atrial flutter were analyzed.

*Results.*—In 54 patients, atrial flutter was identified at a mean of 5.3 years after the operation. Patients who were older at the time of the Fontan operation, had a longer follow-up, had had a previous atrial septectomy or pulmonary artery reconstruction, or had worse New York Heart Association class symptoms were more likely to have atrial flutter and to have it sooner. Sinus node dysfunction was associated with a higher rate of atrial flutter. A lower rate of atrial flutter was seen in patients with a total cavopulmonary anastomosis; these patients had a shorter follow-up. There was no association between increased risk of atrial flutter and anatomical diagnoses, perioperative hemodynamics, or previous palliative operations. Multivariate analysis showed that age at operation, length of follow-up, extensive atrial baffling, and type of repair were associated with atrial flutter.

*Discussion.*—Atrial flutter continues to be a midterm and long-term complication of the Fontan operation. The high rate of this complication is further indication of the palliative nature of Fontan circulation. Performing the Fontan operation in younger patients may lower the rate of atrial flutter, as may earlier identification of sinus node dysfunction and early institution of atrial pacing. Total cavopulmonary anastomosis may be associated with a lower incidence of atrial flutter.

▶ Intra-atrial re-entry tachycardia or atrial flutter was found to increase with age at operation, duration of follow-up, extensive atrial baffling, and, possibly, with type of repair. Although there was great hope that the total cavopulmonary connection might decrease this problem significantly, as seen from Figure 4, it is unclear that this modification is a major factor in preventing atrial tachycardia. Ablation therapy can be useful in some patients, but this arrhythmia remains a difficult clinical problem.

**T.P. Graham, M.D.**

---

## QRS Prolongation Is Associated With Inducible Ventricular Tachycardia After Repair of Tetralogy of Fallot

Balaji S, Lau YR, Case CL, et al (Med Univ of South Carolina, Charleston)
*Am J Cardiol* 80:160–163, 1997                                    4–2

---

*Introduction.*—In patients who have had repair of tetralogy of Fallot, sudden death and ventricular tachycardia are important problems. Adverse arrhythmic events have been associated with QRS prolongation of 180 msec or longer. It is unknown whether electrophysiologically inducible ventricular tachycardia is also associated with QRS duration. In patients with repaired tetralogy of Fallot, various parameters were studied, including QRS duration in relation to inducible ventricular tachycardia.

*Methods.*—There were 135 survivors of tetralogy of Fallot surgery whose age at surgery was 34 days to 37 years in an 11-year period. Patients underwent echocardiography and cardiac catheterization. An electrophysiologic study with programmed ventricular stimulation was performed on all patients who were 1.4–43 years old at the time of study. Multivariate analysis was conducted.

*Results.*—In 9 patients, QRS duration was 180 msec or longer, and it ranged from 80 to 240 msec in all patients. In 22 patients, sustained ventricular tachycardia was induced. QRS duration, right ventricular dimension, H-V interval, and presence of symptoms were related to induced sustained monomorphic ventricular tachycardia. Sustained monomorphic ventricular tachycardia was also related to QRS duration. For induced sustained monomorphic ventricular tachycardia, a QRS duration of 180 msec or longer was 35% sensitive and 97% specific. For detecting clinical ventricular tachycardia, a QRS duration of 180 msec or longer was 100% sensitive and 96% specific.

*Conclusion.*—On the electrophysiologic study, prolonged QRS duration on the electrocardiogram is associated with induced sustained monomorphic ventricular tachycardia. When there is a finding of prolonged QRS duration in patients who have undergone repair of tetralogy of Fallot, further testing is suggested, even if the patients are asymptomatic, so that the risk of adverse arrhythmic events can be determined.

▶ The relatively rare patient who has a significant ventricular arrhythmia after repair of tetralogy of Fallot continues to be a problem in terms of identification and treatment. This finding of a prolonged QRS duration as 1 potential marker for adverse ventricular arrhythmic events could prove useful. Fortunately, this complication is uncommon with early repair, but there are a significant number of adolescent and adult patients with less than optimal repairs who have a potential risk for symptomatic ventricular tachycardia.

**T.P. Graham, M.D.**

---

**Effects of Dual-Chamber Pacing for Pediatric Patients With Hypertrophic Obstructive Cardiomyopathy**
Rishi F, Hulse JE, Auld DO, et al (Egleston Children's Hosp, Atlanta, Ga; Emory Univ, Atlanta, Georgia)
*J Am Coll Cardiol* 29:734–740, 1997                    4–3

---

*Background.*—The management of children with hypertrophic obstructive cardiomyopathy can be difficult. These children have progressive left ventricular hypertrophy and have a higher rate sudden death and overt congestive heart failure than adults. Current treatment includes pharmacologic management or surgical resection of obstructing left ventricular outflow tract muscle for unresponsive patients. These treatments can cause serious side effects and may not change the natural history of the disorder. More effective treatment is needed. Dual-chamber pacing may reduce left ventricular outflow tract gradient and relieve symptoms in pediatric patients.

*Methods.*—There were 10 patients with hypertrophic obstructive cardiomyopathy and a Doppler left ventricular outflow tract gradient of 40 mmHg or more. The patients were between 1.0 and 17.5 years of age. Seven patients had surgical implantation of a permanent dual-chamber pacing system. Evaluation of permanent pacing was made using a questionnaire, Doppler evaluation, treadmill testing, and repeat cardiac catheterization.

*Results.*—At initial cardiac catheterization, 3 patients did not respond to temporary pacing and 7 patients had a significant reduction in left ventricular outflow tract gradient, left ventricular systolic pressure, and pulmonary capillary wedge pressure. After implantation, the 7 patients had a significant reduction in exercise intolerance and dyspnea on exertion. A significant reduction in left ventricular outflow tract gradient was seen on serial Doppler evaluation. In 6 patients, follow-up catheterization at 23 months revealed persistent reductions in left ventricular outflow tract gradient, left ventricular systolic pressure, and pulmonary capillary wedge pressure compared with values before implantation.

*Discussion.*—In these selected patients with hypertrophic obstructive cardiomyopathy, implantation of a dual-chamber pacing system resulted in decreased left ventricular outflow tract gradient. Certain patients who are unresponsive to medications may also improve with permanent pacing. Limitations remain for using this pacing system in younger children with hypertrophic obstructive cardiomyopathy.

▶ These authors show good results in a small number of patients with the use of dual-chamber pacing in reducing left ventricular outflow tract gradients. There has been significant controversy in this area in the adult literature, with considerable doubt placed on the efficacy of this treatment for adult patients. Current therapeutic choices for patients with obstruction include pharmacologic therapy, pacing, surgery, and septal infarction with transcatheter intervention. Each of these may play a role, but, currently, it is not clear which therapy is most useful for different groups of patients.

**T.P. Graham, M.D.**

**Prospective Screening of 5,615 High School Athletes for Risk of Sudden Cardiac Death**
Fuller CM, McNulty CM, Spring DA, et al (Sierra Nevada Cardiology Associates; Washoe Med Ctr; Univ of Nevada, Reno; et al)
*Med Sci Sports Exerc* 29:1131–1138, 1997                     4–4

*Introduction.*—The number of traumatic deaths on the playing field has been reduced among high school athletes (HSA) because of safer game rules and equipment, and nontraumatic deaths now outnumber traumatic deaths by 2:1. Most nontraumatic deaths result from cardiovascular causes, primarily hypertrophic cardiomyopathy. A prospective study sought to determine whether the addition of an ECG to the standard preparticipation history and physical examination would improve the detection of potentially serious cardiac abnormalities in HSA.

*Methods.*—The study was conducted at 30 high schools in northern Nevada. An ECG was added to the usual participation screening, and an echocardiogram and/or treadmill test was performed when results were abnormal. The usual screening included a cardiac history, cardiovascular auscultation/inspection, and blood pressure measurement. Guidelines of the 16th Bethesda Conference, which makes recommendations for competition eligibility among athletes with cardiovascular abnormalities, were followed.

*Results.*—The 5,615 HSA screened included 3,375 boys and 2,240 girls aged 13 to 19 years. Ninety percent had no screening abnormality and were approved for participation in sports. Among the 10% of HSA with abnormalities, 115 of 582 had an abnormal history, 175 had abnormal findings at cardiovascular auscultation/inspection, and 146 had an abnormal ECG; only 20 had abnormal blood pressure. After further evaluation, 22 (0.4%) of the screened HSA were not approved for participation in sports. Sixteen had an abnormal ECG, 5 had severe hypertension, and 1 was found to have severe aortic insufficiency. During the 3-year study period, 1 of the athletes who passed the screening was successfully resuscitated after ventricular fibrillation developed during track practice.

*Conclusion.*—The use of ECG screening for common causes of sudden cardiac death among young athletes had a specificity of 97.4%. Because the ECG was performed on-site by a cardiac technician with computer interpretation and over-read by a qualified physician off-site, the cost of each ECG could be as low as $10. The addition of the ECG to routine screening might reduce sudden cardiac death on high school playing fields.

▶ Screening of high school athletes for risk of sudden death continues to be problematic. Cardiologists usually get the patients referred after screening has suggested a cardiac problem. These authors show the potential value of the ECG as an adjunct to screening when combined with a careful history, physical examination, and blood pressure determination. It is estimated that there are 10 sudden cardiac deaths per year in high school athletes in the United States, and half of these result from hypertrophic cardiomyopathy, which usually can be diagnosed by careful history including family history, physical examination, and ECG. From various population data on the prevalence of hypertrophic cardiomyopathy, it is estimated that this disease process occurs in only 1 of 40,000 high school athletes. It is also estimated that a screening and follow-up study of 120,000 high school athletes would have to be performed to clearly determine the effectiveness of screening. Nevertheless, these data are helpful along with the recommendations from the 26th Bethesda Conference.[1] It is of interest in this 3-year study, only one high school athlete developed serious cardiac abnormalities during sports participation. This was a student who had ventricular fibrillation during track practice and was successfully resuscitated. Subsequent angiography revealed an anomalous right coronary artery with its point of origin adjacent to the ostium of the left coronary artery and its path between the aorta and the pulmonary artery. This student had a normal screening examination, as would virtually all patients with this particular rare abnormality.

**T.P. Graham, M.D.**

*Reference*

1. Mitchell JH, Maron BJ, Raven PB: 26th Bethesda Conference: Recommendations for determining eligibility for competition in athletes with cardiovascular abnormalities. *Med Sci Sports Exerc* 26:223–283, 1994.

## Congenital Heart Disease—Medical

**Are Chest Radiographs and Electrocardiograms Still Valuable in Evaluating New Pediatric Patients With Heart Murmurs or Chest Pain?**
Swenson JM, Fischer DR, Miller SA, et al (Univ of Pittsburgh, Pa)
*Pediatrics* 99:1–3, 1997                                                         4–5

*Introduction.*—The largest group of patients seen by pediatric cardiologists is composed of patients who have been referred for evaluation of heart murmurs and chest pain. There are mixed conclusions regarding the efficacy of routine chest radiographs and ECGs to evaluate these new patients in conjunction with an evaluation by a pediatric cardiologist. Echocardiographic technology has greatly advanced, but so has its cost. In the complete evaluation of new patients with heart murmurs or chest pain referred to the pediatric cardiologist, the value of chest x-ray studies and ECGs was determined.

*Methods.*—There were 106 patients who were categorized as having definite heart disease, no heart disease, or possible heart disease based on physical examination and history. All of the patients then had chest x-ray studies and ECGs. An echocardiogram could be ordered by the examining cardiologist after studies were reviewed.

*Results.*—Solely on the basis of a radiograph or ECG with abnormal results, 4 patients were thought to have no heart disease but had the diagnosis changed to definite heart disease. After review of the chest x-ray films and ECGs, 25 patients thought to have possible heart disease had their diagnosis changed to no heart disease or definite heart disease. Abnormal radiograph or ECG results, or both, and, in some cases, an echocardiogram all confirmed definite heart disease for all 25 patients with a diagnosis of heart disease.

*Conclusion.*—Heart disease was diagnosed in 5 patients thought to have possible heart disease; heart disease was confirmed in 9 patients, heart disease was diagnosed in 4 thought to have no heart disease, and lesions were ruled out in 7 patients with possible heart disease after review of chest x-ray films and ECGs. In the evaluation of patients with heart murmurs or chest pain, routine chest x-ray studies and ECGs continue to be valuable tools for the pediatric cardiologist, even in these days of cost containment.

▶ In this study, it was concluded that ECGs and radiographs can be of value in patients referred for heart murmurs or chest pain. These studies helped to diagnose heart disease in 4 patients thought to have no heart disease and helped to rule in or out heart disease in 21 additional patients. Thus, ECGs and radiographs were believed to be definitely helpful in approximately 25% of these patients. Both the ECG and chest x-ray study cost a fraction of what an echocardiogram costs, but the former are frequently not definitive, and the echocardiogram needs to be added to these other procedures. A study by Danford et al.[1] found that initial consultation with a pediatric cardiologist is the preferred approach when not clearly innocent murmurs are found, and echocardiography is not a cost-effective screen for murmur evaluation. The chest x-ray and ECG should be ordered on an individual basis by the cardiologist as needed.

**T.P. Graham, M.D.**

*Reference*

1. Danford DA, Nasir A, Gumbiner C: Cost assessment of the evaluation of heart murmurs in children. *Pediatrics* 91:365–368, 1993.

## Children With Heart Murmurs: Can Ventricular Septal Defect Be Diagnosed Reliaby Without an Echocardiogram?

Danford DA, Martin AB, Fletcher SE, et al (Univ of Nebraska, Omaha; St Elizabeth Hosp, Lincoln, Neb)
*J Am Coll Cardiol* 30:243–246, 1997                          4–6

*Introduction.*—Some studies have found clinical examination without echocardiography to be sufficient for detecting ventricular septal defect (VSD), but others report a low accuracy of clinical examination for diagnosing congenital heart disease in general. A large group of previously unevaluated children with heart murmurs were enrolled in a study designed to determine the sensitivity and specificity of the pediatric cardiologist's clinical examination for identification of VSD.

*Methods.*—None of the 287 consecutive outpatients had previously undergone echocardiography or had a pediatric cardiology consultation. All were examined with or without the use of chest radiography, ECG, or pulse oximetry. Board-certified pediatric cardiologists prospectively recorded a working diagnosis and their level of confidence in the diagnosis for each child. Any VSD was categorized as small or moderate to large. After echocardiography was performed, VSDs were subcategorized by location and treatment requirement (minor, intermediate, or major).

*Results.*—The study group had a mean age of 2.72 years (median age, 0.71 years). Seventy-three (25%) patients had VSD, which was minor in 52 (71%), intermediate in 10, and major in 11. The area under the receiver operating characteristic curve (1.0 = perfect discrimination, 0.5 = indiscriminate) was 0.92 for recognition of minor VSD vs. 0.69 for intermediate or major VSD, a significant difference. Clinical examination failed to identify 4 of 52 minor VSDs. Fourteen patients without a minor VSD were believed with confidence to have a small VSD, whereas 4 were subsequently determined to have an intermediate VSD, 3 had an innocent murmur, 2 had a major VSD, 2 had pulmonary stenosis, and 1 patient each had subaortic membrane, atrial septal defect, and mitral regurgitation.

*Discussion.*—Although almost all minor VSDs are identified without echocardiography, errors occur even when an experienced pediatric cardiologist is confident of the diagnosis. Intermediate or major VSDs were not recognized with great accuracy at clinical examination. In this series, 30% of the intermediate and 18% of the major VSDs were not included as a VSD of any size in the differential diagnosis.

▶ The findings of this study were a little disappointing to those of us older clinicians who feel that we can recognize small, intermediate, or major VSDs by clinical examination. These investigators clearly shows that there are a small number of patients in whom expert pediatric cardiologists are unable to separate minor VSDs from non-VSD conditions. In addition, there were occasional errors in the diagnosis of intermediate or major VSDs. Although the reference standard for diagnosis of minor VSD should continue to be expert clinical auscultation, the present study suggests that auscultation is not perfect now and may have not been so in the past. Studies such as this are important in attempting to define appropriate use and avoid the misuse of echocardiographic Doppler studies. If echocardiography is needed, it should be done only by those with experience and expertise in pediatric cardiovascular disease. It is a common scenario now for patients to come to the pediatric cardiologist after echocardiography has been performed only to find that it is nondiagnostic and needs repeating. This unfortunate overuse of resources should be eliminated

**T.P. Graham, M.D.**

## Hemodynamic and Clinical Effects of Oral Levodopa in Children With Congestive Heart Failure

Mendelsohn AM, Johnson CE, Brown CE, et al (Univ of Cincinnati, Ohio; Univ of Michigan, Ann Arbor)
J Am Coll Cardiol 30:237–242, 1997                                    4–7

*Introduction.*—There are limited therapeutic options for children with congestive cardiomyopathy and congestive heart failure. Treatment usually includes preload reduction with diuretic agents, afterload reduction with angiotensin-converting enzyme prohibitors, digoxin, and hospital administration of dopamine, dobutamine, and amrinone. These patients would benefit from improved oral medical therapy. A pharmacologically inert form of dopamine that is converted to its parent compound through pyridoxine-dependent aromatic amino acid decarboxylation is levodopa. Adults with congestive heart failure have been shown to benefit from levodopa, but children have not been studied in connection with this form of treatment. In children with congestive heart failure, the safety and efficacy of oral levodopa was studied.

*Methods.*—There were 9 children with congestive cardiomyopathies (age, $10 \pm 1.7$ years) in a 3-year period who participated in this study. They had 2–dimensional and M-mode echocardiography, Holter monitoring, and exercise testing, and surface electrocardiography, when applicable. During a 3-day period, the children had levodopa administered in a dose escalation scale from 8 mg/kg body weight per dose to 20 mg/kg per dose with concomitant metoclopramide and pyridoxine. Measurements of catecholamine levels were taken at the initiation of the trial and throughout dose escalation. The measurements were correlated with electrocardiographic and echocardiographic data. Before and after administration of levodopa after a 24-hour drug washout, cardiac catheterization was performed.

*Results.*—After levodopa administration at $100 \pm 14.8$ minutes, serum dopamine levels rose from $108.5 \pm 59.2$ pg/mL to $1,375.8 \pm 567.9$ pg/mL at cardiac catheterization without a significant change in serum norepinephrine or epinephrine levels. There were also significant increases in stroke volume index, cardiac index, systemic vascular resistance, and oxygen consumption. The daily fluid volume output/input ratio significantly reversed from $0.8 \pm 0.1$ to $1.2 \pm 0.1$. Three patients needed a dose reduction of levodopa because of hypertension or tachycardia or both. One patient had significant gastrointestinal distress. After a median of 19.5 months of drug initiation, there was sustained symptomatic improvement in 7 patients.

*Conclusion.*—In the treatment of congestive heart failure in children, these data support the hemodynamic value of oral levodopa.

▶ The search for improved therapy for chronic congestive heart failure secondary to systolic dysfunction continues. Because IV sympathetic agents have been useful in therapy for congestive heart failure, the use of levodopa, which is converted to dopamine, has theoretical merit. Unfortunately, most studies in adults with oral inotropic agents have shown major side effects, minimal or no benefit, tachyphylaxis, or adverse effects. This early and continuous improvement using outpatient therapy in a small number of patients deserves further follow-up. Excessive sympathetic stimulation as found with chronic congestive heart failure can have deleterious side effects; thus, careful evaluation of this type of therapy is needed. Adults with chronic congestive failure frequently benefit from β-blocker therapy, particularly with third-generation drugs such as carvedilol. These drugs deserve a trial in pediatric patients.

**T.P. Graham, M.D.**

---

**Enalapril Does Not Enhance Exercise Capacity in Patients After Fontan Procedure**
Kouatli AA, Garcia JA, Zellers TM, et al (Univ of Texas, Dallas)
*Circulation* 96:1507–1512, 1997                                                4–8

---

*Background.*—The exercise capacity of many patients who have a Fontan procedure is reduced, a problem attributed in part to a decreased stroke volume response to exercise. These patients also have decreased cardiac output, increased systemic vascular resistance, and abnormal diastolic function. A randomized trial was conducted to test the hypothesis that angiotensin converting enzyme inhibitor therapy, known to increase exercise capacity in cases of left ventricular dysfunction, would have a similar effect in patients who have undergone the Fontan procedure.

*Methods.*—Eligible patients were 7 years or older and had undergone the Fontan procedure 6 or more months before the study. In a double-blind crossover design, patients received a single dose of enalapril (maximum, 15 mg/day) or placebo every morning, each for 10 weeks. At the conclusion of treatment, the patients underwent Doppler echocardiography and an exercise test and completed a questionnaire on potential side effects. Eighteen of 21 enrolled patients completed the study.

*Results.*—Patients who completed the study had a mean age of 14.5 years. Twelve had tricuspid atresia, 2 had pulmonary atresia and hypoplastic right ventricle, 2 had d-transposition of the great arteries and hypoplastic right ventricle, and 2 had complex heart disease. When compared with placebo, enalapril therapy did not affect the heart rate, respiratory rate, systolic or diastolic pressure, cardiac index, or the decrease in systemic vascular resistance measured at maximum exercise. Exercise duration was similar for the enalapril (mean of 6.4 minutes) and placebo (mean of 6.7 minutes) groups. There was a slight but significant decrease in the mean percent increase in cardiac index from rest to maximum exercise after 10 weeks of enalapril therapy vs. placebo (mean of 102% vs. 125%, respectively). Perceived side effects, which were relatively frequent, did not differ between the 2 groups.

*Discussion.*—These patients who had undergone the Fontan procedure denied having cardiorespiratory symptoms during ordinary daily activities, but testing revealed a decreased resting cardiac index and exercise capacity. Ten weeks of enalapril treatment failed to alter these measures or their abnormal systemic vascular resistance and diastolic function.

▶ This well-controlled study indicated that angiotensin converting enzyme inhibition with enalapril was not effective in improving the cardiac index, diastolic function, or exercise capacity in post-Fontan patients. It is interesting that both systolic and diastolic blood pressures were not different between the enalapril and placebo groups, and it is possible that a higher dose of an angiotensin converting enzyme inhibitor might be effective in improving cardiac function in these patients.

**T.P. Graham, M.D.**

---

**Coagulation Factor Abnormalities After the Fontan Procedure and Its Modifications**
Jahangiri M, Shore D, Kakkar V, et al (Royal Brompton Hosp, London)
*J Thorac Cardiovasc Surg* 113:989–993, 1997                    4–9

---

*Introduction.*—In patients with tricuspid atresia, use of the Fontan operation was first reported in 1971. The systemic venous return reaches the pulmonary circulation without being pumped by a ventricle after the Fontan procedure or one of its modifications, and this can be complicated by thromboembolism, protein-losing enteropathy with ascites, or increased right atrial pressure. Some have suggested that coagulation abnormalities may contribute to thromboembolism after this procedure. Coagulation status was examined in a group of patients who were in stable condition in the postoperative period.

*Methods.*—The Fontan procedure and its modifications were performed in 20 children, who were then examined for coagulation factor abnormalities. At the time of the operation, the median age of the children was 6.2 years (range, 17 months to 8 years). Measurements were taken of concentrations of serum albumin, total protein, and liver enzymes. Follow-up continued for up to 4.9 years (range, 18 to 76 months).

*Results.*—The 20 patients who underwent the Fontan-type operations, had significantly lower levels of protein C, protein S, and factor VII than the normal range, but no significant changes in serum albumin or total protein or in factors II, IX, and X. There was no association between the type of heart defect, time of follow-up, or coagulation factor abnormalities. Patients who received a right atrial–pulmonary anastomosis or a total cavopulmonary connection did not demonstrate any significant differences in coagulation factor abnormalities.

*Conclusion.*—The prevalence of thromboembolism after Fontan-type repairs is partly accounted for by a deficiency in protein C, protein S, and factor VII. The best palliative procedure for these patients should be weighed against the risk of long-term anticoagulation. In this group of patients, reduced protein C, protein S, and factor VII levels should be regarded as risk factors, and these patients should be given anticoagulation therapy.

▶ Thromboembolic problems after the Fontan operation continue to be a problem in terms of deciding effective prophylaxis and management. Deficiencies in protein C, protein S, and factor VII could prove to be additional risk factors for thromboembolism to the sluggish venous circulation frequently found in these patients.

**T.P. Graham, M.D.**

---

**Reversal of Protein-losing Enteropathy With Heparin Therapy in Three Patients With Univentricular Hearts and Fontan Palliation**
Donnelly JP, Rosenthal A, Castle VP, et al (Univ of Michigan, Ann Arbor)
*J Pediatr* 130:474–478, 1997                                                4–10

---

*Introduction.*—As a consequence of either abnormal protein leakage across the gut mucosa or diminished protein uptake by intestinal lymphatics, protein-losing enteropathy can occur in a wide variety of disease states. Patients with congenital heart disease often also have protein-losing enteropathy, but there has been no effective therapy for this condition. Heparin therapy has been used to treat patients with protein-losing enteropathy and heart disease. Before and during heparin therapy, 3 children with protein-losing enteropathy in conjunction with univentricular hearts and right atrial to pulmonary artery anastomosis were studied.

*Case Report.*—Several years after undergoing the Fontan surgical procedure at 4 years old, a male was given a diagnosis of protein-losing enteropathy. He was started on a low-fat, high-protein diet but still had enteric protein loss. He was then started on heparin at 4,000 units every 4 hours and showed a marked improvement in his symptoms. The heparin was stopped, and he had the symptoms return. Then he was put on 10,000 units of heparin intravenously every 12 hours. Four months later, back pain developed, which signaled bone toxicity. He was finally started on 5,000 units/m$^2$, which was the same protocol followed for 2 other patients.

*Results.*—Within a few weeks of beginning therapy, each patient showed dramatic improvements in symptoms, marked elevations in serum albumin levels, and quantitative reversal of enteric protein loss. The first 2 patients had complete reversal of enteric protein loss within 3 weeks of starting therapy, and the third patient had a more delayed response because of an intercurrent, viral illness. The doses probably lie well below anticoagulative doses, and are unlikely to cause significant toxic effects.

*Conclusion.*—For this poorly understood condition, heparin may be an important treatment. The anticoagulative properties of heparin may be related to its therapeutic effects on the enteric protein-loss condition.

▶ This is an exciting report of reversal of the hypoalbuminemia associated with protein-losing enteropathy after Fontan repair. It is hoped that this will signal a new approach to this frequently devastating complication. The mechanism by which heparin decreases enteric protein loss is unclear. The authors suggest that it involves the binding of the exogenously administered heparin to enteric endothelial cells where it becomes internalized and stabilizes cell matrix interactions at the capillary endothelium to reduce the leakage of protein in the extravascular space. Further trials of this therapy will be forthcoming, and it is hoped that they will be as successful as this initial report.

**T.P. Graham, M.D.**

# Congenital Heart Disease—Surgical

**Is a High-risk Biventricular Repair Always Preferable to Conversion to a Single Ventricle Repair?**
Delius RE, Rademecker MA, de Leval MR, et al (Great Ormond Street Hosp NHS Trust, London)
*J Thorac Cardiovasc Surg* 112:1561–1569, 1996                4–11

*Background.*—Results of the Fontan operation show an increase in hazard function beginning about 6 years after the procedure. It is often assumed that if the patient has 2 functional ventricles, it is always preferable to perform a biventricular repair than a single ventricle repair. In some cases of congenital heart defect, a complex repair is needed to achieve the physiologic advantages of 2 ventricles. These repairs can result in high morbidity and mortality. The Fontan procedure has recently been modified and has resulted in better short-term and mid-term results.

*Methods.*—There were 50 patients with atrioventricular concordance or discordance, ventriculoarterial discordance, ventricular septal defect, pulmonary stenosis, or atresia, and who had 2 functional ventricles. Group 1 consisted of 34 patients who had biventricular repair, and group 2 consisted of 16 patients who had single ventricle repair with a total cavopulmonary connection because of a straddling atrioventricular valve or a noncommitted ventricular septal defect.

*Results.*—The mean follow up was 3.9 years in group 1 and 3.0 years in group 2. Operative mortality was 14.7% in group 1 and 6.3% in group 2. At 7 years, freedom from reoperation was 45.5% in group 1 and 100% in group 2. At 7 years, survival was 68.0% in group 1 and 93.8% in group 2.

*Discussion.*—In these patients, the short-term and midterm results of total cavopulmonary connection were comparable to results of a complex biventricular repair. Patients who had total cavopulmonary connection had fewer reoperations, possibly better survival, and similar functional status compared with patients who had the biventricular repair. Differences may have resulted from selection bias, although any bias would have been against patients who had total cavopulmonary connection because it was believed the risk of biventricular repair was high in these patients. In selected patients, the risks of biventricular repair may outweigh the long-term disadvantages of total cavopulmonary connection.

▶ These authors' comparison provides interesting food for thought. There is a better outcome with a Fontan vs. a Rastelli-type repair with conduit in patients with certain intracardiac abnormalities. All the patients in this group did have 2 functional ventricles, so ventricular hypoplasia was not a confounding variable. Complex biventricular operations can be associated with outflow obstruction to either ventricle and/or atrioventricular valve abnormalities. Although the Fontan operation seems palliative in most patients, it may be the best operation despite the presence of 2 adequate ventricles in selected patients with complex intracardiac anatomy, particularly unusual ventricular septal defect locations and atrioventricular valve anomalies. Further studies of such comparisons are needed.

**T.P. Graham, M.D.**

---

**Intermediate Results of the Extracardiac Fontan Procedure**
Laschinger JC, Redmond JM, Cameron DE, et al (Johns Hopkins Med Insts, Baltimore, Md; Univ of Maryland, Baltimore)
*Ann Thorac Surg* 62:1261–1267, 1996                                            4–12

---

*Purpose.*—The extracardiac Fontan procedure is a modification of the total cavopulmonary connection in which the bidirectional Glenn shunt is combined with an extracardiac lateral tunnel, which carries the inferior vena caval flow to the pulmonary arteries. The authors believe that this modified procedure can offer the hemodynamic benefits of the total cavopulmonary connection while avoiding the difficulties associated with aortic cross-clamping and intra-arterial baffles or tunnels. The results of the extracardiac Fontan procedure in 15 patients were reported.

*Methods.*—The study included 14 children and 1 adult with complex congenital heart disease who underwent definitive conversion to Fontan circulation. Nine patients underwent placement of a extracardiac lateral tunnel, in most cases constructed with a polytetrafluoroethylene patch. In the other 6 patients, an extracardiac lateral conduit was constructed, using either a polytetrafluoroethylene tube graft or nonvalved homograft. In 12 of the patients, it was possible to avoid aortic cross-clamping completely.

*Results.*—None of the patients died. One had prolonged chest tube drainage. At a mean follow-up of 27.5 months, all patients were in New York Heart Association class I or II and had normal sinus rhythm. One patient had late protein-losing enteropathy, which was successfully treated percutaneously by creation of a stented fenestration from the extracardiac tunnel to the systemic atrium. At cardiac catheterization, the extracardiac lateral tunnels were functional, with pulmonary pressures of 11 to 13 mm Hg.

*Conclusion.*—The extracardiac Fontan procedure has several important benefits for patients undergoing conversion to Fontan circulation. It can usually avoid the need for aortic cross-clamping, atriotomy, and intra-atrial suture lines while preserving the hemodynamic benefits of total cavopulmonary connection. Follow-up shows that patients remain in normal sinus rhythm. The procedure permits drainage of the coronary sinus to low-pressure atrium, permits placement of early or late fenestrations, and prevents baffle leaks and intra-atrial obstruction.

▶ These authors report early results in 15 patients with use of an extracardiac tunnel or conduit for Fontan completion. There are a number of theoretical advantages to this technique including avoidance of aortic cross-clamping in a number of patients, avoidance of atriotomy and intra-atrial suture lines with preservation of sinus rhythm in most patients, and drainage of the coronary sinus to a low-pressure atrium. In addition, there is allowance for growth when a tunnel is used instead of a conduit. Potential problems with the conduit will be all those problems previously associated with conduits, including development of an intimal peel and lack of sufficient size to accommodate growth in younger patients. The place for this choice for completion of the Fontan procedure remains to be determined.

**T.P. Graham, M.D.**

---

### Pulmonary Atresia With Intact Ventricular Septum: Results of the Fontan Procedure

Najm HK, Williams WG, Coles JG, et al (Hosp for Sick Children, Toronto; Univ of Toronto)
*Ann Thorac Surg* 63:669–675, 1997                4–13

*Objective.*—The cardiac findings of children with pulmonary atresia and an intact ventricular septum (PA/IVS) vary significantly. Some children can undergo a biventricular repair, whereas others must have a Fontan procedure or one-and-a-half ventricle repair. One difficult-to-manage group includes children with a right ventricle–to–coronary artery connection, whether or not they have right ventricle–dependent coronary artery blood flow. An experience with the Fontan procedure in children with PA/IVS was reported.

*Methods.*—The experience included 22 children with PA/IVS who underwent a Fontan procedure over a 14-year period. The children's mean age at surgery was 6 years. All had had at least 1 previous palliative procedure, and 19 had had 2 or more palliative procedures. Fifteen of the children had right ventricle–to–coronary artery connections, 5 of whom had right ventricle–dependent coronary artery blood flow. Ten children also underwent thromboexclusion of the right ventricle, 3 at the same time as the Fontan procedure and 7 before. The mean follow-up was 48 months.

*Results.*—The 30-day mortality rate was 14%, with 3 children dying of low cardiac output. Another child died 1 year later during a subsequent operation. The 10-year actuarial survival rate was 80%. Three of the survivors had atrial arrhythmia, and 4 had permanent pacemakers implanted. All survivors were free of signs of myocardial ischemia, ventricular arrhythmias, or progressive left ventricular dysfunction.

*Conclusion.*—The authors report good results with the Fontan procedure for children with PA/IVS. Patients who have right ventricle–to–coronary artery connections without right ventricle–dependent coronary artery flow should undergo thromboexclusion of the right ventricle. However, those with right ventricle–dependent coronary artery flow should not have right ventricular decompression or thromboexclusion. In this group, saturated blood must enter the right ventricle during the Fontan procedure.

▶ These authors produce reasonably good survival rates at 10 years for the Fontan operation in this difficult group of patients. Sixty-eight percent of their patients had right ventricular–coronary artery connections with right ventricular dependence of this circulation in 23% of the total group. Thromboexclusion of the right ventricle was performed in 7 of 10 patients with coronary connections to the right ventricle and no evidence of right ventricular dependence of this circulation; there was only 1 early death in this group. These authors continue to advocate closure of the tricuspid valve with palliative thromboexclusion of the right ventricle in patients with right ventricular coronary artery connections when these connections are not right-ventricle dependent. In those patients with right ventricle-dependent–connections, use of the cavopulmonary connection and creation of a large atrial septal defect allows only oxygenated blood to return to the right ventricle. Further long-term follow-up data are needed in these subgroups with right-ventricular coronary connections to determine optimal management. There is no general agreement that tricuspid valve closure and thromboexclusion of the right ventricle are necessary in the subgroup described above.

**T.P. Graham, M.D.**

---

**Outcome After the Single-stage, Nonfenestrated Fontan Procedure**
Hsu DT, Quaegebeur JM, Ing FF, et al (Columbia Univ, New York)
*Circulation* 96(suppl II):335–340, 1997                    4–14

---

*Introduction.*—Although the Fontan operation and its modifications have been widely adopted since the procedure was developed 30 years ago, many controversies remain regarding its application. Centers differ on the indications for the staged procedure and on whether baffle fenestration should be performed routinely. At the study institution, patients with favorable anatomy and hemodynamics undergo a single-stage, nonfenestrated Fontan. Outcome is reported for a group of such patients.

*Methods.*—The single-stage, nonfenestrated Fontan was performed in 61 of 94 patients who underwent a modified Fontan procedure between May 1990 and October 1996. Patients had a median age of 3.3 years and were followed for a mean of 3.5 years. Five preoperative risk factors were identified: young age (less than 2 years) at operation (18 cases), significant branch pulmonary artery stenosis (20 cases), elevated (more than 15 mm Hg) mean pulmonary artery pressure (16 cases), atrioventricular valve regurgitation (5 cases), and decreased ventricular function (2 cases). These risk factors were compared between patients whose outcome was successful and those in whom the Fontan operation failed and between those who did or did not have significant postoperative effusions.

*Results.*—The most common diagnoses were double-inlet left ventricle (26%) and tricuspid atresia (23%). Forty-four patients had previously undergone cardiac surgery and 25 had additional surgery at the time of the Fontan. The most frequently used type of Fontan connection was the total caval-pulmonary connection (87%). The mean bypass time was 2.3 hours and the median duration of mechanical ventilation was 1 day; patients were hospitalized for a median of 14 days. After the Fontan procedure, mean oxygen saturation rose significantly from 84% to 95%. Three patients died in the early postoperative period and 1 required heart transplant. One- and 5-year actuarial survival was 93%, and 19 patients have survived more than 5 years. Neither survival nor the development of significant postoperative effusions was related to preoperative risk factors.

*Conclusion.*—Forty-one of the 61 patients in this series had 1 or more risk factors associated with increased morbidity and mortality after the Fontan procedure. Nevertheless, their surgical results and intermediate-term outcome after a single-stage, nonfenestrated Fontan was excellent. Many patients with single-ventricle physiology should not require routine baffle fenestration or a 2-stage approach.

▶ Most centers are currently using the bidirectional Glenn followed by a fenestrated Fontan procedure for palliation of patients with various types of single ventricle. Data from the group at Columbia, as well from the Mayo Clinic, have indicated excellent outcomes in patients with single-staged, nonfenestrated Fontan procedures. It will be important to try to determine which subgroups of patients can have optimal therapy with the single stage, nonfenestrated Fontan and avoid the extra operation and which patients will benefit from the staging with a bidirectional Glenn and a Fontan with or without a fenestration. Certainly those with multiple risk factors for Fontan palliation (particularly hypoplastic left heart patients) and those with significant hypertrophy and/or ventricular dysfunction probably will benefit from the 2-stage procedure. Sorting all of this out for each individual patient remains a challenge for even the most experienced clinician.

**T.P. Graham, M.D.**

### Inhaled Nitric Oxide in Patients With Critical Pulmonary Perfusion After Fontan-type Procedures and Bidirectional Glenn Anastomosis

Gamillscheg A, Zobel G, Urlesberger B, et al (Univ of Graz, Austria)
J Thorac Cardiovasc Surg 113:435–442, 1997                                4–15

*Introduction.*—Inhaled nitric oxide (NO) has decreased elevated pulmonary artery pressure, pulmonary vascular resistance, and ventilation-perfusion mismatch in a number of conditions, including adult respiratory distress syndrome and congenital heart disease complicated by pulmonary hypertension. In the cases reported here, inhaled NO was used when critical pulmonary perfusion was present in the early postoperative period after Fontan-type procedures and bidirectional Glenn anastomosis.

*Methods.*—Thirteen patients were included in the study, 5 girls and 8 boys with a mean age of 5.6 years. Four underwent bidirectional cavopulmonary Glenn anastomosis and 9 were treated by total cavopulmonary connection. Indications for treatment with NO were a central venous pressure (CVP) greater than 20 mmHg or a transpulmonary pressure gradient greater than 10 mmHg. Inhaled NO (1.5 to 10 ppm, mean of 4.1 ppm) was administered with the use of a microprocessor-controlled system and delivered at the lowest effective dose to obtain a transpulmonary pressure gradient less than 10 mmHg or a decrease in the transpulmonary pressure gradient of more than 20%. The mean duration of inhaled NO therapy was 106 hours.

*Results.*—Patients had a mean CVP of 22 mmHg and a mean transpulmonary pressure gradient of 14.2 mmHg before the start of NO inhalation therapy. The therapy significantly decreased CVP (mean of 15.3%) and the transpulmonary pressure gradient (mean of 42%) in the 9 patients who underwent total cavopulmonary connection. Left atrial pressure was increased by a mean of 28% and mean systemic arterial pressure by a mean of 12%. Mean arterial and venous oxygen saturations improved in these patients by 8.2% and 14%, respectively. Inhaled NO therapy resulted in a mean 22% decrease in CVP among patients with bidirectional Glenn anastomosis. The transpulmonary pressure gradient decreased by a mean of 55%, and mean improvements in arterial and venous oxygen saturations were 37% and 11%, respectively. There were no toxic side effects.

*Conclusion.*—Even low doses of inhaled NO (1.5 to 10 ppm) improved critical pulmonary perfusion and oxygenation in the early postoperative period after Fontan-type procedures and bidirectional Glenn anastomosis. The use of low doses of inhaled NO and a short treatment duration reduces the risk of toxicity.

▶ Inhaled NO has become an important part of intensive care therapy for patients with increased pulmonary resistance and critical pulmonary perfusion. Post-Fontan and post–bidirectional Glenn anastomosis patients frequently have pulmonary vasoconstriction, usually contributed to by the effects of cardiopulmonary bypass. Nitric oxide can be extremely useful in this situation.

**T.P. Graham, M.D.**

## An Institutional Experience With Second- and Third-stage Palliative Procedures For Hypoplastic Left Heart Syndrome: The Impact of the Bidirectional Cavopulmonary Shunt

Forbess JM, Cook N, Serraf A, et al (Harvard Med School, Boston)
*J Am Coll Cardiol* 29:665–670, 1997                                                          4–16

*Introduction.*—Infants with hypoplastic left heart syndrome (HLHS) are now treated in 3 stages, with first-stage palliation followed by bidirectional cavopulmonary anastomosis before completion of the Fontan operation. A retrospective study was conducted to identify patient- or procedure-specific risk factors related to second-stage palliation and to examine outcome after third-stage modified fenestrated Fontan operations.

*Methods.*—Between 1983 and 1993, 212 consecutive patients underwent stage I reconstruction for HLHS at the study institution; 70 of 114 operative survivors subsequently had palliative procedures and 2 underwent heart transplantation. Anatomic subtypes in the stage II cohort included mitral stenosis and aortic stenosis (44.3%), mitral atresia and aortic atresia (27.1%), and mitral stenosis and atrial atresia (25.7%). Follow-up ranged from 0.5 to 8.0 years after second-stage palliation. Patient-specific factors and features of the stage II operation were analyzed for influence on stage II mortality and survival.

*Results.*—Post–stage I patients underwent a total of 38 interim operative procedures before stage II, including gastrostomy in 12 patients and balloon dilation of the aorta in 10. Stage II operations included bidirectional cavopulmonary shunt in 50 patients and a modified Fontan procedure in 18; two patients had a classic Glenn anastomosis with a left Blalock-Taussig shunt and 2 underwent orthotopic heart transplantation. There were 9 in-hospital deaths (69%) in the 13 patients who had a stage II nonfenestrated Fontan procedure, and this procedure was the only risk factor for stage II mortality. Only 4 early deaths occurred in the group of 50 patients who underwent intermediate superior vena cava–to–pulmonary artery anastomosis at stage II. The anatomic subtype of HLHS had an effect on stage I survival but did not influence stage II mortality. Thirty-two patients had the modified fenestrated Fontan procedure as a third stage at a median age of 28.7 months; 1 died during a median follow-up of 24.5 months.

*Conclusion.*—A second-stage bidirectional cavopulmonary anastomosis for HLHS was confirmed to reduce mortality and allow the modified fenestrated Fontan operation to be performed as the final palliative stage with a low operative risk, stable intermediate survival, and good intermediate cardiac functional outcome in most patients.

▶ These authors show that going directly from stage I palliation for hypoplastic left heart to a nonfenestrated Fontan operation is associated with high mortality. Use of the bidirectional caval pulmonary shunt as an intermediate stage before the Fontan operation for most patients with single-ventricle anatomy of any type has been advocated by a number of groups. It appears to be associated with improved outcome in a number of studies. There are some patients who have very few risk factors for completion of a Fontan procedure, and these can probably go straight for a fenestrated or a nonfenestrated Fontan operation depending on institutional preference. Improved outcomes for the Fontan procedure have been apparent, but there is still debate as to how much of this improvement is due to the use of fenestration in the final stage, the use of the intermediate bidirectional caval pulmonary shunt, and/or improved patient selection and timing of surgery.

**T.P. Graham, M.D.**

---

**Pulmonary AV Malformations After Superior Cavopulmonary Connection: Resolution After Inclusion of Hepatic Veins in the Pulmonary Circulation**
Shah MJ, Rychik J, Fogel MA, et al (Univ of Pennsylvania, Philadelphia)
*Ann Thorac Surg* 63:960–963, 1997                                    4–17

---

*Introduction.*—For palliation of various forms of cyanotic congenital heart disease, the surgical connection of the superior vena cava to the right pulmonary artery was used; however, the late onset of pulmonary arteriovenous malformations contributed to the abandonment of this procedure. For palliation of single-ventricle anomalies, other forms of superior cavopulmonary artery connections have been investigated. Children with polysplenia syndrome and interruption of the inferior vena cava have not benefited from the 2-stage strategy of incorporating inferior vena caval flow and hepatic venous flow into the pulmonary circulation. These children have had successful resolution of pulmonary arteriovenous malformations via operative redirection and inclusion of hepatic venous blood in the pulmonary circulation.

*Methods.*—There were 3 patients with congenital heart disease and polysplenia who had pulmonary arteriovenous malformations. Hepatic vein inclusion was performed in the pulmonary circulation. Two patients had single ventricles of the dominant right ventricular type, and the other patient had the dominant left ventricular type.

*Results.*—No complications occurred in any of the 3 patients who successfully underwent hepatic vein inclusion. Their hospitalizations ranged from 6 to 14 days. At a median duration of 8 months after the operations, pulmonary arterial venous malformations were diagnosed. In the pulmonary circulation, hepatic venous flow was included at the time of the operations. At a median duration of 7 months after the operations, resolution of pulmonary arteriovenous malformations occurred.

*Conclusion.*—The resolution of pulmonary arteriovenous malformations occurs with surgical inclusion of hepatic venous blood in the pulmonary circulation. The development of pulmonary arteriovenous malformations in patients who are at risk may be prevented by electively associating the hepatic veins with the pulmonary vasculature.

▶ The intriguing phenomenon of the development of pulmonary arteriovenous malformations both in patients who have interruption of hepatic venous return to the pulmonary circulation and in patients with severe liver failure has suggested the presence of a putative hepatic factor that protects against or mitigates the development of these malformations. This hypothesis is supported by the disappearance of these malformations in patients with hepatic failure after liver transplantation as well as by the rapid resolution of these malformations after hepatic venous flow is included in the pulmonary circulation via reoperation as reported here.

**T.P. Graham, M.D.**

---

**Takedown of Glenn Shunts in Adults With Congenital Heart Disease With Polytetrafluoroethylene Grafts: Technique and Long-term Follow-up**
Bruckheimer E, Bulbul ZR, Hellenbrand WE, et al (Yale Univ, New Haven, Conn)
*J Thorac Cardiovasc Surg* 113:607–608, 1997                    4–18

---

*Introduction.*—One method of augmenting effective pulmonary blood flow in congenital heart disease is by using the Glenn shunt, a direct end-to-end anastomosis of the superior vena cava to the right pulmonary artery. With time, palliation with Glenn shunts diminishes and a corrective action is required. In 4 adults, successful takedown of Glenn shunts is described.

*Methods.*—Four patients had Glenn shunt operations for palliation of cyanosis at a mean age of 5 years. At a mean age of 29.5 years, the patients underwent Glenn shunt takedown; all patients had cardiac catheterization before their operations. Three patients required aortic cross-clamping and cardioplegia for intracardiac repair or conduit replacement. Two patients had reconstitution of pulmonary arterial continuity to relieve severe unilateral left pulmonary hypertension.

*Results.*—At a mean follow-up of 7.7 years, all patients were alive and free of cyanosis. A marked decrease in pulmonary vascular resistance at follow-up cardiac catheterization was evident in 2 patients with left pulmonary artery hypertension. In patient 3, cardiac catheterization was performed 15 years after the operation to assess subaortic obstruction with normal pulmonary hemodynamic findings. The fourth patient had polytetrafluoroethylene grafts.

*Conclusion.*—Successful takedown and corrective operations were performed on 4 adults with long-standing Glenn shunts. They had good results on follow-up. Glenn shunt takedown is feasible in selected adult patients and obviates the long-term complications of the shunt. Relief of unilateral left pulmonary artery hypertension can be provided with the restoration of pulmonary arterial continuity.

▶ This short communication is an important one. These authors have shown the marked improvement of 2 patients in terms of the relief of severe left pulmonary artery hypertension after takedown of the classic Glenn shunt as a result of allowing pulmonary flow to both left and right lungs. In selected adult patients, this difficult operative procedure is an alternative that should be considered. Patients who might be rejected for further operative procedures or for heart transplantation without lung transplantation might achieve reasonable midterm palliation or become candidates for a heart transplantation without lung transplantation after this procedure.

**T.P. Graham, M.D.**

## Delayed Sternal Closure After Cardiac Operations in a Pediatric Population

Tabbutt S, Duncan BW, McLaughlin D, et al (Harvard Med School, Boston)
*J Thorac Cardiovasc Surg* 113:886–893, 1997                    4–19

*Introduction.*—Delayed sternal closure (DSC) can provide significant hemodynamic and pulmonary stability in infants in whom considerable capillary leak and edema could develop after cardiopulmonary bypass (CPB). The morbidity and mortality associated with delayed sternal closure after pediatric cardiac operations was analyzed.

*Methods.*—During a 3-year period, 239 of 2,559 patients (9%) who underwent CPB had an open sternum. Records of 178 patients with DSC were reviewed retrospectively. All patients received a dressing that was applied once and not changed until final sternal closure or interim procedure. Intravenous antibiotic prophylaxis was administered throughout the perioperative duration. Cephazolin or vancomycin and gentamicin were used until sternal closure. Additional coverage was provided if culture-positive infection developed at other sites. A negative fluid balance for 3 days was viewed as an important indicator for achievement of successful sternal closure.

*Results.*—Forty-nine percent (51 of 104) of all patients with hypoplastic left-heart syndrome and 22% of patients with transposition of the great arteries (42 of 194) underwent DSC. Fourteen patients died at a median of 22 days after sternal closure, and 20 patients died before sternal closure. There were no significant predictors for risk of surgical site infection among bypass time, time the sternum remained open, or number of postoperative sternal explorations. The incidence of surgical site infection was 10% for patients in whom the sternum was opened in the coronary intensive care unit and 6.2% for patients in whom the sternum was left open in the operating room. There was a 3.9% (7 of 178) incidence of mediastinitis.

*Conclusion.*—Delayed sternal closure after pediatric cardiac surgeries may be required because of edema, unstable hemodynamic conditions, or bleeding, or may be used electively to help with hemodynamic and respiratory stability. Findings indicate a low rate of morbidity associated with DSC in pediatric patients.

▶ As younger and more complex patients undergo successful cardiac operations, delayed sternal closure becomes an important component of perioperative and postoperative management. These authors show relative low overall mortality and morbidity rates for this complex management strategy. The increases in atrial pressure, peak inspiratory pressure, and fraction of inspired oxygen should all be expected, with delayed sternal closure and this manuscript offers guidelines for what these changes usually are. Fortunately, infection, including mediastinitis, can be prevented or treated effectively in most patients.

**T.P. Graham, M.D.**

## One-stage Complete Unifocalization in Infants: When Should the Ventricular Septal Defect Be Closed?

Reddy VM, Petrossian E, McElhinney DB, et al (Univ of California, San Francisco)
*J Thorac Cardiovasc Surg* 113:858–868, 1997                    4–20

*Introduction.*—The ultimate goal of surgical management of pulmonary atresia with ventricular septal defect and major aortopulmonary collateral arteries is to achieve a completely separated, in-series, 2–ventricle circulation. Before complete repair is achieved, multiple operations are often necessary. Recently, a single surgery was developed for complete unifocalization with complete repair, including ventricular septal defect and placement of a right ventricle–pulmonary artery conduit; however, proper criteria for its use have not been established. Methods for determining whether ventricular septal defect closure is suitable during one-stage unifocalization were developed.

*Methods.*—Twenty-seven infants with ventricular septal defect, pulmonary atresia, and aortopulmonary collateral vessels underwent treatment. In 25 infants, midline complete unifocalization was performed. In 17 patients the ventricular septal defect was closed, and in 8 it was left open. Staged unifocalization was performed in 2 patients with severe distal collateral stenoses. Preoperative angiograms were used to measure pulmonary artery and collateral vessel diameters and to calculate the indexed cross-sectional area of the total neopulmonary artery bed. In 6 patients an intraoperative pulmonary flow study previously validated with experiments in neonatal lambs was performed. A known flow was used to perfuse the unifocalized neopulmonary arteries with this method, and recordings were made of pulmonary artery pressures.

*Results.*—Patients who underwent ventricular septal defect closure had a neopulmonary artery index that was greater than did patients who did not undergo ventricular septal defect closure. The ventricular septal defect was closed uneventfully at the time of unifocalization in patients with a total neopulmonary artery index greater than 200 $mm^2/m^2$. The postoperative right ventricular/left ventricular pressure ratio correlated with this index. Comparable mean pulmonary artery pressures were obtained during the intraoperative flow study and after bypass. The intraoperative pump flow study was further validated as a method for assessing pulmonary vascular resistance during cardiac operations in 8 additional infants who underwent complete one-stage unifocalization after the original study was submitted for publication.

*Conclusion.*—Postrepair right ventricular/left ventricular pressure ratio correlated with the total neopulmonary artery index. In deciding whether to close the ventricular septal defect in all patients, the pulmonary flow study is helpful, as is measurement of the postsurgical "new" size of the branch pulmonary arteries.

▶ This report on unifocalization for pulmonary atresia and ventricular septal defects in infants is a follow-up of previous studies showing the feasibility of this operation at their institution in a large number of infants and young children. This study indicates that more patients than were originally described can have the ventricular septal defect closed at the time of the initial surgery. The flow studies in the operating room can aid in determining when ventricular septal defect closure is reasonable.

**T.P. Graham, M.D.**

## The Clamshell Incision for Bilateral Pulmonary Artery Reconstruction in Tetralogy of Fallot With Pulmonary Atresia
Luciani GB, Wells WJ, Khong A, et al (Children's Hosp Los Angeles; USC School of Medicine, Los Angeles)
*J Thorac Cardiovasc Surg* 113:443–452, 1997                    4–21

*Objective.*—Underdevelopment or iatrogenic distortion of the pulmonary vasculature sometimes limits the complete surgical repair of complex tetralogy of Fallot/pulmonary atresia (ToF/PA). The results of the bilateral thoracosternotomy (clamshell) approach for completion of repair or of unifocalization in infants and children with complex ToF/PA were retrospectively reviewed.

*Methods.*—Between October 1993 and December 1995, 10 children, aged 4 months to 15 years, with complex ToF/PA underwent the bilateral thoracosternotomy (clamshell) repair. Nine patients had previously undergone 1–4 procedures.

*Results.*—Eight children had complete repair and 2 had complete unifocalization of the pulmonary arterial vasculature, connecting it to the right ventricle. Median duration of ventilatory support was 2 days, median duration of intensive care stay was 4 days, and median duration of hospitalization was 9 days. All patients were discharged from the hospital. There were 2 complications: 1 postoperative hemorrhage necessitating reexploration and 1 transient left phrenic nerve palsy. Both were successfully resolved. There were no late deaths during the 12- to 26-month follow-up period. Average peak right ventricular/left ventricular pressure ratios were 0.44, significantly lower than baseline values. One patient with a pseudoaneurysm of the pulmonary homograft conduit after 14 months who required reoperation recovered uneventfully and had no recurrence. The 2 infants who had unifocalization of the pulmonary arterial vasculature are awaiting complete repair.

*Conclusions.*—The clamshell approach is a safe and effective technique for one-step repair of ToF/PA in infants and children, even if they have had previous surgeries.

▶ Clamshell bilateral thoracotomies for patients with complex pulmonary atresia have not been used by many surgeons because of the fear of excessive pulmonary morbidity. Complete bilateral exposure of both central and peripheral pulmonary arteries and of major aorticopulmonary collateral arteries facilitates reconstruction and unifocalization even in patients with extensive scarring from previous operations, as well as in patients with a heavily calcified conduit. It is important to incorporate as many of the pulmonary arteries into the repair as possible and to provide access to these pulmonary arteries for the interventional cardiologist. These patients require a major collaborative effort between the surgeons and interventionalists to achieve effective treatment.

**T.P. Graham, M.D.**

---

**Biventricular Repair of Conotruncal Anomalies Associated With Aortic Arch Obstruction: 103 Patients**
Lacour-Gayet F, Serraf A, Galletti L, et al (Paris Sud Univ)
*Circulation* 96(suppl II):328–334, 1997                                    4–22

---

*Introduction.*—Infants with conotruncal anomalies associated with aortic obstruction are often able to undergo early, 1-stage total repair, although several complex surgical procedures are involved. Outcome is reported for 103 infants whose treatment combined a cardiac repair and a aortic arch reconstruction.

*Methods.*—From January 1984 to April 1996, 103 infants with combined conal and truncal anomalies with a coarctation of the aorta or an interrupted aortic arch underwent a biventricular repair. Conotruncal anomalies included 15 transpositions of the great arteries (TGAs) with intact ventricular septum, 44 TGAs with ventricular septal defect, 32

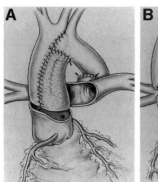
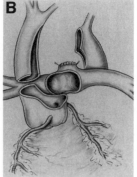
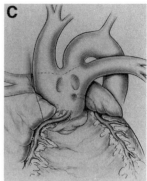

FIGURE 2.—(A) Aspect of a truncus arteriosus type II with interrupted aortic arch type B. (B) The truncal root is transected. A large pulmonary cuff is taken and mobilized to the right. The ascending aorta is incised. (C) The ascending and descending aorta are anastomosed. An ascending aorta patch enlargement corrects the size mismatch between the ascending aorta and the truncal root. (Courtesy of Lacour-Gayet F, Serraf A, Galletti L, et al: Biventricular repair of conotruncal anomalies associated with aortic arch obstruction: 103 patients. *Circulation* 96[supp II] 328–334, 1997. Reproduced with permission *Circulation.* Copyright 1997, American Heart Association.)

double outlet right ventricles with subpulmonary ventricular septal defect, 10 truncus arteriosus, 1 double outlet left ventricle, and 1 tetralogy of Fallot. Coarctation of the aorta was present in 88 patients and interrupted aortic arch in 15.

One-stage repair was performed in 58 infants: 38 with TGA or double outlet right ventricle and ventricular septal defect, 10 with TGA with intact ventricular septum, and all 10 with truncus arteriosus (Fig 2). Two-stage repair was employed in 45 infants. Cardiac repair was achieved

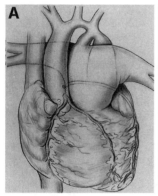
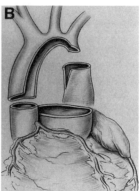
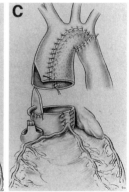

FIGURE 1.—(A) Aspect of a Taussig-Bing heart associated with coarctation and arch hypoplasia with double loop coronary arteries, side-by-side vessels, major great vessels size mismatch, and moderate hypoplasia of the RV. (B) The great vessels are transected. The coarctation is resected, and the ascending and transverse aorta is incised all the way down to the isthmus. (C) The descending aorta is anastomosed to the transverse arch. An ascending aorta patch enlargement corrects the great vessels' size discrepancy. The right coronary artery is relocated above the aortic anastomosis. (Courtesy of Lacour-Gayet F, Serraf A, Galletti L, et al: Biventricular repair of conotruncal anomalies associated with aortic arch obstruction: 103 patients. *Circulation* 96[supp II] 328–334, 1997. Reproduced with permission *Circulation.* Copyright 1997, American Heart Association.)

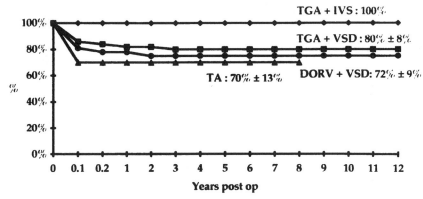

FIGURE 3.—Actuarial survival according to pathology. *Abbreviations: TA,* truncus arteriosus; *IVS,* intact ventricular septum. (Courtesy of Lacour-Gayet F, Serraf A, Galletti L, et al: Biventricular repair of conotruncal anomalies associated with aortic arch obstruction: 103 patients. *Circulation* 96[supp II] 328–334, 1997. Reproduced with permission *Circulation.* Copyright 1997, American Heart Association.)

by 89 arterial switch operations, 2 Kawashima reroutings, 10 truncus arteriosus repairs, a double-outlet left ventricle repair, and 1 tetralogy of Fallot repair. Reconstruction of the aortic arch employed direct anastomosis in 85 neonates; an ascending aortic patch was used in 15 cases (Fig 1), and a Gore-Tex conduit in 3.

*Results.*—Four infants died after the initial palliation, 9 at the second-stage repair, and 7 at the 1-stage repair. There were 6 late deaths. Eleven infants, including 10 with Taussig-Bing, required 12 reoperations for right ventricle outflow tract obstruction after arterial switch. Survivors were followed for a mean period of 6 years, and all but 4 are in class I functional status. Actuarial survival varied according to pathology (Fig 3) and 1–stage vs. 2-stage repair (Fig 4).

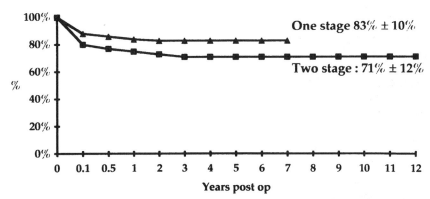

FIGURE 4.—Actuarial survival after 1-versus 2-stage repair. (Courtesy of Lacour-Gayet F, Serraf A, Galletti L, et al: Biventricular repair of conotruncal anomalies associated with aortic arch obstruction: 103 patients. *Circulation* 96[supp II] 328–334, 1997. Reproduced with permission *Circulation.* Copyright 1997, American Heart Association.)

*Conclusion.*—In selected infants, 1-stage biventricular repair of conotruncal anomalies associated with aortic arch obstruction achieved a survival rate of 83% at 7 years. An ascending aortic patch was useful to correct mismatch of the great vessels' diameters.

► These authors show outstanding results for biventricular repair of conotruncal anomalies associated with aortic arch obstruction (see Figs 1 and 2). Their current preference is for a 1-stage repair in these patients, with 2-stage repairs used in the presence of multiple ventricular septal defects, multiorgan failure, or suspicion of CNS hemorrhage detected at transfontanellar ultrasound. Follow-up at 6 years suggests excellent long-term survival as depicted in Figs 3 and 4, with truncus arteriosus and interrupted aortic arch showing the poorest survival at 70%. This is an incredible success story when one considers that this combination of complex defects had very few survivors reported until the last 5 years.

**T.P. Graham, M.D.**

**Modified Damus-Kaye-Stansel Procedure for Single Ventricle, Subaortic Stenosis, and Arch Obstruction in Neonates and Infants: Midterm Results and Techniques for Avoiding Circulatory Arrest**
McElhinney DB, Reddy VM, Silverman NH, et al (Univ of California, San Francisco)
*J Thorac Cardiovasc Surg* 114:718–726, 1997                    4–23

*Introduction.*—A modified Damus-Kaye-Stansel (DKS) procedure has been used successfully for palliation or repair of a number of congenital heart lesions. Results have been disappointing, however, when the procedure is employed for palliation of single ventricle with subaortic obstruction in neonates. Modifications of the DKS procedure described here avoid great vessel distortion and subsequent semilunar valve dysfunction, together with deep hypothermic circulatory arrest and the associated neurologic insult.

*Methods.*—Since 1990, a modified DKS procedure has been performed in 14 neonates and 7 infants. All had a single ventricle and subaortic stenosis, and 15 had arch obstruction. Twelve patients had double-inlet left ventricle, 2 had tricuspid atresia, and 7 had other forms of hypoplastic ventricle with subaortic obstruction. The proximal ascending aorta–main pulmonary artery anastomosis was performed in a side-to-side manner in all cases. Two basic techniques were used. In 12 patients, a V- or L-shaped aortotomy was performed (Fig 1) with one leg parallel to the sinotubular junction and the other angled posterosuperiorly. Nine patients had both the ascending aorta and main pulmonary artery transected above the sinotubular junction, with the proximal stumps anastomosed side to side.

*Results.*—One neonate and 3 of the infants died in the early postoperative period, for an early mortality rate of 19%. No late deaths or neurologic complications had occurred in the remaining patients at a median

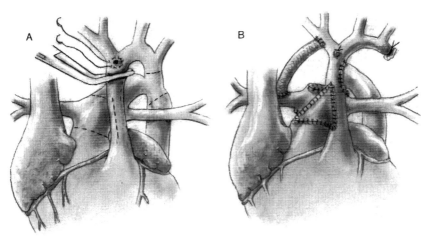

**FIGURE 1.**—Modified technique for performing the DKS procedure in a patient with coarctation of the aorta. The aortic inflow cannula is inserted at the base of the innominate artery, immediately distal to the aortic crossclamp. After institution of bypass, the patent ductus arteriosus is doubly ligated and divided. The pulmonary artery is transected above the sinotubular junction (*dashed lines* in the *left* frame indicate incisions) and at the origin of the ductus. Both defects in the central pulmonary artery are patched with either allograft or pericardium. The ascending aortotomy is performed with an L-shaped incision, and the flap of aortic tissue is retracted posteriorly as a flap for reconstruction of the posterior wall of the main pulmonary artery–ascending anastomosis. The DKS anastomosis is completed anteriorly with a hood of allograft tissue. A longitudinal aortotomy is then made in the opposite side of the ascending aorta (*left side* in this example), all ductal tissue is resected, and arch repair is performed by advancing the descending aorta to the ascending aorta and performing an end-to-side anastomosis. In this manner, circulatory arrest to the brain is avoided. A modified Blalock-Taussig shunt is then placed. *Abbreviation: DKS,* Damus-Kaye-Stansel. (Courtesy of McElhinney DB, Reddy VM, Silverman NH, et al: Modified Damus-Kaye-Stansel procedure for single ventricle, subaortic stenosis, and arch obstruction in neonates and infants: Midterm results and techniques for avoiding circulatory arrest. *J Thorac Cardiovasc Surg* 114:718–726, 1997.)

follow-up of 33 months. Nine patients later underwent bidirectional Glenn anastomosis and 1 required a transplant for cardiomyopathy. All of the remaining 12 patients appear to be good candidates for Fontan completion. Semilunar valvular regurgitation is present in 4 patients, but is mild or trivial in all cases. There has been no recurrent arch obstruction.

*Conclusion.*—In this group of neonates and infants with single ventricle, subaortic stenosis, and arch obstruction, a modified DKS procedure proved to be an effective primary palliation, particularly in neonates. A DKS procedure is recommended whenever the possibility of subaortic obstruction is present, unless there is significant semilunar valvular regurgitation.

▶ Treatment of infants with single ventricle and severe subaortic obstruction has been difficult and frequently the results have been disappointing. This method of palliation using a modified Damus-Kaye-Stansel procedure to treat both subaortic obstruction and coarctation or aortic arch interruption has been shown to produce reasonable early results in the majority of these neonates (see Fig 1). In the discussion of this paper the concern was expressed that anastomosis of the descending aorta to the side of the ascending aorta proximal to the innominate artery could cause compression of the left mainstem bronchus or left pulmonary artery with either respiratory complications or growth limitations of the left pulmonary artery with time. To date, these complications have not surfaced but are potential problems for the future. The authors favor this technique over a modified Norwood stage I in that one can avoid circulatory arrest and eliminate nonnative tissue in the arch repair.

**T.P. Graham, M.D.**

---

### Senning Plus Arterial Switch Operation for Discordant (Congenitally Corrected) Transposition

Karl TR, Weintraub RG, Brizard CP, et al (Royal Children's Hosp, Melbourne, Australia; The Cleveland Clinic, Ohio)
*Ann Thorac Surg* 64:495–502, 1997                                           4–24

---

*Background.*—Patients with congenitally corrected transposition of the great arteries (ccTGA) often exhibit the complications of a large ventricular septal defect and left ventricular (LV) outflow tract obstruction (LVOTO). Even when tricuspid insufficiency (TI) is the only associated anatomical defect, ccTGA may have an unfavorable natural history. The surgical technique reported was used in a subset of patients without LVOTO who underwent the Senning plus the arterial switch operation (ASO).

*Methods.*—Fourteen patients with a median age of 12 months underwent the Senning and ASO for ccTGA between 1989 and 1996. All had discordant atrioventricular and ventriculoarterial connections, and 8 had a large ventricular septal defect. Structural abnormalities of the tricuspid valve were present in 10 and greater than mild TI in 9 of the children. The combined Senning plus ASO was adopted when results of classic repairs proved unsatisfactory. At least 10 of the 14 patients had strong contraindications to classic repair. Criteria for the alternate strategy include unobstructed LV to pulmonary artery and right ventricle (RV) to aortic connections, balanced ventricular and atrioventricular valve sizes, septatable heart, translocatable coronary arteries, current or recent LV/RV pressure ratio greater than 0.7, and a competent mitral valve with good LV function.

*Results.*—There was 1 hospital death, and a second child died 10 months postoperatively. With 389 patient-months of follow-up time, actuarial survival beyond 10 months was 81%. The median postoperative hospital stay was 11 days. Complete heart block developed in 3 of the 10 patients who were in sinus rhythm preoperatively. Permanent pacing was established in these patients at a second operation during the same admission. Another child required reoperation after 7 years for relief of stenosis of the coronary graft. With 1 exception, all survivors are in New York Heart Association class 1 or 2. Detailed long-term neurodevelopmental outcome is not yet available, but survivors have had no permanent gross neurologic, renal, or metabolic sequelae.

*Discussion.*—Selected children with ccTGA may be treated more successfully by the Senning plus ASO than by classic repair. The operation is recommended for those with ccTGA, a systemic LV pressure, and nonobstructed outflow tracts. Features strongly favoring Senning plus ASO include TI, mild to moderate RV hypoplasia, or RV dysfunction.

▶ The use of the so-called double switch (atrial plus arterial switch) for patients with congenitally corrected transposition and no pulmonary stenosis has evolved in a subset of patients usually with significant RV dysfunction. Results have been encouraging. Similar early results have been obtained in patients with congenitally corrected transposition and pulmonary stenosis in whom an atrial switch plus a Rastelli type of conduit operation has been employed. These operations are very long and demanding, and it is unclear how many patients with congenitally corrected transposition will be reasonable candidates. It is important to get follow-up of these patients to determine the best strategy for dealing with this relatively rare condition.

**T.P. Graham, M.D.**

---

**Coronary Artery Fistulas in Infants and Children: A Surgical Review and Discussion of Coil Embolization**
Mavroudis C, Backer CL, Rocchini AP, et al (Northwestern Univ Med School, Chicago)
*Ann Thorac Surg* 63:1235–1242, 1997                                    4–25

---

*Introduction.*—An abnormal direct communication between any coronary artery and any of the cardiac chambers, as well as the superior vena cava, the coronary sinus, the pulmonary artery, and the pulmonary veins, is considered to be a congenital coronary artery fistula. Most infants and children with coronary artery fistulas are asymptomatic; symptoms appear in those older than 20 years who have fatigue, anginas, dyspnea, or congestive heart failure. The comparative therapeutic efficacy of an operation and coil occlusion should be determined by guidelines. A 28-year surgical experience with coronary artery fistulas in children and infants was reviewed to determine the efficacy of transcutaneous catheter coil embolization as an alternative therapy.

*Methods.*—There were 17 patients (mean age, 5.5 years) given diagnoses of coronary artery fistula in a 28-year period. Cardiac catheterization was used to diagnose the problem in all 17 patients, and echocardiography diagnosed the problem in 8 of 12 patients. Despite significant clinical, electrocardiographic, and chest x-ray findings in 10 of 13 patients with isolated coronary artery fistulas, all 13 patients were asymptomatic. Congenital coronary artery fistulas were diagnosed in 16 patients, and 1 patient had a coronary artery fistula after a tetralogy of Fallot repair causing injury of the anomalous left anterior descending coronary artery.

Two patients had tetralogy of Fallot, 1 patient had an atrial septal defect, and 1 patient had patent ductus arteriosus. Eight fistulas originated from the left coronary artery, and 9 originated from the right. Nine patients had drainage to the right ventricle, 4 had drainage to the right atrium, 3 had drainage to the pulmonary artery, and 1 patient had drainage to the left atrium.

*Results.*—A median sternotomy with endocardial or epicardial ligation was found in all patients. Eight patients underwent cardiopulmonary bypass surgery. A distal internal mammary artery bypass graft was required in 1 patient who had an iatrogenic coronary artery fistula. No operative or late deaths were observed. No evidence of recurrent or residual coronary artery fistulas was seen on the follow-up physical examination of the 17 patients, on the echocardiograms of 8 patients, or via catheterization of 2 patients. Coil embolization was possible in, at most, 6 patients, according to a retrospective review of the 16 available cine cardioangiograms.

*Conclusion.*—There is a 100% survival rate and a 100% closure rate using early surgical management of coronary artery fistulas, and it is considered to be a safe and effective treatment. In a very small, select group of patients, transcatheter embolization is a reasonable alternative to standard surgical closure. Transcatheter techniques should be compared against these surgical results, which should be considered the standard.

▶ This rare condition can be treated effectively by surgical techniques, as indicated by this report. There have been reports of transcatheter embolization for this problem also, but, as is pointed out in this article, only a small percentage of patients are candidates for coil embolization.

**T.P. Graham, M.D.**

---

### Effect of Repair Strategy on Hospital Cost for Infants With Tetralogy of Fallot

Ungerleider RM, Kanter RJ, O'Laughlin M, et al (Duke Univ, Durham, NC; Texas Children's Hosp, Houston; Children's Hosp of Philadelphia)
*Ann Surg* 225:779–784, 1997                4–26

---

*Introduction.*—In the field of cardiac surgery, surgical treatment of tetralogy of Fallot provided some of the first great success stories. Although advances in technology have led to the development of pediatric cardiac surgery as a distinct subspecialty, the optimal treatment strategy for tetralogy of Fallot in patients younger than 1 year remains controversial, particularly when it comes to 2-stage repair vs. 1-stage repair. Low early mortality and presumed improved long-term outcome are cited by those who want to justify 2-stage repair. The cost of treatment has emerged as an important determinant in treatment strategies in today's managed care environment. The cost of 1-stage repair was compared with 2-stage repair for infants with tetralogy of Fallot.

*Methods.*—The review included 22 patients younger than 1 year who had tetralogy of Fallot in a 2-year period. One-stage repair was performed on 18 patients and 2-stage repair, initial palliation followed by later repair, was performed on 4 patients. Severe hypercyanotic spells at the time of presentation, anomalous coronary arteries and critical illness were cited as the reasons for needing palliation. All patients were evaluated for the hospital costs in 1996 dollars and hospital length of stay. The cost accounting system used evaluated data on all direct and indirect hospital-based nonprofessional costs.

*Results.*—Neither group had any mortality. The average length of stay in the group having 1-stage repair was $14.5 \pm 11.2$ days, whereas the 2-stage group had an average total length of stay of $43 \pm 30.8$ days. The average cost for 1-stage repair was $\$32,541 \pm \$15,968$, and the average total cost for 2-stage repair was $\$79,795 \pm \$40,625$. A best-case analysis was performed to eliminate cost outliers; thus, 50% of patients were eliminated from each group. In the 1-stage group, the average length of stay was $8.5 \pm 1.4$ days, and for the 2-stage group, the average length of stay was $16.5 \pm 2.1$ days. In this best-case group, the cost for 1-stage repair was $\$22,360 \pm \$3331$, and for 2-stage repair, it was $\$44,660 \pm \$3645$.

*Conclusion.*—Excellent clinical results were found with primary complete repair of tetralogy of Fallot at a lower total cost than for the 2-stage repair. The 2-stage approach may be better for some patients; however, it is more expensive.

▶ As might be expected, the 2-stage repair of tetralogy of Fallot in infants costs about twice as much as the 1-stage repair. There has been an increasing trend toward primary repair in the first 3–9 months of life for most patients with tetralogy of Fallot. This can be accomplished in many patients who have relatively small pulmonary arteries and occasionally in patients whose coronary arteries are anomalous and cross the right ventricular outflow tract. In addition, the length of stay for patients with tetralogy of Fallot who do not have complications can be as little as 3–5 days, which is considerably shorter than was presented in this paper. The most important questions about this approach are brought out in the discussion of this paper; what is quality of outcome for early primary repair? Fortunately, it appears that most infants who have early repair do exceedingly well and have less long-term problems than those who have a 2-stage repair performed.

**T.P. Graham, M.D.**

### Hypertrophic Obstructive Cardiomyopathy in Pediatric Patients: Results of Surgical Treatment

Theodoro DA, Danielson GK, Feldt RH, et al (Mayo Clinic and Found, Rochester, Minn)
*J Thorac Cardiovasc Surg* 112:1589–1599, 1996                4–27

*Introduction.*—An extended left ventricular septal myectomy (LVM) has been offered at the study institution to patients with severe hypertrophic obstructive cardiomyopathy (HOCM) that is unresponsive to medical management. Most reports of this procedure have not included a separate

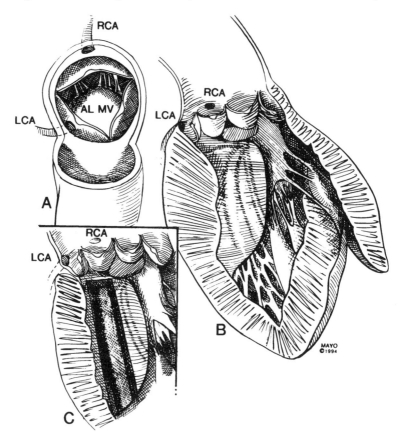

FIGURE 2.—Anatomic characteristics of hypertrophic obstructive cardiomyopathy. **A,** surgeon's view through transverse aortotomy. Right coronary cusp is located anteriorly and left cusp is located posteriorly and to left. Gentle retraction of aortic cusps, combined with posterior displacement of left ventricle as needed, exposes ventricular septum and anterior leaflet of mitral valve (*AL MV*). **B,** sagittal view through opened left ventricle showing membranous septum below commissure between right and noncoronary cusps, distribution of left bundle branches, septal hypertrophy, and anterior leaflet of mitral valve with its subvalvular apparatus. **C,** extent of initial septal resection is shown. Resection is then extended leftward to anterior leaflet of mitral valve and apically to relieve all midventricular obstruction. *Abbreviations: RCA,* right coronary artery; *LCA,* left coronary artery. (Courtesy of Theodoro DA, Danielson GK, Feldt RH, et al: Hypertrophic obstructive cardiomyopathy in pediatric patients: Results of surgical treatment. *J Thorac Cardiovasc Surg* 112:1589–1599, 1996.)

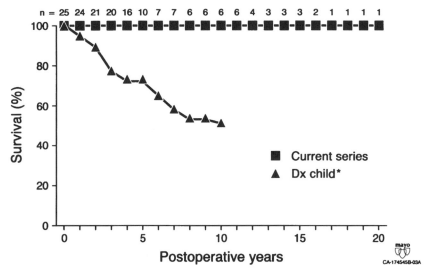

FIGURE 6.—Patient survival in current surgical series compared with survival in pediatric patients with hypertrophic obstructive cardiomyopathy treated nonsurgically (*Dx child*). (From Theodoro DA, Danielson GK, Feldt RH, et al: Hypertrophic obstructive cardiomyopathy in pediatric patients: Results of surgical treatment. *J Thorac Cardiovasc Surg* 112:1589–1599, 1996. Courtesy of McKenna WJ, Deanfield JE, Farugui A, et al: Prognosis in hypertrophic cardiomyopathy: Role of age and clinical, electrocardiographic, and hemodynamic features. *Am J Cardiol* 47:532–538, 1981.)

analysis of results for pediatric cases. In the 20-year series reported here, 25 pediatric patients underwent LVM at a single institution.

*Patients and Methods.*—The 13 boys and 12 girls ranged in age from 2 days to 19 years at diagnosis; median age at operation was 14 years. Seventeen had moderate-to-severe mitral valve insufficiency, and 3 had a history of serious ventricular arrhythmia. All had failed to respond to medical therapy, and 1 showed no improvement after dual-chamber pacemaker implantation. Patients had a mean preoperative left ventricular outflow gradient of 99.9 mmHg. All underwent a primary transaortic extended LVM (Fig 2). Mean aortic crossclamp time was 35.3 minutes. Follow-up ranged from 10 months to 20 years (mean 6.4 years).

*Results.*—Intraoperative left ventricular outflow tract gradients ranged from 20 to 117 mmHg before myectomy and from 0 to 20 mmHg after myectomy. None of the patients required mitral valve replacement. The procedure successfully eliminated moderate or severe mitral regurgitation in 16 of 17 patients. Postmyectomy mitral insufficiency was reduced to a regurgitant fraction of 0% to 12%. The 1 patient who needed a pacemaker because of complete heart block had a return to normal sinus rhythm. There were no early or late deaths and no instances of aortic or mitral valve injury. Freedom from re-operation because of recurrent left ventricular outflow tract (LVOT) obstruction was 94.4% at 5 years. All patients but 1 are in New York Heart Association functional class 1 or 2. Maintenance medical therapy consists of β-adrenergic antagonists alone in 14 patients, calcium channel antagonists alone in 5, and both in 2; 4 patients are on other combination therapies.

*Conclusions.*—Outcome in this series of patients shows extended LVM to be safe and effective in pediatric patients with severe HOCM. Cardiac symptoms are relieved, LVOT reduced, and mitral valve insufficiency corrected. Late survival after extended septal myectomy compares favorably with the expected mortality rate for patients who do not undergo operation (Fig 6).

▶ These authors show outstanding surgical results for patients who failed medical therapy. Gradient reduction was excellent and there have been no late deaths. Although this approach does not cure this muscle disease, it can be a valuable adjunct to treatment. The place for dual-chamber pacing (see (Abstract 4–3) and for intracoronary alcohol injections for "controlled" septal infarction in this group of patients remains to be determined.

**T.P. Graham, M.D.**

## Catheterization: Interventional and Therapeutic Procedures

### Intermediate-term Outcome of Transcatheter Secundum Atrial Septal Defect Closure Using the Bard Clamshell Septal Umbrella

Prieto LR, Foreman CK, Cheatham JP, et al (Cleveland Clinic Found, Ohio; Univ of Nebraska, Omaha)
*J Am Coll Cardiol* 78:1310–1312, 1996                                4–28

*Background.*—Transcatheter techniques for closure of secundum atrial septal defect were introduced in 1976. In 1989, the Bard Clamshell Septal Umbrella was developed. This device was implanted in more than 500 patients in the United States and Canada between 1989 and 1991. Indications included secundum atrial septal defect closure, closure of atrial fenestrations after the Fontan procedure, and closure of patent foramen ovale in patients with paradoxical emboli. Initial results were positive, but the trials were canceled pending further follow-up and possible redesign of the device because of a high rate of device arm fracture. Many patients have now been followed for 6 years, but no information is available on their clinical course.

*Methods.*—The medical records of patients with secundum atrial septal defect who had Clamshell atrial septal defect closure were reviewed. The purpose of the study was to evaluate results in patients with typical secundum atrial septal defect; patients with complex congenital heart disease or a history of stroke were excluded. Transcatheter closure of simple secundum atrial septal defect was done in 31 patients (9 patients were male); the age range was 27 months to 63 years. Evaluations were performed 7 times in the first 24 months after implantation and annually thereafter. Follow-up was 12 to 65 months.

*Results.*—At last follow-up, complete atrial septal defect closure by 1 device was seen in 17 patients, a clinically insignificant leak was seen in 12 patients, and a moderate leak was seen in 2 patients. Information on the size of the right ventricle and the pattern of interventricular septal motion was available in 28 patients. Right ventricular size and septal motion had returned to normal in 23 patients; mild right ventricular enlargement was seen in 4 patients, 2 with flattened septal motion; and moderate right ventricular enlargement with normal septal motion was seen in 1 patient with a moderate residual shunt. At a mean follow-up of 41 months, all patients were asymptomatic, but fractures of 1 arm or more developed in many devices as early as 1 month after atrial septal defect occlusions. These fractures have not been associated with leaks or enlargement of an existing leak. Device displacement has not occurred, and there has been no device-related dysfunction of adjacent structures. There have been no cases of clinically significant arrhythmia.

*Discussion.*—In these patients, transcatheter atrial septal defect occlusion with the Clamshell device has been safe and relatively effective. These findings compare favorably with surgical atrial septal defect closure in cases of small-to-moderate isolated secundum atrial septal defects. The Bard Clamshell Septal Umbrella is currently unavailable for clinical use because of concerns about unexpected device arm fractures. The patients are being monitored for fragment embolization, late device dislodging, and other problems.

▶ All of the data regarding this device are still being evaluated because of the problem with device arm fractures. In this study, 26 of 31 patients have documented device arm fractures, but there has been no documented device embolization in these patients. The presence of residual shunt in 45% is discouraging, but most of these shunts are small and, hopefully, with new modifications of this device, residual shunts and fractures will be rare. There are 4 devices for atrial septal defect closure currently in clinical trials, including a modification of the Bard Clamshell.

**T.P. Graham, M.D.**

---

**Percutaneous Balloon Dilatation of the Atrial Septum: Immediate and Midterm Results**
Thanopoulos BD, Georgakopoulos D, Tsaousis GS, et al (Aghia Sophia Children's Hosp, Athens, Greece; Univ Children's Hosp, Belgrade, New Yugoslavia)
*Heart* 76:502–506, 1996                                                    4–29

---

*Introduction.*—Blade atrial septostomy, which involves a catheter equipped with a knife blade at its tip, was performed to create an atrial septal defect to improve hemodynamics in patients in which a classic balloon atrial septostomy was impossible. As an alternative to blade atrial septostomy, atrial septostomy by percutaneous balloon dilation using valvuloplasty balloons has been used in some patients. The immediate and midterm results from 23 patients who had atrial septal defects created or enlarged by percutaneous balloon dilation of the atrial septum were reported.

*Methods.*—There were 23 patients who had atrial septostomy by percutaneous balloon dilation. In this group of patients, there were 15 boys and 8 girls who were 10 days to 10 years old. Congenital heart defects were seen in 17 patients, and 6 had primary pulmonary hypertension. All were hemodynamically unstable under optimal medical treatment. Fourteen patients had the balloon catheter enter the left atrium through a patent foramen ovale, whereas 9 patients had the balloon catheter enter via a transseptal puncture. There was a range in size of the balloons from 13 to 18 mm.

*Results.*—No complications were seen. After dilation, interatrial communication increased and remained unchanged during a 16-month follow-up period. In patients with transposition and mitral atresia, the transatrial gradient fell and arterial oxygenation improved. In the groups of patients with mitral atresia or stenosis, there were 2 failures—1 early and 1 late. In patients with primary pulmonary hypertension, there was a decrease in arterial oxygenation and an increase in left atrial pressure and cardiac index.

*Conclusion.*—For creating an adequate interatrial communication that can be used as an alternative to blade septostomy, percutaneous balloon dilation is effective and safe.

▶ These authors report good results in 23 patients who underwent balloon dilatation of either an intact atrial septum or a small atrial defect. There were 7 patients with congenital heart disease who showed marked improvement; virtual abolishment of atrial pressure gradients and an improvement in arterial saturations were seen in the majority. In addition, the 6 patients with primary pulmonary hypertension showed the expected decrease in arterial saturation and an increase in left atrial pressure and cardiac index. This technique is useful in all patients who need a larger atrial septal defect to decompress left atrial hypertension and to improve pulmonary venous congestion or in those patients who need a larger atrial septal defect to enhance right-to-left shunting because of primary pulmonary hypertension. It is also useful in patients who have undergone a Fontan procedure and who need an increase in blood flow to the left side of the heart. This technique needs to be available in all centers that deal with patients with complex congenital heart disease and primary pulmonary hypertension.

**T.P. Graham, M.D.**

## Acute Results of Balloon Angioplasty of Native Coarctation Versus Recurrent Aortic Obstruction Are Equivalent

McCrindle BW, for the Valvuloplasty and Angioplasty of Congenital Anomalies (VACA) Registry Investigators (Univ of Toronto; Children's Hosp, Seattle; Wayne State Univ, Detroit; et al)

*J Am Coll Cardiol* 28:1810–1817, 1996                                              4–30

*Introduction.*—Balloon angioplasty for native aortic coarctation is not used in some centers because of concern about an increased risk of acute aortic transmural tear or rupture, vascular complications in neonates and infants, and an increased incidence of late aortic aneurysm formation. To determine whether such concerns are valid, investigators compared acute results from 970 procedures, 422 for angioplasty of native aortic coarctation and 548 for recurrent aortic obstruction.

*Methods.*—The procedures were performed between 1982 and 1995 in 907 patients from 25 centers. Data collected for each procedure included patient selection characteristics, aortic dimensions, associated cardiac lesions, previous procedures, and hemodynamic data from cardiac catheterization. Native coarctation and recurrent aortic obstruction cases were compared for immediate results and risk factors for suboptimal outcomes. An acute suboptimal outcome was defined as a residual systolic pressure gradient of 20 mmHg or greater, residual proximal-to-distal systolic pressure ratio of 1.33 or greater, and/or a major complication.

*Results.*—Both the native and recurrent aortic obstruction groups showed a significantly increased lesion diameter after balloon angioplasty (mean of 128% and 97%, respectively), and the increase was significantly greater in the native group. Reductions in systolic pressure gradients were also significant in both groups, but slightly higher in the native group. Angioplasty-associated death was reported at equivalent rates (0.7%) in patients with native and those with recurrent lesions. The incidence of acute suboptimal outcome, however, was higher in the recurrent lesion group (25%) than in the native obstruction group (19%). Significant independent risk factors for suboptimal outcome included higher pre-angioplasty systolic gradient, earlier date of the procedure, older age, and recurrent obstruction. Suboptimal outcome was more likely to occur at institutions reporting fewer procedures, but this was unrelated to the time over which the number of procedures had been performed.

*Discussion.*—This study, which represents the largest series of patients undergoing percutaneous balloon angioplasty of aortic obstruction, suggests that the acute results and complications of balloon angioplasty of native coarctation are at least equivalent to those of recurrent aortic obstruction. Some outcomes were superior in the native coarctation group.

▶ The debate continues about the results and complications of balloon angioplasty of native coarctation. This report from a large registry indicates that the results are equivalent or slightly superior for native coarctation vs. recurrent coarctation angioplasty. In addition, previous studies, as well as this one have indicated that outside of the neonatal and early infancy age groups, the results for native coarctation appear equivalent to surgical results. There were 7 deaths relatively equally distributed between the native and recurrent coarctation groups. All were critically ill before the procedure and died in the catheterization laboratory. Balloon angioplasty continues to be a useful technique, but a technique like surgery, which is not devoid of complications. These procedures should be performed by experienced interventionalists with surgical backup available as needed.

**T.P. Graham, M.D.**

---

**Evaluation of Superficial Femoral Artery Compromise and Limb Growth Retardation After Transfemoral Artery Balloon Dilatations**
Lee HY, Reddy SCB, Rao PS (Univ of Wisconsin, Madison; St Louis Univ, Mo)
*Circulation* 95:974–980, 1997                                                        4–31

---

*Introduction.*—Retrograde femoral arterial catheterization is sometimes complicated by abnormalities of arterial pulse and limb growth. There have been no studies detailing the magnitude of these complications after transfemoral artery balloon dilation, however. The prevalence of superficial femoral artery (SFA) compromise and limb growth retardation was evaluated in children who have had transfemoral artery balloon dilation.

*Methods.*—Three groups of patients were studied: 43 consecutive patients who had transfemoral artery balloon dilation, 35 patients who had retrograde femoral artery catheterization, and 47 controls. The patients in the balloon dilation group ranged in age from 1 day to 15.5 years and were seen at a mean follow-up of 42 months. The 3 groups were evaluated for interventional ankle/control ankle blood pressure index (AAI), ratio of interventional/control lower limb length (LLI), and leg length difference (LLD). The occurrence of SFA compromise was assessed, together with its effect on limb growth.

*Results.*—The 3 groups were similar in terms of age and weight. The balloon dilation and catheterization groups were similar in age and weight at intervention and in length of follow-up. Patients in the balloon dilation group had an AAI of 0.95, compared with 1.0 in the catheterization group and 1.01 in the control group. Patients in the balloon dilation group were also significantly more likely to have an AAI of 0.9 or less. There were no significant differences in LLI or LLD. In the balloon dilation group, AAI and LLD were unrelated to patient age and weight at the time of the intervention, length of follow-up, or size of the balloon or balloon catheter shaft.

*Conclusion.*—Children undergoing transfemoral artery balloon dilation have some compromise of the superficial femoral artery. However, no significant limb growth retardation is apparent after several years' follow-up. Growth problems may be avoided because of the development of collateral circulation (Fig 2). The authors call for longer-term studies of

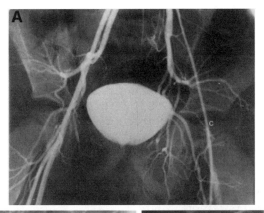

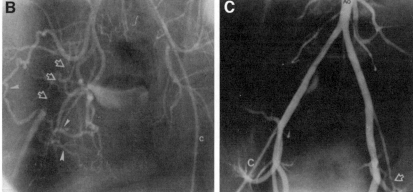

**FIGURE 2.**—Selected frames from descending aortograms during filming of femoral arteries. Balloon dilation had been performed via right (**A** and **B**) or left (**C**) femoral artery 1 year before this study. Catheters (**C**) were introduced via left (**A** and **B**) or right (**C**) femoral artery, and tips of catheters were positioned in lower part of abdominal descending aorta (not shown). Note good opacification of right iliac and femoral arteries (**A**) in a patient without blockage of femoral artery. In another child (**B**), note complete blockage of artery (*open arrows*). Also note good collateral circulation (*arrowheads*) opacifying distal femoral artery. In third child (**C**), there is partial blockage of left femoral artery, which had been used for balloon dilation 1 year before this study. *Abbreviation*: *Ao*, aorta. (Courtesy of Lee HY, Reddy SCB, Rao PS: Evaluation of superficial femoral artery compromise and limb growth retardation after transfemoral artery balloon dilatations. *Circulation* 95:974–980. Reproduced with permission of *Circulation*, copyright 1997, American Heart Association.)

more children to confirm that SFA compromise does not affect limb growth in children undergoing transarterial balloon dilation procedures.

▶ With the use of more interventional catheterization procedures, occasional compromise of femoral arterial circulation is inevitable despite the use of heparin and smaller catheters. Fortunately, most infants and children have excellent collateral vessel formation, and pulses may even be normal or near normal despite complete occlusion of the femoral vessels. Further follow-up studies will be useful to determine incidence of this problem and whether patients need orthopedic evaluation.

**T.P. Graham, M.D.**

## Follow-up Studies

### Cardiorespiratory Response to Exercise After Modified Fontan Operation: Determinants of Performance

Durongpisitkul K, Driscoll DJ, Mahoney DW, et al (Mayo Clinic and Found, Rochester, Minn)

*J Am Coll Cardiol* 29:785–790, 1997                                    4–32

*Objective.*—Patients who have undergone the Fontan procedure have below-normal maximal oxygen uptake and exercise heart rate. However, there is little information on which perioperative variables influence the patient's ultimate response to exercise. Cardiorespiratory responses to exercise and the determinants thereof were studied in patients who had a modified Fontan operation.

*Methods.*—Fifty-nine patients who had a modified Fontan operation and at least 1 postoperative exercise study were analyzed. The patients' median age at the time of the study was 12 years; mean time since surgery was 3 years. All patients underwent spirometry at rest, followed by incremental cycle ergometer exercise testing. Factors associated with oxygen uptake at peak exercise ($VO_2$max), blood oxygen saturation ($O_2$sat), and heart rate at peak exercise were assessed by multiple linear regression analysis.

*Results.*—The patients' $VO_2$max ranged from 29% to 95% of normal, $O_2$sat at peak exercise from 77% to 96%, and HRmax from 40% to 97%

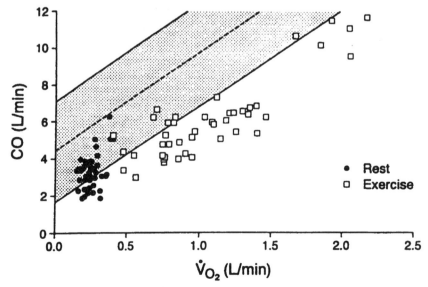

FIGURE 1.—Relation between cardiac output (CO) and $VO_2$. Shaded area, normal range. (Reprinted with permission from the American College of Cardiology from Durongpisitkul K, Driscoll DJ, Mahoney DW, et al: Cardiorespiratory response to exercise after modified Fontan operation: determinants of performance. *J Am Coll Cardiol* 29:785–790, 1997.)

of normal (Fig 1). Factors associated with log $VO_2max/kg^{2/3}$ were age at exercise, male sex, body surface area, preoperative confluent pulmonary arteries, and rest $VO_2max/kg^{2/3}$. Factors associated with $O_2sat$ at peak exercise were preoperative left pulmonary stenosis, classic Glenn anastomosis at exercise, and rest $O_2sat$. Factors associated with HRmax on exercise testing were age, body surface area, heart rate at rest, and diastolic blood pressure.

*Conclusions.*—Patients who have undergone a modified Fontan operation have subnormal $VO_2max$ and HRmax at peak exercise. The study identifies certain perioperative variables as determinants of $VO_2max$ and $O_2sat$ at peak exercise. Patients with a classic Glenn anastomosis have reduced $O_2sat$ at peak exercise, consistent with the presence of intrapulmonary shunting.

▶ Patients with the Fontan operation do have an abnormal cardiac output response to exercise. This study excluded patients with central hypoxia at rest with oxygen saturations less than 85% so that those who would correspond more to a fenestrated Fontan would not have been included. Older patients had a lower $VO_2max$ than younger patients and females had a lower value than males. Ventricular morphology did not affect the $VO_2max$. The presence of a classic Glenn anastomosis was associated with a decrease in $O_2$ sat at peak exercise suggesting extrapulmonary shunting that may be minimal at rest and substantial with exercise.

**T.P. Graham, M.D.**

---

### Fontan Operation in Five Hundred Consecutive Patients: Factors Influencing Early and Late Outcome

Gentles TL, Mayer JE Jr, Gauvreau K, et al (Children's Hosp, Boston; Harvard Med School, Boston)
*J Thorac Cardiovasc Surg* 114:376–391, 1997                                    4–33

---

*Introduction.*—During the almost 3 decades since the Fontan operation was first reported, early survival rates have improved to over 90% despite application of the operation to patients previously considered at higher risk. The 2 large series that have provided information about overall and late outcome have not included many patients operated on in recent years. To determine risk factors influencing early and late outcome after Fontan procedures, investigators reviewed a large, single-center experience of nearly 20 years.

*Methods.*—Databases identified the first consecutive 500 patients treated with various modifications of the Fontan procedure at Children's Hospital, Boston, between April 1973 and July 1991. The patients' medical records, preoperative echocardiographic and cardiac catheterization data, and operative notes were reviewed. Modifications of the Fontan procedure were classified according to the type of atriopulmonary connection. The primary outcome variable was survival with an intact Fontan circulation.

*Results.*—The mean age at surgery declined from 8.6 years in 1973–1984 to 5.1 years in 1990–1991. The operative technique first involved a conduit connecting the systemic venous atrium to the pulmonary artery or to a hypoplastic subpulmonic infundibular chamber and then evolved to a direct atriopulmonary anastomosis. In the last 252 patients, the total cavopulmonary anastomosis was used. The incidence of early failure decreased from 27.1% in the first quartile of the experience to 7.5% in the last quartile. Multivariate analysis identified variables associated with an increased probability of early failure: a mean preoperative pulmonary artery pressure of 19 mmHg or greater, younger age at surgery, heterotaxia syndrome, a right-sided tricuspid valve as the only systemic atrioventricular valve, pulmonary artery distortion, an atriopulmonary connection originating at the right atrial body or appendage, absence of a baffle fenestration, and longer pulmonary bypass time. The presence of a pacemaker before the Fontan operation was associated with an increased probability of late failure. Patients with a morphologically left ventricle and normally related great arteries or a single right ventricle had a lower probability of late failure. The probability of survival in the Fontan state was 84.9% at 1 month, 80.5% at 1 year, 78.5% at 5 years, and 71.4% at 10 years.

*Conclusion.*—Early failure after the Fontan procedure has declined considerably in recent years, in part because of procedural modifications. Late outcome, however, appears to be influenced by patient-related rather than by procedural variables.

▶ The risk factors for early outcome failure of the Fontan operation included young age at surgery, heterotaxia, systemic right-sided tricuspid valve, pulmonary artery distortion, mean pulmonary artery pressure elevation, right atrial/pulmonary connection, and absence of baffle fenestration. All were predictors of early failure. It is of interest that systemic right ventricle did not quite reach significance as a predictor of early outcome, although obviously this variable would be associated with a systemic atrioventricular right-sided tricuspid valve. An increased probability of late Fontan failure could only be associated with the presence of a pacemaker before the operation. A morphological left ventricle with normally related great arteries and a single right ventricle were associated with a decreased probability of late failure. There continues to be controversy about the fate of the systemic right ventricle and the Fontan circulation. Since there are a large number of potential contributing factors to Fontan failure, it is difficult to clarify the independent risk of the systemic right ventricle in this setting. With the further passage of time, I would speculate that a systemic right ventricle will become more and more important in terms of late failure of this form of palliation.

**T.P. Graham, M.D.**

**Patterns of Developmental Dysfunction After Surgery During Infancy to Correct Transposition of the Great Arteries**
Bellinger DC, Rappaport LA, Wypij D, et al (Harvard Med School, Boston; Children's Hosp of Philadelphia)
*J Dev Behav Pediatr* 18:75–83, 1997                                      4–34

*Introduction.*—Most studies of the developmental effects of reparative open heart surgery during infancy have focused on intelligence quotient scores, and little attention has been paid to the specific aspects of development and functioning that are most affected by cardiovascular interventions. A randomized clinical trial compared the incidence of brain injury in 2 groups of children who underwent *d*-transposition of the great arteries (*d*-TGA) with different operative support techniques.

*Methods.*—The prospective trial enrolled 171 infants between April 1988 and February 1992. Inclusion criteria included a birth weight of 2,500 g or more and a diagnosis of *d*-TGA with either an intact ventricular septum or a ventricular septal defect repair scheduled to occur by 3 months of age. Excluded were infants who had undergone previous cardiac surgery or had a recognizable syndrome of congenital anomalies or associated extracardiac abnormalities that were moderate or severe. Randomization was to either predominantly total circulatory arrest or predominantly continuous low-flow cardiopulmonary bypass during *d*-TGA. Standard scales were used to assess behavior and development at 1 and at 2.5 years of age.

*Results.*—Four children died during the follow-up period and 53 did not have at least 1 questionnaire returned at age 2.5 years, which left 114 children (68%) with complete data. Overall, children in both groups developed slower than would be expected. At age 1, children assigned to the circulatory arrest group scored lower on the Bayley Scales of Infant Development than did those assigned to low-flow bypass. Questionnaires completed by parents when the children were 2.5 years old indicated that those in the circulatory arrest group, especially in the subgroup with a ventricular septal defect, showed poorer expressive language and exhibited more internalizing and externalizing problem behavior. There was a strong association between behavioral problems and expressive language delay.

*Discussion.*—In this generally homogeneous group of infants who underwent *d*-TGA in early infancy, developmental delays were common. Children assigned to the circulatory arrest group, especially those with an associated septal defect, were likely to have poorer scores on both motor skills and language development than were children assigned to low-flow bypass.

▶ These studies of developmental outcome following infant repair of transposition by arterial switch are extremely important. One of the most gratifying findings is that the majority of these patients appear to be developing as well or almost as well as any group of patients born with a serious life-threatening disease. There are findings of poorer expressive language and more developmental abnormalities in the domains of motor and language function in the patients with circulatory arrest, particularly in those with an associated ventricular septal defect vs. those with continuous low-flow cardiopulmonary bypass. These authors suggest the advisability of minimizing to the extent possible the duration of circulatory arrest when repairing the complex defects of infants such as these.

**T.P. Graham, M.D.**

---

**Long-term Follow-up of Truncus Arteriosus Repaired in Infancy: A Twenty-Year Experience**
Rajasinghe HA, McElhinney DB, Reddy VM, et al (Univ of Calif, San Francisco)
*J Thorac Cardiovasc Surg* 113:869–879, 1997                4–35

---

*Introduction.*—Few data are available regarding long-term survival and freedom from reintervention after truncus arteriosus repair in infants. Long-term outcomes in 165 patients who survived the early postoperative period after complete repair of truncus arteriosus since 1975 were prospectively evaluated.

*Methods.*—Median age at operation was 3.5 months (range, 2 days to 36 years). Eighty-one percent of the patients underwent surgery at less than 1 year of age. Fifteen patients had undergone pulmonary artery banding, and 2 patients underwent repair of interrupted aortic arch. Significant repairs performed concurrently with truncus repair included 10 truncal valve replacements, 5 truncal valve repairs, and 4 repairs of interrupted aortic arch.

*Results.*—Patients were followed up for a median of 10.5 years (range, 0.1–20.4 years). Thirteen of 23 late deaths occurred within 1 year of truncus repair. Of those, 8 deaths occurred within 6 months of repair. Ten late deaths were associated with reoperation. In infants, actuarial survival was almost identical: 90% at 5 years, 85% at 10 years, and 83% at 15 and 20 years. Moderate to severe truncal valve insufficiency before repair was a significant independent risk factor for poor long-term survival. One hundred thirty-three conduit reoperations were performed in 107 patients at a mean of 5.1 years after initial repair. Smaller conduit size at first operation was significantly associated with shorter time to conduit replacement. Twenty-six patients required 30 truncal valve replacements. Of these, 6 patients required truncal valve replacement before any conduit-related reintervention. Two of the 6 patients died. The 10-year actuarial freedom from truncal valve replacement in patients with no prerepair truncal valve insufficiency was 95%, compared with 63% in patients who had truncal insufficiency before initial repair. All except 3 patients were in New York Heart Association functional class 1.

*Conclusion.*—Long-term survival and functional status are excellent for infants who undergo complete repair of truncus arteriosus. These patients usually require later conduit replacement or revision.

▶ The long-term survival of patients who undergo repair of truncus arteriosus and the first operation is impressively good. These patients do require relatively frequent reoperation, with the median age at time of conduit replacement about 5½ years both for young infants and older patients. Reoperation was tolerated well in this group, and the truncal valve held up well long-term if there was no prerepair truncal valve insufficiency.

**T.P. Graham, M.D.**

**Congenital Aortic Valve Disease: Improved Survival and Quality of Life**
Elkins RC, Knott-Craig CJ, McCue C, et al (Univ of Oklahoma, Oklahoma City)
*Ann Surg* 225:503–511, 1997                                                                4–36

*Introduction.*—In the medical and surgical management of children with aortic valve disease, significant improvement has taken place during the past 40 years, but surgical treatment has proved to be palliative. A retrospective review was of all patients requiring a surgical aortic valve procedure, resection of a discrete subvalvar membrane, or an aortic balloon valvuloplasty to assess the effect of recent trends in surgical management, including the use of the Ross operation, on improved survival and quality of life.

*Methods.*—The retrospective review included 301 patients undergoing surgery during a 36-year period. The patients were 1 day to 26 years old, with a median age of 5 years. All prior and subsequent operations were recorded.

*Results.*—At age 10 years, the survival rate for all patients was 90% ± 2%. At age 25 years, the survival rate was 73% ± 8%. An aortic valve procedure was required in 52% ± 4% by age 5, and by age 15, it was 89% ± 3%. The diagnosis of valvar aortic stenosis had an adverse effect on patient survival 79% ± 6% at age 25, compared with 95% ± 4% for subvalvar aortic stenosis or aortic insufficiency. Patients with a bicuspid or unicuspid valve required operative intervention at an earlier age, but aortic valve morphology did not affect survival. In comparison with other types of valve replacement, survival after autograft replacement of the aortic valve (Ross operation) was significantly better. The use of the Ross operation is favored for quality of life as assessed by need for reoperation. With the Ross operation, there was freedom from reoperation at 9 years of 87% ± 7%, compared with 55% ± 5% in all patients after first aortic valve surgery.

*Conclusion.*—In children requiring a valve replacement as a first operation or after a prior aortic valve procedure, the Ross operation appears to have a significant advantage in survival and quality of life.

▶ Dr. Elkins and his group have been proponents of the pulmonary autograft for aortic valve surgery since 1986. His current results indicate that early mortality for this procedure is not different from that of prosthetic aortic valve replacement, which is an easier operation and requires less cross-clamp time—unless one has extensive experience with the pulmonary autograft. These results are impressive and, hopefully, these valves will hold up over the long haul. Except for avoiding heavy weight lifting and collision sports, the majority of these patients have no restrictions.

**T.P. Graham, M.D.**

**Late Left Ventricular Function After Surgery for Children With Chronic Symptomatic Mitral Regurgitation**
Krishnan US, Gersony WM, Berman-Rosenzweig E, et al (Columbia Univ, New York)
*Circulation* 96:4280–4285, 1997                                           4–37

*Introduction.*—Guidelines for the treatment of children with chronic mitral regurgitation (MR) are not well defined, although mitral valve surgery is often delayed as long as possible. Surgery is undertaken in many cases because of the appearance of severe symptoms. A group of 33 symptomatic children operated on for MR was reviewed for long-term ventricular function and risk factors for adverse outcome.

*Methods.*—The mean age of the patients was 6.7 years (range 6 months to 19 years). All had severe MR as a single hemodynamically significant lesion and underwent surgery at the study institution between July 1976 and September 1996. Excluded were patients with other causes of left ventricular dysfunction and those with significant shunts or involvement of other valves. Three echocardiographic studies were analyzed in each case: the latest preoperative (median 8.5 days before surgery); prehospital discharge (median 7 days after surgery); and the most recent follow-up. Risk factors examined included end-diastolic dimension, end-systolic dimension, shortening fraction (SF), left atrial pressure, pulmonary artery pressure, MR duration, bypass and cross-clamp time, and early vs. recent surgical era.

*Results.*—One patient died during surgery; the remaining 32 patients were followed for a mean 4.5 years. Residual MR was graded qualitatively as absent to mild in 29 patients and moderate in 3. At late follow-up, no patient with moderate mitral insufficiency had elevated end-diastolic dimensions. All but 1 of the 32 patients showed complete recovery of left ventricular function at late follow-up, regardless of pre- or postoperative ventricular performance. Overall, 6 patients were judged to have suboptimal outcome and 27 (82%) to have a good outcome, with no symptoms, no need for medications, and good left ventricular function. Only duration of MR proved to be a risk factor for poor outcome in multivariate analysis.

*Conclusion.*—Children with chronic symptomatic MR who undergo corrective surgery achieve normal late left ventricular function. Although delay of surgery until the onset of severe symptoms does not, as in adult patients, increase the risk for long-term ventricular dysfunction, late atrial arrhythmias may occur in those with prolonged duration of MR before surgery.

▶ The Columbia Group showed the predicted drop in shortening fraction early after repairing mitral regurgitation. In contrast to many adult studies, the majority of patients then showed improvement in systolic function when studied approximately 3 years after operation. Indeed, most patients had normalization of left ventricular size as well as normalization of shortening fraction. One implication of the study emphasized by the authors is that delaying repair or replacement of the mitral valve until children develop significant symptoms usually does not result in long-term ventricular dysfunction. Late atrial rhythm disturbances, however, were encountered in a number of these patients with long-standing regurgitation. Although most of the patients had marked volume overload, the preoperative shortening fraction was normal ($\geq 0.28$) in 30 of 33 patients, and only 1 patient had late left ventricular dysfunction. Correction of severe volume overload as soon as possible usually results in the best long-term functional outcome. Many young pediatric patients have valves that may not be amenable to repair, and valve replacement is carried out at the time of surgery. This invariably leads to the late development of mitral stenosis due to a small prosthetic valve as growth ensues. The utilization of load-independent indices of contractility may be useful in deciding when to intervene surgically in patients with large ventricles and borderline low shortening fractions.

**T.P. Graham, M.D.**

---

**Aortic Valve Prolapse and Aortic Regurgitation Associated With Subpulmonic Ventricular Septal Defect**
Tohyama K, Satomi G, Momma K (Tokyo Women's Med College)
*Am J Cardiol* 79:1285–1289, 1997                                        4–38

---

*Background.*—Patients with subpulmonic ventricular septal defect have a high incidence of associated aortic valve prolapse and aortic regurgitation. Surgery can be necessary to treat aortic regurgitation. Echocardiography allows noninvasive diagnosis and location of ventricular septal defect and aortic valve deformity. The natural development of aortic valve prolapse in patients with subpulmonic ventricular septal defect was examined, with attention to hemodynamic factors associated with early development of aortic regurgitation.

*Methods.*—The medical records of 315 patients with subpulmonic ventricular septal defect were reviewed. Patients were between 20 days and 35 years old. Patients with subpulmonic ventricular septal defect underwent echocardiographic examination on the first visit and every 6 months to 2 years thereafter or in cases of diastolic murmur or bounding pulse.

*Results.*—Of the 315 patients with subpulmonic ventricular septal defect, 218 (69%) developed aortic valve prolapse. The prevalence of aortic valve prolapse and aortic regurgitation increased with age. The prevalence of mild to moderate aortic regurgitation peaked between 5 and 7 years of age. A large left to right shunt was noted in patients with early onset of aortic regurgitation. More than 50% of patients younger than 7 years had

(Qp/Qs) greater than 1.5, and all these patients except 1 infant had mild to moderate aortic regurgitation. All patients except 1 older than 7 years had a Qp/Qs less than 1.5 and mild to slight aortic regurgitation. More severe aortic regurgitation was associated with higher Qp/Qs.

*Discussion.*—Early detection of aortic valve prolapse and aortic regurgitation may be critical, because early surgical closure of the defect may prevent the development or progression of aortic regurgitation. In about 40% of patients with subpulmonic ventricular septal defect, associated aortic valve prolapse progressed to aortic regurgitation within 1 year. Surgery early after the development of aortic valve prolapse may be advantageous.

▶ These authors have vast experience with subpulmonic ventricular septal defect and have carefully analyzed the prevalence of aortic valve prolapse and subsequently of aortic regurgitation with follow-up. The onset of regurgitation can occur as early as the first 2 years of life, but most commonly between ages 5 and 10 years. With the advent of echocardiography and Doppler flow studies, the prevalence of aortic regurgitation has been detected prior to the development of a diastolic murmur. Although this point could be debated, I favor surgical repair of subpulmonic defects even when aortic regurgitation is silent but can be detected easily with color Doppler studies.

**T.P. Graham, M.D.**

---

## Natural Course of Isolated Pulmonary Valve Stenosis in Infants and Children Utilizing Doppler Echocardiography

Rowland DG, Hammill WW, Allen HD, et al (Ohio State Univ, Columbus; Univ of Virginia, Charlottesville)
*Am J Cardiol* 79:344–349, 1997                                   4–39

---

*Background.*—Valvular pulmonary stenosis with intact ventricular septum occurs in about 9% of all cases of congenital heart disease. Most of the information on the natural history of pulmonary stenosis was gathered from studies of cardiac catheterization conducted 15 to 20 years ago, and selection bias sometimes excluded infants and patients with mild disease. Today, Doppler echocardiography has become a common method of measuring stenotic lesions in all patients.

*Methods.*—Patients with pulmonary stenosis between 1985 and 1994 were identified through a database review. Medical records and echocardiography reports were examined. Patients with other cardiac anomalies were excluded.

*Results.*—Of 269 patients identified, 147 met inclusion criteria. At initial echocardiogram, patients were between 2 days and 15 years of age. The mean follow-up was 2.4 years. Of 56 newborns evaluated at under 1 month of age, 16 had an increase in peak systolic pressure gradient of 20 mmHg or more; in 8 of these 16 infants the increase developed in 6 months or less. Of 89 patients initially evaluated after 1 month of age, only 7 had an increase in peak systolic pressure gradient of 20 mmHg or more. Severe pulmonary stenosis did not develop in any patient older than 2 years who had an initial gradient less than 50 mmHg. Progression to moderate or severe pulmonary stenosis was seen in 11 of 40 newborns with mild obstruction compared with 10 of 68 infants initially evaluated after 1 month of age. The rate of progression from moderate pulmonary stenosis was higher in infants than in older children.

*Discussion.*—These findings suggest that mild pulmonary stenosis is not static, especially in young infants. Rapid and significant progression in obstruction was seen in a small percentage of infants initially evaluated in the first month of life. Follow-up evaluation is recommended within 2 to 3 months for infants who are initially evaluated at age 1 month of age or younger.

▶ These interesting natural history data indicate the likelihood that a significant increase in gradient requiring treatment is much more common in the newborn and young infant than in older patients. Of interest is the fact that in no patient older than 2 years with an initial gradient less than 50 mmHg, did severe pulmonary stenosis develop. There is a small but significant percentage of infants seen under 1 month of age who can have a rapid and progressive obstruction; therefore, follow-up within 2 to 3 months for an infant initially seen at under 1 month of age is recommended.

**T.P. Graham, M.D.**

---

**Pulmonary Valve Replacement Late After Repair of Tetralogy of Fallot**
Yemets IM, Williams WG, Webb GD, et al (Hosp for Sick Children, Toronto; Toronto Congenital Cardiac Centre for Adults)
*Ann Thorac Surg* 64:526–530, 1997                                                    4–40

*Introduction.*—Some patients who have undergone repair of tetralogy of Fallot (TOF) later experience increasing fatigue, dyspnea, and arrhythmias, signs of progressive right heart failure resulting from pulmonary valve incompetence. The results of pulmonary valve replacement (PVR) in a group of 85 such patients are presented in this review.

*Methods.*—The 31 female and 54 male patients had undergone TOF repair at a mean age of 8 years; their mean age at the time of PVR was 19.6 years. Most were experiencing diminished tolerance for exercise and had evidence of progressive right ventricular enlargement. Operative records were reviewed for prior palliative procedures, initial repair, indications for PVR, and subsequent clinical course. At the initial repair, a transannular patch was used to treat right ventricular outflow tract obstruction in 56 (66%) patients; the pulmonary valve annulus was preserved in the remaining patients. Additional procedures at the time of PVR were required in 56 patients.

*Results.*—One patient, a 5-year-old child, died within 1 month of PVR. The remaining patients had an uneventful postoperative course with no PVR-related complications. During a mean follow-up of 5.8 years there were 3 late deaths, but none were related to the PVR. Actuarial survival was 95% at 10 years and 87% at 15 years. Most patients showed improvement in symptoms after PVR, and 90% are in New York Heart Association class 1. By actuarial analysis, 86% of the survivors have not had a reoperation 10 years after PVR. Although there was no statistically significant difference in survival free of reoperation between the porcine valve and pericardial valve implant groups, the trend suggests that porcine valves will prove more durable.

*Discussion.*—Almost all patients who have undergone TOF repair will experience some degree of pulmonary valve incompetence, but those without important residual lesions can often tolerate the condition for many years. Pulmonary valve replacement can be performed in patients with increasing fatigue and dyspnea with low operative risk, good intermediate-term survival, and symptomatic improvement.

▶ The decision to replace the pulmonary valve in postoperative tetralogy patients with relatively severe pulmonary insufficiency is a difficult one. Those patients who clearly have reduced exercise capacity and moderate right ventricular enlargement will usually benefit from this operation. One can, however, wait too long to apply this procedure, and right ventricular dysfunction may be irreversible. These authors show very low operative risk and a markedly improved functional classification after surgery.

**T.P. Graham, M.D.**

# Doppler Echocardiography/Magnetic Resonance Imaging

## Comparison of Patterns of Pulmonary Venous Blood Flow in the Functional Single Ventricle Heart After Operative Aortopulmonary Shunt Versus Superior Cavopulmonary Shunt

Rychik J, Fogel MA, Donofrio MT, et al (Univ of Pennsylvania, Philadelphia)
*Am J Cardiol* 80:922–926, 1997                                          4–41

*Introduction.*—Little is known about pulmonary venous blood flow in the single-ventricle heart. To better understand the determinants of transpulmonary blood flow, Doppler transesophageal echocardiography (TEE) was used to examine patterns of pulmonary venous flow in 68 children with functional single ventricles.

*Methods.*—The children all underwent TEE in the operating room before proceeding to the next stage of their planned surgery. Pulmonary arterial blood flow was derived from an aortopulmonary shunt in 34 patients (group I) and from a semi-Fontan in 34 (group II). Two group II patients also underwent simultaneous evaluation of superior vena caval flow. Forty-four children had functional single ventricles of right ventricular morphology and 25 of left ventricular morphology. At the time of TEE, all group I and 28 group II patients were in normal sinus rhythm.

*Results.*—All patients in normal sinus rhythm had biphasic forward flow in the pulmonary veins. The 6 group II patients with transient junctional rhythm exhibited significant early systolic reversal of flow. Both the S- and D-wave velocity-time intervals were greater in group I than in group II. Although pulmonary venous flow was predominantly systolic in both groups, the proportion of flow during ventricular systole was significantly greater in group II. When superior vena caval flow was analyzed in group II patients, a single predominant wave was observed with onset at early systole and peak in late systole at a mean of 150 ms after the pulmonary venous S-wave peak.

*Discussion.*—In patients with a functional single ventricle, pulmonary venous blood flow was found to be skewed slightly towards systole in those with aortopulmonary shunt and became predominantly systolic with diminished diastolic flow after superior cavopulmonary connection. Thus atrial relaxation and systolic properties of the ventricle, in addition to diastolic properties, play a significant role on generating the impetus for transpulmonary flow in such patients. Preservation of systolic ventricular performance and maintenance of sinus rhythm appear to be essential for optimal physiology in the functional single ventricle anatomy.

▶ The patterns of pulmonary venous inflow into the heart as determined with echo Doppler studies represent a fascinating window into the dynamics of filling the left heart. These authors show variations in these patterns in patients with single ventricle with aortic/pulmonary shunt physiology vs hemi-Fontan physiology, as well as alterations in flow with junctional vs. sinus rhythm. These methods could be clinically useful as another means for assessing post-operative hemodynamics in this complex group of patients. Of particular interest is the marked change in flow patterns with junctional rhythm, which can prove deleterious to maintaining adequate systemic blood flow.

**T.P. Graham, M.D.**

---

**Right Ventricular Diastolic Function in Children With Pulmonary Regurgitation After Repair of Tetralogy of Fallot: Volumetric Evaluation by Magnetic Resonance Velocity Mapping**
Helbing WA, Niezen RA, Le Cessie S, et al (Leiden Univ, The Netherlands; Interuniversity Cardiology Inst, Utrecht, The Netherlands)
*J Am Coll Cardiol* 28:1827–1835, 1996                                4–42

---

*Background.*—Early complete surgical correction is currently the favored approach to repair of tetralogy of Fallot, but can lead to high transanular patch rates and pulmonary regurgitation. Recent reports have suggested pulmonary regurgitation could be reduced and exercise capacity increased by restricting late diastolic filling of the right ventricle, as indicated by diastolic forward flow in the pulmonary artery after atrial contraction. There are few data on right ventricular diastolic function in patients undergoing repair of tetralogy of Fallot. This issue was addressed in a study using volumetric evaluation by magnetic resonance imaging (MRI) with flow velocity mapping.

*Methods.*—The study included 19 children (mean age, 12 years) who had undergone repair of tetralogy of Fallot at a mean age of 1.5 years, and 12 healthy children. In both groups, right ventricular time-volume curves were determined by summation of MR velocity mapping of pulmonary and tricuspid volume flow curves. Tomographic MRI was performed to determine ventricular size. Some patients performed a graded exercise test.

*Results.*—Six of the patients who had undergone tetralogy of Fallot repair had no late diastolic forward pulmonary flow (group I), whereas in 13 such flow contributed 1% to 14% to RV stroke volume (group II). The patients had a significantly greater right ventricular end-diastolic volume index than did control subjects. The right and left ventricular ejection fractions were lower in patients than in the control group. Patients in group I had a pulmonary regurgitation volume of 33% of right ventricular stroke volume, compared with 42% in group II. On exercise testing, tolerance was significantly lower in patients in group II than in control subjects or patients in group I. Although exercise capacity was weakly associated with pulmonary regurgitation, it was unrelated to right or left ventricular volume or ejection fraction.

*Conclusion.*—This study found abnormal right ventricular diastolic function in children with residual pulmonary regurgitation after repair of tetralogy of Fallot. Restriction to filling leads to increased early filling rates and decreased deceleration times. Exercise performance is reduced in the presence of predominantly restrictive right ventricular physiology. Magnetic resonance imaging with flow velocity mapping can be used to measure right ventricular diastolic function in patients with pulmonary regurgitation.

▶ The authors performed some elegant MRI studies to determine time-volume curves and diastolic function in patients following repair of tetralogy of Fallot. They conclude that restrictive right ventricular physiology is associated with decreased exercise function but could not relate exercise performance to degree of pulmonary regurgitation. These studies are in contrast to studies published by the group at the National Heart Institute in London, which suggested that restrictive physiology can decrease the degree of pulmonary regurgitation and be associated with superior exercise performance.[1] The small number of patients in this study makes their conclusion somewhat tenuous; hopefully, these authors will continue their studies with increased numbers of patients. These studies did show that right ventricular volume was significantly greater in the group with poor exercise performance. Increased right ventricular volume usually is associated with pulmonary regurgitation in this group of patients, but with the relatively small numbers in this study, these two factors could not be associated statistically.

**T.P. Graham, M.D.**

*Reference*

1. Gatzoulis MA, Clark AL, Cullen S, et al: Right ventricular diastolic function 15 to 35 years after repair of tetralogy of Fallot. Restrictive physiology predicts superior exercise performance. *Circulation* 91:1775–1781, 1995.

## Transplant

### Long-term Survivors of Pediatric Heart Transplantation: A Multicenter Report of Sixty-Eight Children Who Have Survived Longer Than Five Years

Sigfússon G, Fricker FJ, Bernstein D, et al (Univ of Pittsburgh, Pa; Stanford Univ, Calif; Columbia Univ, New York)

*J Pediatr* 130:862–871, 1997                                    4–43

*Introduction.*—Pediatric and adult heart transplantation became more common after the introduction of cyclosporine in 1980, the first drug that selectively inhibited T-cell function. Improved survival has occurred among the pediatric heart transplantation group because of better donor organ preservation, increased experience with immunosuppressive therapy, and lower perioperative mortality rates. Throughout the world, about 400 children have heart transplants each year, and little is known about long-term survival, complications of immunosuppression, and the quality of life. Children who survived longer than 5 years after heart transplantation were studied.

*Methods.*—A retrospective review was conducted of patients who had heart transplants in a 14-year period and who survived more than 5 years after receiving their transplants. A review of the records showed that 48 children had dilated cardiomyopathy, 3 had hypertrophic cardiomyopathy, and 1 had restrictive cardiomyopathy, and 15 had end-stage congenital heart disease. The most common form of maintenance immunosuppression was triple-drug immunosuppression with cyclosporine, azathioprine, and corticosteroids.

*Results.*—Five-year survival after transplantation was found among 68 children, and at the median follow-up of 6.8 years, 60 children (88%) were still alive. Ten-year survival after transplantation was seen with 13 children. Late renal transplantation was required by 2 patients, and renal dysfunction caused by immunosuppressive agents was common. Twelve patients had lymphoproliferative disease or other neoplasms, but none resulted in death. Thirteen patients (19%) had coronary artery disease, and 8 patients needed retransplantation. In 5 of 8 patients, death after 5 years was related to acute or chronic rejection. Noncompliance with immunosuppressive medication accounted for 2 of the deaths. New York Heart Association class 1 was evident in all of the survivors.

*Conclusion.*—Although complications of immunosuppression remain common, long-term survival with good quality of life can be achieved after heart transplantation in childhood. The main factor that limits long-term graft and patient survival is posttransplantation coronary artery disease.

All survivors were doing age-appropriate activities and were without significant limitations. Prospective studies are needed to examine psychosocial adjustment to heart transplantation, particularly among adolescents who have shown noncompliance, depression, anxiety, disruptive behavior, and drug abuse after heart transplantation.

▶ In this multicenter study, 88% of 68 children who survived more than 5 years after transplantation (median follow-up, 7 years) are currently alive. Renal dysfunction is common, and lymphoproliferative disease or neoplasms have resulted but have been successfully treated. Coronary artery disease was diagnosed in 13 patients or (19%, which led to retransplantation in 8. Good quality of life can be achieved by the majority of children receiving heart transplants. Immunosuppressive complications and posttransplantation coronary artery disease are major factors that continue to plague this patient population. Nevertheless, for those patients and parents who can effectively deal with the treatment regimens required, this form of therapy can provide excellent palliation for a variety of complex heart problems in children.

**T.P. Graham, M.D.**

---

**Posttransplantation Lymphoproliferative Disorders in Pediatric Thoracic Organ Recipients**
Boyle GJ, Michaels MG, Webber SA, et al (Univ of Pittsburgh, Pa)
*J Pediatr* 131:309–313, 1997                                                        4–44

---

*Introduction.*—Posttransplantation lymphoproliferative disorders (PTLDs) cause significant morbidity and mortality in survivors of organ transplantation. In adults, primary Epstein-Barr virus (EBV) after transplantation is associated with an increased risk of having PTLD, and children are at higher risk of acquiring primary EBV posttransplantation because of their lower rate of exposure to the virus. A retrospective review of 120 pediatric thoracic organ recipients examined the frequency, clinical findings, predisposing factors, and outcome of PTLD.

*Methods.*—Included in the study were 61 girls and 59 boys who ranged in age from 1 day to 21 years at organ transplantation. There were 78 heart, 22 heart-lung, 18 double-lung, 1 single lung, and 1 heart-liver transplant recipients. Medical records were reviewed for EBV serologic findings, immunosuppressive regimen, and the prevalence and treatment of rejection. Charts of those in whom PTLD developed were further examined. Follow-up ranged from 1.5 months to 11.6 years.

*Results.*—Among the 103 children with documented pretransplantation EBV serologic status, 58 were seronegative and 45 were seropositive. Donor EBV serologic status, known for 30 patients, was positive in 11 and negative in 19. Fourteen children had a diagnosis of PTLD: 7.7% of the heart and 19.5 of the heart-lung/lung transplant recipients (not a statistically significant difference). Thirty (52%) of the previously seronegative children acquired primary EBV infection, and PTLD developed in 10 (33%) of them. In contrast, none of the children with evidence of past EBV infection had PTLD. Four additional patients had PTLD, including 2 with unknown pretransplantation EBV status and 2 who were found to have EBV IgM seropositivity on the day of transplantation. The signs of PTLD varied from asymptomatic lung nodules on chest radiography to diffuse multiorgan failure. Resolution of PTLD was achieved in 8 patients after a reduction in immunosuppressive therapy and the institution of antiviral therapy. Among the 8 patients who died, PTLD contributed to death in 5.

*Discussion.*—In this group of pediatric thoracic organ transplant recipients, there was a significant association between primary EBV infection posttransplant and the development of PTLD. Children in whom primary EBV infection develops posttransplant should be carefully observed for signs of PTLD and managed with a reduction in immunosuppression.

► As more heart and lung transplantations are carried out in the pediatric age group, familiarity with the potential complications is mandatory for the pediatric cardiologist. Posttransplantation lymphoproliferative disorders were found in 12% of this group of 120 children, with the higher percentage found in heart-lung or lung recipients. Patients who are seronegative for EBV before transplantation are at significantly greater risk for this complication. Chest radiography and CT (see Figures 1 and 2 in the article) can usually strongly suggest this diagnosis, but biopsy is required to provide specific data for treatment.

**T.P. Graham, M.D.**

## Epidemiology

**Periconceptional Multivitamin Use and the Occurrence of Conotruncal Heart Defects: Results From a Population-based, Case-Control Study**
Botto LD, Khoury MJ, Mulinare J, et al (Ctrs for Disease Control and Prevention, Atlanta, Ga)
*Pediatrics* 98:911–917, 1996                                                  4–45

*Background.*—Conotruncal heart defects are malformations of the cardiac outflow tract and a major cause of infant morbidity and mortality. There have been recent advances in medical and surgical treatment of these defects, but not all infants can be treated surgically. Also, the treatment itself is associated with substantial personal and economic costs and uncertain outcome. Studies have indicated that the use of multivitamins or folic acid alone around the time of conception can prevent neural tube defects and possibly some types of heart and other birth defects. The effect of periconceptional multivitamin use on the incidence of conotruncal defects was examined.

*Methods.*—A subset of the Atlanta Birth Defects Case-Control Study population was analyzed. A total of 158 infants with conotruncal defects and 3,026 unaffected, control infants were identified. The use of multivitamins from 3 months before pregnancy through the first 3 months of pregnancy was determined from telephone interviews. The relative risk of conotruncal defects associated with use of multivitamins was calculated.

*Results.*—The infants of mothers who reported taking multivitamins around the time of conception had a 43% lower risk of conotruncal defects than infants whose mothers did not take multivitamins. Of the relative risks for isolated conotruncal defects and defects associated with noncardiac defects or a recognized syndrome, the relative risk for isolated conotruncal defects was the lowest. The risk of anatomical subgroups of defects was also analyzed. The greatest reduction in risk was for transposition of the great arteries.

*Discussion.*—In these individuals, the use of multivitamins around the time of conception was associated with a lower risk of infant conotruncal defects. The protective effect was strongest for transposition of the great arteries, and somewhat less strong for tetralogy of Fallot. A lower risk of conotruncal defects was seen in mothers who used multivitamins around the time of conception, but not in those who began taking multivitamins at or after the second month of pregnancy. Increasing the use of multivitamins during this critical time before and during pregnancy may prevent conotruncal defects and significantly lower infant morbidity and mortality. Large doses of vitamin A during pregnancy may be associated with birth defects and should be avoided.

▶ There is a definite lower risk of a conotruncal defect in infants whose mothers received periconceptional multivitamins. These defects represent a major cause of infant morbidity and mortality and have been the subject of interesting new information regarding a gene defect and abnormalities of the neural crest. The 21st century hopefully will bring further enlightenment on cause and prevention of congenital heart disease.

**T.P. Graham, M.D.**

---

**Viral Infection of the Myocardium In Endocardial Fibroelastosis: Molecular Evidence for the Role of Mumps Virus as an Etiologic Agent**
Ni J, Bowles NE, Kim Y-H, et al (Baylor College of Medicine, Houston)
*Circulation* 95:133–139, 1997                                    4–46

---

*Background.*—Endocardial fibroelastosis is usually seen in infants and young children with signs of congestive heart failure. The incidence of endocardial fibroelastosis was about 1 in every 5,000 live births in the past but has recently declined. It was previously believed that myocarditis caused by viral infection of the myocardium was the first step in the pathogenesis of endocardial fibroelastosis. Enteroviruses and mumps virus were the suspected causes, but there was limited direct evidence for this. Polymerase chain reaction was recently shown to be a sensitive technique for identifying the viral genome in the myocardium of patients with myocarditis and dilated cardiomyopathy.

*Methods.*—Polymerase chain reaction or reverse transcriptase–polymerase chain reaction was used to analyze myocardial samples from 29 patients aged 26 weeks' gestation to 7 years with endocardial fibroelastosis at autopsy. Samples were analyzed for viral genome (enterovirus, adenovirus, mumps, cytomegalovirus, parvovirus, influenza, and herpes simplex virus). Samples from 65 control patients with no evidence of endocardial fibroelastosis or myocarditis were also examined.

*Results.*—The viral genome was amplified in 90% of samples. More than 70% of samples were positive for mumps viral RNA and 28% were positive for adenovirus. Only 1 of 65 control samples amplified a virus (enterovirus). Positivity for 2 regions of mumps virus was seen; these were the nucleocapsid gene and the polymerase-associated protein gene. Only 3 of 21 samples positive for mumps RNA showed positivity with both sets of primers. This suggested that the persistence of mumps virus in the myocardium may be associated with the selection of defective virus mutants.

*Discussion.*—Mumps virus genome in the myocardium was found in a significant number of these patients with endocardial fibroelastosis. These findings suggest that endocardial fibroelastosis is a complication of myocarditis caused by mumps virus rather than enterovirus. More research is needed to define the role of defective interfering viruses in the pathogenesis of disease.

▶ "This is deja vu all over again," as Yogi Berra would say. I remember mumps being considered the possible causal agent for endocardial fibroelastosis during my internship, which was so long ago I am having trouble remembering the year. With improved recognition of viral genomes, further evidence for a viral cause of many cardiomyopathies is becoming available.

**T.P. Graham, M.D.**

## Miscellaneous

### Restrictive Cardiomyopathies in Childhood: Etiologies and Natural History

Denfield SW, Rosenthal G, Gajarski RJ, et al (Texas Children's Hosp, Houston; Baylor College of Medicine, Houston)
*Tex Heart Inst J* 24:38–44, 1997                                          4–47

*Background.*—Children rarely have restrictive cardiomyopathy. What little is known about pediatric restrictive cardiomyopathy comes from a few small studies in which less than half of patients were alive at 2 years. Management is often extrapolated from that for adults, which may not be appropriate. Twelve cases of restrictive cardiomyopathy in children were reviewed to gain insight into the causes and natural history of this condition.

*Methods.*—The children were identified through a 27-year review of patient records. They were selected through echocardiographic and cardiac catheterization criteria. The patients were 6 boys and 6 girls (mean age, 4.6 years). The records were reviewed for information on age, sex, cause of restrictive cardiomyopathy, right- and left-sided cardiac hemodynamics, pulmonary vascular resistance index, shortening fraction, treatment, and outcome.

*Findings.*—The cause of restrictive cardiomyopathy was hypertrophic cardiomyopathy in 3 patients, cardiac hypertrophy with restrictive physiology in 3, idiopathic in 2, familial in 2 patients who were twins, "chronic eosinophilia" in 1, "postinflammatory" in 1, and no definitive cause in 1. The mean shortening fraction at initial evaluation was 33%. Right ventricular pressures averaged 44/13, whereas left ventricular pressures averaged 88/25. During 1 to 4 years' follow-up, the mean pulmonary vascular resistance index increased from 3.4 to 9.9 U · m². Embolic events occurred in 4 patients, including 2 with cerebrovascular accidents. Medical treatments included diuretics, verapamil, propranolol, digoxin, and captopril. Nevertheless, 9 of the 12 patients died within 6 years.

*Conclusion.*—Pediatric restrictive cardiomyopathy is a rare condition that is commonly idiopathic or is seen in association with cardiac hypertrophy. The prognosis is poor, with high rates of embolic events and death. Pulmonary vascular resistance often becomes very high within a few years after diagnosis, so early transplantation should be considered.

▶ Restrictive cardiomyopathy remains a rare and, unfortunately, usually fatal childhood problem. Many patients appear to have a fulminant course and require rapid consideration for heart transplantation, as medical therapy has not been helpful. Other patients appear to have a more indolent course and may remain stable with minimal symptoms for a number of years.

**T.P. Graham, M.D.**

---

**Cardiac Troponin I in Pediatrics: Normal Values and Potential Use in the Assessment of Cardiac Injury**
Hirsch R, Landt Y, Porter S, et al (Washington Univ, St Louis; State Univ of New York, Syracuse)
*J Pediatr* 130:872–877, 1997                                                    4–48

---

*Introduction.*—The diagnosis of myocardial injury in adults has markedly improved with the recent development of sensitive and specific assay procedures. Identification of myocardial cell damage either in isolated conditions or associated with other pathologic conditions through a sensitive and specific test is necessary in pediatrics. It is still not known what the clinical utility is of measuring serum cardiac troponin I for diagnostic or screening purposes in a pediatric population because normal values have not been established. Children with cardiac disease and those with no apparent cardiac disease had measurements taken of cardiac troponin I.

*Methods.*—There were 120 ambulatory children with no apparent cardiac disease, 96 patients in stable condition with known congenital or acquired cardiac abnormalities, 16 patients admitted to ICUs with normal echocardiograms, 36 with abnormal echocardiograms, and 7 patients with blunt chest trauma who were thought to have cardiac contusions. These children had measurements taken of the concentrations of their cardiac troponin I values.

*Results.*—In the normal children and in those in stable condition, the cardiac troponin I concentrations were generally less than 2.0 ng/mL and were frequently below the level of detection for the assay; these 2 groups of children showed no statistical differences. Cardiac troponin I values were greater than 2.0 ng/mL in the 9 patients in the ICU. Values less than 7.7 ng/mL were found in 6 of these patients, all of whom had abnormal echocardiograms. These patients showed improvement and normal cardiac troponin I concentrations. The other 3 patients who had values greater than 8.0 ng/mL did not survive; 2 had trauma and sepsis, and 1 had severe pulmonary hypertension. Cardiac troponin I concentrations were greater than 2.0 ng/mL in 3 of 4 patients with a high likelihood of cardiac contusions, and 1 of these patients died.

*Conclusion.*—In children with stable cardiac disease or general pediatric conditions, cardiac troponin I values are generally not elevated. Significant elevation of cardiac troponin I values may be an indicator of poor outcome in the context of severe short-term illness. In cases in which cardiac contusions are suspected, elevation of cardiac troponin I values may also have diagnostic value.

▶ The establishment of normal values for serum cardiac troponin I in children is a laudable goal. It appears that the vast majority of patients without clinical evidence of cardiac disease have values less than the normal lower limit, and these values are frequently below the level of detection for the current assay. Although cardiac troponin is apparently found only in cardiac muscle, there are a few false positives. Nevertheless, the data provided here will aid in finding more sensitive markers for the assessment of cardiac injury in children.

**T.P. Graham, M.D.**

---

### Is Mitral Valve Prolapse a Congenital or Acquired Disease?

Nascimento R, Freitas A, Teixeira F, et al (Unidade de Cardiologia Pediátrica, Funchal, Portugal)
*Am J Cardiol* 79:226–227, 1997                                    4–49

---

*Introduction.*—An examination of a large consecutive series of newborns was undertaken to determine the prevalence of mitral valve prolapse (MVP) at birth. This abnormality is generally considered to be acquired, although some authors have suggested that MVP is a congenital disease.

*Methods.*—During the period from January to June 1994 and in June and July 1995, 1,752 newborns were examined for evidence of MVP. This group of infants represented 95% of all live births at the study institution for the period; all but 1 of the 902 female and 850 male newborns were

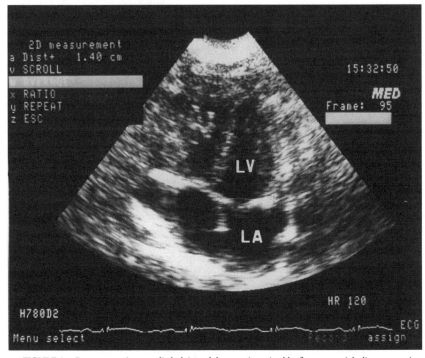

FIGURE 1.—Posterosuperior systolic bulging of the anterior mitral leaflet to a straight line connecting the annular leaflet hinge points as seen in the apical transition from 4- to 2-chamber views. *Abbreviations: LA,* left atrium; *LV,* left ventricle. (Reprinted by permission of the publisher from Nascimento R, Freitas A, Teixeira F, et al: Is mitral valve prolapse a congenital or acquired disease? *American Journal of Cardiology,* vol. 79, pp. 226–227, copyright 1997 by Excerpta Medica, Inc.)

white. Auscultatory signs of MVP were sought and echocardiographic studies requested when mothers reported a positive family history. Color flow and pulsed Doppler were performed to determine the timing and severity of mitral regurgitation. A second independent observer reviewed the echocardiograms for MVP identification.

*Results.*—Eighteen of the 1,752 newborns were excluded because of congenital structural heart disease. Eleven parents with MVP were identified, all with typical auscultatory and echocardiographic findings. None of the 1,734 infants without congenital heart disease had auscultatory signs of MVP. There were 19 infants with mild systolic bulging confined to the anterior leaflet (Fig 1), but none had posterosuperior displacement of the mitral leaflets to the line connecting the annular leaflet hinge points in the parasternal long-axis and apical 5- and 4-chamber views. The second observer's evaluation yielded no evidence of MVP.

*Discussion.*—Although 19 of 1,734 newborns had some bulging of the anterior leaflet beyond the reference line, none had altered papillary muscle systolic motion, pathologic mitral regurgitation, or abnormal thickening of mitral leaflets. Findings support the hypothesis that MVP is an acquired rather than a congenital disease.

▶ There continues to be a mild degree of controversy as to whether or not MVP is a congenital or acquired disease. There are rare newborns with severe connective tissue abnormalities, usually Marfan syndrome, who have obvious mitral prolapse and mitral regurgitation. These authors studied 1,752 normal newborns, including newborns in whom 11 parents had MVP by auscultation and echocardiography. They found no evidence of definite mitral prolapse in the infants. The presence of some mild bulging of the anterior leaflet beyond the annular leaflet hinge points in the apical 2-chamber view or in the transition from the 4- to 2-chamber view is common and not felt to be a definite sign of mitral prolapse (see Fig 1). Although the propensity for mitral prolapse is undoubtedly present in newborns, it is extremely uncommon for definite clinical or echocardiographic signs of this abnormality to be present in newborns other than those with severe connective tissue disorders.

**T.P. Graham, M.D.**

# 5 Cardiac Surgery

## Introduction

During the more than 40 years since the introduction of the heart-lung machine, there has been a continuing effort to introduce changes in operative technique, instrumentation, and equipment, and management protocols for pre- and postoperative care for cardiac surgical patients.

Progress in these very important areas necessitates change. Change, however, does not necessarily connote progress. The trick is to recognize those changes which provide an advantage without producing loss of simplicity, inordinate expense, or unforeseen risk.

The first section in this selection of cardiac surgical publications illustrates the variety of changes from which progress may eventually be distilled. The routine postoperative chest roentgenogram is questioned, while intraoperative echocardiography finds more and more utility. Even the ultimate diagnostic study, autopsy, is questioned.

One of the areas in which a great deal of activity has existed for several years is the use of antifibrinolytic agents. Some believe such agents should be used routinely, others prefer use only in reoperations or other special conditions, and there is the question of whether aprotinin (expensive) or ethylenediaminetetraacetic acid (EDTA) (less expensive) should be used. Then there are those who use hetastarch infusion, which seems to be associated with more bleeding.

The section on coronary artery surgery is still concerned with the selection of conduits and the development of techniques for minimally invasive operations. The section on aortic valve surgery reflects continuing interest in tissue valve replacement techniques. Comparison of the long experience with mechanical valves vs. tissue valves preserves the place of each in a comprehensive management program. Mitral valve surgery continues to be more concerned with reparative operations than replacements. In the section that follows, the question of whether implantable left ventricular assist devices may become an alternative to transplantation is debated. Intraluminal operations, as pointed out in the following section, are gradually receiving more interest and, in certain patients, appear to have substantial advantages. The Fontan and Mustard operations continue to occupy a most important area of pediatric cardiac surgical attention.

The last section consists only of two articles discussing management of pedicled intracavitary thrombi. This is an interesting area and the approach should perhaps not always be an open operation.

This collection of publications, I think, illustrates quite nicely what is happening in scientific cardiac surgery. There has been a particular attempt not to involve the question of cost vs. benefit ratios or management of contracts, insurance, or various payment packages. There is no doubt that these considerations have a substantial impact upon the practice of surgery, but it does seem tiresome that so much time and so much emphasis should occupy so many people to the exclusion of humanitarian or scientific consideration.

John J. Collins, Jr., M.D.

## General Problems in Open Heart Surgery

### Routine Chest Roentgenography on Admission to Intensive Care Unit After Heart Operations: Is It of Any Value?

O'Brien W, Karski JM, Cheng D, et al (Univ of Toronto)
*J Thorac Cardiovasc Surg* 113:130–133, 1997                                  5–1

*Bacgkround.*—Many hospitals still perform routine postoperative chest radiography after heart operations. However, some authors have questioned the need for this practice. The effects of routine postoperative chest radiography on ICU treatment of patients undergoing heart operations were analyzed.

*Methods.*—The study included a random sample of 404 patients admitted to the cardiovascular ICU after heart operations performed through a median sternotomy. All patients underwent a standard clinical assessment, including the positioning of the endotracheal tube, nasogastric tube, pulmonary artery catheter, and laboratory assessment of oxygenation. After these assessments were done, a chest radiograph was obtained and the findings were reviewed by the same cardiovascular ICU physician. Any abnormalities noted on the chest radiographs, and the required treatments, were recorded on the study form.

*Results.*—The chest radiograph detected conditions that required intervention but were not predicted by the protocol assessments in 4.5% of patients. Five patients required repositioning of the endotracheal tube, 8 had unexpected distal positioning of the pulmonary artery catheter, and 1 had pulmonary edema requiring diuretic treatment. None of these conditions were life-threatening, however.

*Conclusions.*—The findings question the need for routine chest radiography in patients who have undergone heart operations. Chest radiographs should be obtained only in patients whose postoperative assessments suggest a pathologic condition that can only be confirmed or excluded by radiography. It is estimated that this policy can reduce the number of chest radiographs taken at the study hospital by 83%, with attendant cost savings.

▶ The finding by Dr. O'Brien and his associates in Toronto that routinely obtaining a chest roentgenogram on return of a patient to the ICU may not be necessary is hardly arguable. Unfortunately, the reason that a routine chest roentgenogram is not an absolute necessity relates to the fact that careful examination of the patient may serve in lieu of the chest roentgenogram. Many personnel caring for patients in ICUs are not nearly so observant, and it may not be possible in many institutions to eliminate routine chest roentgenograms so safely. In procedures so simple and relatively inexpensive, what risk of major complication is tolerable to achieve the elimination of chest radiographs?

**J.J. Collins, Jr., M.D.**

### The Use of Transesophageal Echocardiography to Guide Sternal Division for Cardiac Operations via Mini-Sternotomy

Sardari FF, Schlunt ML, Applegate RL II, et al (Loma Linda Univ, Calif)
*J Card Surg* 12:67–70, 1997                                                   5–2

*Objective.*—The mini-sternotomy technique reduces pain and decreases the hospital stay. Transesophageal echocardiography (TEE) can be used to correctly position the sternal incision.

*Technique.*—A TEE probe is inserted into the endotracheal tube, and the right atrial-superior vena cava junction is imaged using a 90° scan plane. Depth of insertion in centimeters is marked on the probe scale and measured from the incisors or alveolar ridge. Distance from the incisors or alveolar ridge to the angle of the mandible is subtracted. The difference is the distance from the angle of the mandible to the midline of the sternum, or the site of incision. The "T" of the sternotomy is located just below this site over the right atrial appendage.

*Conclusion.*—Because patient anatomy may alter the extent of sternotomy, TEE can be useful in reliably predicting the level of the right atrium.

### Intraoperative Echocardiography Is Indicated in High-risk Coronary Artery Bypass Grafting

Savage RM, Lytle BW, Aronson S, et al (Cleveland Clinic Found, Ohio)
*Ann Thorac Surg* 64:368–374, 1997                                             5–3

*Objective.*—Intraoperative echocardiography has improved surgical results in valvular operations, congenital heart operations, and postoperative management. The effect of intraoperative echocardiography in the management of high-risk patients undergoing coronary artery bypass grafting and on clinical outcomes was examined.

*Methods.*—Between March and November 1995, intraoperative echocardiography was performed on 82 high-risk patients, with a preoperative severity score of more than 4, undergoing coronary artery bypass grafting.

The surgical and anesthesia team's management plans were documented without the assistance of intraoperative echocardiography. Alterations to the plans as a result of intraoperative echocardiography before cardiopulmonary bypass, before cardiopulmonary bypass separation with the heart filled and ejecting, after cardiopulmonary separation, and after chest closure were also documented. Perioperative morbidity and mortality were documented.

*Results.*—Alterations were triggered by significant arteriosclerotic or atheromatous disease, regional wall motion abnormalities, and global ventricular dysfunction. Coronary artery bypass grafting was performed without cardiopulmonary bypass in 3 patients with a severely calcified ascending aorta. When echocardiography detected anterior wall motion hypokinesia, 1 patient was placed on femoral artery-femoral vein cardiopulmonary bypass.

*Discussion.*—One study evaluating the diagnostic value of intraoperative transesophageal echocardiography assessed the technique as valuable or essential in 12% of patients and informative in 22%. Whereas intraoperative echocardiography is not yet routine, any management strategy for its use should require techniques that provide structural, functional, and hemodynamic information about the heart and large vessels. Patient risk is directly related to events involving cardiac operation, anesthesia, and extracorporeal circulation. Because intraoperative echocardiography is capable of assessing aortic pathology, valvular dysfunction, and ventricular function or segmental wall motion before and after bypass grafting, its influence on surgical and anesthesia decisions and ultimate patient outcome is significant.

*Conclusion.*—The use of intraoperative echocardiography in high-risk patients is safe and provides important information that has a significant impact in the intraoperative decision-making process.

▶ Advantages of intraoperative transesophageal echocardiography have been remarkable. In most units the anesthesiologists have become very skillful echocardiographers, and it is rarely necessary to send outside the operating room for appropriate expertise for interpretation of echocardiographic studies. The usefulness in high-risk coronary artery surgery is well known and the report by Sardari (Abstract 5–2) of the use of echocardiography for guidance in sternal incision making is previously unknown, at least to me.

**J.J. Collins, Jr., M.D.**

---

**The Autopsy: Still Important in Cardiac Surgery**
Zehr KJ, Liddicoat JR, Salazar JD, et al (Johns Hopkins Hosp, Baltimore, Md)
*Ann Thorac Surg* 64:380–383, 1997                                    5–4

---

*Background.*—Although autopsy has traditionally been used to determine the cause of in-hospital death, fewer autopsies are performed these days. In large part this is because, given the accuracy of current diagnostic tests, many physicians believe autopsies are unnecessary. Whether the current utilization of autopsy in cardiac surgery is appropriate was examined.

*Methods.*—Of 600 cardiac surgery patients who died in the hospital during an 11-year period, 147 (25%) received a postmortem examination. Autopsy results were compared with mortality conference notes prepared before the autopsy results were known, and agreement or disagreement was noted.

*Findings.*—The mortality conference notes and the autopsy results agreed in 76 (52%) of cases, but disagreed in 14 (0.5%). In 20 cases (14%), autopsy provided a definitive diagnosis when clinical signs could not, and in 37 (25%), even autopsy could not identify a definitive diagnosis. Findings that might have altered clinical management had they been recognized were revealed in 57 (39%) of the autopsies. Common causes of death determined by autopsy differed somewhat from those determined by clinical signs: cardiac (27% vs. 42%, respectively), sepsis (14% vs. 15%), stroke (9.9% vs. 9.5%), adult respiratory distress syndrome (4.1% vs. 4.8%), and unknown cause (25% vs. 14%). Autopsy also revealed cholesterol embolism (4%) and pulmonary embolism (4%) to be common causes of death. In 20 patients (14%), autopsy identified a cause of death that had not been suspected clinically.

*Conclusions.*—The need for autopsy is clear: In more than 20% of patients, results of the autopsy differed significantly enough from the clinical impressions to warrant its utility. Autopsy confirmed or revealed the cause of death in 75% of cases, and its utility may be greatest in examining suspected cases of technical error so that such errors can be avoided in the future. Ultimately, the autopsy is an important part of quality assurance.

▶ I am surprised that autopsy examinations showed significant difference from the final clinical impression in more than 20% of cases. One hopes that the majority of patients who did not have autopsy examination had that examination omitted because of certainty of the final clinical impression.

**J.J. Collins, Jr., M.D.**

---

### Prevention of the Hypoxic Reoxygenation Injury With the Use of a Leukocyte-depleting Filter

Bolling KS, Halldorsson A, Allen BS, et al (Univ of Illinois, Chicago)
*J Thorac Cardiovasc Surg* 113:1081–1090, 1997                    5–5

---

*Background.*—As the successful repair of cyanotic heart defects in infancy became more common, it was noted that postoperative myocardial dysfunction was a major cause of morbidity and mortality. Chronic cyanosis appears to make the immature heart more susceptible to oxygen-mediated injury. The polymorphonuclear leukocyte can produce oxygen-derived free radicals and is believed to be a major contributor to this reoxygenation injury. This suggests that reoxygenation injury could be decreased by utilizing a leukocyte filter in the cardiac bypass circuit. This method of preventing reoxygenation injury was explored in a newborn piglet model of cardiovascular hypoxia.

*Methods.*—Fifteen neonatal piglets were subjected to 60 minutes of ventilator hypoxia followed by reoxygenation with cardiopulmonary bypass for 90 minutes. In the 9 piglets of group 1, a routine bypass circuit was used. In the 6 piglets of group 2, a leukocyte-depleting filter was added in the arterial line. Six control piglets underwent bypass without hypoxia. Myocardial and pulmonary function was evaluated after bypass by pressure volume loops, arterial/alveolar ratio, and pulmonary vascular resistance index. Results were expressed as a percentage of control values.

*Results.*—Hypoxic newborn piglets who underwent reoxygenation with a leukocyte-depleting filter (group 2) had significantly better myocardial systolic function, diastolic compliance, preload recruitable stroke work, better preservation of the arterial/alveoalr ratio, and less increase in pulmonary vascular resistance than the piglets in group 1 who underwent the standard procedure. Leukocyte filtration also prevented adenosine triphosphate depletion and tissue antioxidant level changes. The results of bypass were very similar for group 2 piglets and control piglets.

*Conclusions.*—The results of this study employing a piglet model of reoxygenation of the hypoxic heart demonstrate that oxygen radicals produced by white blood cells are a major source of reoxygenation injury. This injury appears to be preventable with the use of a leukocyte-depleting filter during the bypass. When this injury is avoided, postbypass myocardial and pulmonary function are improved. This suggests that leukocyte depletion should be standard procedure for all children undergoing operation for cyanotic heart disease.

▶ It would appear from this experimental study that very serious consideration should be given to the use of a leukocyte-depleting filter for children with complex congenital heart disease. Perhaps adults also should be candidates when prolonged ischemic intervals are expected.

**J.J. Collins, Jr., M.D.**

---

**Antifibrinolytic Drugs and Perioperative Hemostasis**
Slaughter TF, Greenberg CS (Duke Univ, Durham, NC)
*Am J Hematol* 56:32–36, 1997                                    5–6

---

*Introduction.*—Excessive bleeding is a frequent complication of cardiac surgery. Antifibrinolytic drugs have been successful prophylactic hemostatic agents, but such treatment is not well known outside the surgical literature. The cause of coagulopathy after cardiac surgery involves multiple factors, but the success of antifibrinolytic drugs as hemostatic agents indicates that fibrinolysis contributes to the bleeding. There is a need for better awareness of the risks and benefits of perioperative antifibrinolytic therapy because of the increasing use of these drugs.

*Antifibrinolytic Drugs.*—Epsilon-aminocaproic acid and tranexamic acid are synthetic lysine analogues that suppress fibrinolytic activity by inhibiting the binding of plasminogen and plasmin to fibrin. Many studies have shown that aprotinin is effective in reducing blood loss after cardiac surgery. It has been shown that a high dose of aprotinin can consistently reduce bleeding by 30% to 50%. Aprotinin also reduces blood loss in cases of reoperation, bacterial endocarditis, patients receiving aspirin, and other high-risk settings.

*Comparisons of Antifibrinolytic Drugs.*—It is unknown if one antifibrinolytic drug provides better hemostasis than another. The current wholesale cost for a standard high-dose regimen of aprotinin is just over $1,000 per patient, compared with $11 per patient for ε-aminocaproic acid. There is evidence that both synthetic antifibrinolytic drugs and aprotinin reduce bleeding after cardiac surgery. Most prospective, randomized trials have not shown a significant difference in blood loss in patients given one drug or the other. A meta-analysis of antifibrinolytic drugs in cardiac surgery has shown that both synthetic antifibrinolytic drugs and aprotinin significantly reduce bleeding and the need for transfusion.

*Discussion.*—Synthetic antifibrinolytic drugs and aprotinin can inhibit fibrinolytic activity and bleeding during cardiac surgery without increasing the risk of perioperative thrombosis. The relative safety of antifibrinolytic drugs in cardiac surgery may be related to platelet dysfunction and trace levels of circulating heparin postoperatively. Although one advantage of aprotinin over synthetic antifibrinolytic drugs may be platelet protection and serine protease inhibitory activity, the best form of antifibrinolytic therapy in cardiac surgery has not been determined.

▶ Controversy over the use of antifibrinolytic drugs and their effect on postoperative bleeding continues (see the following 2 abstracts, Abstracts 5–7 and 5–8). I think it has been established that fibrinolysis is a significant contributor to postoperative bleeding, particularly in patients who have had complex reoperative surgery. There seems to be no evidence, however, to suggest that every patient undergoing cardiopulmonary bypass should receive antifibrinolytic therapy.

**J.J. Collins, Jr., M.D.**

---

**Tranexamic Acid Reduces Blood Loss and Transfusion in Reoperative Cardiac Surgery**
Dryden PJ, O'Conner JP, Jamieson WRE, et al (Univ of British Columbia, Vancouver)
*Can J Anaesth* 44:934–941, 1997                                                5–7

---

*Background.*—The benefits of reducing blood loss and the need for transfusion in cardiovascular surgery include less potential transmission of viral infections, improved outcome, shorter operating room time, and cost containment. There has been interest in using medication to help reduce surgical blood loss. Reoperative cardiac surgery carries a high risk of blood loss and need for transfusion. The antifibrinolytic agent tranexamic acid forms a reversible complex with plasminogen and removes it from the fibrin surface, thereby retarding fibrinolysis.

*Methods.*—In a randomized, double-blind, placebo-controlled study, 41 patients having reoperative valve replacement were given intravenous tranexamic acid 10 g in 500 mL of saline or placebo for 30 minutes after anesthesia induction and before incision. Intraoperative and postoperative blood loss were measured. A standardized protocol was used for transfusion of blood products.

*Results.*—The 2 patient groups were similar in age, weight, sex, surgical time, extracorporeal circulation time, cross-clamp time, complications, hospital stay, mortality, and number of valves replaced. Tranexamic acid reduced intraoperative blood loss from a median of 1,656 mL to 720 mL and postoperative blood loss from a median of 1,170 mL to 538 mL. The total red blood cells needed for transfusion was reduced from a median of 1,500 mL to 480 mL in patients given tranexamic acid. There was no reduction in complications or mortality rates in patients given tranexamic acid.

*Discussion.*—In patients undergoing reoperative valve replacement, tranexamic acid reduced blood loss and the need for transfusion. In patients undergoing complicated cardiac surgery involving repeat sternotomy and valvular surgery, prophylaxis with antifibrinolytic agents appeared to be effective.

## Antithrombin III During Cardiac Surgery: Effect on Response of Activated Clotting Time to Heparin and Relationship to Markers of Hemostatic Activation

Despotis GJ, Levine V, Joist JH, et al (Washington Univ, St Louis; St Louis Univ)
*Anesth Analg* 85:498–506, 1997

5–8

*Background.*—This study investigated the effect of antithrombin III concentrations on the response of the activated clotting time to heparin at levels used in cardiac surgery. Also, the relationship between concentrations of antithrombin III and markers of activation of coagulation during cardiopulmonary bypass was characterized.

*Methods.*—In phase 1, blood samples from 8 healthy subjects were used to measure the response of kaolin- and celite-activated clotting time to heparin after antithrombin III 200 U/dL was added in vitro, and after dilution with antithrombin III-deficient plasma to yield concentrations of 20, 40, 60, 80, and 100 U/dL antithrombin III. In phase 2, blood samples obtained before heparin was administered and before cardiopulmonary bypass was discontinued were used to determine the response of the kaolin-activated clotting time to heparin, antithrombin III levels, and various coagulation assays in 31 patients having repeat or combined cardiac surgeries.

*Results.*—In phase 1, there were strong linear relationships between kaolin- and celite-activated clotting time slopes and antithrombin III levels less than 100 U/dL. In the precardiopulmonary bypass period of phase 2, multivariate analysis showed that only factors V and VIII were independently associated with heparin-derived slope. Antithrombin III and fibrinopeptide A levels were inversely related at the end of cardiopulmonary bypass.

*Discussion.*—These findings show that the responsiveness of whole blood to heparin at the high levels used during cardiopulmonary bypass progressively decreases when the level of antithrombin III falls below 80 U/dL. Because antithrombin III is variably reduced in many patients during cardiopulmonary bypass, supplementing antithrombin III may help reduce excessive thrombin-mediated consumption of labile hemostatic blood components, excessive microvascular bleeding, and transfusion. Heparin is not as effective at anticoagulation during cardiac surgery at reduced levels. These findings indicate that antithrombin III may help preserve hemostasis during cardiopulmonary bypass.

---

**Prospective, Randomized, Double-blind Study of High-dose Aprotinin in Pediatric Cardiac Operations**
Davies MJ, Allen A, Kort H, et al (Great Ormond Street Hosp for Children, London; Harefield Hosp, Middlesex, England; Bayer PLC, Newbury, England)
*Ann Thorac Surg* 63:497–503, 1997                                             5–9

---

*Background.*—In adults, high-dose aprotinin can reduce perioperative bleeding during cardiac procedures with cardiopulmonary bypass. In children, the use of aprotinin may be warranted during cardiac operations because of the friability of tissue, proportionately long suture lines, poor tolerance to postoperative hemorrhage, complex surgical procedures with hypothermic cardiopulmonary bypass, and a high rate of reoperation. There is little information about the effectiveness of aprotinin in pediatric patients.

*Methods.*—There were 42 patients younger than 16 years undergoing open heart procedures with cardiopulmonary bypass. Patients were randomly assigned to high-dose aprotinin or placebo. Patients given aprotinin received a loading dose of 140 KIU/m², a priming dose of 240 KIU/m², and a continuous infusion of 56 KIU · m² · hr⁻¹. The time from protamine administration to skin closure, postoperative blood and hemoglobin loss, postoperative transfusion, and measures of fibrinolysis and platelet preservation were evaluated.

*Results.*—No significant differences were seen in any blood loss or transfusion parameters between the groups. Fibrin degradation product levels at 4 hours after operation were significantly increased in patients given placebo, but were unchanged in patients given aprotinin. In patients given placebo, beta-thromboglobulin levels increased faster during cardiopulmonary bypass than in patients given aprotinin.

*Discussion.*—In these patients, high-dose aprotinin had no benefit during cardiac procedures. At the study institution, the use of aprotinin is now restricted to reoperations because of the potential for reduced loss of hemoglobin, to first-time arterial switch operations, and to patients likely to hemorrhage.

▶ We have also concluded that aprotinin provides no clinical benefit in routine adult cardiac operations. We have discontinued its use under those circumstances. We still use either aprotinin or amicar in patients undergoing reoperative surgery, and we have the impression that this affords some reduction of postoperative bleeding. It is not easy to demonstrate, however, any significant advantage of one or the other.

**J.J. Collins, Jr., M.D.**

---

**Intraoperative Autologous Blood Donation Preserves Red Cell Mass But Does Not Decrease Postoperative Bleeding**
Helm RE, Klemperer JD, Rosengart TK, et al (New York Hosp-Cornell Med Ctr)
*Ann Thorac Surg* 62:1431–1441, 1996                                          5–10

---

*Objective.*—One method of blood conservation in cardiac surgery, intraoperative autologous donation (IAD), involves removal of some of the patient's blood before cardiopulmonary bypass (CPB) and reinfusing it after CPB. Whereas this technique is simple and cost-effective, results have been inconsistent. An optimized 3-principle IAD technique was developed that involved removal and preservation of a safe maximum volume of autologous blood, adherence to the lowest safe transfusion trigger during CPB, and use of IAD blood before banked blood for hematocrit values below this trigger. This technique was tested in a randomized, prospective, controlled trial.

*Methods.*—Ninety patients undergoing coronary artery bypass grafting ($n=60$) or valvular procedures ($n=30$) were randomly allocated to receive calculated maximum volume IAD or not to receive IAD. Transfusion guidelines are provided and were uniformly applied.

*Results.*—An average of 1540 ml of blood was removed from and reinfused in IAD patients. Crystalloid requirements in the IAD and control groups were similar. Homologous red blood cell transfusions were required for 17% of IAD patients and 52% of control patients ($P < 0.01$). The average number of units transfused per patient were 0.28 for IAD patients and 1.14 for control patients. The total number of allogenic red blood cell units transfused were 13 in the IAD group and 45 in the control group. At 4 and 12 hours postoperatively, hematocrit levels were significantly higher in the IAD group than in the control group (32.5% vs.

29.8% and 30.7% vs. 28.2%, respectively). Volume of chest tube drainage, incidence of increased bleeding after the first postoperative hour, incidence of excessive bleeding, and use of platelets, fresh frozen plasma, and cryoprecipitates were similar between groups.

*Conclusion.*—Maximum volume IAD preserved red cell mass and decreased dependence on homologous transfusion. The incidence of postoperative bleeding and transfusion requirements were not affected.

▶ This very nice paper by Dr. Robert Helm and his associates suggests that intraoperative autologous blood donation is probably not very useful for most patients.

**J.J. Collins, Jr., M.D.**

---

**Intraoperative Hetastarch Infusion Impairs Hemostasis After Cardiac Operations**
Cope JT, Banks D, Mauney MC, et al (Univ of Virginia, Charlottesville)
*Ann Thorac Surg* 63:78–83, 1997                                    5–11

---

*Objective.*—A bleeding outbreak occurred at 1 institution after cardiac operations when hetastarch (HES) was substituted for 5% albumin, which was in short supply. Whereas HES is an effective perioperative volume expander, its influence on coagulation has not been studied. Results of a retrospective review to evaluate the effects of intraoperative HES infusion shortly after termination of cardiopulmonary bypass (CPB) on hemostasis following a cardiac operation and the role of perioperative HES administration on the bleeding outbreak were discussed.

*Methods.*—Between April 1994 and April 1995, a bleeding outbreak occurred among 189 patients undergoing coronary artery bypass grafting. Patients were divided into those who received an average of 796 ml HES in the OR shortly after CPB was terminated (HIO, $n=68$), those who received an average of 856 ml HES during the 8-hour postoperative period (HPO, $n=59$), and those who did not receive HES (NH, $n=62$). Hematological parameters, mediastinal blood loss, and transfusion requirements were recorded.

*Results.*—Preoperative ASA was administered to approximately 50% of patients in each group. Postoperatively, 4 HIO patients had significantly lower hematocrit and platelet count, prolonged prothrombin time, but a similar partial thromboplastin time. Patients in this group also had significantly higher rates of chest tube drainage during the postoperative period. HES dose was significantly correlated with the rate of mediastinal blood loss in the HIO group. Significantly more patients in this group required administration of hemostatic agents to control chest tube drainage and had a greater need for postoperative transfusions and reexploration for mediastinal hemorrhage. Three patients in this group appeared to have generalized coagulopathy.

*Conclusion.*—Administration of HES shortly after discontinuing CPB increases the risk of bleeding after coronary artery bypass grafting.

▶ Our experience with Hetastarch is similar to what was observed by Dr. Cope and his associates.

**J.J. Collins, Jr., M.D.**

---

**Technical and Economic Feasibility of Reusing Disposable Perfusion Cannulas**
Bloom DF, Cornhill JF, Malchesky PS, et al (Cleveland Clinic Found, Ohio; STERIS Corp, Mentor, Ohio)
*J Thorac Cardiovasc Surg* 114:448–460, 1997                5–12

---

*Background.*—Although a perfusion cannula was often reused in the past, the current availability of single-use, disposable cannulas has promoted their use. However, disposable cannulas are more expensive, and finding a way to reuse them safely would be expected to result in cost savings. The safety, logistical, and economic issues of reusing disposable perfusion cannulas were examined.

*Methods.*—Single- and dual-stage perfusion cannulas were tested in 3 conditions: new, used once clinically, or used once clinically + 9 times in simulations. Reused catheters were rinsed with tap water, sonicated in a detergent solution, rinsed with deionized water, dried with compressed air, and sterilized by liquid chemicals before simulated reuse. Simulated use consisted of flexing the cannula, connecting it to the blood tubing adaptor, and soaking it in plasma. To verify sterilization, *Bacillus subtilis* was swabbed onto the cannulas and growth was monitored for 5 consecutive sterilization cycles. Sterilization was defined as the absence of growth in all 5 cycles. Physical and functional changes, biocompatibility, and in vivo testing (in sheep) were assessed.

*Findings.*—Sterilization was successful in each instance. A slight yellowing of the cannula was noted after reuse, and scarring increased at the site of the connector with repeated use. The internal diameters and the hardness of the cannula did not change with repeated use, although a 20% increase in stiffness occurred. However, a cardiac surgeon pronounced that none of these physical changes would have clinical significance. The cathethers remained biocompatible with repeated (simulated) reuse, and they performed adequately during in vivo tests. Reusing a cannula up to 5 times would result in a 65% savings (from $53.13 to $18.64 per procedure), or $110,364 during the course of a year.

*Conclusions.*—Perfusion cannulas can be safely reused without incurring clinical risks. The insignificance of the physical changes after reuse indicates that the cannulas could continue to be used safely. The few physical changes that occurred were easily identified by visual inspection, and the surgeon could eliminate these cannulas. Although the incremental cost savings were small, these savings would add up over the long-term.

Further studies are needed to assess the greater economic and clinical impacts of reusing perfusion cannulas.

▶ This study reported by Bloom et al. is very interesting indeed. I can't help but wonder whether the question of liability and the long trail directly back to the manufacturer of the plastic material involved in perfusion cannulas is not going to generate enough risk to discourage the concept of multiple-use perfusion cannulas. I think it must be of some concern when it is necessary to make a judgment as to whether perfusion cannulas should be used one more or two more times.

**J.J. Collins, Jr., M.D.**

---

**Higher Hematocrit Improves Cerebral Outcome After Deep Hypothermic Circulatory Arrest**
Shin'oka T, Shum-Tim D, Jonas RA, et al (Harvard Med School, Boston)
*J Thorac Cardiovasc Surg* 112:1610–1621, 1996                    5–13

---

*Background.*—Hemodilution is used during hypothermic cardiopulmonary bypass to counteract the negative rheologic sequelae of deep hypothermic circulatory arrest (DHCA). Hemodilution also reduces the oxygen-carrying capacity of the blood and may limit oxygen delivery to neurons. Direct evaluation of the sufficiency of oxygen delivery to cerebral cells is now possible with magnetic resonance spectroscopy (MRS) and near infra-red spectroscopy (NIRS). A piglet model was employed with simultaneous MRS and NIRS to examine the neurologic effects of perfusate hematocrit during DHCA.

*Methods.*—Seventeen piglets were randomly assigned to receive either colloid and crystalloid prime with a hematocrit of less than 10%, blood and crystalloid prime with a hematocrit of 20%, or blood prime with a hematocrit of 30% during DHCA. All piglets were subjected to 60 minutes of DHCA with continuous MRS and NIRS. Neurologic recovery was observed for 4 days, and then the animals were euthanized for histologic analysis.

*Results.*—The 10% hematocrit group had significant phosphocreatine loss and intracellular acidosis during early cooling. The final recovery was the same for all groups. Cytochrome $aa_3$ was more reduced in the low hematocrit group during DHCA than in the other 2 groups. The neurologic deficit score was best preserved in the high hematocrit group on the first postoperative day. All animals were neurologically normal at 4 days postoperation. Histologic assessment was the poorest in the neocortex of the low hematocrit group on day 4.

*Conclusions.*—During deep hypothermic circulatory arrest, extreme hemodilution is associated with evidence of inadequate oxygen delivery to neurons. Whole-blood priming is associated with optimal preservation of both mitochondrial redox state and high-energy phosphates, as well as better early neurologic and histologic scores. Higher hematocrit is associated with improved cerebral recovery after DHCA.

▶ In another experimental study from the Children's Hospital in Boston, it appears that higher hematocrits may result in better neurologic protection during deep hypothermia. I think the data suggest that higher hematocrit should be better in small children.

**J.J. Collins, Jr., M.D.**

## Coronary Artery Surgery

**Coronary Artery Bypass Grafting "On Pump": Role of Three-Day Discharge**
Ott RA, Gutfinger DE, Miller MP, et al (Univ of California Irvine Med Ctr, Orange)
*Ann Thorac Surg* 64:478–481, 1997                                         5–14

*Background.*—"Off-pump" coronary artery bypass grafting (CABG) has been touted as a method of reducing CABG-associated morbidity and reducing the length of postoperative hospital stay. These authors maintain that CABG with "on-pump" cardiopulmonary bypass (CPB) can achieve the same level of revascularization and reduced postoperative stay as the "off-pump" approach. Their experience was reported, as well as recommendations regarding which cases are most appropriate for such a rapid-recovery regimen.

*Methods.*—Isolated CABG with "on-pump" CPB was used in 104 patients. The recovery protocol focused on reduced CPB time (goal of 75 minutes), early extubation (12–24 hours after surgery), perioperative administration of corticosteroids and thyroid hormone, and aggressive diuresis. At the end of the first day, the goals were extubation, a negative fluid balance, and a lack of postoperative bleeding. On the second day, chest drains were removed and the patient started walking. On the third day, if the patient was walking without assistance, had normal bowel function, and had no atrial fibrillation, then he was discharged. Patients were followed up within 72 hours of discharge.

*Findings.*—Of the 102 survivors, 30 (29%) were discharged within 3 days after surgery (mean stay 3.0 ± 0.2 days) and 72 (71%) were discharged later (mean stay 5.5 ± 2.5 days). Patients who achieved early discharge differed from the others in significant ways: they were younger (61.8 years vs. 66.4 years), they were less likely to have diabetes (7% vs 28%), and they had a lower Parsonnet score (6.9 vs. 11). The early discharge group also tended to have fewer comorbidities such as congestive heart failure, symptomatic vascular disease, chronic obstructive pulmonary disease, ambulatory difficulties, and the need for a preoperative intra-aortic balloon pump. Patients with a longer hospital stay had a greater readmission rate than those discharged early (6.9% vs. 3.3%).

*Conclusions.*—Although ambitious, discharge 3 days after CABG with CPB is safe and cost-effective in a substantial percentage of patients.

Understanding the patient factors that increase the likelihood of a shorter hospital stay can ensure that this rapid-recovery regimen optimizes hospital stay and recovery. The reduction in CPB time is a key factor, particularly considering the morbidity associated with CPB.

▶ Dr. Ott has had a long interest in efficiency of cardiac surgical care. This report emphasizes that very early discharge is possible in patients who have had full sternotomy and CPB. I am sure this is true. When considering reports such as this, it is difficult to avoid concern about whether other units might be strongly tempted to discharge patients before they have achieved "maximum hospital benefit."

**J.J. Collins, Jr., M.D.**

---

**Troponin I Release During Minimally Invasive Coronary Artery Surgery**
Birdi I, Caputo M, Hutter JA, et al (Univ of Bristol, England)
*J Thorac Cardiovasc Surg* 114:509–510, 1997                    5–15

---

*Background.*—Increasingly, conventional left anterior descending artery (LAD) grafting with cardiopulmonary bypass (CPB) is being replaced by revascularization access through a left anterior small thoracotomy (LAST) without CPB. Although foregoing CPB may result in lower costs, the effects of LAD occlusion on the active myocardium have not been adequately characterized. Levels of troponin I, a specific marker for myocardial injury, were compared in patients undergoing LAST and in patients undergoing conventional LAD grafting with CPB.

*Methods.*—Two groups of 14 patients each underwent either the LAST approach (13 men, mean age 58 years) or the conventional CPB approach (12 men, mean age 57 years). All surgeries were elective, and left ventricular function was preserved. Troponin I levels were measured in blood samples drawn before the operation and at regular intervals up to 48 hours thereafter.

*Findings.*—Cardiopulmonary bypass lasted an average of 49 ± 8 minutes, with ischemic times in the LAST and conventional CPB groups of 37 ± 8 and 24 ± 5 minutes, respectively. In the conventional CPB group, troponin I was detected 4 hours after surgery, and levels remained significantly elevated compared with baseline up through 48 hours. In the LAST group, troponin I levels were measurable at 4 hours, but they declined thereafter and were much lower than those in the conventional CPB group.

*Conclusions.*—Myocardial injury, as indicated by troponin I release, may not be a significant consideration when the LAST approach is used. The fact that troponin I levels were lower in the LAST group than in the conventional CPB group lends further support for the development of minimally invasive cardiac surgical procedures.

▶ The finding of higher levels of troponin I release in patients who have had coronary bypass operations utilizing CPB compared with those having no use of the heart-lung machine comes as a surprise to me. I would not have thought there would be much difference.

**J.J. Collins, Jr., M.D.**

---

### Minimally Invasive Coronary Bypass for Protected Left Main Coronary Stenosis Angioplasty

Mack MJ, Brown DL, Sankaran A (Columbia Hosp at Medical City, Dallas)
*Ann Thorac Surg* 64:545–546, 1997                                              5–16

*Introduction.*—Coronary artery bypass grafting with cardiopulmonary bypass for circulatory support comprises conventional management of left main coronary artery disease. For management of "unprotected" left main coronary artery disease, percutaneous transluminal coronary angioplasty has not been acceptable because of the hazards of vessel occlusion during or after the procedure. A patient with left main coronary artery stenosis and significant comorbidities was successfully managed with minimally invasive direct coronary artery bypass as protection before percutaneous transluminal coronary angioplasty.

> *Case.*—Woman 73, with known coronary artery disease had unstable rest angina. She had cardiac catheterization and was turned down for surgical consideration because of comorbidities such as presenile dementia, scleroderma of the esophagus, and pulmonary hypertension. She then had a combined surgical and catheter intervention with a minimally invasive direct coronary artery bypass procedure.

*Results.*—A favorable outcome resulted with this "hybrid" approach for the management of a high-risk patient. This hybrid approach involved placing the left internal mammary artery to the left anterior descending coronary artery to serve as protection that allowed a safe catheter intervention to be performed on the left main coronary artery. Three days after the combined procedure, she was asymptomatic and was discharged. At 10-month follow-up, she was well and free of angina.

*Discussion.*—Minimally invasive coronary artery bypass grafting eliminates the median sternotomy incision and cardiopulmonary bypass, which are significant risk factors that add to the morbidity of conventional surgery. Through a limited left anterior thoracotomy, there is successful surgical revascularization of the left anterior descending coronary artery.

▶ The "hybrid" approach for management of patients with coronary artery disease is not very appealing to me. There may be instances where an inadequate operation should be combined with percutaneous transluminal coronary angioplasty, but these must be quite rare. Perhaps this patient illustrates the point.

**J.J. Collins, Jr., M.D.**

## Aortic Atheroma Is Related to Outcome but Not Numbers of Emboli During Coronary Bypass

Barbut D, Lo Y-W, Hartman GS, et al (Cornell Univ, New York)
*Ann Thorac Surg* 64:454–459, 1997       5–17

*Introduction.*—In substantial numbers of patients, coronary artery bypass grafting is associated with neurologic deficits. Several studies have found a correlation between severe aortic atheroma and stroke or death; however, the association between atheroma severity and nonneurologic indices of clinical outcome has not been determined. The impact of severe aortic atheromatosis on a number of outcome variables was determined, and its relation to numbers of emboli was defined.

*Methods.*—In 84 patients having operations, the severity of atheroma was determined in the ascending, arch, and descending aortic segments with transesophageal echocardiography. Transcranial Doppler ultrasonography was used to monitor 70 patients.

*Results.*—Among 74 patients with nonmobile plaque of the arch, the incidence of stroke was 2.7%; and among 9 patients with mobile plaque of the arch, the incidence of stroke was 33.3%. There was no significant relationship between cardiac complications and atheroma severity in any aortic segment. In the aortic arch and descending segment, atheroma severity was significantly related to length of stay. Significantly longer hospital stays were associated with the presence of severe atheroma in the arch and descending segments, compared with the hospital stays of patients with severe atheroma in neither segment. Patients with severe atheroma at clamp placement had greater numbers of emboli, but there was no statistical significance in the differences.

*Conclusions.*—Stroke and duration of hospitalization after coronary artery bypass grafting are related to aortic atheroma severity. There is a suggestion that many emboli may be nonatheromatous in nature because of the lack of correlation between numbers of emboli and atheroma severity. A strong association has been established between mobile plaque and stroke in patients having cardiac procedures. The increased procedural cost of transesophageal echocardiography in those patients with unidentified, severe aortic atheromatosis must be weighed against the cost-effectiveness of performing preoperative transesophageal echocardiography on all candidates for cardiac procedures in an attempt to identify those at high risk for increased length of stay and multisystem complications.

▶ Transesophageal echocardiography is better for imaging lesions in the descending aorta and the arch. An epicardial probe is more sensitive for atheromata of the ascending aorta.

**J.J. Collins, Jr., M.D.**

## Pathology of the Radial and Internal Thoracic Arteries Used as Coronary Artery Bypass Grafts

Kaufer E, Factor SM, Frame R, et al (Montefiore Med Ctr, Bronx, NY)

*Ann Thorac Surg* 63:1118–1122, 1997                                    5–18

*Background.*—In the 1970s, the use of the radial artery as a coronary artery bypass graft was proposed by Carpentier et al. This was abandoned after a short time because about a third of the radial artery grafts were occluded, and another third had severe stenosis. There has been renewed interest in the radial artery as a coronary artery bypass graft after it was discovered that 3 radial artery grafts from the Carpentier study believed to have early postoperative occlusion were patent and free of atherosclerotic lesions 15 years later. Refinement of harvesting and preparation techniques and the use of calcium channel blockers have contributed to current high early patency rates. The incidence and degree of atherosclerosis in radial artery and internal thoracic artery segments after coronary artery bypass grafting were compared.

*Methods.*—Histologic analysis was done in 170 specimens from 102 patients. There were 106 radial artery specimens, 62 left internal thoracic artery specimens, and 2 right internal thoracic artery specimens.

*Results.*—The mean degree of atherosclerosis in the radial artery was 0.89 on a scale of 0–4. The mean grade of atherosclerosis for the internal thoracic artery was 0.30. There was a correlation between presence of diabetes, aortofemoral disease, femoral-popliteal disease, age, and male gender and an increase in radial artery pathology. There was no correlation between flow in the in situ radial artery and degree of pathology.

*Discussion.*—Analysis of the excess radial artery and internal thoracic artery segments after coronary artery bypass grafting showed that a higher degree of atherosclerosis was present in the radial artery than in the internal thoracic artery at the time of harvest. Overall, the degree of disease in the radial artery was low. Long-term performance of these grafts will determine if this degree of atherosclerotic disease is clinically significant. The finding that grafts that are patent at 5 years are likely to remain patent indicates that early occlusion results from intimal hyperplasia, which can be avoided by harvesting the radial artery with its vena comitantes and avoiding mechanical luminal dilatation.

▶ These data, reported by Kaufer and associates, suggest that radial artery grafts may be less efficacious than many believe. Time will tell.

**J.J. Collins, Jr., M.D.**

## Use of Cardiac Procedures and Outcomes in Elderly Patients With Myocardial Infarction in the United States and Canada

Tu JV, Pashos CL, Naylor CD, et al (Inst for Clinical Evaluative Sciences, Ont, North York, Canada; Univ of Toronto; Abt Associates, Cambridge, Mass; et al)
*N Engl J Med* 336:1500–1505, 1997                                      5–19

*Introduction.*—Medical care in Canada and the United States is often compared during the debate over health care reform because the 2 countries have different methods of financing care. Previous studies have found that the higher rates of revascularization in the United States than in Canada just after the postinfarction period had slightly improved the quality of life; however, survival benefits were less convincing. The use of cardiac procedures and mortality were compared between U.S. and Canadian cohorts of elderly patients with new acute myocardial infarctions.

*Methods.*—There were 9,444 elderly patients in Ontario, Canada, and 224,258 elderly Medicare beneficiaries in the United States with a new acute myocardial infarction in 1991. The use of invasive cardiac procedures and the mortality rates were compared in these 2 groups.

*Results.*—Coronary angiography was performed more often for U.S. patients than Canadian patients (34.7% vs. 6.7%) (Fig 1). Percutaneous transluminal coronary angioplasty was also performed more often for U.S. patients than for Canadian patients (11.7% vs. 1.5%), as was coronary-artery bypass surgery (10.6% vs. 1.4%) (Fig 2). These were found during

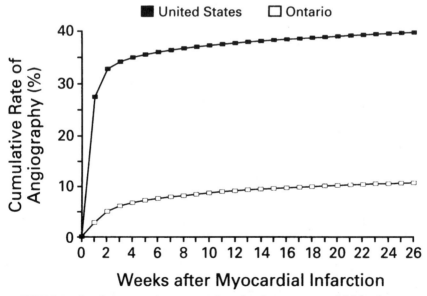

**FIGURE 1.**—Cumulative rates of coronary angiography after acute myocardial infarction among elderly patients in the United States and Ontario, 1991. (Courtesy of Tu JV, Pashos CL, Naylor CD, et al: Use of cardiac procedures and outcomes in elderly patients with myocardial infarction in the United States and Canada. *N Engl J Med* 336:1500–1505. Copyright 1997, Massachusetts Medical Society. Reprinted by permission of *The New England Journal of Medicine.* All rights reserved.)

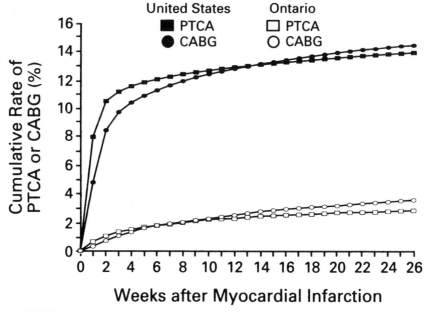

FIGURE 2.—Cumulative rates of percutaneous transluminal coronary angioplasty and coronary-artery bypass grafting after acute myocardial infarction among elderly patients in the United States and Ontario, 1991. (Courtesy of Tu JV, Pashos CL, Naylor CD, et al: Use of cardiac procedures and outcomes in elderly patients with myocardial infarction in the United States and Canada. *N Engl J Med* 336: 1500–1505. Copyright 1997, Massachusetts Medical Society. Reprinted by permission of *The New England Journal of Medicine*. All rights reserved.)

the first 30 days after the index infarction. Through 180 days of follow-up, these differences narrowed but persisted. For the U.S. patients, the 30-day mortality rates were slightly lower than for Canadian patients (21.4% vs. 22.3%). There were virtually identical 1-year mortality rates (34.3% in the United States and 34.4% in Canada) (Fig 3).

*Conclusion.*—In the United States, short-term mortality after an acute myocardial infarction was slightly lower than in Ontario; but at 1-year follow-up, these differences did not persist. Better long-term survival rates for elderly U.S. patients with acute myocardial infarction are not evident, despite cardiac procedures being performed at strikingly higher rates in U.S. patients than in Canadian patients. The long-term survival rates of elderly U.S. patients with acute myocardial infarction are not improved with the greater use of revascularization procedures. Before firm conclusions can be drawn, additional population-based studies with more detailed data on medical treatments and patients' characteristics are required.

▶ The study reported by Tu and associates has to be of great interest. I think the obvious next question would relate to lifestyle among the survivors of myocardial infarction. These data are not presented in the reported study. Nevertheless, this study is certainly provocative and perhaps this is evidence

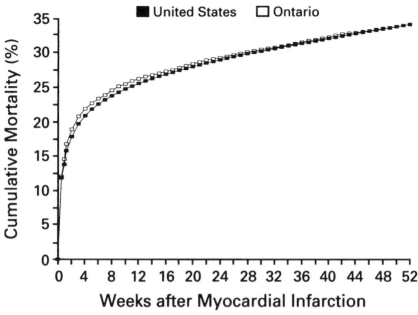

■ United States   □ Ontario

**Weeks after Myocardial Infarction**

FIGURE 3.—Cumulative mortality after acute myocardial infarction among elderly patients in the United States and Ontario, 1991. (Courtesy of Tu JV, Pashos CL, Naylor CD, et al: Use of cardiac procedures and outcomes in elderly patients with myocardial infarction in the United States and Canada. *N Engl J Med* 336:1500–1505. Copyright 1997, Massachusetts Medical Society. Reprinted by permission of *The New England Journal of Medicine*. All rights reserved.)

that we do use coronary bypass in more than the minimally necessary number of patients.

**J.J. Collins, Jr., M.D.**

---

**Bilateral Thoracotomy and Inferior Sternotomy for Bypass Grafting After Esophagostomy**
Smedira NG, Eng J, Rice TW (Cleveland Clinic Found, Ohio)
*Ann Thorac Surg* 63:847–849, 1997                                                   5–20

---

*Introduction.*—In cardiac surgical procedures, the median sternotomy incision is the most common approach to the heart. However, for some patients, an alternative approach is necessary. By using a modified bilateral thoracotomy before esophageal reconstruction, coronary artery bypass grafting was performed in a patient with cervical esophagostomy.

*Case Report.*—Man, 69, had atypical anginal chest pain, a history of dyspnea on exertion, and ischemia. He had lower esophageal perforation, and the left pleural space was grossly contaminated at left thoracotomy. A thoracic esophagectomy was performed. After the operation, he had septicemia, atrial fibrillation,

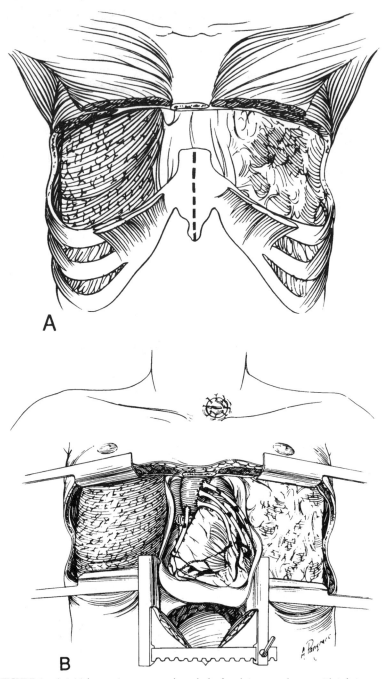

FIGURE 1.—A, initial operative exposure through the fourth intercostal space with inferior sternotomy. B, excellent exposure to the heart and pleural space for coronary artery bypass grafting. (Courtesy of Smedira NG, Eng J, Rice TW: Bilateral thoracotomy and inferior sternotomy for bypass grafting after esophagostomy. *Ann Thorac Surg* 63:847–849, 1997. Reprinted with permission from the Society of Thoracic Surgeons.)

and required prolonged ventilation. Before esophageal reconstruction, he needed myocardial revascularization.

*Bypass Grafting.*—A bilateral thoracotomy incision was used to avoid jeopardizing the esophageal stoma on the lower and medial left side of his neck. The lower sternum was divided in the midline to improve exposure of the inferior part of the heart (Fig 1). Aortocoronary bypass grafts were performed with segments of reversed saphenous vein. Esophageal reconstruction was performed.

*Discussion.*—Maneuvers that might jeopardize the esophagostomy were avoided by confining the surgical field to the lower part of the chest. Bilateral lung transplantation and other bilateral pulmonary procedures have been associated with the bilateral anterior thoracotomy incision, and its familiarity allows it to be adapted for cardiac surgical procedures.

▶ Coronary bypass surgery after either tracheostomy or esophagostomy can be a problem. This approach by Smedira and associates at the Cleveland Clinic may be useful. We have also utilized development of a flap at the upper portion of the sternotomy incision and dissecting beneath the flap for a distance of 2 or 3 inches to allow placing a saw in the sternal notch as usual. This works well in our hands. In addition, it may perhaps be simpler for most surgeons.

**J.J. Collins, Jr., M.D.**

---

**Surgical Resection of Right Coronary Artery Stenoses**
Zingone B, Dreas L (Ospedale Maggiore, Trieste, Italy)
*J Card Surg* 12:77–80, 1997                                            5–21

---

*Background.*—The technique of segmental resection of right coronary artery lesions followed by end-to-end anastomosis artery reconstruction has been used as an alternative to bypass grafting.

*Technique.*—Short, isolated focal obstructions within a relatively healthy right coronary artery were selected for resection. The artery was inspected and the lesion located. The artery was divided downstream from the stenosis and then opened until normal wall was observed. Up to 20 mm of diseased artery could be resected. End-to-end reconstruction was performed with continuous sutures. The operation was completed with additional internal thoracic artery grafts as needed. The procedure was performed on 8 patients with angina and multivessel coronary artery disease.

*Results.*—The average number of coronary arteries revascularized was 3 per patient. All patients recovered from the procedure uneventfully and were discharged home after 7–13 days. No myocardial infarction or angina was experienced by these patients with up to 15 months of follow-up.

*Conclusions.*—This report describes surgical resection of right coronary artery stenoses followed by end-to-end reconstruction to restore a patent arterial lumen lined with normal intima without resorting to bypass grafting. With proper selection criteria, this technique is a viable alternative to bypass grafting in the right coronary artery. Further follow-up is necessary to evaluate the long-term efficacy of this procedure.

▶ Resection of localized coronary artery obstructions is a reasonable option when the coronary artery can be sufficiently mobilized for a comfortable primary anastomosis. I think this is probably often true in the right coronary artery, but I rather doubt that it will frequently be found to be the case in the left coronary branches.

**J.J. Collins, Jr., M.D.**

---

**New Approach to Patency and Flow Assessment After Left Internal Thoracic Artery Hypoperfusion Syndrome With Additional Saphenous Vein Graft to the Left Anterior Descending Artery With Phase-Contrast Magnetic Resonance Angiography**
Zünd G, Hauser M, Vogt P, et al (Zurich Univ Hosp, Switzerland)
*J Thorac Cardiovasc Surg* 114:428–433, 1997                    5–22

---

*Background.*—The left internal thoracic artery (LITA) is the most popular conduit for revascularization. However, spasms, steal phenomena, a small LITA, or excessive myocardial flow demand in a hypertrophied ventricle can lead to LITA hypoperfusion syndrome, a rare but potentially fatal complication. Some surgeons advocate adding another vein graft to the distal left anterior descending artery (LAD) to improve myocardial perfusion and prevent myocardial infarction, whereas others believe that a high-flow LAD graft could lead to concurrent or backward LITA flow. Postoperative flow rates in both LITA and LAD grafts were examined.

*Methods.*—Left anterior descending artery grafts were used in 21 patients in whom LITA hypoperfusion syndrome developed (1.8% of all patients undergoing myocardial revascularization at the authors' institution). Of these, 19 underwent phase-contrast magnetic angiography to determine early (less than 6 months) and late (greater than 12 months) flow rates in the 2 grafts.

*Findings.*—All grafts were patent at both early and late measurements; mean flow rates were 49.2 mL/min for the LAD graft and 72.6 mL/min for the LITA graft. Coronary flow was always in the appropriate direction for the graft, with diastolic perfusion the most prominent finding. Angiography revealed no concurrent flow, flow reversal, or steal phenomena.

*Conclusions.*—Early diagnosis and treatment of the LITA hypoperfusion syndrome is imperative, and the addition of an LAD graft resulted in satisfactory flow rates with no flow abnormalities whatsoever. Furthermore, obstruction was not a problem because all the conduits were patent. Flow in the conduits adapted early, moving to the diastolic predominance within 6 months after surgery. Based on their results, the authors recommend creating a distal LAD graft during cardiac revascularization in patients with LITA hypoperfusion syndrome.

▶ Most surgeons, when confronted with apparent hypoperfusion of the anterior descending coronary artery after grafting with the left internal mammary artery, proceed directly to saphenous vein grafting of the distal anterior descending coronary artery. They will be comforted to see this study.

**J.J. Collins, Jr., M.D.**

---

## Simvastatin Reduces Graft Vessel Disease and Mortality After Heart Transplantation: A Four-Year Randomized Trial

Wenke K, Meiser B, Thiery J, et al (Univ Hosp, Munich-Grosshadern, Germany)
*Circulation* 96:1398–1402, 1997                                                    5–23

*Introduction.*—The most critical long-term complication of heart transplantation is accelerated graft vessel disease (GVD). It is possible that progressive coronary vascular disease is the result of posttransplantation hypercholesterolemia. The efficacy of primary antihypercholesterolemia with simvastatin was compared with that of general dietary therapy in a 4-year prospective, randomized trial of 72 patients who underwent orthotopic heart transplantation.

*Methods.*—The goal was to maintain posttransplant low-density lipoprotein (LDL) cholesterol levels at below 120 mg/dL. All patients received triple immunosuppression therapy. Patients were randomized to an active treatment group that received a low-cholesterol diet and simvastatin (10 mg/day initially, depending on their LDL cholesterol level, then increased to 10 mg/day at 6 weeks if needed) or a control group that was treated with dietary measures alone.

*Results.*—During the course of the trial, the mean serum cholesterol level in the simvastatin group was significantly lower than that of the control group (Fig 1). Patients in the simvastatin group also had significantly better long-term survival (Fig 2) and a decreased incidence of GVD in coronary angiographic findings (16.6% vs. 42.3%). At 4 years, 88.6% of patients in the simvastatin group and 70.3% of patients in the control group were alive. There were no significant between-group differences in the occurrence of graft rejections, but there was a decreased tendency toward serious rejections in the simvastatin group, compared with the control group (2.8% vs. 13.5%). In a subgroup of 10 patients from the simvastatin group and 17 patients from the control group, patients with an LDL cholesterol level less than 110 mg/dL had significantly less intimal thickening and a significantly lower intimal index than patients with higher cholesterol levels.

*Conclusion.*—Compared with dietary measures alone, patients in a treatment group of simvastatin and diet who underwent heart transplan-

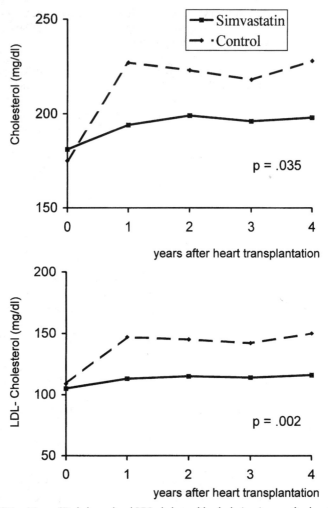

FIGURE 1.—Mean ±SD cholesterol and LDL cholesterol levels during 4 years after heart transplantation (to convert values to mmol/L, multiply by 0.02586). (Courtesy of Wenke K, Meiser B, Thiery J: Simvastatin reduces graft vessel disease and mortality after heart transplantation: A four-year randomized trial. *Circulation* 96:1398–1402, 1997. Reproduced by permission of *Circulation*. Copyright 1997 American Heart Association.)

tation had a significant reduction in cholesterol levels, a significantly higher long-term survival rate, and a lower incidence of GVD.

▶ These data strongly suggest that simvastatin or a similar antihypercholesterolemic drug should be used in patients following cardiac transplantation.

**J.J. Collins, Jr., M.D.**

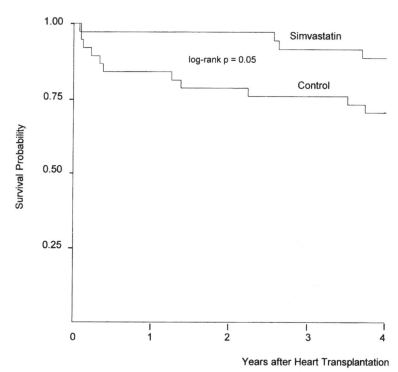

FIGURE 2.—Kaplan-Meyer curves for survival 4 years after heart transplantation in the study patients. (Courtesy of Wenke K, Meiser B, Thiery J: Simvastatin reduces graft vessel disease and mortality after heart transplantation: A four-year randomized trial. *Circulation* 96:1398–1402, 1997. Reproduced by permission of *Circulation*. Copyright 1997 American Heart Association.)

## Angiographic Features of Vein Grafts Versus Ungrafted Coronary Arteries in Patients With Unstable Angina and Previous Bypass Surgery

Chen L, Théroux P, Lespérance J, et al (Montreal Heart Inst)
*J Am Coll Cardiol* 28:1493–1499, 1996                                    5–24

*Objective.*—Whereas the pathogenesis of vein graft atherosclerosis is known to differ from that of coronary artery atherosclerosis, the angiographic features associated with unstable angina have not been systematically studied. Progression of atherosclerosis and the angiographic features of the culprit lesions are compared for grafts and native coronary arteries in patients with unstable angina and previous coronary artery bypass graft surgery (CABG).

*Methods.*—Between December 1991 and September 1993, 95 patients (16 women), aged 40 to 80, with unstable angina or non-Q wave myocardial infarction (MI) who had undergone CABG at least 6 months before, were entered into a randomized, double-blind, placebo-controlled trial. The trial qualitatively and quantitatively assessed disease progression and angiographic features of vein grafts and ingrafted and grafted coronary arteries within 8 days of admission. Culprit lesions were defined by the location of stenosis progression corresponding to ECG abnormalities and new wall motion abnormalities.

*Results.*—Streptokinase was given to 46 patients and placebo to 49. There was angiographically documented 1-, 2-, and 3-vessel disease in 6%, 28%, and 65% of patients. Functionally, 34% had 0- or 1-vessel disease, and 66% had 3-vessel disease. The culprit vessel was identified in 77 patients, as a vein graft in 51, as an ungrafted native coronary artery in 17, and as a grafted coronary artery in 9. There was total occlusion in 49% of vein grafts and 24% of ungrafted coronary arteries. A thrombus was detected in 37% of culprit vein grafts and 12% of ungrafted coronary arteries. Within the first 5 years after CABG, vein grafts and native arteries were approximately equally responsible for episodes of unstable angina. After 10 years, culprit lesions were found in a graft in 22 of 24 patients. Six culprit vein grafts and no ungrafted coronary arteries were shown to have intravessel thrombi and total occlusion. Streptokinase had no influence on the development of total occlusion or thrombus.

*Conclusion.*—Unstable angina in patients with previous CABG is mainly the result of graft disease. These patients also have an increased incidence of thrombus that does not respond to therapy.

▶ This very interesting paper by Dr. Lijia Chen and associates confirms the observation that recurrence of unstable angina in patients after coronary surgery is usually due to graft obstruction rather than progression of native arterial disease. Native arterial disease becomes progressive more commonly with increasing age and the time since operation.

**J.J. Collins, Jr., M.D.**

---

**A Profile of Candidates for Repeat Myocardial Revascularization: Implications for Selection of Treatment**
Brener SJ, Loop FD, Lytle BW, et al (Cleveland Clinic Found, Ohio)
*J Thorac Cardiovasc Surg* 114:153–161, 1997                    5–25

---

*Introduction.*—Both coronary artery bypass grafting (CABG) and percutaneous transluminal coronary angioplasty (PTCA) are associated with increased risk and decreased efficacy in patients who have undergone prior bypass surgery. Differences between patients with prior bypass grafts referred for surgery or angioplasty were assessed to determine the clinical and angiographic findings that correlated best with either choice and to find clues that could help in selecting 1 treatment over another.

*Methods.*—During a 2-year period, 870 patients who underwent first isolated reoperation and 793 patients who underwent first balloon angioplasty after a previous operation were assessed to compare the following: angiographic and echocardiographic data and jeopardy scores. The jeopardy scores of 0–8 are based on the proportion of myocardium supplied by native coronary arteries or bypass grafts with flow-limiting stenosis.

*Results.*—Forty-two (4.8%) patients with repeat CABG died, compared with 4 (0.5%) patients with repeat PTCA. The rate of Q-wave myocardial infarction was 1.4% (11 patients) for the PTCA group and 3.7% (32 patients) for the CABG group. Patients referred for repeat CABG had a larger proportion of myocardium that could be revascularized, compared with patients referred for repeat PTCA. Progression of native coronary atherosclerosis caused new symptoms in two thirds of patients who underwent PTCA. This progression, rather than vein graft disease, caused a shorter interval between revascularization in the PTCA group, compared with the CABG group. There was an independent association between CABG and higher jeopardy score, diabetes, and coexisting valvular disease with referral to CABG for revascularization. A patent arterial graft to the left anterior descending coronary artery and a higher number of functional grafts were related to PTCA as a revascularization strategy. Age, gender, and severe left ventricular systolic dysfunction were not significantly related to either surgical approach.

*Conclusion.*—When large regions of myocardium were in jeopardy, reoperation was the preferred procedure. Angioplasty was chosen more frequently with patent arterial graft to the left anterior descending coronary artery or multiple functioning bypass grafts. Increased risk of in-hospital complications was associated with reoperation, compared with angioplasty.

▶ This interesting study from the Cleveland Clinic examines a large group of patients who underwent either angioplasty or open reoperation following previous coronary surgery.

The criteria used to prescribe one or the other procedure are similar in many other institutions, I'm sure.

**J.J. Collins, Jr., M.D.**

---

**Effect of Cardiac Surgery Patient Characteristics on Patient Outcomes From 1981 Through 1995**
Warner CD, Weintraub WS, Craver JM, et al (Emory Healthcare, Atlanta, Ga)
*Circulation* 96:1575–1579, 1997                                                5–26

---

*Introduction.*—There is an increasing trend toward performing coronary artery bypass graft (CABG) surgery on patients who are older and high risk. Outcome of this trend is not well documented. Patients from 3 different periods were evaluated to determine if the trend toward higher risk patients is continuing and to evaluate the effect risk has on in-patient outcomes.

*Methods.*—The 3 periods were 1981–1987 (group I), 1988–1992 (group II), and 1993–1995 (group III). Data were collected prospectively and compared using univariate and multivariate analyses.

*Results.*—Group characteristics changed significantly over the 3 periods. High-risk characteristics increased with each period, with the greatest increase in risk noted between groups I and II. The mean age and percentage of patients over age 65 years were significantly higher in group II than they were in group I. This change was slight between group II and group III. There was a significant increase in the number of patients 80 years and older from group I to group II and from group II to group III. There was an association between increased risk and increased mortality in group II, but there was a decline in group III, despite continued increase in patient risk. Actual mortality for group III was lower than what was predicted. Complications increased in group II but not in group III.

*Conclusion.*—Although there has been a trend toward performing CABG on high-risk patients, in-hospital mortality rates have been decreasing. This decrease may reflect improved technology and greater expertise on the part of health care providers. Patient complexity and complications increase the length of stay, but economic pressures have not caused a preferred selection of low-risk patients.

▶ This study once again documents the remarkable improvement in surgical care for high-risk patients. This cannot continue forever.

**J.J. Collins, Jr., M.D.**

## Aortic Valve Surgery

**Geometric Mismatch of the Aortic and Pulmonary Roots Causes Aortic Insufficiency After the Ross Procedure**
David TE, Omran A, Webb G, et al (Toronto Hosp; Univ of Toronto)
*J Thorac Cardiovasc Surg* 112:1231–1239, 1996                    5–27

*Introduction.*—A patient's diseased aortic valve is replaced with the normal pulmonary valve in a complex operation called the Ross procedure. Postoperative aortic insufficiency is common, regardless of the operative technique used to implant the pulmonary valve in the aortic position. Aortic insufficiency may be caused by geometric mismatch between the diseased aortic valve and the normal pulmonary valve. By adjusting the diameter of the aortic anulus and of the sinotubular junction of the aortic root to those of the pulmonary root during implantation of the pulmonary valve in the aortic position, aortic insufficiency may be prevented.

*Methods.*—Within a 5-year period, the Ross procedure was performed in 81 patients. In 77 patients, the diameters of the aortic and pulmonary roots were measured. In 27 patients, reduction of the aortic anulus and of the sinotubular junction was necessary. In 12 patients, reduction of the aortic anulus alone was necessary, and in 10 patients, reduction of the sinotubular junction alone was necessary. In 2 patients, the pulmonary autograft was implanted in the subcoronary position in the aortic root. In 58 patients, the pulmonary autograft was implanted as a complete root replacement. In 21 patients, the pulmonary autograft was implanted as an inclusion root. Patients were followed up for a mean of 15 months, and a range of 2 to 64 months.

*Results.*—Myocardial infarction caused 1 operative death. One patient did not have measurement and reduction of the aortic anulus, and aortic insufficiency developed, making it necessary to have aortic root replacement 2 weeks later. One patient had pulmonary artery stenosis and another had a false aneurysm between the autograft and the mitral valve, and both of these patients required late reoperations. Ten percent of patients have mild aortic insufficiency, and 90% have only trace or no aortic insufficiency, according to the most recent Doppler echocardiographic study.

*Conclusion.*—To prevent aortic insufficiency after the Ross procedure, adjustment of the diameter of the aortic anulus or of the sinotubular junction of the aorta may be important, as are intraoperative measurements of both semilunar valves.

---

**Pulmonary Autograft Versus Homograft Replacement of the Aortic Valve: A Prospective Randomized Trial**
Santini F, Dyke C, Edwards S, et al (Harefield Hosp, Middlesex, England)
*J Thorac Cardiovasc Surg* 113:894–900, 1997                    5–28

---

*Background.*—If aortic valve disease is left untreated, ventricular hypertrophy or dilatation can result, and ventricular failure is inevitable. The pulmonary autograft has many theoretical advantages over homograft aortic valve replacement, such as the potential for growth in children, greater cellular viability, and better durability and possible internal innervation of the cusps. These advantages are offset by greater surgical complexity, longer surgical time, potential for coronary arterial injury, the effect of dissection on right ventricular function, and the disadvantages of 2 valves at risk.

*Methods.*—Aortic valve replacement was performed with aortic homograft in 37 patients (group A) and pulmonary autograft in 33 patients (group B). The age of patients ranged from 3 to 64 years. Of the 70 patients, 61 were male. Eighteen patients had previous aortic valve surgery.

*Results.*—Mean cardiopulmonary bypass time was 113 minutes in group A and 151 minutes in group B. Mean aortic cross-clamp time was 85 minutes in group A and 109 minutes in group B. The aortic homograft was implanted as a root with coronary reimplantation in 32 patients. All pulmonary autografts were implanted as a root. At a mean follow-up of 16 months, there were no early or late deaths. In each group, 1 patient had re-exploration for bleeding. There were no significant differences in ventilatory support, total blood loss, ICU stay, or hospital stay between groups. After the procedures, all patients were in New York Association class I or II. There was no significant change in ejection fraction in either group during follow-up. Left ventricular mass and diastolic diameter had similar progressive regression in both groups. At 6 months, echocardiographic examination of aortic valve function revealed good valve function in 100% of patients and no evidence of aortic regurgitation in 80% of patients. During follow-up, the right ventricular outflow gradient was less than 15 mm Hg in group B. Holter monitoring was available in 44 patients and showed that most of the arrhythmias were grade 0–1 of the modified Lown grading system.

*Discussion.*—The pulmonary autograft procedure is technically more complex than aortic homograft implantation, but the risk of complications and mortality is low for both procedures. Continued evaluation of patients for evidence of long-term valve degeneration and right ventricular function and arrhythmias is recommended.

▶ Dr. Santini's report (Abstract 5–28) of the experience of Sir Magdi Yacoub and his associates is a very useful publication. Sir Magdi is a very skilled surgeon, and I think there is no better technical group in the world at present. Their excellent results justify a prospective randomized trial. We will await further results with great interest. The report by Tirone E. David (Abstract 5–27), also an excellent surgeon, and his group suggests a cautionary concern for geometric mismatch in patients undergoing the Ross procedure.

**J.J. Collins, Jr., M.D.**

---

**Results of Allograft Aortic Valve Replacement for Complex Endocarditis**
Dearani JA, Orszulak TA, Schaff HV, et al (Mayo Clinic and Found, Rochester, Minn)
*J Thorac Cardiovasc Surg* 113:285–291, 1997                               5–29

---

*Introduction.*—The incidence of infective endocarditis is increasing in the United States, perhaps as a result of an aging population with structural valvular abnormalities, more immunosuppressed or immunodeficient patients, and more patients with prosthetic heart valves or indwelling catheter/pacing systems. The surgeon may be confronted with extensive annular destruction and perivalvular ring abscesses that complicate insertion of a standard aortic valve prosthesis because the operation is often accompanied by the presence of active infection for uncontrolled sepsis, congestive heart failure, septic emboli, and prosthetic valve or fungal endocarditis. Aortic valve replacement with an allograft is said to result in a lower rate of subsequent infection than when mechanical prostheses or other bioprostheses are used. Recent experience with allografts for aortic valve endocarditis were reviewed to determine the early outcome of allograft aortic valve replacement for complex infections.

*Methods.*—Allograft aortic valve replacement was performed on 36 patients, with a mean age of 53 years, in a 10-year period. After valve replacement, follow-up occurred for a mean of 2.6 ± 2.8 years. In 69% of patients, *Staphylococcus* and *Streptococcus* species were seen, and 6% had fungi. Twenty-five patients had valvular vegetations, 25 had annular abscesses, and 13 had cusp destruction. Twenty-five patients required complex reconstruction of the aortic anulus, 2 had mitral valve repair, 3 had

## A Aortic valve allograft

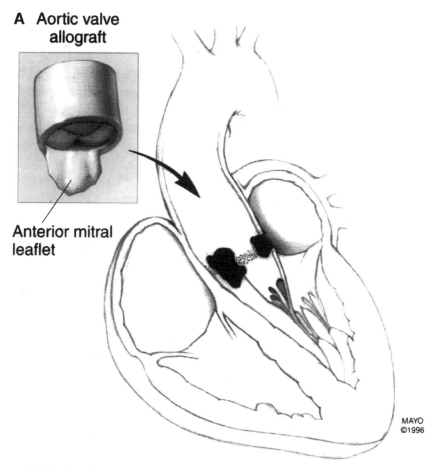

Anterior mitral leaflet

MAYO
©1996

FIGURE 3A.—Four-chamber view demonstrating 2 defects from endocarditis, 1 annular defect involving the anterior leaflet of the mitral valve and the other a left ventricular outflow tract defect involving the ventricular septum. (Courtesy of Dearani JA, Orszulak TA, Schaff HV, et al: Results of allograft aortic valve replacement for complex endocarditis. *J Thorac Cardiovasc Surg* 113:285–291, 1997.)

mitral valve replacement, 8 had coronary artery bypass grafting, 4 had repair of the ventricular septal defect, 1 had left ventricular aneurysmectomy, and 1 had repair of atrial septal defect. The scalloped technique was used in 7 patients to perform the allograft valve insertion. The intra-aortic cylinder technique was used in 19 patients, and 10 had allograft aortic root replacement (Figs 3A and B).

*Results.*—Ten patients had low cardiac output; 2 had bleeding; 1 had myocardial infarction; 1 had stroke; 2 had renal insufficiency; 3 had respiratory insufficiency; and 8 had heart block. Operative mortality was 13.8%. In 5 patients, grade III/IV aortic regurgitation was seen with late echocardiography at a mean of 2.6 ± 1.8 years. Seven late deaths occurred, with 2 noncardiac deaths and 5 that were cardiac-related but not valve-

**B**

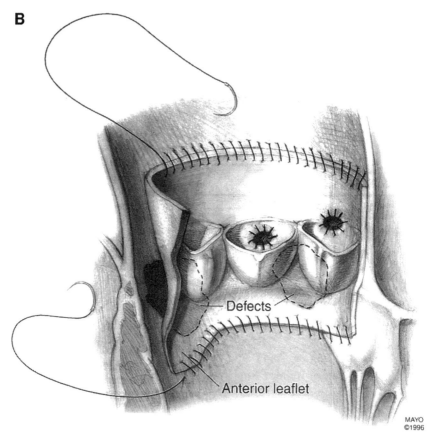

Defects

Anterior leaflet

MAYO
©1996

**FIGURE 3B.**—Circumferential reconstruction of the aortic root with the allograft aortic valve being used as an intra-aortic cylinder. Note that the allograft anterior mitral leaflet is used to repair the ventricular septal defect and a portion of the allograft aortic wall is attached to the recipient anterior mitral leaflet. (Courtesy of Dearani JA, Orszulak TA, Schaff HV, et al: Results of allograft aortic valve replacement for complex endocarditis. *J Thorac Cardiovasc Surg* 113:285–291, 1997.)

related. Endocarditis did not recur in any patient. At 5 years, actuarial survival was 53.1% ± 11.5%. Late survival was adversely affected by prosthetic valve endocarditis. At 5 years, the cumulative risk of reoperation was 8% ± 5.6%.

*Conclusion.*—Reconstruction of complex aortic valve endocarditis was facilitated by allograft aortic valve replacement with a low reoperation rate and no recurrent endocarditis.

▶ Dr. Dearani and associates report excellent results in the use of allograft aortic valves for complex endocarditis of the aortic root. Their results are remarkably good. I think such complex problems are very difficult to deal with, and the surgical mortality rate of about 14% is really quite fine.

**J.J. Collins, Jr., M.D.**

### Coronary Artery Problems During Homograft Aortic Valve Replacement: Role of Transesophageal Echocardiography

Koh TW, Ferdinand FD, Jin XY, et al (Royal Brompton Hosp, London)
*Ann Thorac Surg* 64:533–535, 1997                                    5–30

*Overview.*—Two patients undergoing homograft aortic valve and root replacement could not be weaned from cardiopulmonary bypass. In 1, intraoperative transesophageal echocardiography (TEE) showed aliasing on color-flow mapping in the proximal right coronary artery (CA) and severely depressed right ventricular (RV) function. In the other, TEE showed left main CA aliasing and severely depressed left ventricular anterior wall function. In both, CA bypass grafting successfully corrected the condition.

> *Case 1.*—Man, 59, underwent reoperative aortic valve replacement, with a cryopreserved homograft aortic root and reimplantation of the CAs, for bacterial endocarditis. Heavy inotropic support was required for bypass weaning, and RV enlargement and poor contraction were noted. Normally functioning aortic homograft, good left ventricular systolic function, severe RV impairment with an almost akinetic free wall, and narrowing of the right CA were seen on TEE.

*Discussion.*—In both cases, TEE easily demonstrated the proximal left and right CAs. Aliasing within a CA and severely depressed wall motion in that vessel's perfusion region suggest compromised coronary blood flow, as with CA atherosclerosis. Such CA problems may not be recognized by conventional means. In patient 1, ECG changes were absent and the RV was involved, but left ventricular function was preserved. In a recent series of 9 acute RV failures from right CA involvement after aortic valve replacement, the diagnosis was established only postmortem in 1 case; TEE might have led to timely intervention. In the 2 cases described, had the root cause of impaired cardiac function not been promptly identified with intraoperative TEE and immediately corrected, deterioration would probably have progressed.

▶ Transesophageal echocardiography has many well-documented uses during cardiac surgery in adults (as well as in children).

**J.J. Collins, Jr., M.D.**

### Thirty-Year Results of Starr-Edwards Protheses in the Aortic and Mitral Position

Gödje OL, Fischlein T, Adelhard K, et al (Ludwig-Maximilians-Univ, Munich)
*Ann Thorac Surg* 63:613–619, 1997                                          5–31

*Introduction.*—The modern era of heart valve replacement began more than 3 decades ago with the Starr-Edwards ball valve. Thirty years of long-term results were reviewed in a group of patients who received the Starr-Edwards ball valve between 1963 and 1977.

*Methods.*—There were 416 patients with a mean age of 40.1 ± 10.1 years who had an operation in which a Starr-Edwards ball valve was used. There were 286 aortic valve replacements and 130 mitral valve replacements, and most patients were in New York Heart Association class III.

*Results.*—After aortic valve replacement, the 10-year survival rate was 62.3%; the 20-year survival rate was 39.4%; and the 30-year survival rate was 19.9%. After mitral valve replacement, the 10-year survival rate was 75%; the 20-year survival rate was 36.5%; and the 30-year survival rate was 22.6%. Freedom from all valve-related complications, reoperations, and valve-related death after aortic valve replacement was 66.4%, 43.3%, and 23.8%, respectively, and after mitral valve replacement was 73.4%, 35.4%, and 14.3%, respectively. Of the surviving patients, 82% of those who received aortic valves are in New York Heart Association class I or II, and 76% of those who received mitral valves are in New York Heart Association class I or II. The pressure gradients of the mitral valves were between 9 and 30 mm Hg, and those of the aortic valves were between 20 and 73 mm Hg. No echocardiographic peculiarities were seen in 52% of aortic valves and 68% of mitral valves.

*Conclusions.*—After 30 years of use, the Starr-Edwards valve represents a standard that still needs to be achieved by newer prostheses, according to the long-term results and the echocardiographic results. Only 2 of the valve models used in this study are still available today.

### Event Status of the Starr-Edwards Aortic Valve to 20 Years: A Benchmark for Comparison

Orszulak TA, Schaff HV, Puga FJ, et al (Mayo Clinic and Found, Rochester, Minn)
*Ann Thorac Surg* 63:620–626, 1997                                          5–32

*Introduction.*—The treatment of valvular heart disease was revolutionized with Starr's pioneering insertion of the caged-ball valve. It is still not known whether significant improvements in design resulted in better patient event-free survival in the 30 years since this prosthesis was first introduced. Since 1965, the Starr-Edwards aortic model 1260 has been implanted unchanged and can be used as a comparison for other devices. This prosthesis was reviewed.

*Methods.*—Using the 1260 Starr-Edwards caged-ball prosthesis, aortic valve replacement with or without coronary artery bypass grafting was performed on 1,110 patients in a 22-year period. There were 838 men and 194 women with a median age of 57 years. Aortic valve replacement plus coronary artery bypass grafting was performed on 136 patients, and aortic valve replacement alone was performed on 964 patients.

*Results.*—There was a 6.2% operative mortality. Small valve size of 19–21 mm, presence of atrial fibrillation, recent operative interval, age greater than 56 years, and female sex were predictive of early mortality. Five-year survival rate was 76.6%; 10-year survival rate was 59.6%; 15-year survival rate was 44.9%; and 20-year survival rate was 31.2%. Age older than 56 years, New York Heart Association class III or IV, and lower ejection fraction were operative variables predictive of poor late survival. At 5 years, freedom from thromboemboli was 90.8%, and freedom from anticoagulation-related bleeding was 98.7%. Age older than 56 years, New York Heart Association class III or IV, and female sex were risk factors for late thromboemboli. No valve failures were found.

*Conclusions.*—In the aortic position, the Starr-Edwards valve provides an excellent, safe, durable alternative and is a benchmark against which to compare other prostheses. There were excellent late results of survival and freedom from thromboemboli or anticoagulant-related bleeding, particularly in patients with larger sizes (9A/23 mm or above). In patients who have an aortic root diameter of 21 mm or less, serious consideration should be given to an annulus-enlarging procedure.

▶ Orszulak and associates at the Mayo Clinic (Abstract 5–32) have reported on this large group of patients who have undergone aortic valve replacement with a Starr-Edwards valve with very satisfactory results. This valve certainly does have a long and honorable history. The 30-year results reported by Godje and associates (Abstract 5–31) adds weight to that history.

**J.J. Collins, Jr., M.D.**

**An Analysis of Valve Re-replacement After Aortic Valve Replacement With Biologic Devices**
McGiffin DC, Galbraith AJ, O'Brien MF, et al (Univ of Queensland, Brisbane, Australia; Univ of Alabama, Birmingham)
*J Thorac Cardiovasc Surg* 113:311–318, 1997                    5–33

*Introduction.*—In the treatment of valvular heart disease, biological valve replacement devices (xenograft and allograft valves) have an important and complementary role in conjunction with mechanical valve devices. Biological valves provide freedom from anticoagulant-related hemorrhage and a low incidence of thromboembolic events when compared with mechanical devices. However, their disadvantage is that they tend to fail because of leaflet degeneration and geometric distortion and changing mechanical properties of leaflets. The probability of re-replacement of a biological valve is an important factor for the surgeon when deciding between a mechanical and biological valve replacement device. In a series of patients who had aortic valve replacement, biological valve re-replacement was examined in the context of the competing risks of valve re-replacement before death.

*Methods.*—There were 1,343 patients who had aortic valve replacement with a xenograft valve or a cryopreserved or 4°C stored allograft. To simultaneously model the competing risks of death and re-replacement before death, a parametric model approach was used.

*Results.*—A first re-replacement was performed in 111 patients, of whom 60 had xenograft valves, 28 had 4°C stored allograft valves, and 14 had cryopreserved allograft valves. Xenograft, 4°C stored allograft, and cryopreserved allograft valve replacement was associated with younger age at operation. However, older patients have a decreased survival time, and this reduces their probability of requiring valve re-replacement, whereas younger patients have a longer survival time, increasing their exposure to the risk of re-replacement. The probability of re-replacement before death was similar for xenograft and cryopreserved allograft valves in patients older than 60 at the time of aortic valve replacement. The probability of re-replacement was higher for 4°C stored valves for patients older than 60 years. However, compared with the xenograft valve and 4°C

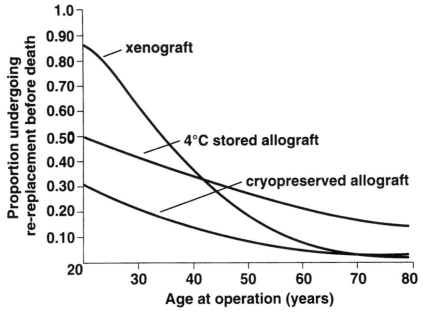

FIGURE 4.—Nomogram of the probability of re-replacement before death for any reason for patients with xenograft, 4°C stored, and cryopreserved allograft valves as a function of age at initial valve replacement. The *solid lines* are the parametric estimates. (Courtesy of McGiffin DC, Galbraith AJ, O'Brien MF, et al: An analysis of valve re-replacement after aortic valve replacement with biologic devices. *J Thorac Cardiovasc Surg* 113:311–318, 1997.)

stored allografts, the probability of re-replacement at any time during the remainder of the life of a patient younger than 60 years was lower with the cryopreserved allograft valve (Fig 4).

*Conclusion.*—The probability of re-replacement may be reduced by the current preference for the cylindric or root replacement technique of allograft valve insertion by decreasing geometric distortion and improving leaflet coaptation, as opposed to the subcoronary technique, the method most frequently used in this series. This study must be repeated in the future to evaluate the efficacy of using the cylindric or root replacement technique.

▶ This excellent article by McGiffin and associates emphasizes that cryopreserved allografts in patients younger than age 60 did somewhat better than xenograft or 4°C allografts. These differences were, however, not terribly great. One thing that was not discussed is whether the second round of valves fared any better or worse than the first round. There may not actually be a very large number of patients who have been through the entire course of 2 separate biological valves. It would be interesting to know whether earlier calcification or any other type of premature valvular deterioration has been observed in these repeat bioprostheses.

**J.J. Collins, Jr., M.D.**

---

**Results of Valve Replacement With Mechanical and Biological Prostheses in Chronic Renal Dialysis Patients**
Lucke JC, Samy RN, Atkins BZ, et al (Duke Univ, Durham, NC)
*Ann Thorac Surg* 64:129–133, 1997                                    5–34

---

*Background.*—The value of biological or mechanical valves in patients receiving chronic dialysis has not been defined clearly. The results of valve replacement in such patients were investigated, and biological and mechanical valves were compared.

*Methods.*—Nineteen consecutive patients with end-stage renal disease receiving chronic peritoneal or hemodialysis were studied retrospectively. Twelve were undergoing aortic valve replacement; 5, mitral; and 2, aortic-mitral. Nine patients had biological valves, and 10 had mechanical ones.

*Findings.*—The groups with biological and mechanical valves were similar in age and cardiovascular risk factors. Overall estimated Kaplan-Meier survival was 60% at 12 months and 42% at 60 months. The rate of postoperative cerebrovascular accidents or bleeding complications was significantly higher in patients with mechanical valves. No repeat surgery was needed for biological valve failure at a mean 32 months after surgery.

*Conclusions.*—The use of mechanical valves in patients with end-stage renal disease is associated with a significant risk of complications. Biological valve failure from prosthetic dysfunction in this population is unusual. Both groups have a poor overall survival.

▶ The report of Dr. Lucke and associates from Duke University Medical Center presents a relatively small group of persons with a need for dialysis who have undergone valve replacement with mechanical or tissue valves. Their conclusion that tissue valves are safer in this group is the opposite of ours. We have been impressed with premature calcification in tissue valves used in patients requiring dialysis and have been less impressed with the possible occurrence of substantial bleeding in patients requiring Warfarin.

**J.J. Collins, Jr., M.D.**

---

**Oral Disease Burden in Patients Undergoing Prosthetic Heart Valve Implantation**
Terezhalmy GT, Safadi TJ, Longworth DL, et al (Cleveland Clinic Found, Ohio)
*Ann Thorac Surg* 63:402–404, 1997                                             5–35

---

*Background.*—Valvular heart disease predisposing to endocarditis and requiring prosthetic valve implantation is often encountered in the elderly. This population also has been found to have a disproportionate percentage of oral disease among adults in the United States. Spontaneous bacteremia associated with oral and odontogenic infections may carry a much higher risk for endocarditis than do occasional health care procedures. The oral disease burden in patients having mechanical or bioprosthetic heart valve implantation was determined.

*Methods.*—A comprehensive clinical and radiographic regional examination was performed in 156 consecutive patients with valvular heart disease requiring mechanical or bioprosthetic valve implantation. Acute and chronic oral and odontogenic infections and conditions were identified.

*Results.*—There were 59 women and 97 men, and the mean patient age was 62.8 years. All patients had aortic valve, mitral valve, or multiple valve replacement. The mean number of remaining teeth in these patients was 19.32. Of these, 107 were carious, involving a mean of 2.51 tooth surfaces. Evidence of acute or chronic periapical abscesses was noted in 15.38% of patients. Evidence of past root canal treatment was seen in 30.76% of patients. Type I periodontitis was seen in 4.5% of patients, type II in 50%, type III in 26.9%, and type IV in 16.7% of patients.

*Discussion.*—The prevalence of oral disease in these patients was substantial, although it was not determined if these patients had a higher rate of oral disease than other populations. These findings indicate that a routine preoperative dental examination should be part of a multidisciplinary evaluation because of the substantial morbidity and mortality associated with prosthetic valve endocarditis and because of the high incidence of dental disease in this study group. Appropriate treatment should be performed when possible before valve implantation. Third-party payors should consider such evaluations a medical necessity.

▶ Dr. Terezhalmy and associates at the Cleveland Clinic have brought up a very important point for preoperative preparation of patients about to undergo valve replacement surgery. I think that at the present time the Clinic requires a dental examination before admission for valve surgery. Whether this is an absolute prerequisite, I can't say for sure. A dental examination is probably a useful investment for any patient about to undergo cardiac valve replacement surgery.

**J.J. Collins, Jr., M.D.**

---

**Drawback of Aortoplasty for Aneurysm of the Ascending Aorta Associated With Aortic Valve Disease**
Mueller XM, Tevaearai HT, Genton CY, et al (Centre Hospitalier Universitaire Vaudois, Lausanne, Switzerland)
*Ann Thorac Surg* 63:762–767, 1997                                     5–36

---

*Introduction.*—Frequently, an associated ascending aortic aneurysm must be dealt with during aortic valve replacement. It is unknown whether these aortic changes are the result of underlying intrinsic wall weakness or turbulent flow related to valvular pathology. The more common approach is to use graft replacement to repair the ascending aortic aneurysm. A more conservative approach involves unsupported aortoplasty with excision of a segment of the aortic wall to decrease the diameter of the aneurysm and remodel the ascending aorta. This technique was reviewed and aneurysm recurrence was evaluated.

*Methods.*—A total of 17 patients with unsupported aortoplasty were studied. Five patients had stenosis and 12 had aortic valve regurgitation. In 14 patients, the aortic wall was analyzed histologically. There was a mean follow-up of 6 years, with a range of 2.3–10.5 years. The operative technique involves using the usual median sternotomy to approach the ascending aorta. An aortic cannula is placed, and the aorta was cross-clamped distal to the aneurysm. An aortotomy was performed and was carried into the noncoronary sinus. A prosthesis was used to replace the excised aortic valve.

*Results.*—Among the 15 hospital survivors, 2 patients died of causes unrelated to aortic pathology during follow-up. At 7 years, survival was 87.7%. After a mean of 63 months, 4 patients had recurring aortic aneurysms, with an event-free survival rate of 41% at 7 years. Cystic medial necrosis and aortic valve regurgitation were found in all 4 of these patients.

*Conclusions.*—In patients with aortic regurgitation, the recurrence rate of aneurysms after unsupported aortoplasty and aortic valve replacement is high. These patients have an aortic dilatation that is related to an underlying wall deficiency associated with aortic valve pathology. Early echocardiographic follow-up should be conducted in all patients who had aortoplasty without wall support to detect aneurysm recurrences. Aortoplasty is likely to suffice in patients with aortic stenosis.

▶ The report of Mueller and associates emphasizes the possibility of recurrent and serious aortic dilatation in patients having unsupported aortoplasty. Certainly that has been the experience of a number of surgeons. I think the problem of management of such aneurysms is very well discussed by Dr. Francis Robicsek in his invited commentary about the article by Mueller et al.

**J.J. Collins, Jr., M.D.**

## Mitral Valve Surgery

**Early Surgery in Patients With Mitral Regurgitation Due to Flail Leaflets: A Long-term Outcome Study**
Ling LH, Enriquez-Sarano M, Seward JB, et al (Mayo Clinic and Mayo Found, Rochester, Minn)
*Circulation* 96:1819–1825, 1997                                            5–37

*Objective.*—Although surgical correction of mitral regurgitation (MR) results in improved cardiac symptoms, there is disagreement on the timing of such surgery. Whether early surgery or conservative management improved the long-term outcome of patients with MR as a result of flail leaflets by reducing overall mortality, cardiovascular mortality, and cardiovascular morbidity was investigated.

*Methods.*—Between January 1, 1980 and December 31, 1989, 221 patients (64 women), average age 65, diagnosed with flail leaflets were operated on within a month of diagnosis (group I, $n = 63$) or treated conservatively (group II, $n = 158$). Patients were followed until February 1995. Mortality and complications were recorded. Group statistical comparisons were performed.

*Results.*—Group I patients were younger, had more serious symptoms including atrial fibrillation, and a lower comorbidity index than group II patients. In group II, 80 patients had delayed surgery. There were 9 (14%) deaths in group I and 47 (30%) in group II. Overall survival at 5 and 10 years was 89% and 79%, respectively, in group I and 78% and 65% in group II. One group I patient and 5 group II patients died during surgery. Early surgery significantly improved overall survival, decreased cardiovascular mortality, decreased the incidence of congestive heart failure, and decreased development of new chronic atrial fibrillation. Early surgery also significantly lowered the incidence of endocarditis.

*Conclusion.*—Early surgery for patients with MR as a result of flail leaflets improves long-term survival, decreased cardiac mortality, and decreased morbidity compared with delayed surgery or conservative management.

▶ In this study by Ling and associates from the Mayo Clinic, early surgical repair of severe mitral regurgitation is strongly supported. The practice of "conservative" management awaiting worsening of symptoms was, in this study, shown to be distinctly inferior to prompt surgery.

**J.J. Collins, Jr., M.D.**

▶ This is a follow-up to the authors' 1996 publication (Ling LH, Enriquez-Sarano M, Seward JB, et al. Clinical outcome of mitral regurgitation due to flail leaflet. *N Engl J Med* 335:1417–1423, 1996).

We would agree that early surgery should be recommended for most patients with degenerative diseases such as flail leaflets. Early surgery should probably be done only in medical centers that have a less than 2% risk of mitral valve surgery and a high success (more than 90%) with mitral valve repair.

**R.C. Schlant, M.D.**

---

**Surgery for Acquired Heart Disease: Reoperation for Failure of Mitral Valve Repair**
Gillinov AM, Cosgrove DM, Lytle BW, et al (Cleveland Clinic Found, Ohio)
*J Thorac Cardiovasc Surg* 113:467–475, 1997                    5–38

---

*Objective.*—Although mitral valve repair is the treatment of choice for mitral regurgitation (MR), approximately 10% of patients require late reoperation. Little information about the mechanism of recurrent dysfunction is available. Results of a study of the causes of failed mitral valve repair are presented.

*Methods.*—Between January 1986 and December 1994, 81 patients (26 women), average age 59.2, had 86 reoperations at the Cleveland Clinic for recurrent MR. The primary mitral valve repair was made for disease that was degenerative in 48 patients, rheumatic in 16, ischemic in 13, endocarditis in 3, and congenital in 1. Time to reoperation averaged 15.6 months, and at reoperation all patients had recurrent MR of grade 3+ or 4+. Seventy-two of 74 hospital survivors were followed for an average of 45.9 months.

*Results.*—Causes of failed mitral valve repair were procedure-related in 50 patients, valve-related in 33, and unknown in 3. Procedure-related failures resulted from suture dehiscence in 21 patients, ruptured chordae in 19, and incomplete in 10. Valve-related repair failures were caused by progressive disease in 27 patients, endocarditis in 5 patients, and leaflet retraction in 1 patient. Valve failures were procedure-related in 70% of patients with degenerative disease and valve-related in 87% of patients with rheumatic disease. Valve failures in patients with ischemic MR were 54% procedure-related and 39% valve-related. Time to reoperation was significantly longer for patients with procedure-related failures than for valve-related failures (22.5 vs. 12.8 months). At reoperation, 64 patients had mitral valve replacement and 17 had repeat repair. Of these, 6 later required mitral valve replacement. There were 14 late deaths at an average of 45.9 months.

*Conclusion.*—The failure mechanism was predominantly procedure-related in patients with degenerative disease resulting in recurrent MR. In patients with rheumatic disease, the failures were primarily valve-related. Careful patient selection and close attention to technique can reduce late failure rates. Intraoperative use of echocardiography can eliminate incomplete mitral valve repair. Most patients at reoperation will require mitral valve replacement.

▶ The group at the Cleveland Clinic have a substantial experience with mitral valve repair. Their conclusion that most mitral valve repair failures are procedure-related in degenerative disease and valve-related in rheumatic disease is an important observation with which we are in full agreement.

**J.J. Collins, Jr., M.D.**

---

**Malfunctioning Starr-Edwards Mitral Valve 21 Years After Installation**
Sakata K, Ishikawa S, Ohtaki A, et al (Gunma Univ, Maebashi, Japan)
*J Cardiovasc Surg* 38:81–82, 1997                                    5–39

---

*Introduction.*—Two rare cases of malfunctioning Starr-Edwards cloth-covered mitral valve prostheses that required reoperation are described. Both patients had successful surgical repair of the prosthesis 21 years after valve replacement. The malfunctions were caused by a disturbance of the poppet during the opening phase because of excessive tissue ingrowth in one valve and a paravalvular leak associated with a tear of the valve seat in the other valve. There are no other reports of replacement of a Starr-Edwards valve prosthesis more than 20 years after initial placement.

*Case Report.*—Woman, 51, had valve replacement with a Starr-Edwards cloth-covered mitral valve prosthesis for mitral stenosis in 1972. She was hospitalized because of increasing dyspnea and abdominal distention. Examination showed remarkable ascites and a grade 2 systolic murmur and diastolic rumble. Two-dimensional transthoracic echocardiograms indicated a severely enlarged left atrium and a left ventricle of normal size and with normal ejection fraction. Tricuspid regurgitation was noted on color Doppler echocardiography. Pulmonary artery wedge pressure was 17 mm Hg, pulmonary artery pressure was 80/35 mm Hg, and mean right atrial pressure was 16 mm Hg. Cardiac fluoroscopy was performed and showed a well-anchored prosthesis ring and smooth poppet, but the poppet motion had slight transverse oscillations during the valve-opening movement. In 1993, the Starr-Edwards valve was replaced with a 25 mm CarboMedics valve. Tricuspid annuloplasty also was performed. The Starr-Edwards valve showed excessive fibrin deposition on the valve seat and one of the struts. A lack of cloth covering and exposed metal was seen on the inner surface of the valve ring and all the struts. No ball variance was noted. The patient has been asymptomatic for 2 years.

*Discussion.*—Early models of the Starr-Edwards valve prosthesis were not cloth covered and resulted in a high rate of thromboembolism. The cloth-covered model was introduced to cause tissue encapsulation of the base and struts and had a lower rate of thromboembolism. The cloth-covered model, however, had problems with hemolysis and cloth wear. Complications from cloth wear include fiber emboli in the systemic circulation and severe hemolytic anemia with or without regurgitation across the prosthesis. In these 2 patients, there were no signs of cloth wear and only mild hemolytic anemia.

▶ In a case report, Dr. Sakata et al. point out that very late pannus accumulation may affect prosthetic valve performance. I think this applies to all prosthetic valves, although in this instance, a Starr-Edwards valve was involved.

**J.J. Collins, Jr., M.D.**

---

**Obstruction of Mechanical Mitral Prostheses: Analysis of Pathologic Findings**
Vitale N, Renzulli A, Agozzino L, et al (Univ of Bari, Italy; Univ of Naples, Italy)
*Ann Thorac Surg* 63:1101–1106, 1997                                    5–40

---

*Background.*—The design and structure of mechanical mitral prostheses have improved through the years, and the prostheses are now often preferred to bioprostheses. However, their use still carries a risk of complications, the most serious of which is thrombosis. There is little information about the mechanisms of prosthetic obstruction. The incidence of pannus formation and thrombosis, and the time to occurrence of pannus and thrombosis were compared.

*Methods.*—Pathologic and echocardiographic findings in 87 patients with mitral valve obstruction were examined. Studied were 25 men and 62 women aged 17 to 71 years. The findings included pannus morphology, its location on the valve, and presence and relationship of associated thrombi. The time from valve replacement to development of obstruction was compared for pannus and thrombosis.

*Results.*—Ten caged-ball valves, 65 tilting-disk valves, and 12 bileaflet valves were used. Prosthetic replacement was performed in 72 patients, and thrombolysis was performed in 15 patients. Pannus alone occurred in 27 patients, pannus and thrombus in 39, and thrombus alone in 21 patients. Primary thrombosis developed earlier than pannus in patients with bileaflet valves and tilting-disk valves. The location of pannus was atrial in 19.7% of patients, ventricular in 21.2%, and atrioventricular in 59.1%. Pannus morphology was concentric in 22.7% of patients and eccentric in 77.3% of patients. Patients with atrioventricular pannus had a higher rate of atrial secondary thrombi. Reobstruction occurred in 8 patients. This resulted from pannus formation in 5 patients and thrombosis in 3 patients. Five patients had reoperation and 3 had thrombolysis. The time to reobstruction was shorter than the time to initial obstruction.

*Discussion.*—In these patients, the prevalence of pannus formation was much higher than the prevalence of thrombus formation. Thrombosis had an earlier onset than pannus. Thrombosis results from deposition of clots on the prosthesis and a pannus results from an inflammatory reaction on both valve surfaces. About 94% of prostheses with eccentric pannus were tilting-disk valves with protruding edges of the pannus localized over the minor orifice area. This area is the site of low flow, which may have a role in the development of pannus. These findings indicate a significant relationship between atrioventricular pannus and atrial secondary thrombi. This may result from the obstruction and the interactions between inflammation and thrombosis. The comparable incidence of secondary thrombi in association with both types of pannus suggest that either type may activate a thrombotic mechanism, especially when inadequate anticoagulation occurs.

▶ Dr. Vitale and associates have written an interesting paper on the modes of prosthetic valve obstruction. In my experience, symptomatic or hemodynamically significant prosthetic valve obstruction from accumulation of pannus is much more likely in small valves than it is in larger ones. This may be intuitively obvious, but it has not received much attention in the literature.

**J.J. Collins, Jr., M.D.**

## Transplantation and Mechanical Ventricular Assistance

**Bridge Experience With Long-term Implantable Left Ventricular Assist Devices: Are They an Alternative to Transplantation?**
Oz MC, Argenziano M, Catanese KA, et al (Columbia-Presbyterian Med Ctr, New York)
*Circulation* 95:1844–1852, 1997                                5–41

*Background.*—The shortage of hearts for transplantation has led to the development of "bridging" therapy with left ventricular assist devices (LVADs). If these devices can be successfully used over the long term, it will be possible to consider permanent LVAD implantation instead of transplantation. A medium-term experience with LVADs—including both pneumatically and electrically powered ThermoCardiosystems devices—was evaluated.

*Patients.*—The analysis included prospectively recorded data on 58 patients undergoing insertion of a Heartmate LVAD in a 5-year period. The patients were 45 men and 13 women, with a mean age of 50. The major causes of end-stage heart failure were ischemic cardiomyopathy (52%) and idiopathic cardiomyopathy (41%). A scoring system based on criteria obtained at initial evaluation was developed to select patients

TABLE 1.—Association Between Scale Risk Factors and Mortality

| Risk Factor | Relative Risk | Weight |
|---|---|---|
| Urine output <30 mL/h | 3.9 | 3 |
| Central venous pressure | 3.1 | 2 |
| Mechanical ventilation | 3.0 | 2 |
| Prothrombin time >16 | 2.4 | 2 |
| Reoperation | 1.8 | 1 |
| Leukocyte count >15000 | 1.1 | 0 |
| Temperature >101.5° | 0 | 0 |

(From Oz MC, Argenziano M, Catanese KA, et al: Bridge experience with long-term implantable left ventricular assist devices: Are they an alternative to transplantation? *Circulation* 95:1844–1852, 1997. Reproduced with permission from *Circulation*. Copyright 1997, American Heart Association.)

(Table 1). A pneumatically driven LVAD was implanted in 76% of patients and a vented electric type in 24% (Fig 1).

*Outcomes.*—With a mean duration of support of 98 days, overall survival was 74%. Thirty patients had successful cardiac transplantation, 11 were still waiting for transplantation, and 2 were weaned off LVAD support. Pre-existing infection and infection during LVAD support were common problems; however, they did not lead to any increase in mortality or reduction in the successful transplant rate. Even though the patients did not receive anticoagulation, the rate of thromboembolic complications was only 5%. Except for patients with early perioperative right ventricular failure, ventricular arrhythmias were well tolerated, causing no deaths. One third of patients had right ventricular failure. Most of these patients were managed with inotropic support, while others were managed with a right ventricular assist device or inhaled nitric oxide therapy or both methods. The patients required a number of different noncardiac operations, which were successfully performed with no major morbidity or mortality.

*Conclusions.*—Promising medium-term results are reported for patients with heart failure, managed by implantable LVAD support. The good experience is attributed to current patient selection and management techniques, along with device improvements that have lowered the incidence of thrombosis while facilitating rehabilitation. A prospective, randomized trial to assess LVADs as a possible alternative to medical management is needed.

▶ Dr. Oz and his group have achieved excellent results with long-term implantable ventricular assist devices. I think they, as well as others in this field, are questioning whether we may not already have the capability for implanting permanent assist devices with reasonable long-term outcome. If this should (and it probably will) become an acceptable therapeutic alternative, the cost of management of such patients may become a heavy burden.

**J.J. Collins, Jr., M.D.**

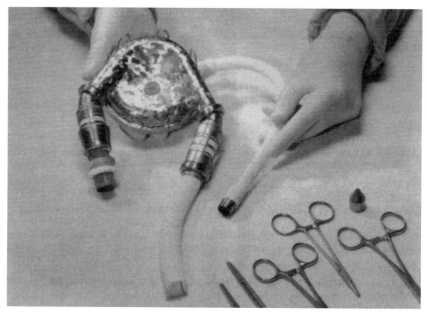

FIGURE 1.—The TCI pneumatic device demonstrating the titanium housing, inflow and outflow valves with attached Dacron graft, and Dacron-coated driveline. (From Oz MC, Argenziano M, Catanese KA, et al: Bridge experience with long-term implantable left ventricular assist devices: Are they an alternative to transplantation? *Circulation* 95:1844–1852, 1997. Reproduced with permission from *Circulation*. Copyright 1997, American Heart Association.)

## Clinical Status of Patients Removed From a Transplant Waiting List Rivals That of Transplant Recipients at Significant Cost Savings

Levine TB, Levine AB, Goldberg AD, et al (Henry Ford Hosp, Detroit)
*Am Heart J* 132:1189–1194, 1996                                        5–42

*Introduction.*—For patients who are severely symptomatic and have a poor prognosis, heart transplantation has been proposed, but long transplant waiting list periods occur because of the limited availability of donor hearts. Improved therapeutic modalities have resulted for these potential transplant recipients while they wait, and in some instances, the therapy leads to the removal of the patient from the transplant list, which was once thought to be impossible. Patients who required transplantation were compared with patients who were removed from the waiting list to determine their clinical characteristics and the efficacy of their therapies.

*Methods.*—There were 60 patients awaiting transplantation for at least 3 months; 18 were removed from the list, while 42 required transplant or died. All patients received diuretics, vasodilating agents, and digitalis. Nitrates were used for continued pulmonary hypertension. Patients had intense dietary counseling and were encouraged to participate in an exercise program.

*Results.*—Significant improvement was seen in exercise oxygen uptake, ejection fraction, and hemodynamics in patients removed from the list. Both groups had comparable symptoms—New York Heart Association class I or II—for more than 2 years after transplantation or delisting. For the delisted group, 1 of 18 patients died of cardiovascular causes, and 3 of 32 patients died in the transplant group. The number of hospitalizations was lower in the delisted group when compared with that in the transplant group. There was $2.2 million in savings for delisting

*Conclusions.*—Clinical improvement is sustained for 1–3 years at significant cost savings with transplant recipient list removal because of advanced medical therapy. Patients who respond to augmented vasodilator therapy should have transplantation delayed, whereas early transplantation should be encouraged for those who are clinically unstable and who do not respond to medical therapy. Some delisted patients required subsequent transplantation.

▶ Levine and associates from Detroit published this very interesting paper describing the favorable course of patients who are taken off a transplant waiting list. This really should not be surprising. The reason the patients were removed from the list is that they made remarkably good progress toward a more normal cardiovascular status. The likelihood that they would immediately deteriorate again is actually pretty small. If that were not so, they would have remained on the list, wouldn't they? Nevertheless, this is a very interesting commentary.

**J.J. Collins, Jr., M.D.**

## Management of Left Ventricular Assist Device Infection With Heart Transplantation

Prendergast TW, Todd BA, Beyer AJ III, et al (Temple Univ, Philadelphia)
*Ann Thorac Surg* 64:142–147, 1997                                      5–43

*Background.*—Left ventricular assist devices are being used as a bridge to heart transplantation. Infection of such devices is a grave complication because removal of the device or delay of heart transplantation can result in death. Heart transplantation was performed in patients with left ventricular assist device infection to help improve outcome.

*Methods.*—Left ventricular assist devices were implanted in 22 patients, but 4 patients developed complications unrelated to the device and did not undergo transplantation. The remaining 18 patients had heart transplantation. Left ventricular assist device infection was present in 8 patients and absent in 10 patients. Treatment was similar in both groups, except for modification of immunosuppression in patients with infection.

*Results.*—Both groups of patients had similar infectious and noninfectious complications. Intraoperative deaths, long-term survival, wound complications, and mean hospital stay after transplantation were similar in both groups.

*Discussion.*—Although the presence of left ventricular assist device infection is considered to contraindicate heart transplantation, such treatment was effective in patients with left ventricular assist device infection. There has been concern that active infection increases postoperative risk because immunosuppression may increase the infection. However, patients with left ventricular assist device infection are too ill for the device to be removed or for heart transplantation to be delayed. In such cases, the benefits of heart transplantation outweigh the risks of immunosuppression. The immunosuppression protocol in this study excluded induction therapy and delayed administration of cyclosporin A for 48–72 hours to avoid renal failure. Also, azathioprine was withheld to improve leukocyte availability and the ability to fight infection. It should be noted that no patient required postoperative dialysis. Left ventricular assist device infection did not increase the risk of postoperative infection in this small series. The incidence of rejection in the first year was similar in both groups of patients.

▶ Dr. Prendergast and associates have had an excellent experience with cardiac transplantation in patients who have infection of ventricular assist devices. This is very useful information.

**J.J. Collins, Jr., M.D.**

---

**Relation of Donor Age and Preexisting Coronary Artery Disease on Angiography and Intracoronary Ultrasound to Later Development of Accelerated Allograft Coronary Artery Disease**
Gao S-Z, Hunt SA, Alderman EL, et al (Stanford Univ, Calif)
*J Am Coll Cardiol* 29:623–629, 1997                                  5–44

---

*Background.*—It is generally accepted that organs used for transplantation should be healthy and have a good prognosis for long-term functioning. Selection criteria for donor hearts have included freedom from cardiac disease and an upper age limit of 35–40 years. As the demand for donor hearts has increased in some settings, attempts have been made to expand the donor pool by increasing the upper age limit for donor hearts. The effect of donor age and preexisting donor coronary artery disease on later development of allograft coronary artery disease, ischemic events, and survival was examined.

*Methods.*—Analysis was done of 223 consecutive patients who had heart transplantation and who had baseline early postoperative and follow-up coronary angiograms. A subset of 47 patients with baseline intracoronary US recordings also was analyzed. Mean follow-up was 3.8 years. Patients were classified according to presence of donor coronary artery disease on baseline angiograms and donor age younger or older than 40 years.

*Results.*—There were 219 patients without preexisting coronary artery disease on baseline angiograms. These patients were significantly less likely

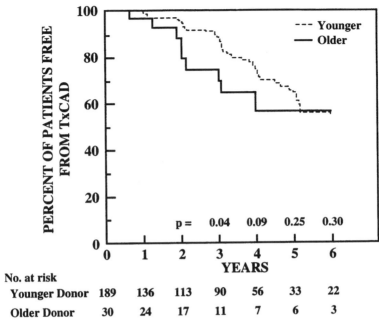

FIGURE 2.—Graph showing comparison of time-related percent freedom from new allograft coronary artery disease in patients receiving hearts from younger (< 40 years) and older (≥ 40 years) donors in patients with normal baseline angiograms. *Abbreviation*: *TxCAD*, allograft coronary artery disease. (Courtesy of Gao S-Z, Hunt SA, Alderman EL, et al: Relation of donor age and preexisting coronary artery disease on angiography and intracoronary ultrasound to later development of accelerated allograft coronary artery disease. *J Am Coll Cardiol* 29:623–629, 1997. Reprinted with permission from the American College of Cardiology.)

to develop new disease than the 14 patients with pre-existing coronary artery disease. At 3 years, older donors had earlier coronary artery disease than younger donors, but there was no difference at 5 years (Fig 2). Both groups had similar survival and probability of developing ischemic events. Baseline US showed significant disease in 7 of 9 older donor hearts and in 7 of 38 younger donor hearts. Significant predictors of allograft coronary artery disease were preexisting coronary artery disease, non-use of calcium channel blockers, older donor age, posttransplantation cytomegalovirus infection, higher very low density lipoprotein levels, and prior ischemic heart disease in the recipient.

*Discussion.*—These findings indicate that older heart donors and donors with angiographic evidence of preexisting coronary artery disease have a higher incidence of new allograft coronary artery disease by 3 years postoperatively. In these patients, no difference in survival or freedom from ischemic events was seen between younger and older donors at 3.8 years.

▶ The observation by Gao and his associates suggests that the use of older donors should not be a major risk factor for early coronary disease if donors are otherwise carefully selected.

**J.J. Collins, Jr., M.D.**

**Management of Cardiac Allograft Vasculopathy by Transmyocardial Laser Revascularization**
Malik FS, Mehra MR, Ventura HO, et al (Ochsner Med Institutions, New Orleans, La)
*Am J Cardiol* 80:224–225, 1997                    5–45

*Background.*—Transmyocardial laser revascularization (TLR) involves the creation of transmural channels in ischemic myocardium. Evidence suggests that it effectively relieves anginal symptoms and improves myocardial perfusion in native coronary disease unsuitable for revascularization. This intervention may be of value for improving myocardial perfusion in diffuse cardiac allograft vasculopathy (CAV). Transmyocardial laser revascularization was used successfully in 4 recipients of orthotopic heart transplants as treatment for symptomatic diffuse advanced CAV.

*Patients and Findings.*—The patients were 3 men and 1 woman, mean age 52 years, with progressively worsening symptoms of exertional chest pressure and dyspnea with resolution at rest. Symptoms were refractory to anti-ischemic medications. Coronary angiography showed diffuse epicardial CAV in all 3 vessels with no focal stenoses. Acute myocardial infarction was ruled out before elective thoracotomy and TLR were done. Lateral thoracotomy was performed in 3 patients and a median sternotomy in 1. The pericardium was opened vertically, and transmyocardial channels were created in predefined ischemic territories using holmium yttrium aluminum garnet laser from a 1-mm optical fiber. Each channel, 1 mm in diameter, was placed approximately in a 1 cm²-diameter region of the left ventricle. Transesophageal echocardiography was used to confirm channel placement. Direct pressure was applied to control epicardial bleeding, and the pericardium was approximated after securing hemostasis. All but 1 patient had an uneventful postoperative course. Four and 8 weeks postoperatively, all patients were ambulatory with no symptoms of ischemia while performing activities of daily living. At the 8-week follow-up, anginal class was found to have improved from class IV to II in all patients. Allograft function was unchanged. There was also significant improvement in myocardial perfusion at rest, with minimal stress redistribution in all patients compared with images before TLR. At 3 months, all 4 patients continue to be free of angina.

*Conclusions.*—Transmyocardial laser revascularization appears to be a unique, effective method for treating diffuse CAV. This procedure provides symptomatic relief and reduces ischemic burden in diffuse CAV.

▶ Transmyocardial revascularization of the heart is one of the more mystical types of surgical therapy. I do not understand why blood should flow through the tiny channels made by the laser when the gradient promoting flow occurs only during systole and when the channels cannot be demonstrated to be patent more than a month after the procedure. I think we will eventually see the disappearance of this type of revascularization.

**J.J. Collins, Jr., M.D.**

## Intraluminal Operations

### Intentional Asystole During Endoluminal Thoracic Aortic Surgery Without Cardiopulmonary Bypass

Baker AB, Bookallil MJ, Lloyd G (Royal Prince Alfred Hosp, Sydney, Australia; Univ of Sydney, Australia)
*Br J Anaesth* 78:444–448, 1997            5–46

*Introduction.*—The anesthetic management of patients undergoing endoluminal grafting of the aorta is challenging, especially during balloon expansion of the aortic stents when arterial pressure has to be decreased to prevent misplacement of the stent and damage to the proximal aorta or heart. Reported are 3 patients who received intravenous bolus doses of adenosine to arrest the heart without cardiopulmonary bypass during endoluminal repair of thoracic aortic aneurysms.

> *Case 1.*—Female, 38, received adenosine during endoluminal repair of an aneurysm of the thoracic aorta. There were no adverse complications resulting from use of adenosine. At 6 days after surgery, she underwent a right brachial artery thrombectomy, which was most likely related to the brachial artery sheath used for access in the arm. She was discharged 10 days after initial surgery. A 6-month follow-up period revealed the aneurysmal sac was isolated.
>
> Case 2.—Male, 66, underwent reoperation for recurrent thoracic aortic aneurysm distal to the site of an open repair under cardiopulmonary bypass 3 years earlier. There were no adverse effects from the procedure or the use of adenosine. At 6-month follow-up, the aneurysmal sac was isolated.
>
> Case 3.—Male, 51, with Marfan's syndrome had undergone 2 aortic valve replacements 17 and 12 years earlier. He was seen for a rapidly expanding thoracic aortic aneurysm. The defect underwent endoluminal repair using adenosine. He experienced no adverse effects and was discharged on postoperative day 5.

*Conclusion.*—The use of adenosine during endoluminal repair enhances the management of balloon inflation of the graft stent and allows better expansion to match the aortic diameter. This approach helps control transient hypotension and may help protect the brain and heart. Adenosine must be used with caution in patients with bronchial asthma and patients with sick sinus syndrome or second- or third-degree heart block, unless a pacemaker is inserted.

▶ Baker et al. describe a very useful and novel approach using adenosine-induced cardiac arrest for short intervals in specialized vascular surgery. I think this type of innovation reduces the hazard of simple maneuvers performed on the myocardium or, as in this report, on the great vessels. We have often used temporary ventricular fibrillation for patients not on cardiopulmonary bypass to place sutures carefully in coronary arterial anastomoses that have bled after the discontinuance of cardiopulmonary bypass. It looks a bit shocking but works extremely well.

**J.J. Collins, Jr., M.D.**

---

**Monitoring Considerations for Port-Access Cardiac Surgery**
Siegel LC, St Goar FG, Stevens JH, et al (Stanford Univ, Calif; Palo Alto Veterans Affairs Health Care System, Calif)
*Circulation* 96:562–568, 1997                                                      5–47

---

*Background.*—As the techniques for port-access cardiac surgeries have developed, so too has the need for methods to monitor such operations. Port-access cardiac monitoring via an endovascular cardiopulmonary bypass (CPB) system was evaluated.

*Methods.*—Patients with coronary artery disease ($n = 15$) or mitral valve disease ($n = 10$) underwent CPB via femoral cannulas. Four cannulas were used (Fig 1): a venous cannula in a femoral vein for drainage, a balloon-tipped catheter (Endoaortic Clamp Heartport) to occlude the ascending aorta, a single-lumen pulmonary artery vent catheter (Endopulmonary Vent Heartport), and a triple-lumen catheter (Endosinus Catheter Heartport) to administer cardioplegic solution. Catheters were inserted under transesophageal echocardiographic or fluoroscopic guidance, and these 2 methods plus pulsed-wave Doppler were used to monitor pressures, flows, and catheter positioning throughout the procedure.

*Findings.*—The monitoring methods used effectively measured catheter insertion and positioning. Transesophageal echocardiography readily imaged that, as cardioplegia was delivered, the balloon cathether migrated toward the aortic arch; thus, flow of the solution could be stopped to allow proper reorientation of the catheter. Visualization of the aortic root showed the presence of cardioplegic solution and the appropriate pressure responses to cardioplegia administration. Balloon volume was appropriate, indicating a stable cathether position.

*Conclusions.*—The technique described for monitoring endovascular CPB was successful. The authors note that minimal-access coronary artery bypass grafting without CPB has complications similar to those of open-chest surgery without CPB, and that performing cardiac surgery without

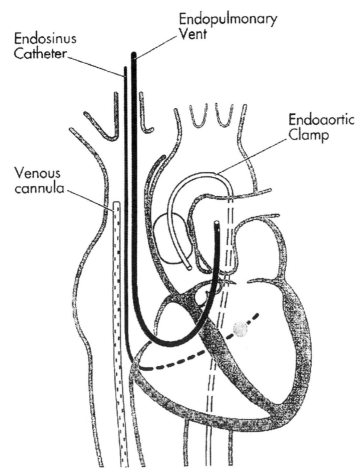

**FIGURE 1.**—Endovascular cardiopulmonary bypass system catheters. (Courtesy of Siegel LC, St Goar FG, Stevens JH, et al: Monitoring considerations for port-access cardiac surgery. *Circulation* 96:562–568. Copyright 1997, American Heart Association. Reproduced with permission.)

circulatory support can be problematic. The current technique provides similar myocardial protection as used in open cardiac surgery with CPB, yet with the reduced morbidity associated with a minimal access procedure.

### Video-assisted Minimally Invasive Mitral Valve Surgery: The "Micro-Mitral" Operation

Chitwood WR Jr; Elbeery JR, Chapman WHH, et al (East Carolina Univ, Greenville, NC)
*J Thorac Cardiovasc Surg* 113:413–414, 1997                    5–48

*Background.*—Minimally invasive procedures such as coronary surgery and cardiac valve repairs are becoming more popular. The replacement of a mitral valve via a minimally invasive approach under video assistance was reported.

*Case Report.*—Man, 43, underwent valve repair for type II severe mitral insufficiency. An endotracheal tube was positioned and cardiopulmonary support was prepared. A 2-inch incision was made in the midaxillary line over the fifth rib, and a small part of this rib was removed. The pericardium was cut and a thoracoscopic port was placed for insertion of a camera to visualize the surgical field. A transthoracic aortic crossclamp was used to occlude the ascending aorta. Surgeons exclusively used the camera to excise the anterior leaflet, suture the valve, position the prosthesis, and tie knots. The procedure took 2 hours and 45 minutes, and after extubation the next morning the patient reported no pain at the incision site.

*Conclusions.*—This video-assisted microaccess mitral valve replacement is the first reported in the United States. The transthoracic aortic cross-clamp was not impeded by a port or incision entrance site, thus allowing better placement and visualization of clamping. The authors recommend this simple and cost-effective approach for patients with a pliable aorta.

▶ The paper by Siegel et al. (Abstract 5–47) on monitoring considerations for port-access and the recent report by Chitwood et al. (Abstract 5–48) are simply indicative of the continuing interest in port-access cardiac surgery. Perhaps I am too old, but I really am concerned about operations that are greatly more complex than necessary to achieve a small skin incision. I am aware that there is great hope that along with a small skin incision, a lower operative mortality and morbidity, a shorter hospital stay, and a less expensive hospitalization will be achieved. I'm not yet convinced that this is the case.

**J.J. Collins, Jr., M.D.**

## Congenital Heart Disease

### Arrhythmia and Mortality After the Mustard Procedure: A 30-Year Single-center Experience

Gelatt M, Hamilton RM, McCrindle BW, et al (Hosp for Sick Children, Toronto; Toronto Gen Hosp; Univ of Toronto)
*J Am Coll Cardiol* 29:194–201, 1997                                                5–49

*Objective.*—The Mustard procedure to correct transposition of the great vessels is being performed less often now because of frequent late-term complications including right ventricular failure, loss of sinus rhythm, and development of atrial flutter. The incidence and risk factors for late mortality, sinus node dysfunction, and atrial flutter in patients treated by the Mustard procedure were investigated.

*Methods.*—Electrocardiographic, demographic, diagnostic, and outcome records of 534 children aged 0–18.6 years who underwent the Mustard procedure between May 1963 and December 1993 at The Hospital for Sick Children in Toronto were reviewed. Risk factors for long-term adverse outcome were determined.

*Results.*—There were 52 deaths during the operative (duration of hospitalization or 30 days, whichever was longer) period, and significantly more patients dying during the first decade of surgical experience. Data were available for survival analysis at a median of 11.5 years for 478 of 482 early survivors. There were 77 late deaths, 31 of which were sudden and unexpected (Fig 1). Ventricular septal defect and atrial tachycardia during the operative period were independent risk factors for late death.

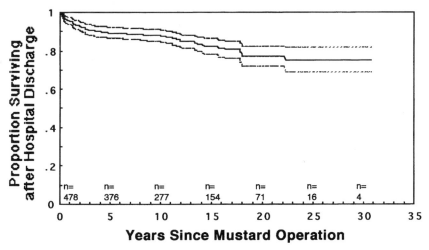

**FIGURE 1.**—Kaplan-Meier estimates of late survival after hospital discharge after the Mustard procedure. *Top and bottom lines* indicate 95% confidence intervals. (Reprinted with permission from the American College of Cardiology, from Gelatt M, Hamilton RM, McCrindle BW, et al: Arrhythmia and mortality after the Mustard procedure: A 30-year single-center experience. *Am Coll Cardiol* 29:194–201, 1997.)

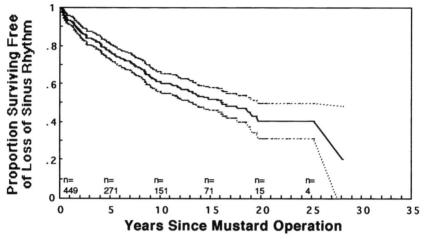

FIGURE 3.—Kaplan-Meier estimates of late survival free of loss of sinus rhythm after the Mustard procedure. *Top and bottom lines* indicate 95% confidence intervals. (Reprinted with permission from the American College of Cardiology, from Gelatt M, Hamilton RM, McCrindle BW, et al: Arrhythmia and mortality after the Mustard procedure: A 30-year single-center experience. *J Am Coll Cardio* 29:194–201, 1997.)

Smaller size at operation, presence of atrial tachycardia during operative period, and presence of permanent heart block were independent risk factors for unexpected sudden death. The presence of preoperative arrhythmia, bradycardia during the operative period, and the presence of late atrial flutter were independent risk factors for loss of sinus rhythm. Sinus rhythm was present in 77% of survivors at 5 years, 61% at 10, 52% at 15, and 40% at 20 years (Fig 3). Presence of bradycardia during the operative period, permanent heart block, need for reoperation, and loss of sinus rhythm were independent risk factors for atrial flutter. Freedom from atrial flutter was found in 92% of survivors at 5 years, 89% at 10, 83% at 15, and 76% at 20 years. Atrial flutter is an increasing risk that peaks at later years.

*Conclusion.*—Because of the late risk of death, loss of sinus rhythm, and atrial flutter, patients undergoing the Mustard procedure require continued follow-up. Perioperative bradycardia and atrial tachycardia are increased risk factors for death.

▶ This report by Dr. Gelatt and multiple associates details the Toronto experience with long-term follow-up after Mustard operations in children. This series is among the largest and best and deserves careful study.

**J.J. Collins, Jr., M.D.**

## The Fontan Procedure in Adults

Gates RN, Laks H, Drinkwater DC, et al (Univ of California, Los Angeles)
*Ann Thorac Surg* 63:1085–1090, 1997                                    5–50

*Background.*—The Fontan procedure has undergone many modifications since it was first performed successfully in 1971. There have been many studies of risk factors for this procedure. Current selection criteria suggest that the ideal patient age for this procedure is between 18 months and 6 years. Occasionally, the Fontan procedure is performed in adults who have had only simple palliation or no surgery at all. The clinical course of adult patients who had the Fontan procedure was examined in a retrospective study.

*Methods.*—There were 21 adults aged 18–40 years who underwent a Fontan procedure. Nine patients had tricuspid atresia, 4 patients had a double-inlet left ventricle, and 8 patients had various single ventricles. A right atria–right ventricle connection was done in 4 patients, a right atria–pulmonary artery connection was done in 13 patients, and a lateral-tunnel Fontan procedure was done in 4 patients. Of the 4 latter patients, 3 had a snare-adjustable atrial septal defect. Preoperative risk factors were left ventricular end-diastolic pressure greater than 10 mm Hg, ejection fraction lower than 0.45, mean pulmonary artery pressure higher than 15 mm Hg, transpulmonary gradient greater than 10 mm Hg, pulmonary artery abnormalities, and atrioventricular valve regurgitation. The mean preoperative risk score was 1.6 and the mean New York Heart Association class was 2.6.

*Results.*—Operative mortality was 5%. Major complications, including prolonged effusions, occurred in 6 patients. Twenty patients were monitored for a mean of 7.4 years; 1 patient was lost to follow-up. The mean New York Heart Association class was 1.7 at follow-up. There was 1 late death at more than 9 years, which may have resulted from ventricular arrhythmia. Three patients had reoperation and survived. Freedom from reoperation was 94% at 3 years, 87% at 6 years, and 69% at 12 years. Atrial arrhythmias requiring medication developed in 7 patients, 2 of whom have been treated for ventricular arrhythmias.

*Discussion.*—Carefully selected adult patients can undergo the Fontan procedure with low morbidity and mortality. The potential for late-developing arrhythmias, reoperation, and decreasing ventricular function require careful follow-up. Morbidity was generally related to prolonged pleural drainage and was seen only early in these patients. Prolonged drainage was not seen in the 3 recent patients who had a lateral-tunnel, snare-adjustable atrial septal defect Fontan procedure, or in the 2 patients who had reoperation with a lateral-tunnel, snare-adjustable atrial septal defect Fontan procedure. This probably results directly from the lower right atrial pressure. Atrial arrhythmias have been the most serious long-term complication of this procedure. Atrial arrhythmias requiring medical treatment occurred in 7 of these study patients. Older adults who develop atrial arrhythmias should be screened for atrial enlargement, atrial thrombosis, ventricular function, and valvular regurgitation. In patients with acceptable surgical risk and reduced functional status because of recent development of atrial arrhythmias, valvular repair or atrial reduction with conversion to a lateral-tunnel Fontan procedure should be seriously considered.

▶ These authors have considerable experience in the use of the Fontan procedure in adults. I think their observations in this unusual group are very useful.

**J.J. Collins, Jr., M.D.**

---

**Orthotopic Pulmonic Valve Replacement With a Pulmonary Homograft as an Interposition Graft**
Balaguer JM, Byrne JG, Cohn LH (Brigham and Women's Hosp, Boston)
*J Card Surg* 11:417–420, 1996                                                    5–51

---

*Introduction.*—Pulmonary regurgitation is usually well tolerated after nonvalved reconstruction of the right ventricular outflow tract in tetralogy of Fallot or other congenital heart disease associated with pulmonary atresia or stenosis. Because of chronic pulmonary valve regurgitation that overloads the right ventricle, a small percentage of patients have right ventricular dilatation and right heart failure develop. Pulmonic valve replacement may offer relief for these patients, particularly with the advent of cryopreserved homograft valves. Two patients who have been operated on for severe pulmonary valve insufficiency and right heart failure who received cryopreserved pulmonary homografts were described, along with the technique of pulmonic valve replacement using a pulmonary homograft as an orthotopic root replacement.

*Case 1.*—Woman, 40, had pulmonary and infundibular stenosis repair by pulmonic valve and hypertrophic parietal and septal band excision 14 years ago. Ten years after her surgery, she had right ventricular dysfunction, dyspnea, and peripheral edema. After her pulmonary valve replacement with a 2-mm cryopreserved pulmonary homograft and primary closure of the recurrent secundum atrial septum defect, she had an uneventful recovery.

*Case 2.*—Man, 52, had complete correction of tetralogy of Fallot 23 years earlier. He then had right ventricular failure with right ventricular dilatation 5 years before reoperation. He had pulmonary valve replacement with a 27-mm pulmonary homograft, and 24 months later, he was found to still have some residual right ventricular failure.

*Operative Technique.*—A longitudinal incision along the main pulmonary artery was made, and the upper part of the old pericardial patch used during the initial repair was excised (Fig 1). The pulmonic valve leaflets were removed, and the annulus was

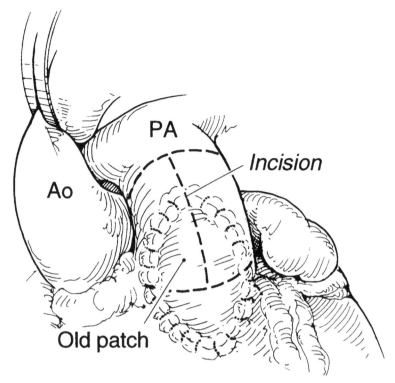

**FIGURE 1.**—A longitudinal incision along the main pulmonary artery (*PA*) was made, and the upper part of the old pericardial patch used at the time of the initial repair was excised. *Abbreviation: Ao*, aorta. (Courtesy of Balaguer JM, Byrne JG, Cohn LH: Orthotopic pulmonic valve replacement with a pulmonary homograft as an interposition graft. *J Card Surg* 11:417–420, 1996.)

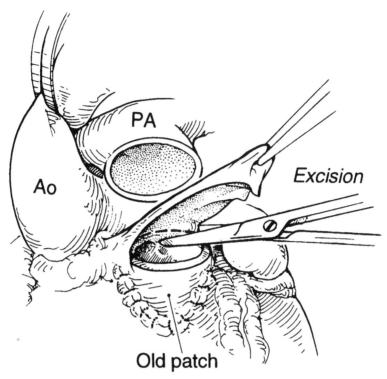

**Old patch**

FIGURE 2.—The pulmonic valve leaflets were removed and the annulus trimmed and débrided. The lower aspect of the patch at the previous right ventricular outflow tract reconstruction was left in place. The pulmonary artery (*PA*) was excised to the bifurcation. *Abbreviation: Ao*, aorta. (Courtesy of Balaguer JM, Byrne JG, Cohn LH: Orthotopic pulmonic valve replacement with a pulmonary homograft as an interposition graft. *J Card Surg* 11:417–420, 1996.)

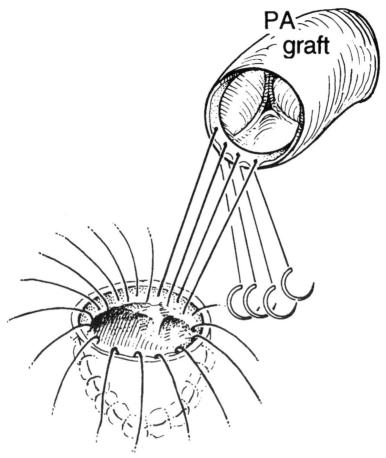

**FIGURE 3.**—The annulus is sized and the cryopreserved pulmonary homograft (CryoLife) is thawed. A series of simple 4–0 Ethibond sutures were placed through the pulmonic annulus and through the lower end of the pulmonary homograft without telescoping it inside the right ventricular outflow tract. The homograft is lowered down to the pulmonic annulus and the sutures tied. *Abbreviation: PA*, pulmonary artery. (Courtesy of Balaguer JM, Byrne JG, Cohn LH: Orthotopic pulmonic valve replacement with a pulmonary homograft as an interposition graft. *J Card Surg* 11:417–420, 1996.)

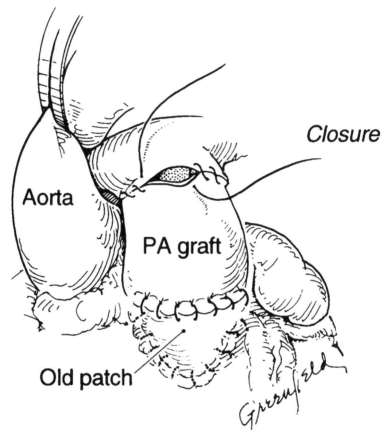

FIGURE 4.—The anastomosis between the upper end of the pulmonary homograft and the main pulmonary artery (*PA*) is performed at the level of bifurcation with a running 4-0 Prolene. (Courtesy of Balaguer JM, Byrne JG, Cohn LH: Orthotopic pulmonic valve replacement with a pulmonary homograft as an interposition graft. *J Card Surg* 11:417–420, 1996.)

trimmed and débrided. The pulmonary artery was excised (Fig 2). Sutures were placed through the pulmonic annulus, and the homograft was lowered to the pulmonic annulus (Fig 3). Anastomosis was performed at the level of bifurcation (Fig 4).

*Discussion.*—The optimal choice for pulmonary valve replacement may be the cryopreserved pulmonary homograft. The pulmonary homograft in orthotopic position has a very low gradient, ensuring optimal hemodynamics, and is a simple technique to perform. It also seems to have a lower long-term morbidity than other valved conduits.

▶ Pulmonic valve replacement is uncommonly necessary, but this technique appears to be an excellent alternative when patients are symptomatic from pulmonary valve dysfunction.

**J.J. Collins, Jr., M.D.**

## Miscellaneous Surgical Topics

**Calcified Pedicled Thrombus in the Left Ventricle: The Fine Art of Nature**
Morales C, Bernal JM, Rabasa JM, et al (Universidad de Cantabria, Santander, Spain)
*J Thorac Cardiovasc Surg* 114:491–492, 1997                    5–52

*Background.*—Cardiac thrombi within the ventricles are rare, and fixed calcifications are rarer still. The first case of a calcified pedicled thrombus in the left ventricle was reported.

*Case Report.*—Man, 46, with no symptoms of cardiac disease was evaluated for generalized discomfort and asthenia of 6 months' duration. Doppler echocardiography revealed a mass connected to the apex of the left ventricle, and a left ventriculogram revealed apical akinesia in the area of the mass. Cardiac catheterization confirmed the presence of 2-vessel disease and the need for coronary revascularization. During the revascularization procedure, the left ventricle was opened and a fixed, pearly mass was removed. The histologic features indicated a calcified thrombus, 5 × 1.8 cm. The patient's recovery was uneventful.

*Conclusions.*—This fixed, calcified thrombus in the left ventricle is the first report of its kind. How long the thrombus had existed is unknown. Also unknown is how the thrombus formed, although the presence of apical akinesia in this same area may be more than a coincidence.

▶ This is an interesting short report by Morales and associates. I think one can assume that a calcified pedicled mass in the left ventricle must have been there for a very long while. It is not so perfectly clear to me that an operation to resect such a mass should have been performed had it not been necessary to perform coronary revascularization surgery. It is extremely difficult for surgeons and even harder for physicians to tolerate a pedicled mass in whatever chamber of the heart it is encountered. I think there may not always be an indication for removal of such masses when the very nature of the mass suggests a very long residence—particularly in the left ventricle.

**J.J. Collins, Jr., M.D.**

## Management of Mobile Right Atrial Thrombi: A Therapeutic Dilemma

Shah CP, Thakur RK, Ip JH, et al (Univ Hosp, London, Canada; Michigan State Univ, Lansing)

*J Card Surg* 11:428–431, 1996                                                5–53

*Introduction.*—An uncommon finding on routine echocardiography is right-sided cardiac thrombi. Enlarged right atrium, decreased cardiac output, and relative stasis of blood are conditions associated with immobile right-sided thrombi. Echocardiographically mobile thrombi are thought to represent emboli from venous structures downstream. The poor prognosis of mobile thrombi may be explained by the postulate that only very large emboli arising from pelvic or proximal leg veins become lodged in the right heart. Six patients with mobile right atrial thrombus during a 3-year period were described.

*Methods.*—The 6 patients, 4 men and 2 women with a mean age of 63 years, had a combined total of 6,000 echocardiograms during a 3-year period. Five patients had progressive dyspnea and chest pain, and 1 patient had syncope with chest pain, which were the indications for echocardiography.

*Results.*—All patients had a mobile thrombus in the right atrium. Ventilation-perfusion mismatch was confirmed in all patients. Absence of the thrombus suggesting pulmonary embolization was seen in 3 patients with subsequent echocardiography. One patient died during transesophageal echocardiography. A large pulmonary embolization in the main pulmonary artery was seen on autopsy. Three patients were treated with heparinization, and 1 patient was treated with systemic thrombolysis. One patient had surgical removal of the right atrial thrombus, which was long and serpiginous and was tethered to a fenestrated eustachian valve. A total of 3 patients died; worsening of hypoxia and hypotension preceded the deaths. Two of 3 patients treated with heparin survived, as well as 1 patient who had surgical removal of the thrombus.

*Conclusions.*—The unusual echocardiographic finding of mobile thrombus in the right atrium portends a poor prognosis, with death resulting from pulmonary embolism. For most patients, initial therapy should be based on the mobility and size of the thrombus, whether pulmonary embolism has already occurred, and the hemodynamic status of the patient. Treatment options consist of systemic or local infusion of thrombolytic agents, anticoagulation, or surgical thromboembolectomy.

▶ There is very little information in the literature about mobile right atrial thrombi. I think this report of 6 cases is very interesting. I would not have guessed that the outlook was so poor for these patients.

**J.J. Collins, Jr., M.D.**

### Regression of Metastatic Carcinoid Tumor After Valvular Surgery for Carcinoid Heart Disease

Rayson D, Pitot HC, Kvols LK (Mayo Clinic and Mayo Found, Rochester, Minn)
*Cancer* 79:605–611, 1997                                                    5–54

*Objective.*—Carcinoid heart disease causes formation of valvular lesions. Although at least 38 cases of carcinoid heart disease requiring valvular surgery since 1966, few reported postoperative tumor status. Reports of tumor regression in 4 patients after valvular heart surgery for severe carcinoid heart disease are discussed.

*Discussion.*—After valvular replacement, all patients had improved cardiac function, regression of their metastatic disease, and a reduction in size of liver metastases. Carcinoid syndrome, characterized by flushing and diarrhea, occurs in patients with long-standing metastatic disease and in as many as 56% of patients with carcinoid syndrome. Patients with the syndrome have a 3-year, 31% survival rate compared with a survival rate of 68% for patients with no heart involvement. Average duration of symptoms before diagnosis was 57 months, and the mean urinary 5-HIAA concentration was 270 mg. Of the 34 patients who died during 1 study, 14 died from congestive heart failure. The 4 patients in this report had significantly elevated urinary 5-HIAA, liver metastases, and incapacitating congestive heart failure. The presence of carcinoid heart disease was confirmed with echocardiography and Doppler ultrasonography. Patients treated with a somatostatin analogue had symptomatic relief from carcinoid syndrome but experienced cardiac failure while taking the drug. Whereas valve replacement has resulted in improvement for these patients, this is the first report of metastatic regression after heart surgery. Cardiac involvement is thought to arise either from increased levels of serotonin secreted into right-sided circulation by liver metastases or from the release of atrial natriuretic peptide (ANP) by cardiac myocytes. Increasing ANP levels are associated with congestive heart failure.

*Conclusion.*—Regression of metastatic carcinoid disease after valvular replacement in 4 patients is reported for the first time.

▶ Dr. Rayson has observed what appears to be regression of metastatic carcinoid tumor after valve surgery for the carcinoid heart syndrome. We have had a modest experience with carcinoid tumors, but we certainly have not recognized regression of tumor afterward. We will carry out a retrospective review of these patients.

**J.J. Collins, Jr., M.D.**

## What is the Appropriate Size Criterion for Resection of Thoracic Aortic Aneurysms?

Coady MA, Rizzo JA, Hammond GL, et al (Yale Univ, New Haven, Conn)
*J Thorac Cardiovasc Surg* 113:476–491, 1997                               5–55

*Objective.*—Rupture is the most common cause of death in patients with atherosclerotic aneurysms of the ascending aorta. Because the size-rupture correlation does not hold for the thoracic aorta, it is important to understand the risk factors that influence the natural course of the disease to select patients for whom the risk of operation is justified. Criteria for surgical intervention based on a study of 230 patients with thoracic aortic aneurysms are presented.

*Methods.*—Between October 1985 and March 1996, of the 230 patients (92 female), aged 16 to 92, including 25 patients with Marfan's syndrome, followed at the Yale Center for Thoracic Aortic Disease, 136 were operated. There were 67 elective and 69 emergency surgeries. Complication rates and operative mortality were recorded, and 5-year survival estimates were calculated.

*Results.*—Aneurysms ranged in size from 4.0 to 8.0 cm and averaged 5.2 cm. The estimated annual growth rate was 0.12 cm with larger aneurysms growing at a greater rate. The growth rate for ascending aortic aneurysms was 0.10 cm and for descending aortic aneurysms was 0.29 cm. Acute dissection or rupture incidence ranged from 7.1% to 45.2% for aortic sizes from less than 4 cm to greater than 6.0 cm. Overall, emergency, and nonemergency operative mortality rates were 15.4%, 21.7%, and 9.0%. One- and 5-year survival for patients with and without aortic dissection were 83% and 46% and 89 and 71%, respectively. Median sizes at rupture or dissection for ascending and descending arteries were 6.0 and 7.2 cm. Ascending aneurysms greater than 6.0 cm had a 32.1% increased risk of rupture or dissection (p=0.005). Descending aneurysms greater than 7.0 cm had a 43.0% increased risk of rupture or dissection (p=0.006). Criteria for preemptive surgical intervention should be based on size smaller than the median rupture or dissection sizes above.

*Conclusion.*—Surgical intervention is recommended for descending aneurysms of 6.5 cm and for ascending aneurysms of 5.5 cm.

▶ This is an excellent study by Dr. Coady. While one may have differences with the precise recommendation of the size constituting an acceptable choice for elective resection, I think the discussion of the paper as presented by Dr. Coady at the American Association for Thoracic Surgery in San Diego in the spring of 1996 is very useful. I highly recommend study of the original article and consideration of the remarks of the discussers as well.

**J.J. Collins, Jr., M.D.**

# 6 Cardiac Arrhythmias, Conduction Disturbances, and Electrophysiology

## Introduction

As expected, this field continues to grow in important ways. In particular, we continue to see the impact of clinical trials on patient care. The past year has seen the publication of the first clinical trial (Antirrhythmics vs. Implantable Defibrillators [AVID]) demonstrating that the implantable cardioverter defibrillator improves outcome significantly better than anti-arrhythmic drug therapy in treatment of patients with ventricular fibrillation or with ventricular tachycardia and syncope or hypotension or left ventricular ejection fraction less than 40-plus symptoms. This is the first secondary prevention trial that has shown such a result, and clearly has already had great impact. We continue to see data from important trials in the treatment of atrial fibrillation as well. Clinical trials will continue to be a very important source of data, and we are always better when we provide evidence-based medical care.

The reader will note that atrial fibrillation studies are at the most plentiful in this year's review. Atrial fibrillation remains the "frontier" of clinical cardiac electrophysiology, with the biggest gains in this field coming from studies using device therapy. Of particular interest, we are beginning to see the slow but, in this editor's judgment, real emergence of the implantable atrial defibrillator in the treatment of patients with atrial fibrillation. While this treatment remains investigational, low-energy defibrillation is now available from two different companies (InControl—the implantable atrial defibrillator, Medtronic, Inc.—the combined implantable atrial and ventricular defibrillator).

Interestingly enough, there is not a whole lot new in the field of radiofrequency ablation except for the documentation of ablation of a single focus rapidly firing as a cure of atrial fibrillation. The latter, of course, is an important advance, but of limited impact. It is widely acknowledged that there are not large numbers of such patients compared with the total number of patients who suffer from atrial fibrillation. Nevertheless, aggressive approaches to the treatment of atrial fibrillation are avidly being pursued, and we can expect a flood of interesting data, perhaps as soon as the next YEAR BOOK OF CARDIOLOGY review. For now, there is still much to absorb from this year's reported studies.

Albert L. Waldo, M.D.

## Atrial Fibrillation

CLINICAL TRIALS

---

**Acute Stroke With Atrial Fibrillation: The Copenhagen Stroke Study**
Jørgensen HS, Nakayama H, Reith J, et al (Bispebjerg Hosp, Copenhagen)
*Stroke* 10:1765–1769, 1996                                                   6–1

---

*Introduction.*—Atrial fibrillation (AF) is an important risk factor for stroke. The characteristics and prognosis of stroke in patients with AF were evaluated prospectively.

*Methods.*—This trial was part of the Copenhagen Stroke Study, a community-based investigation of 1,197 patients with acute stroke treated in a stroke unit from acute admission to end of rehabilitation. The Scandinavian Neurological Stroke Scale (SSS) was used to determine initial stroke severity. The SSS and Bartel Index were used to assess neurologic and functional outcomes.

*Results.*—Two hundred seventeen (18.3%) of 1,185 patients had AF on admission. The incidence of AF rose steeply with age, from 2% in patients under age 50, 28% in patients in their 80s, to 40% in stroke patients older than age 90. Atrial fibrillation was positively correlated with age, ischemic heart disease, previous stroke, and systolic blood pressure. It was not correlated with gender, diabetes, hypertension, previous transient ischemic attack, or silent infarction on CT. Atrial fibrillation was associated with a higher mortality rate, longer hospital stay, and a lower discharge rate to home. Patients with AF had markedly worse neurologic outcomes, compared with patients who did not have AF. A poorer outcome was related to initially more severe strokes.

*Conclusion.*—Patients with AF tend to have more severe strokes and markedly poorer outcome, compared with patients with sinus rhythm. These findings stress the importance of anticoagulant treatment of patients with AF. Lower blood pressure during the acute stroke phase may contribute to increased stroke severity in patients with AF.

► The Copenhagen Stroke Study is the first to measure in detail the consequences of stroke in patients with AF. Atrial fibrillation was associated with a 70% increase in mortality, a 40% decrease in the relative chance of discharge to a patient's own home, a 20% increase in the length of hospital stay, and a marked increase in impairment and disability in survivors. As the study states, "These detrimental effects were explained exclusively by one factor: Patients with AF had more-severe initial strokes." In addition, these studies confirmed the previous observations from the Framingham study that a significant percentage of strokes in the elderly are associated with AF and that this increases with age. Thus, in this study, 15% of patients in their 70s, 28% of patients in their 80s, and 40% of patients in their 90s had AF. The point once again to be emphasized from these sobering data is that despite the risks, elderly patients with AF should receive warfarin to achieve an international normalized ratio between 2–3, if at all possible.

**A.L. Waldo, M.D.**

**Cardioversion Guided by Transesophageal Echocardiography: The ACUTE Pilot Study: A Randomized, Controlled Trial**
Klein AL, for the ACUTE Investigators (Cleveland Clinic Found, Ohio)
*Ann Intern Med* 126:200–209, 97                                                     6–2

*Background.*—Successful electrical cardioversion performed for the restoration of sinus rhythm in patients with atrial fibrillation is associated with an increased risk for embolic stroke. To reduce this risk, conventional therapy consists of 7 weeks of treatment with warfarin before cardioversion is undertaken. Screening for thrombi in the left atrial appendage by means of transesophageal echocardiography (TEE) may permit cardioversion to be done earlier and more safely. A randomized, multicenter pilot clinical trial was designed to assess the feasibility and safety of TEE-guided early cardioversion.

*Methods.*—The ACUTE (Assessment of Cardioversion Using Transesophageal Echocardiography) Pilot Study enrolled 126 patients from 10 hospitals in the United States, Europe, and Australia. Eligible patients had atrial fibrillation (or atrial flutter with a history of atrial fibrillation) lasting longer than 2 days and had not received anticoagulant therapy for more than 7 days. Randomization was to a conventional or a TEE-guided approach to cardioversion. Patients in the TEE group began receiving anticoagulation therapy at their initial visit; heparin was used for inpatients and warfarin for outpatients. When stable therapeutic anticoagulation was assured, TEE was scheduled with subsequent cardioversion immediately or within 24 hours. Cardioversion was postponed and warfarin continued for 4 weeks if thrombi were detected, with TEE repeated to confirm freedom from thrombi.

*Results.*—Fifty-six of the 62 patients randomized to TEE-guided cardioversion had TEE done. Cardioversion was postponed in 7 patients when atrial thrombi were detected. Thirty-eight (84%) of the 45 patients having cardioversion had successful cardioversion without embolization. Of the 11 patients who had TEE but not cardioversion, 7 had thrombi, 3 spontaneously reverted to sinus rhythm, and 1 converted to sinus rhythm after overdrive pacing. Cardioversion was performed in 37 of the 64 patients receiving conventional therapy, and was successful in 28 (76%). One patient had a peripheral embolism to an upper extremity 3 days after cardioversion. Mean time to cardioversion was shorter in the TEE group (0.6 weeks) than in the conventional therapy group (4.8 weeks). There was a tendency toward a greater incidence of clinical hemodynamic instability and bleeding complications in the conventional therapy group.

*Conclusion.*—Preliminary findings in this pilot study of patients with atrial fibrillation suggest that TEE-guided cardioversion with short-term anticoagulation therapy is feasible and safe. Compared with conventional therapy, TEE may allow cardioversion to be done sooner, decrease the risk for embolism, and be associated with less clinical instability.

▶ With the completion of this pilot study, the important full-scale study is ongoing and has much to recommend it. We need to know the potential beneficial role of TEE, if any, in the acute management of patients with atrial fibrillation. There are accumulating data that suggest prompt cardioversion of atrial fibrillation with restoration of sinus rhythm is a very effective and important part of the treatment of atrial fibrillation. This study will help us to know if we can cardiovert fibrillation safely using TEE techniques in patients who have not been therapeutically anticoagulated for 3 weeks or more, but who have no evidence of left atrial clot on TEE. The pilot study clearly demonstrates that we will have much to learn from the full-scale trial.

**A.L. Waldo, M.D.**

---

**Atrial Fibrillation in the Setting of Acute Myocardial Infarction: The GUSTO-I Experience**
Crenshaw BS, for the GUSTO-I Trial Investigators (Duke Clinical Research Inst, Durham, NC)
*J Am Coll Cardiol* 30:406–413, 1997                                    6–3

---

*Introduction.*—Most investigations of atrial fibrillation (AF) in patients with myocardial infarction (MI) were conducted in the prethrombolytic era. The large Global Utilization of Streptokinase and TPA (alteplase) for Occluded Coronary Arteries (GUSTO-I) trial studied this topic during the thrombolytic era. The incidence of AF in acute MI was evaluated, and the clinical and angiographic risk factors related to its development and association with in-hospital, 30-day, and 1-year outcomes was determined.

*Methods.*—Of 4,278 patients with AF and acute MI, 1,026 had AF on admission electrocardiography and 3,254 had postadmission AF. The primary end point was death from any cause within 30 days. Baseline clinical characteristics, short-term clinical and angiographic outcomes, and 1-year mortality were compared.

*Results.*—The overall incidence of AF in this cohort was 10.4%. Compared with patients without AF, the incidence of 3-vessel coronary artery disease and initial Thrombolysis in Myocardial Infarction (TIMI) grade less than 3 flow was greater in patients with AF. Patients with AF were significantly more likely to experience in-hospital stroke (especially ischemic stroke), compared with patients without AF. Significant predictors of later AF were advanced age, higher peak creatine kinase levels, worse Killip class, and increased heart rate. Patients with AF had significantly higher unadjusted mortality rates at 30 days and 1 year, compared with patients without AF. The adjusted 30-day mortality rate was significantly higher in patients with postadmission or overall AF, but not baseline AF.

*Conclusion.*—Atrial fibrillation with acute MI is an independent predictor for stroke and 30-day mortality. More aggressive treatment strategies may be needed for these patients. Further investigation is warranted.

▶ The incidence of 10.4% of AF in the present study indicates that AF continues to be a significant complication of acute myocardial infarction. Also, AF was a marker of higher risk based on clinical and angiographic feature. This editor would like to emphasize the authors' conclusions that "because of their lower ejection fraction, more severe coronary artery disease and greater frequency of incomplete reperfusion, patients with this arrhythmia [atrial fibrillation] should be considered for early angiography and revascularization. These patient, particularly those who develop atrial fibrillation after admission, also have a more complicated hospital course and tend to have worse outcomes (including stroke and overall mortality). A more aggressive approach to management, including close monitoring, anticoagulation, and cardioversion, [seems] warranted."

**A.L. Waldo, M.D.**

---

**Atrial Fibrillation: Maintaining Stability of Sinus Rhythm or Ventricular Rate Control? The Need For Prospective Data: The PIAF Trial**
Hohnloser SH, Kuck K-H (JW Goethe Univ, Frankfurt, Germany; Allgemeines Krankenhaus St Georg, Hamburg, Germany)
*PACE* 20(Pt. 1):1989–1992, 1997                                    6–4

---

*Introduction.*—No prospective, controlled trials have been conducted to compare the benefits and risks of maintaining sinus rhythm or controlling ventricular rate in patients with atrial fibrillation (AF). The rationale and design of the Pharmacological Intervention in Atrial Fibrillation (PIAF) trial was described. The purpose of this multicenter trial is to analyze the benefits and risk of these 2 treatment approaches.

*Rationale.*—The incidence of recurrent AF after successful pharmacologic or electric cardioversion is high. There are hemodynamic advantages to restoration and maintenance of sinus rhythm, but the potential risks of treatment need to be weighed against its benefits. In addition, there has been no prospective controlled study comparing the risks and benefits of maintaining sinus rhythm vs. controlling ventricular rate.

*Study Design.*—This trial is designed as a feasibility (pilot) study that might be followed by a full-sized trial, with the primary end point being all-cause mortality. A large sample size will be needed to have adequate power with mortality alone as the primary end point, so the (pilot) study will use the occurrence of symptomatic recurrences of tachyarrhythmic AF in patients treated with heart rate control only as the primary end point. Secondary end points will include hemodynamic consequences of therapy, thromboembolic events, and mortality. Data will be analyzed on an intention-to-treat basis and on actual treatment.

*Therapeutic Modalities.*—The first-line medication for patients with persistent AF will be diltiazem. It will be up to the treating physician's discretion to modify therapy if diltiazem alone is not effective. A second group will receive amiodarone for restoration and maintenance of sinus rhythm. High efficacy rates are expected with amiodarone.

*Conclusion.*—There is a need for data from controlled trials evaluating the risk-benefit ratios of various therapeutic modalities for AF. Patient enrollment in the PIAF trial began early in 1995. If the trial can confirm the feasibility of the outlined study design, a full-sized mortality trial will be conducted.

▶ This trial has much in common with the NIH trial Atrial Fibrillation Follow-up Investigation of Rhythm Management (AFFIRM). It points, once again, toward the considerable need to resolve the questions relating to efforts to maintain sinus rhythm vs. efforts to simply control ventricular response rate during atrial fibrillation while administering warfarin. This trial is much narrower in scope than AFFIRM, as it is only using amiodarone as treatment to maintain sinus rhythm, and diltiazem as treatment to maintain rate control. Nevertheless, we look forward to its outcome.

**A.L. Waldo, M.D.**

---

**Atrial Fibrillation and Dilated Cardiomyopathy: Therapeutic Strategies When Sinus Rhythm Cannot Be Maintained**
Saxon LA (Univ of California, San Francisco)
*PACE* 20:720–725, 1997                                                                    6–5

---

*Introduction.*—The current and investigational treatments for chronic atrial fibrillation (AF), the problem of discovering the optimal ventricular rate control, and the potential independent adverse effects of an irregular ventricular response to AF are discussed. For patients with heart failure whose normal sinus rhythm (SR) is not restored by amiodarone therapy, alternative strategies for controlling ventricular rate response and symptoms are available.

*Defining Adequate Rate Control.*—Tachycardia-mediated cardiomyopathy may be reversed with successful ventricular rate control using cardioversion, atrioventricular nodal (AV) blocking drugs, or radiofrequency (RF) catheter ablation of the AV junction (AVJ) and pacemaker implantation. Although β-blockers and amiodarone slow the heart rate, they may result in inadequate sinus rhythm or ventricular rate control. The Atrial Fibrillation Follow-up Investigation of Rhythm Management (AFFIRM) Trial will examine if maintaining normal SR is beneficial.

*Role of Rate Regularity.*—Improvements in left ventricular (LV) function have been observed after AVJ ablation and pacemaker implantation. A beat-to-beat ventricular irregularity in AF patients resulting from changes in ventricular filling may lead to LV dysfunction that is independent of rate.

*Radiofrequency Ablation.*—Rate Control and Regularity.—Radiofrequency ablation is now a safer procedure since pacemakers are programmed to higher rates during the implantation process. Atrioventricular junction ablation can produce rate regularity in AF patients with dilated cardiomyopathy.

*The DCAF Trial.*—The Dilated Cardiomyopathy and Atrial Fibrillation (DCAF) trial will compare outcomes of rate control using AV nodal blocking agents vs. AVJ ablation and pacing.

*Anticoagulation-Cornerstone Therapy.*—Warfarin therapy reduces embolic risk and is especially indicated in this patient population.

*Conclusion.*—Optimal treatment of AF patients with dilated cardiomyopathy is uncertain. The DCAF and AFFIRM trials should shed new light on the management of patients with AF and cardiomyopathy.

▶ This is a concise review of the management of two important problems that may come together in one patient, namely, atrial fibrillation and dilated cardiomyopathy. The dilated cardiomyopathy and atrial fibrillation trial (DCAF), a multicenter trial designed to assess the outcomes of pharmacologic rate control vs. antrioventricular junction ablation and physiologic ventricular pacing in the management of atrial fibrillation in the setting of dilated cardiomyopathy, will go a long way torward helping understand this problem. The AFFIRM trial similarly should be helpful, as it is assumed that a fair number of patients who enter the trial will be patients with atrial fibrillation and dilated cardiomyopathy.

**A.L. Waldo, M.D.**

PHARMACOLOGIC THERAPY

**Value of Single Oral Loading Dose of Propafenone in Converting Recent-onset Atrial Fibrillation**

Azpitarte J, Alvarez M, Baún O, et al (Hosp Universitario Virgen de las Nieves, Granada, Spain; Med Dept of Laboratorios Knoll, Madrid)

*Eur Heart J* 18:1649–1654, 1997                                    6–6

*Objective.*—There are reports that a single loading dose of propafenone is highly effective for converting atrial fibrillation to sinus rhythm. The safety and efficacy of a single oral loading weight-titrated dose of propafenone in converting recent-onset atrial fibrillation to sinus rhythm were evaluated in a randomized, double-blind, placebo-controlled trial.

*Methods.*—Oral propafenone ($n = 29$) or placebo ($n = 6$) was administered to 55 consecutive patients treated for acute atrial fibrillation in the emergency department of the Hospital Universitario Virgen de las Nieves, Granada, Spain. Dosages of 450 mg were given to patients weighing 65 to

85 kg and 750 mg to patients weighing 85 kg or more. Patients were observed for 24 hours and then sent for echocardiographic examination.

*Results.*—At 2 hours, significantly more propafenone patients ($n = 12$) than control patients ($n = 2$) had converted to sinus rhythm (41% vs. 8%). The comparisons at 6 were 65% vs. 31% and at 12 hours were 69% vs. 42%. Differences at 24 hours were no longer significant (79% vs. 73%). Atrial flutter was reported by 1 placebo and 1 propafenone patient. Four propafenone patients experienced hypotension. There were too few patients in the study to resolve the safety question.

*Conclusion.*—A single dose of propafenone restored sinus rhythm significantly faster than placebo, although the effect was lost after 24 hours.

---

**Oral Propafenone to Convert Recent-Onset Atrial Fibrillation in Patients With and Without Underlying Heart Disease: A Randomized, Controlled Trial**

Boriani G, Biffi M, Capucci A, et al (Università degli Studi di Bologna, Italy; Ospedale Civile di Piacenza, Italy; Ospedale S Anna, Como, Italy; et al)
*Ann Intern Med* 126:621–625, 1997                                      6–7

---

*Introduction.*—Previous controlled studies have confirmed the effectiveness of oral propafenone in converting recent-onset atrial fibrillation to sinus rhythm, but the benefits and safety of this antiarrhythmic agent in patients with structural heart disease have not been investigated. A randomized, single-blind, controlled study evaluated oral propafenone in patients with and without underlying heart disease.

*Methods.*—Eligible patients were hospitalized with recent-onset ($\leq 7$ days) atrial fibrillation. Among the exclusion criteria were heart failure greater than New York Heart Association (NYHA) class II, recent (within 6 months) myocardial infarction, and long-term digoxin or antiarrhythmic therapy. The study group consisted of 240 patients, 104 with and 136 without structural heart disease. Randomization was to either oral propafenone, 2 tablets of 300 mg each, taken as a single dose (119 patients) or placebo (121 patients). Patients were monitored for blood pressure and 12-lead ECG findings after administration of the study drug. After 8 hours, physicians could continue the initial treatment or switch to a different option. Conversion was defined as a stable sinus rhythm lasting at least 1 hour.

*Results.*—The propafenone and placebo groups were comparable in mean age, sex, cause of atrial fibrillation, NYHA class, left atrial dimension, structural heart disease, hypertension, and duration of atrial fibrillation before randomization. At 3 hours, conversion to sinus rhythm had occurred in 45% of the propafenone group, vs. 18% of the placebo group. Propafenone also was more effective at 8 hours; 76% of patients receiving propafenone and 37% of patients given placebo had converted to sinus rhythm by this time. Among patients without underlying heart disease, 78% of those treated with propafenone and 56% given placebo converted to sinus rhythm within 8 hours. Patients with hypertension and those with structural heart disease benefited similarly from propafenone therapy (8-hour conversion rates of 70% and 81%, respectively). In contrast, patients in these subgroups who were randomized to placebo had 8-hour conversion rates of only 27% and 17%, respectively.

*Conclusion.*—Oral propafenone brought about conversion to sinus rhythm within a few hours in patients with recent-onset atrial fibrillation. The drug was safe and effective in patients with and without underlying heart disease. The rate of spontaneous conversion in patients randomized to placebo was significantly higher, however, among those without structural heart disease.

---

**Propafenone For Conversion and Prophylaxis of Atrial Fibrillation**
Stroobandt R, for the Propafenone Atrial Fibrillation Trial Investigators (St-Jozef Hosp, Oostende, Belgium)
*Am J Cardiol* 79:418–423, 1997                                             6–8

---

*Introduction.*—Antiarrhythmic drugs are the mainstay of treatment for most patients with atrial fibrillation, though few clinical trials have evaluated the safety and efficacy of these agents. A prospective, multicenter trial was designed to assess the ability of propafenone hydrochloride to restore sinus rhythm and prevent recurrences of atrial fibrillation.

*Methods.*—The study was conducted at 23 centers in Belgium and The Netherlands. Eligible patients had atrial fibrillation, either recent-onset (lasting not more than 2 weeks) or chronic (lasting more than 2 weeks), occurring either as a first episode or as a recurrent episode. None had symptoms of heart failure, recent myocardial infarction or cardiac surgery, or other serious cardiac or pulmonary conditions. The 136 patients who met entry criteria were randomized in a double-blind manner to propafenone (2 mg/kg over 30 minutes, followed by oral propafenone 150 mg 3 times daily) or matching placebo. Patients who failed to respond to IV therapy underwent direct-current cardioversion. Follow-up to determine maintenance of sinus rhythm continued for 6 months.

*Results.*—The patient group had a mean age of 62; 99 were men and 37 were women. No underlying cardiac disease was present in 36%, but 46% had previous episodes of atrial fibrillation documented by ECG. Randomization was 3:1, with 101 patients in the propafenone group and 35 in the placebo group. Conversion to sinus rhythm after IV therapy was achieved in 29% of patients taking propafenone and in 17% randomized to placebo, not a significant difference. Direct-current cardioversion was equally successful (70%) for nonresponders in both groups. At 6-month follow-up, 67% of patients treated with propafenone were free from recurrent symptomatic arrhythmia. Only 35% of the placebo group, however, had maintained sinus rhythm without relapse. The propafenone group also had a more favorable outcome in time to atrial fibrillation relapse. Drug-related side effects occurred at similar rates in propafenone (10%) and placebo (14%) groups.

*Conclusion.*—Although a "slow" infusion of propafenone was of limited value in terminating atrial fibrillation, the drug was effective in maintaining sinus rhythm when given orally at a low dosage over a 6-month period.

► These 3 studies (Abstracts 6–6 to 6–8) used different doses of propafenone in conversion of atrial fibrillation. Two studies (Abstracts 6–6 and 6–7) used oral doses and 1 (Abstract 6–8) started with an intravenous dose and then 1 or 2 low oral doses. The point to be made is that probably the best conversion rate to sinus rhythm is obtained with a single 600 mg dose of propafenone. Smaller doses were not as effective, and since the 600 mg dose does not have an incidence of side effects that is different from lower doses, it is the recommended dose. One should note that data from other studies also suggest that flecainide, 300 mg in a single dose, is as effective as propafenone in a single dose of 600 mg. And finally, the last of these studies indicates that on a relatively low dose of propafenone, 150 mg every 8 hours, the atrial fibrillation recurrence rate was significantly lower than with placebo.

In the study, the recurrence rate was in the 40% range, typical of the many prior studies with other drugs to treat atrial fibrillation. The point to emphasize is that recurrence is not failure, it is the frequency of recurrence that is the measure of efficacy. In this regard, Abstract 6–8 also showed that the interval between subsequent episodes of atrial fibrillation was significantly better on propafenone than on placebo. Thus, dear reader, please do not change medication because of a single recurrence. Rather, expect it, cardiovert the patient if need be, and observe the interval to the next episode, if it recurs.

**A.L. Waldo, M.D.**

---

**Efficacy, Safety, and Determinants of Conversion of Atrial Fibrillation and Flutter With Oral *Amiodarone***
Tieleman RG, Gosselink M, Crijns HJGM, et al (Univ Hosp Groningen, The Netherlands)
*Am J Cardiol* 79:53–57, 1997                                                      6–9

---

*Objective.*—The safety of amiodarone in outpatients for controlling heart rate or bradyarrhythmias during atrial fibrillation (AF) has not been tested. Results of a prospective efficacy and safety study of amiodarone for pharmacologic conversion of AF in patients with refractory arrhythmia and of the relation of drug plasma levels to the conversion rate are presented.

*Methods.*—Amiodarone (600 mg/day) was administered for 4 weeks to 129 patients (48 women) with refractory AF or flutter who had failed previous drug therapy. All antiarrhythmic drugs were withdrawn for at least 5 half-lives before amiodarone therapy was initiated. The main outcome was conversion to sinus rhythm within 1 month of beginning treatment.

*Results.*—During the loading phase, 23 patients converted to sinus rhythm. Electrical conversion was successful in 92 of the 106 patients. Multivariate analysis showed that desethylamiodarone plasma level, arrhythmia duration, left atrial area, and treatment with verapamil were significant predictors of conversion. Patients who converted after amiodarone treatment tended to have higher plasma levels of amiodarone and desethylamiodarone than patients who did not convert. After 1 month on amiodarone therapy, the 106 patients who did not convert during the loading period had a significant decrease in at-rest heart rate from 100 to 87 beats/min. The relation between rate reduction and amiodarone serum concentration was significant. Three patients experienced minor gastrointestinal distress.

*Conclusion.*—Amiodarone is a safe and effective treatment for refractory atrial fibrillation. Pharmacologic conversion is related to plasma levels of desethylamiodarone.

▶ This study is of interest because, in a patient population resistant to treatment with other drugs, and with many risk factors for maintenance of AF including duration of AF and left atrial size, 18% of patients converted spontaneously to sinus rhythm. Nevertheless, this editor would remind the reader that endocardial cardioversion techniques using low-energy shocks are safe and effective in converting AF in patients who are otherwise resistant to it. This point should be strongly considered. Data from previous such studies indicate that patients do remarkably well in maintaining sinus rhythm, although they often may require antiarrhythmic drug therapy.

**A.L. Waldo, M.D.**

---

## Effectiveness of Verapamil–Quinidine Versus Digoxin–Quinidine in the Emergency Department Treatment of Paroxysmal Atrial Fibrillation

Innes GD, Vertesi L, Dillon EC, et al (Royal Columbian Hosp, New Westminster, BC, Canada)
*Ann Emerg Med* 29:126–134, 1997                                                 6–10

---

*Background.*—Patients with paroxysmal atrial fibrillation (PAF) are commonly seen in the emergency department (ED). Prompt, appropriate treatment is always desirable. The evidence suggests that digoxin is inappropriate for acute AF—some treatment that offers quicker and more reliable control of the ventricular response could lead to faster conversion of PAF. This would permit faster discharge from the ED and avoid unnecessary hospitalization. The combination of verapamil-quinidine was compared with digoxin-quinidine for the ED treatment of PAF in a double-blind, randomized, controlled trial.

*Methods.*—The study included 54 adult patients up to 75 years of age with new-onset AF. Patients with a ventricular response rate lower than 100 or higher than 200 beats/min were excluded, as were those with allergy to the study drugs, hypotension with signs of end-organ hypoperfusion, and conduction abnormalities. Initially, 1 group of patients received digitalis, 1.0 mg over 2 hours, while the other received IV verapamil, given in sequential 5-mg boluses up to 20 mg. Once the ventricular rate fell below 100 beats/min, all patients received oral quinidine sulfate, 200 mg. Quinidine administration was repeated every 2 hours until normal sinus rhythm was restored, the patient had received a total of 1 g of quinidine, or adverse effects developed.

*Results.*—After withdrawal, there were 19 patients in the verapamil-quinidine (VER-Q) group and 22 in the digoxin-quinidine (DIG-Q) group. Conversion to normal sinus rhythm occurred within 6 hours in 84% of patients in the VER-Q group vs. 45% in the DIG-Q group. The mean time to conversion was 185 and 368 minutes, although the difference was not significant. Sixty-three percent of patients in the VER-Q group were discharged from the ED compared with only 27% of those in the DIG-Q group. Patients receiving VER-Q were more likely to have adverse effects but only minor ones. None of the patients died or experienced significant morbidity.

*Conclusions.*—At the doses used in this study, the sequential combination of verapamil and quinidine appears to be an effective ED treatment for PAF. It is more effective than the combination of digoxin and quinidine. The results may not apply to postcardiac surgery or critical care patients.

▶ The effectiveness of the quinidine-verapamil combination for the cardioversion of atrial fibrillation in this group of patients is impressive. Nevertheless, this editor would like to emphasize that quinidine is no longer often recommended for such use for 2 reasons. First, there is an incidence of torsades de pointes which is quite important. In addition, about 30% of patients get important gastrointestinal side effects from quinidine. Rather, per the above-mentioned studies, propafenone and flecainide should be considered because they have equal efficacy, less side effects, and no incidence of torsades de pointes.

**A.L. Waldo, M.D.**

---

**Effect of Verapamil and Procainamide on Atrial Fibrillation-induced Electrical Remodeling in Humans**
Daoud EG, Knight BP, Weiss R, et al (Univ of Michigan, Ann Arbor)
*Circulation* 96:1542–1550, 1997                                    6–11

---

*Introduction.*—In response to brief or chronic episodes of pacing-induced atrial fibrillation, a progressive shortening of atrial refractoriness has been demonstrated in previous studies. Verapamil has been shown to block the shortening of the atrial effective refractory period, whereas hypercalcemia has been shown to accentuate it, suggesting that this type of atrial electrical remodeling may be caused by calcium loading. The effects of IV verapamil and procainamide on the atrial electrophysiologic changes induced by atrial fibrillation in humans were determined.

*Methods.*—There were 37 patients without structural heart disease who had atrial effective refractory period measured before and after atrial fibrillation. The patients were divided into 3 groups to receive pharmacologic autonomic blockade of verapamil, procainamide, or saline. Rapid pacing was used to induce atrial fibrillation. Using alternating drive cycle lengths of 350 and 500 msec, post-atrial fibrillation effective refractory period measurements were taken immediately upon atrial fibrillation conversion.

*Results.*—At the 350-msec drive cycle length in the saline group, the pre-atrial fibrillation effective refractory period was 206 ± 19 msec and the first post-atrial fibrillation effective refractory period was 179 ± 27 msec. In the saline group, the pre-atrial fibrillation effective refractory period was 217 ± 16 at the 500 msec drive cycle length; it was 183 ± 23 msec at the first post-atrial fibrillation effective refractory period. In the procainamide group, there was a similar significant shortening of the first post-atrial fibrillation effective refractory period. No difference was seen, however, in the verapamil group between the pre-atrial fibrillation and first post-atrial fibrillation effective refractory period at the 350-msec and 500-msec drive cycle length. In 12% of verapamil patients, secondary episodes of atrial fibrillation were unintentionally induced during determinations of the post-atrial fibrillation effective refractory period, compared with 80% of the procainamide patients and 90% of the saline patients.

*Conclusion.*—There is marked attenuation of acute, atrial fibrillation-induced changes in atrial electrophysiologic properties with pretreatment with the calcium channel antagonist verapamil, but not with the sodium channel antagonist procainamide. Atrial fibrillation-induced electrical remodeling may be partially caused by calcium loading during atrial fibrillation.

▶ We now appreciate that there are pathophysiologic changes in the atria that occur during atrial fibrillation because of a sustained rapid rate (about 350 bpm), and that these changes are conducive to the maintenance of atrial fibrillation. This study in patients indicates that verapamil is a good choice for therapy in patients with atrial fibrillation because it will not only provide good ventricular rate control, but also, it appears that it will attenuate some of the adverse remodeling effects that result from the rapid atrial rhythm. We look forward to further studies to learn how better to deal with this aspect of atrial fibrillation.

**A.L. Waldo, M.D.**

### Emergency Management of Atrial Fibrillation and Flutter: Intravenous Diltiazem Versus Intravenous Digoxin

Schreck DM, Rivera AR, Tricarico VJ (Muhlenberg Regional Med Ctr, Plainfield, NJ; Robert Wood Johnson Med School, Piscataway, NJ)

*Ann Emerg Med* 29:135–140, 1997                                                6–12

*Introduction.*—Digoxin has historically been the drug of choice for treating atrial fibrillation and flutter (AFF) in the emergency setting. Intravenous diltiazem was approved for treatment of AFF in 1992 by the United States Food and Drug Administration. No direct comparison trial of IV digoxin and IV diltiazem in the treatment of AFF has been made. The heart rate response to IV digoxin vs. IV diltiazem was compared in patients with acute stable AFF.

*Methods.*—Thirty consecutive patients with AFF were randomized to receive either IV digoxin, 0.25 mg at 0 and 30 minutes; IV diltiazem, 0.25 mg/kg over 2 minutes followed by 0.35 mg/kg at 15 minutes and then titrate ventricular rate with 10 to 20 mg/hour; or IV digoxin plus IV diltiazem. The heart rate response for each treatment regimen was examined at baseline and at 5, 10, 15, 30, 60, 120, and 180 minutes. Heart rate control was considered to be a rate lower than 100 beats per minute.

*Results.*—At baseline, the heart rates were 150 and 144 beats/min for the diltiazem and digoxin groups, respectively. The mean decrease in heart rate at 5 minutes was significant for diltiazem, but not digoxin (111 vs. 144 beats/min). The reduction in heart rate did not reach significance in the digoxin group until 180 minutes. At 180 minutes, heart rates were 90 for diltiazem and 117 for digoxin.

*Conclusion.*—A significant drop in ventricular heart rate was observed within 5 minutes of IV diltiazem administration, compared with 3 hours of treatment with IV digoxin. The treatment group that received IV diltiazem and IV digoxin had no advantage over the group treated with digoxin alone. Intravenous diltiazem was superior to IV digoxin in the emergency treatment of ventricular rate in acute AFF. It should now be considered the drug of choice for managing ventricular rate in acute AFF.

▶ This study presents data that have already been established for some time. However, it serves to emphasize a few points. First, there are many times when intravenous digoxin may be the drug of choice or should be part of the therapy. This includes patients who have atrial fibrillation and a rapid ventricular response rate in the presence of ventricular dysfunction, particularly in patients immediately after open heart surgery. Aggressive use of digitalis can slow the ventricular rate quickly without the negative ionotropic effects of a calcium-channel blocker, the latter being undesirable in certain circumstances. In the current study, the dose of digoxin given was remarkably low and could not be expected to be very effective. Giving half of a digitalizing dose as an initial bolus followed by frequent additional appropriate doses as needed[1] can provide quite satisfactory ventricular rate control.

**A.L. Waldo, M.D.**

*Reference*

1. Waldo AL, Maclean WAH: *Diagnosis and Treatment of Arrhythmias Following Open Heart Surgery—Emphasis on the Use of Epicardial Wire Electrodes.* Futura Publishing Co, Mt. Kisco, New York, 1980.

## Pharmacokinetic Interactions of Moricizine and Diltiazem in Healthy Volunteers

Shum L, Pieniaszek HJ Jr, Robinson CA, et al (Dupont Merck Pharmaceutical Company, Newark and Wilmington, NJ; Pharmaceutical Evaluation Services, Englewood Cliffs, NJ)

*J Clin Pharmacol* 36:1161–1168, 1996             6–13

*Objective.*—Moricizine hydrochloride and diltiazem are metabolized by the liver, subject to a significant first pass effect, rapidly absorbed, and very bioavailable. Because patients with cardiovascular disease may receive both drugs, and both drugs undergo extensive hepatic metabolism and are known to affect the disposition of other drugs, a substantial pharmacokinetic or metabolic interaction is possible. The steady-state pharmacokinetics of concurrent administration of moricizine and diltiazem were studied in healthy male volunteers.

*Methods.*—In a single center, open-label, nonrandom, 3 sequential treatment phase study, 24 healthy male volunteers, aged 18 to 40 years, were given 250-mg doses of oral moricizine every 8 hours during phase I (days 1 to 8), 60 mg of oral diltiazem every 8 hours during Phase II (days 21 to 28), and both medications every 8 hours during Phase III (days 29 to 36), with 12-day washout periods between phases. Plasma drug concentrations were determined on days 8, 28, and 36 at 0.25, 0.5, 0.75, 1, 1.5, 2, 3, 4, 6, and 8 hours. Two additional diltiazem plasma concentrations were determined at 12 and 24 hours.

*Results.*—Sixteen volunteers completed all phases. The frequencies of adverse events were significantly higher during diltiazem and moricizine-diltiazem administration. Plasma concentrations of moricizine were significantly higher and of diltiazem were significantly lower during coadministration than when either drug was administered alone. The mean increase in $C_{max}$ for moricizine was 89%, and the mean decrease in $Cl_o$ was 54%. The mean decrease in $C_{max}$ for diltiazem was 36%, the mean decrease in $AUC_T$ values was 36%, and the mean increase in $Cl_O$ was 52%. The half-life of moricizine was not affected by coadministration of diltiazem, but the half-life of diltiazam was shortened by coadministration of moricizine.

*Conclusion.*—Coadministration of moricizine and diltiazem results in an increase in plasma concentration of moricizine and a decrease in plasma concentration of diltiazem. Dosages may have to be adjusted to achieve optimum therapeutic benefit from each.

▶ Interestingly enough, moricizine's most common use these days is in the treatment of atrial fibrillation. Since diltiazem is also used in atrial fibrillation, this drug interaction is important to appreciate. It may permit a twice-daily dosing of moricizine and either a need for increased diltiazem or the addition of digoxin to the diltiazem regimen to assist in control of the ventricular response rate. And, of course, an alternative to diltiazem may well be indicated.

**A.L. Waldo, M.D.**

RADIOFREQUENCY CATHETER ABLATION THERAPY OF ATRIAL FIBRILLATION AND FLUTTER

**Radiofrequency Catheter Ablation of Common Atrial Flutter in 200 Patients**
Fischer B, Jaïs P, Shah D, et al (Universitaire de Bordeaux, France; Univ of Arizona, Tucson)
*J Cardiovasc Electrophysiol* 7:1225–1233, 1996                    6–14

*Introduction.*—Common (type I) atrial flutter is an often disabling and drug-resistant supraventricular tachycardia. Three recently published articles report the effects of treatment by radiofrequency (RF) ablation with either anatomic or electrophysiologic targets. Three different approaches to targeting the site were used in 200 cases.

*Methods.*—Patients were 172 men and 28 women, with a mean age of 60. All had symptomatic, drug-resistant atrial flutter; 47% had structural heart disease. The flutter was permanent in 45% of patients and paroxysmal in 55%; documented episodes of paroxysmal atrial fibrillation had occurred in 21.5%. In the first 50 patients, a combined anatomic and electrophysiologic approach was used to localize the target sites for RF ablation. The anatomic landmarks were between the tricuspid valve and inferior vena cava orifice (area 1), between the tricuspid valve and coronary sinus ostium (area 2), and between the inferior vena cava and coronary sinus (area 3). Radiofrequency ablation was delivered at the area where the most stable catheter position was first obtained. The next 30 patients had a single line of RF energy applied to each of the 3 areas. For the remaining 120 patients, RF energy was applied only in area 1, with repeated applications. The end point of the RF ablation procedure was interruption and noninducibility of common atrial flutter in the first 110 patients; bidirectional isthmal block was an end point in 48 of the last 90 patients. Mean follow-up was 24 months.

*Results.*—Atrial flutter was interrupted and rendered noninducible after a single session in 43 of the first 50 patients but could not be interrupted in 7. The mean number of applications given to those with noninducible atrial flutter was 16; a single application of RF energy was effective in 2 patients. The next 30 patients had RF applied at various sites. The first targeted area was unsuccessful in 18, but atrial flutter was successfully interrupted at subsequent sites in 17 patients. A mean of 10 applications interrupted atrial flutter in 119 of the last 120 patients. At follow-up, atrial flutter had recurred in 31 patients; second or third RF ablation sessions were successful in 25 cases. Eleven patients had atrial fibrillation at follow-up, that had not been documented before ablation.

*Conclusion.*—Overall, a single session of RF catheter ablation interrupted and rendered atrial flutter noninducible in 95% of these patients. Additional sessions were required, however, in 15.5% who had recurrences. The highest success rate was obtained when RF energy was applied in the isthmus between the inferior vena cava orifice and the tricuspid valve.

▶ These data from a superb clinical group in Bordeaux, France, confirm that if one identifies that the atrial flutter reentrant circuit includes an isthmus between the inferior vena cava, eustachian ridge, coronary sinus, and tricuspid valve annulus, placement of a line of block in this isthmus to provide bidirectional block will provide cure. The expectation is that 95% of patients will be cured with this procedure. It is important to document that the circuit does indeed utilize this isthmus, and that bidirectional block is obtained as a result of the radiofrequency ablation. Simply assuming that the patient has typical atrial flutter, and, therefore, the isthmus must be critically involved, is a potentially fatal flaw. Mastering the techniques of demonstrating achievement of bidirectional block in the isthmus after radiofrequency ablation is also critical.

**A.L. Waldo, M.D.**

---

**A Focal Source of Atrial Fibrillation Treated by Discrete Radiofrequency Ablation**
Jaïs P, Haïssaguerre M, Shah DC, et al (Hôpital Cardiologique de Haut-Lévêque, Bordeaux-Pessac, France)
*Circulation* 95:572–576, 1997                                          6–15

---

*Objective.*—Atrial fibrillation (AF) is usually attributed to multiple migratory re-entrant waves rather than a focal mechanism. A report of 9 patients with paroxysmal AF produced by a focal source is presented.

*Methods.*—Electrophysiologic studies of 9 patients (4 women), average age 38 years, with symptomatic drug-refractory AF demonstrated a focal source of activation during atrial arrhythmias characterized by a consistent and centrifugal pattern of activation.

*Results.*—An ablation procedure, using an average of 4 radiofrequency (RF) pulses, was performed on the earliest bipolar activity site relative to a stable atrial electrogram reference during AF. Ablation sites included 3 in the right atrium, 2 near the sinus node, 1 in the ostium of the coronary sinus, 1 between the right superior and inferior pulmonary veins, 4 at the ostium of the right superior pulmonary vein, and 1 at the ostium of the left superior pulmonary vein. A second ablation procedure was performed 7 days later on 1 patient who had recurrent AF. Neither AF nor atrial tachycardia recurred in any patient during a follow-up period averaging 10 months.

*Conclusion.*—Episodes of monomorphic irregular atrial tachycardia or extrasystoles, particularly in young patients without structural heart disease, are features of focal-source AF and should trigger an early electrophysiologic study during spontaneous episodes of tachycardia. Limited RF ablation can cure these patients.

▶ This fine paper documents very nicely that if one understands the mechanism of an arrhythmia, and a vulnerable, ablatable target is identified, ablation should be expected to provide cure. Thus, the old notion that atrial fibrillation may be caused by a single focus rapidly firing has now been definitively confirmed in patients. The difficulty is first in finding such patients. This etiology seems most likely to occur in young patients with lone atrial fibrillation. However, one should always consider that this may be present in older patients as well. Furthermore, we have known for a long time that atrioventricular reciprocating tachycardia (AVRT) and atrioventricular nodal reentrant tachycardia (AVNRT) can cause atrial fibrillation. This is simply one more variation on the same theme that tachycardia can induce tachycardia. Much as ablation of AVRT and AVNRT will prevent atrial fibrillation in the latter instances, so, too, with an ectopic atrial focus firing rapidly. It seems that one of the best ways to identify these patients is with a Holter monitor, which shows runs of nonsustained atrial tachycardia (i.e., short runs [5–10 beats] of supraventricular tachycardia in which the QRS complexes are preceded by ectopic P-waves) or by documenting a similar rhythm which leads to sustained atrial fibrillation.

**A.L. Waldo, M.D.**

---

### Right and Left Atrial Radiofrequency Catheter Therapy of Paroxysmal Atrial Fibrillation

Haïssaguerre M, Jaïs P, Shah DC, et al (Université de Bordeaux II, France)
*J Cardiovasc Electrophysiol* 7:1132–1144, 1996                6–16

---

*Introduction.*—Extensive surgical incisions of the atria are the only curative techniques available for most atrial fibrillation (AF). The staged creation of ablation lines by sequential applications of radiofrequency (RF) energy was evaluated in 45 consecutive patients with daily episodes of paroxysmal AF.

*Methods.*—Linear lesions were placed to divide the atrial anatomy during progressive anatomically directed ablation. Sequential applications of RF current were applied to the right atrium, then the left atrium, if required (Fig 1). The procedure was considered successful when the episodes of AF were either elimated or recurred at a rate of no more than 1 episode lasting less than 6 hours in 3 months. Patients were considered

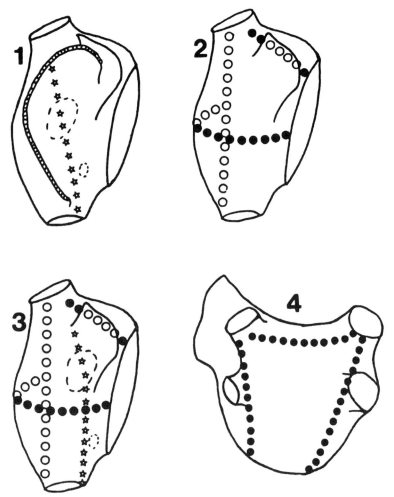

FIGURE 1.—Diagram of the ablation schema used in the right atrium (1, 2, 3, Anterior view) and left atrium (4, Posterior view). Group 1 (15 patients) underwent only a single septal right atrial line: group 2 (15 patients) underwent 2 lines longitudinal and transverse in the right atrial free wall; and group 3 (15 patients) underwent an additional septal line. Diagram 4 shows the left atrial lines performed in the group of 9 failures from the above 3 groups. (Courtesy of Haïssaguerre M, Jaïs P, Shah DC: Right and left atrial radiofrequency catheter therapy of paroxysmal atrial fibrillation. *J Cardiovasc Electrophysiol* 7:1132–1144, 1996.)

improved if they had no more than 1 episode per month. The RF energy was delivered during AF and sinus rhythm in 41 and 4 patients, respectively.

*Results.*—In 18 of 45 patients, ablation lines converted the fibrillatory activity to organized activity and stable sinus rhythm. Atrial pacing was able to induce sustained AF in 40 of 45 patients after ablation. The lesions did not produce evidence of a significant linear conduction block/delay in 41 patients. Complications included 2 transient sinus node dysfunctions.

The average procedure duration was 248 minutes. The average fluoroscopic time was 53 minutes. Nineteen patients required additional sessions to treat sustained right atrial flutter or arrhythmias. At a mean follow-up of 11 months, right atrial ablation was successful in 15 patients (33%) and 9 patients (20%) were improved. Ten patients with unsuccessful outcomes underwent linear ablation in the left atrium. Of these, 1 patient experienced hemopericardium, 2 patients required reablation to treat ectopic atrial foci, left atrial ablation was terminated in 8 patients, and sustained AF was not inducible in 5 patients. Subsequent success was accomplished in 6 patients and 1 patient was improved.

*Conclusion.*—Right and left atrial RF catheter therapy has low morbidity and can improve or cure a significant number of patients with drug-refractory paroxysmal AF. This approach is promising, but more work is needed to shorten procedure duration and optimize lesion characteristics.

▶ This editor agrees with the Bordeaux group that this procedure is highly investigational.The reader is reminded that the procedure is difficult in the first instance, that there is a significant incidence of stroke despite anticoagulation, and now there is a reported incidence of pulmonary hypertension. In addition, it is probably good to realize that the catheter ablation does not make a fine line of block, but rather a lesion which is a band rather than a line of block. Thus, making many of these lesions should be expected to "cook" considerable portions of the atria. In short, it is not yet clear that this is going to become a standard technique to treat atrial fibrillation. Understanding mechanisms of atrial fibrillation (there are probably several) and improving radiofrequency technology are surely important before treating atrial fibrillation with this approach. We look forward to future studies to clarify these issues.

**A.L. Waldo, M.D.**

---

**Exercise Capacity After His Bundle Ablation and Rate Response Ventricular Pacing for Drug Refractory Chronic Atrial Fibrillation**
Buys EM, van Hemel NM, Kelder JC, et al (St Antonius Hosp, Nieuwegein, The Netherlands)
*Heart* 77:238–241, 1997                                        6–17

---

*Introduction.*—His bundle ablation followed by long-term cardiac pacing is often performed in patients with atrial fibrillation who cannot tolerate or have insufficient response to antiarrhythmic drugs. This prospective study examined the long-term effects on exercise capacity of His bundle ablation followed by ventricular rate–responsive pacing (VVIR).

*Methods.*—Twenty-five consecutive patients with chronic symptomatic atrial fibrillation took part in the study. All had been receiving antiarrhythmic drugs before undergoing His bundle ablation and pacemaker implantation. Exercise testing was performed with an upright bicycle ergometer and an automated breath-by-breath system to obtain respiratory gas variables. Exercise capacity, including measurements of oxygen consumption, was evaluated before and a mean of 7 months after His bundle ablation. All patients received the Telectronics Meta III (Telectronics, Lane Cove, Australia), a device that uses changes in minute ventilation as the sensed variable for adjusting pacing rate.

*Results.*—Right-sided His bundle ablation was successful at the first procedure in all cases. All patients were receiving antiarrhythmic drugs at baseline exercise testing and not at the second testing. The mean exercise capacity improved significantly, from 109 W at baseline to 118 W after the intervention. Mean exercise duration increased from 7.2 minutes to 8.2 minutes, but this change was not significant. No improvement was noted in peak oxygen uptake, defined as oxygen uptake at peak exercise (19.0 ml/min/kg at baseline vs. 18.9 ml/min/kg at follow-up). Mean maximum heart rate was significantly reduced, from 153 beats/min to 130 beats/min. Maximum exercise capacity at follow-up was achieved with a maximum driven heart rate significantly lower than the spontaneous heart rate before His ablation.

*Conclusion.*—During a mean follow-up of 7 months after His bundle ablation followed by VVIR pacing, all but 1 of 25 patients had stable (12 patients) or improved (12 patients) exercise capacity. The greatest improvement was seen in patients who had the lowest exercise capacity during drug-treated atrial fibrillation.

▶ The data from this paper really speak for themselves. The notion that all patients will benefit from improved ventricular function and exercise capacity when one performs a His bundle ablation to control ventricular rate during atrial fibrillation is not true, as evidenced by this report. In addition, we have known for a long time that sometimes ectopic pacing from the right ventricle can result in decreased cardiac output. The main indication and benefit from His bundle ablation in patients with atrial fibrillation at this time should be in those patients with uncontrollable rapid ventricular response rates, as we can expect either prevention and/or reversal of a tachycardia-mediated cardiomyopathy. Whether regularization of ventricular response rate that occurs in pacing has a favorable outcome when compared to a controlled ventricular response rate with an irregular R-R interval during atrial fibrillation remains to be demonstrated.

**A.L. Waldo, M.D.**

---

**Use of Intracardiac Echocardiography in Interventional Electrophysiology**

Kalman JM, Olgin JE, Karch MR, et al (Royal Melbourne Hosp, Australia; Krannert Research Inst, Indianapolis, Ind; Univ of California, San Francisco)
*PACE* 20(Pt I):2248–2262, 1997                                    6–18

---

*Introduction.*—The long-term role of intracardiac echocardiography in interventional electrophysiology has yet to be determined, but it has a number of potential benefits. The potential benefits of intracardiac echocardiography during radiofrequency (RF) catheter ablation were discussed.

*Uses of Intracardiac Echocardiography in Interventional Electrophysiology.*—Potential advantages of direct endocardial visualization during RF ablation may include precise anatomical localization of the ablation catheter tip in relation to important endocardial structures not visible on fluoroscopy; decreased fluoroscopy time; assessment of catheter tip contact; immediate identification of complications; and use as a research tool for understanding the critical role played by specific endocardial structures in arrhythmogenesis.

*Arrhythmias.*—Most work with arrhythmias has been limited to the right atrium. Recent animal trials have assessed the feasibility of modifying sinus pacemaker function using catheter-based applications of RF energy at ablation sites along the long axis of the crista terminalis or superior cristal sites. Successful RF modification of the sinus pacemaker complex has already been achieved in 10 patients with drug refractory and clinically incapacitating inappropriate sinus tachycardia. Other arrhythmias being investigated by this approach include ectopic or "focal" atrial tachycardia, atrioventricular node re-entry tachycardia, and typical atrial flutter. Intracardiac echocardiography has been helpful in highlighting the important role of endocardial anatomy in some arrhythmias. It has recently been used to guide placement of mapping and stimulating catheters on 2 sites on each side of the crista terminalis and 6 sites on either side of the eustachian ridge; both structures are difficult to identify on fluoroscopy alone.

*Conclusion.*—The initial work with intracardiac echocardiography has demonstrated its use in understanding arrhythmia mechanisms and its potential utility during mapping and ablation of a wide range of cardiac arrhythmias.

▶ The intracardiac echocardiogram has been used by several laboratories as an investigational tool to help place electrodes, and in particular, to help deliver radiofrequency energy to the desired location. It is even being used experimentally to make lesions to treat atrial fibrillation. These authors present a state-of-the-art review of this subject. A reading of the complete article is recommended.

**A.L. Waldo, M.D.**

---

**Electrophysiological Properties in Patients Undergoing Atrial Compartment Operation for Chronic Atrial Fibrillation With Mitral Valve Disease**
Lo H-M, Lin F-TY, Lin J-L, et al (Taiwan Provincial Tao-Yuan Gen Hosp; Natl Taiwan Univ, Taipei)
*Eur Heart J* 18:1805–1815, 1997                    6–19

---

*Objective.*—Sinus rhythm governing ventricular rate can now be restored surgically to patients with chronic atrial fibrillation using the corridor operation, the Maze operation, or the atrial compartment operation to reduce the critical atrial mass necessary to sustain atrial fibrillation. The chronic electrophysiological properties of patients converted from atrial fibrillation to sinus rhythm as a result of atrial compartment operation were determined.

*Methods.*—Between October 1988 and June 1995, 44 symptomatic patients (20 men), age 14 to 69, underwent the atrial compartment operation. At 11 to 51 months, 20 patients, age 16 to 69, underwent electrophysiologic assessment of sinus node function, atrial conduction, atrial refractoriness, atrioventricular conduction function, and inducible arrhythmias using programmed electrical stimulation delivered via quadripolar electrocatheters placed at various positions in the right and left atria.

*Results.*—There were no deaths. Long-term conversion of atrial fibrillation was achieved in 31 (70%) patients. The 3-compartment operation as significantly more successful than the 2-compartment operation (82% vs. 50%). At assessment, all patients were in sinus rhythm with the earliest atrial activity arising from the high right atrium. The mean sinus cycle length was 750 ms. Eighteen (90%) patients had a normal sinus node recovery time, and 2 had an abnormal sinus recover time, a prolonged corrected sinus node recovery time, and a delayed sino-atrial conduction time. The effective refractory period was significantly longer in the left atrial compartment than in the high right atrium and the right atrial appendage (242 vs. 224 vs. 219 ms). High right atrial appendage conduction times were not impaired in patients having the 2-compartment operation, but were seriously impaired in 12 of 15 patients having the 3-compartment operation. In 13 patients, the left atrial compartment was driven by the sinus node; 11 had a normal or mildly prolonged conduction time; 2 patients had significantly prolonged conduction times; and in 7 the left atrial compartments were dissociated from the rest of the heart. Atrial fibrillation could not be induced in any patient.

*Conclusion.*—Atrial compartment operation preserves sinus node function in most patients and results in conversion to sinus rhythm.

▶ This paper presents yet another example of the application of the Maze operation in patients undergoing open heart surgery for reasons other than atrial fibrillation. If a patient with atrial fibrillation is undergoing open heart surgery, it presents an opportunity to do the Maze operation to restore sinus rhythm. There have been several Maze procedure modifications. This paper shows yet another modification with what appears to be a good result. One would like to see either a multicenter study or some sort of meta-analysis to really put in perspective what the morbidity, mortality, and efficacy of the Maze procedure is.

**A.L. Waldo, M.D.**

### Video Assisted Thoracoscopic and Cardioscopic Radiofrequency Maze Ablation

Inoue Y, Yozu R, Mitsumaru A, et al (Keio Univ, Tokyo; NEC Med System Co Ltd, Tokyo; Johnson & Johnson Med Co Ltd, Tokyo)
*ASAIO J* 43:334–337, 1997                                        6–20

*Introduction.*—Surgical treatment of atrial fibrillation is usually performed with the Maze procedure. An alternative could be transvenous catheter ablation, currently used for Wolff-Parkinson-White syndrome because it is less invasive. Few studies have been done on transvenous linear ablation to treat atrial fibrillation, in part because of the difficulty of identifying anatomical landmarks. Using video-assisted thoracoscopy and cardioscopy, the feasibility of transthoracic radio frequency Maze ablation of atrial fibrillation was studied using porcine hearts.

*Methods.*—A video-assisted thoracoscopy system was used to view the left atrium of 6 pigs under general anesthesia. Using a radiofrequency ablation catheter inserted through a trocar port, radiofrequency linear ablation of the left atrial wall was performed. Under a video-assisted thoracoscopy system, the right atrium was also ablated in the same manner. A cardioscopic catheter device was used to perform transvenous radiofrequency ablation in 6 other pigs. Acetylcholine injection and rapid atrial pacing were used to provoke atrial fibrillation. A thoracoscope and cardioscope were used to monitor the process and document it with a video system

*Results.*—A transthoracic approach was used in the thoracoscopic visual field for radiofrequency catheter ablation. A transvenous approach was used with the cardioscopic visual field. Linear ablation of the atrium was obtained with safe position of the ablation catheter device on the atrial epicardium and endocardium. Per each ablation, the optimal setting for ablation was 70°C to 80°C per 30-second duration

*Conclusion.*—The combination of transthoracic radiofrequency catheter ablation with video-assisted thoracoscopic and cardioscopic linear ablation of atrial fibrillation was found to be safe and potentially useful. This system might eliminate the need for open heart Maze surgery.

▶ At the onset, it is not clear that the Maze operation performed with radiofrequency catheter ablation is a desirable therapeutic strategy. Nevertheless, application of the radiofrequency energy from the epicardium via a limited thoracotomy has been suggested, particularly since there are reported epicardial applications of radiofrequency energy that have prevented induction of atrial fibrillation in the canine model. This study presents some interesting data using this technique. We must await the outcome of systematic studies, but this directed approach is of considerable interest.

**A.L. Waldo, M.D.**

## Origin of Junctional Rhythm During Radiofrequency Ablation of Atrioventricular Nodal Reentrant Tachycardia in Patients Without Structural Heart Disease

Boyle NG, Anselme F, Monahan K, et al (Harvard Med School, Boston)
*Am J Cardiol* 80:575–580, 1997                     6–21

*Background.*—Currently, radiofrequency catheter ablation is the most successful means for treating atrioventricular nodal re-entrant tachycardia (AVNRT). This method is also used to gain knowledge about the atrioventricular (AV) node. In patients with AVNRT, the AV node has been thought to have a "slow" and a "fast" pathway. This notion has been modified from anatomical to functionally defined pathways. Junctional rhythm is a marker of successful ablation of AVNRT. Atrial activation during junctional rhythm was compared with that during AVNRT using high-density catheter mapping in an effort to better understand the relationship of the anatomy and physiology of the AV junction.

*Methods.*—Sixteen patients with confirmed AVNRT in the sedated postabsorptive state were treated with catheter ablation, and the retrograde atrial activation sequence was mapped during the procedure.

*Results.*—Only five of 16 patients had concordance of the earliest site of atrial activation during junctional rhythm and AVNRT. Only 1 patient was noted to have a single breakthrough site during AVNRT. Most patients had numerous atrial activation breakthrough sites scattered throughout the triangle of Koch. During junctional rhythm, multiple breathrough sites were seen in 13 of 16 patients. During AVNRT and junctional rhythm, only 10 of 16 patients had concordant activation patterns.

*Conclusion.*—The multiple breakthrough sites seen in this study do not support the conventional theory that a dual AV nodal anatomical pathways are associated with AVNRT. Rather, they are functionally defined pathways.

▶ This short but provocative paper does not answer the question of origin of the junctional rhythms seen during radiofrequency ablation of AVNRT, but it does force us to rethink some of the notions about slow and fast pathways in AVNRT. Worth the read.

**A.L. Waldo, M.D.**

CARDIOVERSION

Left Atrial Appendage "Stunning" After Electrical Cardioversion of Atrial Flutter: An Attenuated Response Compared With Atrial Fibrillation as the Mechanism for Lower Susceptibility to Thromboembolic Events
Grimm RA, Stewart WJ, Arheart KL, et al (Cleveland Clinic Found, Ohio)
*J Am Coll Cardiol* 29:582–589, 1997                                                    6–22

*Introduction.*—Left atrial appendage stunning may play a key role in the thromboembolic events occurring after cardioversion in patients with atrial fibrillation. Atrial flutter has been thought to carry a low risk of such events; thus, patients with this dysrhythmia do not usually receive anticoagulation before and after cardioversion. The occurrence of left atrial stunning in patients with atrial flutter was studied, including an assessment of left atrial appendage function after cardioversion.

*Methods.*—The study included 19 patients with atrial flutter and 44 with atrial fibrillation. Just before and after electric cardioversion, each patient was studied by transesophageal echocardiography. The 2 groups were compared for the occurrence of thrombi and spontaneous echo contrast. In addition, pulsed wave Doppler and 2-dimensional echocardiography were used to measure the emptying velocity of the left atrial appendage and to calculate shear rates.

*Results.*—Before cardioversion, the mean left atrial appendage flow velocity was 42 cm/sec in patients with atrial flutter vs. 28 cm/sec in those with atrial fibrillation. Left atrial appendage shear rates were 103 vs. 59 sec$^{-1}$, respectively, for those with atrial flutter and for those with atrial fibrillation. The postcardioversion measurements showed that left atrial appendage flow velocity had decreased to 19 cm/sec in the atrial flutter group and to 15 cm/sec in the atrial fibrillation group. Shear rates decreased to 65 and 30 s$^{-1}$, respectively, for those with atrial flutter and for those with atrial fibrillation. Seventy-four percent of patients with atrial flutter and 82% of those with atrial fibrillation had a reduction in flow velocity from before to after cardioversion. Twenty-one percent of the atrial flutter group vs. 50% of the atrial fibrillation group had new or increased spontaneous echo contrast after cardioversion.

*Conclusions.*—Although not as marked as in patients with atrial fibrillation, left atrial appendage stunning does occur in patients with atrial flutter. Thus, patients with atrial flutter appear to be at risk for postcardioversion thromboembolic events. However, because left atrial appendage function is better maintained in patients with atrial flutter, their thromboembolic risk is probably not as high as that for those with atrial fibrillation.

### Recovery of Atrial Systolic Function After Pharmacological Conversion of Chronic Atrial Fibrillation to Sinus Rhythm: A Doppler Echocardiographic Study

Jović A, Troskot R (Zadar Gen Hosp, Croatia)
*Heart* 77:46–49, 1997                                        6–23

*Introduction.*—Assessment of recovery of atrial mechanical function is important in patients being treated for atrial fibrillation (AF). The dynamics of recovery and restoration of atrial systolic function after pharmacologic conversion to sinus rhythm was evaluated by measuring transmitral diastolic flow via Doppler echocardiography in patients with chronic AF.

*Methods.*—The mean patient age was 61 years in 21 patients with chronic AF. Sinus rhythm was achieved with quinidine. Patients underwent serial transmitral pulsed Doppler echocardiography within the first 24 hours after cardioversion and on days 8, 15, and 30.

*Results.*—The A wave of transmitral flow emerged immediately after pharmacologic conversion of AF to sinus rhythm. The peak A-wave velocity and integrated late atrial velocities increased significantly between day 1 and day 8, and gradually increased thereafter. The atrial contribution to total transmitral flow increased significantly immediately after AF conversion from 26% to 34% on day 30, demonstrating the hemodynamic benefit of sinus rhythm restoration. There was a nonsignificant decrease in left atrial diameter from 4.11 cm to 3.98 cm.

*Conclusion.*—The slow and gradual restoration of atrial mechanical function is similarly slow and gradual for patients undergoing either pharmacologic or electric DC shock cardioversion. This time course is important in making clinical decisions regarding how long treatment with anticoagulants and antiarrhythmic agents needs to continue. It also impacts assessment of the hemodynamic benefits of restoring sinus rhythm in patients with chronic AF.

### Clinical Variables Affecting Recovery of Left Atrial Mechanical Function After Cardioversion From Atrial Fibrillation

Harjai KJ, Mobarek SK, Cheirif J, et al (Ochsner Med Insts, New Orleans, La)
*J Am Coll Cardiol* 30:481–486, 1997                          6–24

*Introduction.*—Patients undergoing cardioversion are usually anticoagulated for extended periods because normal atrial contraction is thought to lag behind conversion to sinus rhythm for up to several weeks. The role of clinical variables on recovery of effective mechanical atrial function (EMAF) was evaluated in 52 patients who underwent cardioversion for atrial fibrillation.

*Methods.*—Of 52 patients, 40 underwent electric cardioversion (group I). Of 12 patients in group II, 10 were cardioverted with medications and 2 converted spontaneously. After cardioversion, serial transmitral inflow Doppler variables were recorded until EMAF with an atrial filling velocity of greater than 0.50 m/sec was observed. Age, duration of atrial fibrillation, left ventricular ejection fraction, left atrial diameter, underlying cardiovascular disease, antiarrhythmic drug therapy, and mode of cardioversion were assessed for correlation with the outcomes of recovery of atrial function by day 3 and day 7.

*Results.*—By days 3 and 7 after cardioversion, 68% and 76% of patients, respectively, achieved recovery of EMAF. Group I patients took significantly longer to recover atrial function than group II patients. Group I patients had a significantly lower peak atrial filling velocity and a higher early filling to atrial filling velocity ratio after cardioversion, compared with group II patients. Recovery of atrial function by day 3 was significantly associated with mode of cardioversion. Recovery by day 7 was not.

*Conclusion.*—Most patients recovered EMAF within 7 days after cardioversion. Patients undergoing electric cardioversion experienced a greater degree and longer duration of mechanical atrial dysfunction, compared with patients who were cardioverted with medications or cardioverted spontaneously.

▶ Various laboratories have looked at atrial function following conversion, either by DC shock or drug therapy, of atrial fibrillation to sinus rhythm. And now following conversion of atrial flutter, the story is the same. There is mechanical dysfunction following cardioversion if atrial fibrillation has been present for any length of time. For reasons that are unclear and as shown in several previous studies of atrial fibrillation, DC cardioversion seems to have a more protracted recovery course than pharmacologic cardioversion. Nevertheless, atrial function is depressed in both groups of patients. Although a lesser degree of stunning is seen following conversion of atrial flutter than in patients with atrial fibrillation, it clearly is a real potential. In short, these data simply reinforce the need for adequate anticoagulation in these patients.

**A.L. Waldo, M.D.**

---

**Risk for Clinical Thromboembolism Associated With Conversion to Sinus Rhythm in Patients With Atrial Fibrillation Lasting Less Than 48 Hours**
Weigner MJ, Caulfield TA, Danias PG, et al (Harvard Med School, Boston; Univ of Connecticut, Farmington)
*Ann Intern Med* 126:615–620, 1997                                                6–25

---

*Introduction.*—Patients with atrial fibrillation who undergo cardioversion to sinus rhythm may be at risk for thromboembolism if cardioversion is not preceded by several weeks of warfarin therapy. The risk for thromboembolism is thought to be quite low, however, when cardioversion is performed within 2 days or less of the onset of atrial fibrillation. To provide clinical data to support this assumption, the incidence of clinical thromboembolism was recorded in a large consecutive series of patients with atrial fibrillation that had lasted less than 48 hours.

*Methods.*—A prospective screening of 1,822 adults admitted with a diagnosis that included atrial fibrillation, yielded 375 patients whose symptoms were of less than 48 hours' duration. Excluded were patients who were receiving long-term warfarin treatment. Data on cardioversion and thromboembolism were obtained prospectively from hospital and outpatient records. Only clinical embolic events that occurred during the index hospitalization and within 1 month after conversion were recorded.

*Results.*—During the index hospitalization, 357 (95.2%) patients converted to sinus rhythm. Conversion was spontaneous in 250 (66.7%) and active in 107 (28.5%). The most common underlying systemic disorder was hypertension (41.7%); 30.4% of patients had a clinical history suggestive of coronary artery disease and 48.3% had a history of atrial fibrillation. Clinical thromboembolic events (a stroke, a transient ischemic attack, and a peripheral embolus) occurred in 3 patients (0.8%), all of whom had converted spontaneously to sinus rhythm. All 3 had normal left ventricular systolic function and none had a history of atrial fibrillation or thromboembolism.

*Conclusion.*—Patients admitted with atrial fibrillation that had lasted less than 48 hours and who underwent early cardioversion, without prolonged warfarin therapy or screening by transesophageal echocardiography, had a very low (0.8%) clinical rate of thromboembolism. All 3 patients with embolic events were women older than 75 years, but the group was too small to identify any factors that may dispose to clinical thromboembolism in such populations. Data support the recommendation for early cardioversion when atrial fibrillation is known to have lasted less than 48 hours.

► An incidence of thromboembolism of 0.8% in patients with atrial fibrillation of less than 48 hours is remarkably low, but one would prefer it to be 0%. Thus, the importance of the ACUTE study. We simply do not know when the threshold is crossed for the increased risk of stroke associated with cardioversion. While it is remarkably low if the atrial fibrillation is less than 48 hours, 0.8% is still an incidence that is worrisome for a serious clinical problem which is probably preventable with adequate anticoagulation. The role of transesophageal echocardiography (TEE) in such patients continues to be studied, and needs more resolution. It is probable that after 12 hours of atrial fibrillation, the potential for stroke begins to increase, and perhaps that is where there is a role for TEE. But, clearly, there is a need for data.

**A.L. Waldo, M.D.**

## Is the Automatic Atrial Defibrillator a Promising Approach?

Griffin JC, Ayers GM, Adams J, et al (InControl Inc, Redmond, Wash)
*J Cardiovasc Electrophysiol* 7:1217–1224, 1996                                    6–26

*Background.*—Atrial fibrillation, the most common cardiac rhythm disorder requiring hospitalization, is prevalent in the elderly and strongly associated with other cardiovascular diseases. Antiarrhythmic drugs are often ineffective in patients with the condition. Animal experiments and some small clinical studies suggest that a small implanted device might benefit patients with recurring episodes of persistent, drug-refractory atrial fibrillation.

*The Implantable Atrial Defibrillator.*—A device for managing atrial fibrillation that is recurrent and drug refractory should be small—allowing implantation in the infraclavicular area—safe, and provide several years of implant life. Other desirable characteristics include low thresholds using only transvenous electrodes and freedom from ventricular proarrhythmia. The key to safe delivery of shocks is a very robust and conservative system for R wave synchronization. Such a system should be able to avoid special situations, such as short R-R intervals and long-short sequences, and to completely withhold therapy when there is any question of accurate synchronization. Data redundancy and tests for electrogram quality should be included, together with enhanced systems for noise rejection and R wave recognition. Postshock pacing is important, for some patients have brief pauses after conversion.

*Conclusion.*—Low-energy shocks have been found to be effective in converting atrial fibrillation. Such shocks appear to be safe if delivered synchronous to the R wave in the absence of a short preceding R-R interval. Cost-effectiveness will be a critical issue in determining whether a small, implanted automatic atrial defibrillator will be developed and used. Because the care of patients with complicated refractory atrial fibrillation is costly, device therapy could decrease the need for hospitalization and reduce the incidence of drug-induced and other preventable complications. Most importantly, an implantable atrial defibrillator could improve quality of life in symptomatic, drug-refractory patients.

▶ The implantable atrial defibrillator has been placed in 124 patients at the time of this reviewer's comments. There has not been a single ventricular proarrhythmic event. Twenty-two patients have been using the device safely in automated or patient-activated mode since it has been approved by the Food and Drug Administration. The device has been shown to effectively cardiovert atrial fibrillation without any ventricular proarrhythmia or important morbidity and with no mortality in all these patients with well over 5,000 shocks. Furthermore, these patients have all been cardioverted with less than 6 joules, and most with less than 3 joules. Early data also suggest that the interval between recurrences prolongs as a result of early cardioversion to sinus rhythm. In addition, many patients with persistent atrial fibrillation seem to have their atrial fibrillation revert to paroxysmal atrial fibrillation. These sorts of data make it probable that this technology is here to stay. No doubt, it will continue to improve, and will find a clear niche in patient care. Furthermore, if this technology continues to be widely accepted by patients, continues to improve quality of life, and continues to favorably impact remodeling of the atria and, thereby, helps prevent atrial fibrillation, the therapy will be widely applied. This therapy clearly will not be for everyone, but this editor believes the indications will be many and will continue to grow.

**A.L. Waldo, M.D.**

---

**Cardioversion of Atrial Fibrillation in the Elderly**
Carlsson J, for the ALKK-Study Group (Klinikum Lippe-Detmold, Germany)
*Am J Cardiol* 78:1380–1384, 1996                                6–27

*Introduction.*—There is a strong relationship between increasing age and the prevalence of atrial fibrillation. About 70% of patients with atrial fibrillation are between 65 and 85 years of age, and this group has a higher stroke rate than younger patients, creating therapeutic problems. Because physicians are reluctant to prescribe anticoagulants for this group of patients, they may turn to cardioversion to help in the long-term maintenance of sinus rhythm; however, there is still some controversy over whether age is correlated with success rate of cardioversion or maintenance of sinus rhythm. Complications and success rates of elective cardioversion in elderly patients with atrial fibrillation were studied.

*Methods.*—In 61 cardiology clinics, there were 1,152 patients included in this prospective study. They were divided into 2 groups: 570 were younger than 65 years and 582 were 65 years or older. Demographic, procedural, and outcome data on patients who had cardioversion of atrial fibrillation were recorded.

*Results.*—In the group younger than 65 years, the overall success rate of cardioversion was 76.1%, and in the 65 years or older group, it was 72.7%. Predictors of success were left atrial size and New York Heart Association functional class before cardioversion. The elderly had a larger left atrial size than the younger patients (44.0 ± 6.4 mm vs. 42.8 ± 6.4 mm). The elderly had a greater prevalence of a New York Heart Association functional class II than the younger group (48.6% vs. 29.6%). Between the 2 groups, the overall complications rates were not significantly different, with the younger group having a rate of 4.2% and the older group having a rate of 5.3%. The younger group had a 56.9% frequency of those who were adequately anticoagulated for cardioversion, whereas the frequency for the older group was 39.6%. The same trend for age-dependent underuse of anticoagulation was seen in chronic atrial fibrillation.

*Conclusion.*—Cardioversion success could not be predicted by age itself. In older patients, cardioversion should be considered with the same criteria and emphasis as in younger patients. Particularly in elderly patients, anticoagulation and antithrombotic medication is underused for cardioversion and for treating chronic atrial fibrillation.

▶ This useful paper serves to reinforce 2 fundamental concepts in the treatment of atrial fibrillation. The elderly are at highest risk for systemic embolism and stroke. It is unfortunate that warfarin therapy seems underutilized in these patients. Once again, we see that in this study, emphasizing the need to provide warfarin therapy for these patients. In addition, the efficacy of cardioversion is no different in the elderly than in other patients, and it is generally well tolerated and effective in the elderly as in other patients. Thus, appropriately aggressive treatment which includes cardioversion of recurrent atrial fibrillation should be considered in the elderly. This simple maxim is well supported by several articles presented this year and reviewed here in this section of the YEAR BOOK.

**A.L. Waldo, M.D.**

## Failure of Single- and Multisite High-frequency Atrial Pacing to Terminate Atrial Fibrillation

Paladino W, Bahu M, Knight BP, et al (Univ of Michigan, Ann Arbor)
*Am J Cardiol* 80:226–227, 1997                                        6–28

*Introduction.*—To terminate atrial fibrillation has been thought to be unlikely, although at least 1 report suggested it could occur. However, no studies have confirmed that this is possible, nor have there been studies of atrial pacing at multiple sites to terminate atrial fibrillation (AF). The efficacy of single and multisite atrial pacing for terminating episodes of AF induced in an electrophysiology laboratory was assessed in 28 patients. The patients underwent a catheter ablation procedure for treatment of paroxysmal supraventricular tachycardia.

*Methods.*—Pacing was performed at the high right atrium in 10 patients and simultaneously at the high right atrium, midseptum, and coronary sinus in 18 patients at a pacing cycle length of 20 msec for 1, 2, and 5 seconds. Each pacing burst was repeated 3 times, separated by at least 10 seconds. The pacing protocol was used only during episodes of AF persisting at least 10 minutes.

*Results.*—Four patients had type I AF (mean AF cycle length, 171 msec) and 24 had type II, III, or IV AF, with a mean cycle length of 141 msec. Patients with type I AF experienced transient shortening of the AF cycle length with 1-second bursts of pacing at 10 mA and with 2-second bursts of pacing at 10 mA. Bursts of pacing at 0.1 A at the high right atrium did not affect the AF cycle length. Atrial fibrillation did not terminate in response to simultaneous 1-second bursts with current strengths of 10 or 0.1 mA. With current strengths of 10 mA and 0.1 mA, AF terminated in 7% and 28% of patients, respectively, during 5-second bursts of multisite pacing. Patients with type I AF had notable shortening of the high right atrial cycle length in response to 1- and 5-second bursts of multisite pacing at 10 mA. Atrial fibrillation cycle length was not affected by multisite pacing at 0.1 mA.

*Conclusion.*—Rapid atrial pacing at 1 and 3 sites was not effective in terminating AF. Simultaneous pacing at more than 3 sites has not been tested, so it has yet to be determined whether increasing the number of sites can capture enough atrial myocardium to terminate AF.

▶ The notion that rapid atrial pacing can terminate AF is an interesting one. This editor has thought it highly unlikely that this would work because the rapid pacing may capture a small area, but it generates fibrillatory conduction to the rest of the atria, and, thereby, continues the fibrillation. Simultaneous pacing from several sites at the same time has been suggested. As this editor expected, and as is evident from this paper, it did not work. So, while this editor remains skeptical that such techniques will work, at least theoretically, there is the possibility that with certain mechanisms of AF, rapid atrial pacing from several sites simultaneously may destabilize the AF with resulting restoration of sinus rhythm, but healthy skepticism still seems warranted. Nevertheless, as always, we should be data driven. This paper provides data which support continued healthy skepticism.

**A.L. Waldo, M.D.**

---

**Low-energy Cardioversion of Spontaneous Atrial Fibrillation: Immediate and Long-term Results**
Lévy S, Ricard P, Gueunoun M, et al (Univ of Marseilles, France)
*Circulation* 96:253–259, 1997                                6–29

---

*Introduction.*—Hemodynamic impairment and a decreased life expectancy are associated with atrial fibrillation. The treatment of choice has been antiarrhythmic therapy, but some patients have intolerable side effects, and there is a search for nonpharmacologic therapy for atrial fibrillation. A 2–catheter electrode system with a voltage ranging from 0 to 400 V has been suggested to terminate atrial fibrillation. Several advances have been made with the implanted atrial defibrillator. In patients with spontaneous chronic and paroxysmal atrial fibrillation, the efficacy and safety of low-energy cardioversion were evaluated.

*Methods.*—Low-energy electrical cardioversion was performed on 42 consecutive patients with spontaneous atrial fibrillation. In 28 patients, atrial fibrillation was chronic (1 month or more) with a mean duration of 9 ± 19 months. In 14 patients, atrial fibrillation was paroxysmal with a history of recurrent attacks and a mean duration of the current episode of 7 ± 16 days. In 28 patients, there was an underlying heart disease. In 32 patients, a 3/3-msec biphasic shock was delivered between catheters positioned in the right atrium and the coronary sinus. The left pulmonary artery branch was used in 10 patients. A custom external defibrillator was connected to the catheters. There was synchronization of the shocks to the

R wave. Energy was increased in 40-V steps after a test shock of 60 V, then increased until a maximum of 400 V or restoration of sinus rhythm.

*Results.*—By using a mean leading-edge voltage of 223 ± 41 V, sinus rhythm was restored in 22 of 14 patients (78%) in the paroxysmal group. The energy required for terminating paroxysmal atrial fibrillation was significantly lower than for terminating chronic atrial fibrillation. Successful voltage was significantly affected by the duration of atrial fibrillation. One patient with atrial flutter had ventricular proarrhythmia caused by an unsynchronized shock. Sinus rhythm was restored in 22 patients in the chronic group, and of these, 14 (63%) remained in sinus rhythm with a mean follow-up of 9 ± 3 months. There was a correlation between increasing voltage and pain level.

*Conclusion.*—In patients with persistent spontaneous atrial fibrillation, atrial defibrillation using low energy between 2 intracardiac catheters with an electrical field between the right and left atrium and the protocol used is feasible. Provided synchronization to the R wave is achieved, the technique is safe. In patients in whom sinus rhythm was restored, a low recurrence rate of atrial fibrillation was seen.

▶ This report of 42 consecutive patients treated with low-energy intraatrial defibrillation clearly demonstrates that when this technique is applied properly, the technique is effective, safe, and well tolerated. This study was a prelude to the implantation of a permanent device. In fact, we are aware that over 100 patients have had the low-energy atrial defibrillator implanted permanently with safe delivery of low-energy shocks to convert atrail fibrillation to sinus rhythm. This technique holds promise of providing another important tool in the management of patients with atrial fibrillation. We look forward to the publication of long-term results with this device.

**A.L. Waldo, M.D.**

---

**Clinical Shock Tolerability and Effect of Different Right Atrial Electrode Locations on Efficacy of Low Energy Human Transvenous Atrial Defibrillation Using an Implantable Lead System**
Lok N-S, Lau C-P, Tse H-F, et al (Queen Mary Hosp, Hong, Kong, People's Republic of China; InControl Inc, Redmond, Wash)
*J Am Coll Cardiol* 30:1324–1330, 1997                                    6–30

---

*Objective.*—Because patients with atrial fibrillation (AF) are conscious during their arrhythmia, their ability to tolerate defibrillation shocks is a concern when considering implanting atrial defibrillator devices. The position of electrodes and starting energy level may have an effect on patient acceptance. Defibrillation thresholds were determined using different atrial electrode locations with an implantable lead system, and patient acceptance was assessed using a higher intensity starting shock closer in intensity to the predicted defibrillation threshold.

*Methods.*—Transvenous atrial defibrillation was performed in 28 patients (11 women), average age 62, with AF of duration 1 month or more and a mean left atrial diameter of 4.5 cm. An electrode with a transvenous passive fixation lead was placed in the coronary sinus. An active fixation screw-in lead was placed in the right atrium. Electrodes were placed in the high right atrial appendage, anterolateral right atrium, and inferomedial right atrium. The leads were connected to an external defibrillator. The right atrial electrode was placed in the anterolateral and inferomedial right atrial positions in 9 patients, in the anterolateral right atrial and high right atrial appendage position in 10 patients, and in all 3 locations in 9 patients. Defibrillation thresholds were determined using a step-up protocol design. Pain perception was assessed on a 0 (not felt) to 10 (extremely uncomfortable) scale.

*Results.*—Sinus rhythm was restored in 26 patients. Conversion was successful in 50% of patients using the inferomedial right atrial electrode, in 89% using the high right atrial appendage, and in 81% using the anterolateral right atrial electrode. The latter 2 conversion rates were not significantly different. The respective mean energy defibrillation thresholds, 6.0, 3.9, and 4.6 vs, and the respective mean voltage defibrillation thresholds, 396, 317, and 348 V, were significantly different. The tolerability threshold in most patients (*n* = 22) averaged 2.5 J, 255 V, and 3.4 shocks before cardioversion was achieved or sedation was requested.

*Conclusion.*—Low-energy transvenous atrial defibrillation is effective for treating AF. If electrodes are placed in the coronary sinus and the high right atrial appendage, most patients can tolerate 3 shocks delivered at 255 V without sedation.

▶ The importance of this paper is yet another lab shows that low-energy shocks can be given safely and effectively and, particularly important, that they are well tolerated. The early data suggest that patients will tolerate about 3 low-energy shocks without difficulty. But we will need to evaluate this over the long term to help us evaluate the role of this new technology. This reviewer is optimistic.

**A.L. Waldo, M.D.**

---

**Internal Cardioversion of Chronic Atrial Fibrillation in Patients**
Neri R, Palermo P, Cesario AS, et al (Hosp GB Grassi, Rome)
*PACE* 20:2237–2242, 1997                                              6–31

---

*Introduction.*—The use of high-energy internal cardioversion is often successful in treating patients with atrial fibrillation (AF), but general anesthesia is needed and it can cause significant complications. Recent animal trials have shown that paroxysmal AF can be interrupted with low-energy biphasic shocks lower than 1.0 J. Trials in humans have indicated that transvenous low-energy biphasic shocks with a mean defibrillation threshold of 2.0 J can be effective. The safety, efficacy, and tolerability of internal cardioversion of chronic AF using biphasic shocks up to 34 J was evaluated in 11 patients with long-lasting AF using a right atrium (RA) to skin patch "unipolar" configuration.

*Methods and Findings.*—Biphasic R wave synchronous shocks were delivered between a large defibrillating surface area electrode in the RA and a skin patch placed in the left prepectoral position. The defibrillation protocol was initiated with a test shock of 0.4 J, then repeated and increased until termination at a maximum of 34 J. Patients were sedated when they complained of painful shocks. The mean patient age was 67 years and the mean duration of AF was 11 months. All patients had underlying heart disease. The mean left atrial dimension was 43 mm. Ten of 11 patients experienced termination of AF. The mean delivered energy of successful shocks was 18.7 J and the mean leading edge voltage was 564 V. At the defibrillator threshold, the mean shock impedance was 71 Ω. Of 131 total shocks delivered, there were no complications or proarrhythmia episodes.

*Conclusion.*—Low-energy "unipolar" internal cardioversion may be considered safe and effective in the termination of chronic AF in patients with heart disease. Light sedation is usually all that is needed for this procedure.

▶ This paper of is interest because, unlike the paper from Levy et al.,[1] these authors found that a shock delivered between the right atrium and the chest wall in patients who had had AF for up to 1 month could be used to deliver relatively low energy shocks (less than 20 joules) and successfully cardiovert the rhythm to sinus. Again, the application here is clear. From time to time, there are patients who merit DC cardioversion to restore sinus rhythm, but in whom the standard transthoracic or precordial shock delivery does not accomplish this. Clearly, there are techniques available which have a high likelihood of restoring sinus rhythm. This paper presents a simple and effective and well-tolerated technique.

**A.L. Waldo, M.D.**

*Reference*

1. Levy S, Lacombe P, Cointe R, et al: High energy transcatheter cardioversion of chronic atrial fibrillation. *J Am Coll Cardiol* 12:514–518, 1988.

---

**Changes in Intracardiac Atrial Cardioversion Threshold at Rest and During Exercise**

Santini M, Pandozi C, Toscano S, et al (San Filippo Neri Hosp, Rome; La Sapienza Univ, Rome)

*J Am Coll Cardiol* 29:576–581, 1997

6–32

---

*Objective.*—Low-energy intracardiac transcatheter cardioversion is potentially an alternative to transthoracic cardioversion for patients with chronic atrial fibrillation (AF). Animal studies have shown that such low energy shocks synchronized on the R wave can sometimes induce ventricular tachyarrhythmias if the shock is delivered on the T wave of the preceding beat due to a short R-R interval (less than 300 ms). No similar human studies have been conducted. The change in the intracardiac atrial defibrillation threshold (ADT) at rest and during exercise was analyzed, the effective risk of this procedure in patients with chronic AF was quantified, and the ADTs of chronic and reinduced AF were compared.

*Methods.*—Low-energy endocavitary cardioversion was used to treat 16 patients (6 men), age 43 to 78, with chronic AF of 10 or more days' duration. Two custom-made temporary catheters were used to deliver the shock, and 1 USCI tetrapolar lead was used for ventricular synchronization. Patients randomly received 2 sequences of shocks to determine the ADT at rest and during isometric leg exercises when the heart rate increased at least 20% above baseline. Atrial fibrillation was reinduced by burst atrial pacing and then restored after 1.5 minutes with a second series of shocks. Patients graded shock discomfort on a 1 (not felt) to 5 (severe discomfort) scale. An electrocardiogram was performed within 24 hours of the test to detect pericardial effusion or contractile defects.

*Results.*—Group A (*n* = 9) patients underwent first cardioversion during exercise, and group B (*n* = 7) patients underwent first cardioversion at rest. The mean ADTs at exercise and at rest for group A were 7.10 and 6.42 J and for group B were 6.19 and 7.79 J, respectively. The overall mean ADTs during exercise and at rest, 6.70 and 7.02 J, respectively, were not significantly different, and the individual group values were not significantly different. The ADT in the second shock was significantly lower than the ADT in the first shock (6.32 vs. 7.40 J). The average ADT values for group A and group B were not significantly different (6.76 vs. 6.99 J). The average discomfort scores were 3.25 at rest and 2.94 during exercise. No pericardial effusion or contractile deficits were observed.

*Conclusion.*—Low-energy intracardiac cardioversion is safe, well tolerated, and restores sinus rhythm in almost all chronic AF patients, both at rest and during exercise. The ADT is higher in chronic AF than in reinduced AF.

▶ Still another piece of the pie regarding low-energy internal atrial cardioversion. These data show that in activities of daily living which include exercise, shocks were delivered safely and effectively, and that the atrial defibrillation threshold was not influenced by exercise.

**A.L. Waldo, M.D.**

## Internal Cardioversion of Atrial Fibrillation: Marked Reduction in Defibrillation Threshold With Dual Current Pathways

Cooper RAS, Smith WM, Ideker RE (Univ of Alabama, Birmingham)
*Circulation* 96:2693–2700, 1997                                     6–33

*Introduction.*—One of the most commonly encountered arrhythmias in clinical medicine continues to be atrial fibrillation. A recently demonstrated effective technique for terminating atrial fibrillation is biphasic-waveform shocks delivered via transvenous defibrillation electrodes. The ventricular defibrillation threshold has been shown to be reduced with sequential shocks delivered over dual current pathways. The efficacy of a second shock delivered through a second current pathway was studied to encompass the parts of the atria that would be predicted to be in the low potential gradient area produced by the first current pathway and shock.

*Methods.*—In 12 adult sheep, sustained atrial fibrillation was induced with rapid pacing. There was positioning of defibrillation electrodes in the right atrial appendage, proximal coronary sinus, distal coronary sinus, right ventricular apex, and main/left pulmonary artery junction. Through combinations of these electrodes, single-capacitor biphasic waveforms (3/1 msec) were delivered. Single shocks with a single current pathway were compared with sequential shocks with either single- or dual-current pathways.

*Results.*—For the dual current pathway involving right atrial appendage to distal coronary sinus then proximal coronary sinus to main/left pulmonary artery junction, the $ED_{50}$ for delivered energy was $0.36 \pm 0.13$ J. This was significantly lower than the $ED_{50}$ of the standard single current pathway right atrial appendage to distal coronary sinus ($1.31 \pm 0.3$ J). It was also significantly lower than all other tested configurations.

*Conclusion.*—Compared with the standard single shock delivered over a single current pathway or with sequential shocks delivered over a single current pathway, internal atrial defibrillation thresholds can be markedly reduced with 2 sequential biphasic shocks delivered over 2 current pathways. It still remains to be determined whether discomfort is sufficiently decreased to justify adding 2 more electrodes.

▶ This paper serves to illustrate that this field of internal arial cardioversion of atrial fibrillation continues to evolve. Undoubtedly, the technology will continue to improve. In this editor's judgment, the technology already appears equal to the task. Now that it is being used successfully in patients, we will have an opportunity to be data driven with regard to its continued efficacy, safety, and tolerance by patients. In addition, the indications and applications for this technique will continue to evolve, but are clearly already present.

**A.L. Waldo, M.D.**

**Video Imaging of Atrial Defibrillation in the Sheep Heart**
Gray RA, Ayers G, Jalife J (State Univ of New York, Syracuse; InControl Inc, Redmond, Wash)
*Circulation* 95:1038–1047, 1997                                        6–34

*Introduction.*—Although the mechanisms of ventricular defibrillation have been studied for many years, investigation of atrial defibrillation is relatively recent and its mechanisms are not well understood. Experiments with high-resolution video imaging were conducted to examine the events that precede, accompany, and follow the application of atrial defibrillatory shocks in the sheep heart.

*Methods.*—Hearts from young sheep of either sex were rapidly removed and connected to a Langendorff system for investigation of the sequence of activation on the surface of the atria. Transmembrane potentials were recorded simultaneously from more than 20,000 sites on the epicardium. Recordings were obtained during atrial fibrillation (AF) and also during and after biphasic shocks applied by a programmable atrial defibrillator. The right atrium was divided into 9 areas to study regional effects. Success or failure of defibrillation was determined by monitoring the bipolar surface ECG. Isochrone maps were generated from the sequence of video images of electric activity.

*Results.*—Sheep hearts were connected to the Langendorff apparatus for 4 to 5 hours. Defibrillation thresholds were determined during the first 2 to 3 hours, and optical experiments were performed during the last 2 hours of the experiment. Video recordings obtained during biphasic defibrillation shocks from 17 episodes in 5 animals were analyzed. Defibrillatory shocks depolarized all epicardial regions of the atria and led to 4 types of response: (1) immediate cessation of epicardial activity, (2) a single postshock activation, (3) organized activation for 0.8 to 1.5 seconds followed by termination, and (4) organized activity followed by degeneration back into AF. Of the 17 episodes, 7 were unsuccessful attempts, 4 caused immediate cessation of epicardial activity, 3 resulted in a single postshock activation, and 3 led to delayed termination of epicardial activation. Response types 2 through 4 involved a quiescent period immediately after the shock (mean duration 110 msec), followed by an activation sequence similar to those observed during sinus rhythm. For response types 3 and 4, the first cycle length after the shock was longer than during AF. Mean repolarization time was significantly longer for successful shocks than for unsuccessful shocks.

*Discussion.*—A number of new results were obtained in these experiments. Mean repolarization time was found to be longer for successful shocks. Defibrillation shocks applied to the sheep atrium led to an organization of the activation sequence, after a mean quiescent period of 110 msec. The first cycle length after the shock was longer than during AF. There was no association between synchronous repolarization and successful defibrillation shocks. Finally, after a brief hyperpolarization of tissue near the right atrium electrode, defibrillation shocks depolarized all tissue on the atrial epicardium.

▶ This paper provides an explanation, using contemporary physiologic techniques, to explain the efficacy of low-energy cardioversion.

**A.L. Waldo, M.D.**

MISCELLANEOUS

**A Survey of Atrial Fibrillation in General Practice: The West Birmingham Atrial Fibrillation Project**
Lip GYH, Golding DJ, Nazir M, et al (City Hosp, Birmingham, England; Cape Hill Med Centre, Birmingham, England; Lee Bank Med Centre, Birmingham, England)
*Br J Gen Pract* 47:285–289, 1997                                          6–35

*Introduction.*—Optimal investigation and treatment have not been determined for atrial fibrillation (AF), the most frequently observed disorder of cardiac rhythm. The prevalence, clinical features, and management of patients with AF were assessed in 2 general practice settings.

*Methods.*—A cross-sectional survey of patients with AF was conducted by reviewing clinical records and treatment prescriptions of 2 general practices serving 16,519 research subjects, 4,522 of whom were age 50 years or greater.

*Results.*—The mean age of 111 patients found to be in AF who were over age 50 years was 76.6 years. Age ranges of patients with AF were as follows: 5.4% aged 50–60 years, 16.2% aged 61–70 years, 20.7% aged 71–75 years, 20.7% aged 76–80 years, 24.3% aged 81–85 years, and 12.6% aged over 85 years. Female patients were significantly older than male patients. Of the 111 patients mentioned above, 81 (73%) had chronic AF and 30 (27%) had paroxysmal AF. The most common associated factors for AF were as follows: hypertension in 41 patients (36.9%), associated cardiac failure in 34 patients (30.9%), previous stroke in 20 patients (18%), and transient cerebral ischemic attack in 9 patients (8.1%). Forty patients in this series had a last-recorded blood pressure measurement of greater than 160/90 mmHg, but only 20 had received a diagnosis of or were being treated for hypertension. Only 20 (18%), 26 (23.4%), and 58 (52.3%) patients, respectively, had had an echocardiogram, chest X-ray, or thyroid function test.

Forty patients were receiving warfarin that was monitored by a general practitioner in 3 patients, a hospital clinic in 30 patients, or both in 7 patients. Only 12 of 71 patients not receiving anticoagulation medication had contraindications to warfarin therapy. Patients who received warfarin were significantly younger than patients who were not receiving warfarin. Twenty-one patients were taking aspirin, primarily because of previous myocardial infarction. Cardioversion had been attempted on 5 patients.

*Conclusion.*—Atrial fibrillation is frequently encountered in general practice and is often associated with hypertension, ischemic heart disease, and heart failure. Clinical workup, antithrombotic therapy, and attempted cardioversion are at suboptimal levels. Guidelines for management of this arrhythmia in general practice are needed.

---

**Physician Attitudes Concerning Warfarin for Stroke Prevention in Atrial Fibrillation: Results of a Survey of Long-term Care Practitioners**
Monette J, Gurwitz JH, Rochon PA, et al (Harvard Med School, Boston; Meyers Primary Care Inst, Worcester, Mass; Fallon Healthcare System, Worcester, Mass; et al)
*J Am Geriatr Soc* 45:1060–1065, 1997                                    6–36

---

*Introduction.*—Surveys have been conducted to determine physicians' attitudes regarding anticoagulation for stroke prevention in patients with atrial fibrillation (AF), but none have directly evaluated the decision-making of physicians practicing in the long-term care setting. Because the incidence of AF increases dramatically with increasing age, it is common in the long-term care setting. The knowledge and attitudes of physicians regarding the use of warfarin for stroke prevention in patients with AF in long-term care facilities was examined.

*Methods.*—Two hundred sixty-nine physicians providing primary care to patients in 30 long-term care facilities in New England, Quebec, and Ontario were asked to complete a structured questionnaire regarding the use of warfarin therapy for stroke prevention in patients with AF residing in long-term care facilities. The physicians were presented with 2 clinical scenarios designed to present striking contrasts in patient characteristics, including underlying co-morbidity, functional status, bleeding risk, and stroke risk.

*Results.*—Of 269 physicians asked to participate, 182 (67.7%) returned the questionnaire. The benefits "greatly outweighed the risks," "slightly outweighed the risks," or "risks outweighed benefits," according to 47%, 34%, and 17%, respectively, of physicians answering the questions. Physicians reported that the most important contraindications to warfarin were excessive risk of falls (71% of physicians), history of gastrointestinal bleeding, (71%), history of other non-CNS bleeding (36%), and history of cerebrovascular hemorrhage (25%). Estimates of risk of an intracranial hemorrhage with and without warfarin therapy varied widely.

*Conclusion.*—Findings indicate that there is considerable uncertainty regarding the decision to prescribe warfarin and the appropriate level of warfarin therapy in elderly patients in the long-term care setting. Risks of bleeding events are of foremost concern when physicians consider anticoagulation therapy. It may be that physicians prefer the responsibility of risk of an embolic stroke rather than major bleeding events, even though it is more likely that the patient will have a stroke without warfarin.

▶ This is a truly worrisome study. It indicates that warfarin is grossly underused by the practicing physician (Abstract 6–36). The message should be clear. Warfarin should be used in patients who have an indication, regardless of age, if at all possible. It is a simple and strong message. In the West Birmingham Atrial Fibrillation Project (Abstract 6–35), only 36% of patients with AF received warfarin, and of the 71 patients who were not anticoagulated, only 12 had an apparent contraindication to warfarin therapy. Again, the message is clear.

**A.L. Waldo, M.D.**

---

**Risk of Thromboembolism in Chronic Atrial Flutter**
Wood KA, Eisenberg SJ, Kalman JM, et al (Univ of California, San Francisco)
*Am J Cardiol* 79:1043–1047, 1997                                    6–37

---

*Objective.*—Patients with chronic atrial fibrillation are at increased risk of thromboembolus formation. Although the incidence of thromboembolus formation is not known, conventional anticoagulation therapy has generally not been recommended. The frequency of, and potential risk factors for, thromboembolic events were examined in a retrospective study of patients with chronic atrial flutter referred for radiofrequency ablation treatment.

*Methods.*—Between May 1988 and December 1995, 86 consecutive patients (24 women), average age 60 years, without prior congenital heart surgical repair, were evaluated at the University of California, San Francisco, for ablation of clinical atrial flutter. Atrial flutter was classified as typical clockwise ($n = 5$), typical counterclockwise ($n = 59$), or atypical ($n = 7$).

*Results.*—The duration of flutter ranged from 2 weeks to more than 40 years. Concomitant conditions included coronary artery disease ($n = 24$), systemic hypertension ($n = 23$), ischemic or hypertrophic cardiomyopathy ($n = 20$), mitral valve prolapse ($n = 12$), and congenital heart disease ($n = 5$). Twelve patients (14%) had a history of embolic events. No clear risk factors could be found for thromboembolic events. In the univariate analysis, hypertension was a significant predictor of thromboembolic risk, but multivariate analysis failed to establish any significant risk factors. When patients with transient ischemic attacks or pulmonary emboli were excluded from the analysis to facilitate comparison with other atrial fibrillation studies, the overall risk was 7%, with an annual risk of 4.5 years of 1.6%.

*Conclusion.*—Because the risk of thromboembolus formation in patients with atrial fibrillation is higher that previously thought, treatment with anticoagulant therapy should be considered.

▶ This retrospective study is really quite important. It is really the first study which focuses on the risk of thromboembolism in patients with chronic atrial flutter. More and more, the recommendation is that we anticoagulate patients with atrial flutter just as we do with patients with atrial fibrillation. To this editor, it is logical and reasonable because if atrial remodeling is rate related, the adverse effects of rapid atrial rate for prolonged periods of atrial flutter should be expected to resemble that associated with atrial fibrillation. In addition, one is reminded that atrial flutter and atrial fibrillation often go back and forth. In sum, strongly consider anticoagulating inpatients with atrial flutter just as one would with atrial fibrillation.

**A.L. Waldo, M.D.**

---

**Epicardial Right Atrial Free Wall Mapping in Chronic Atrial Fibrillation: Documentation of Repetitive Activation With a Focal Spread—A Hitherto Unrecognised Phenomenon in Man**
Holm M, Johansson R, Brandt J, et al (Univ Hosp, Lund, Sweden)
*Eur Heart J* 18:290–310, 1997                                                    6–38

---

*Objective.*—Atrial fibrillation appears to arise from a varying number of simultaneous activation waves, re-entering either themselves or each other. Using a new technique of studying the activation of the right atrial free wall in patients with chronic atrial fibrillation, the authors have observed a new phenomenon: repetitive atrial activations with focal spread. The findings of mapping studies of right atrial activation during chronic atrial fibrillation are reported.

*Methods.*—The study included 16 patients with chronic atrial fibrillation. In each, multiple 8-sec epicardial recordings were made at the right atrial posterior free wall and at the appendage. All studies were done with a 20- × 35-mm electrode array and 56 bipolar measurement points. For each recording, the preferable activation pattern was determined; for each individual activation wave, the propagation direction, cycle length, and conduction velocity were established.

*Results.*—Analysis showed an unorganized pattern of activation, with several activation waves present at the same time. Five patients showed an inconsistent preferable activation pattern, with mainly organized activation. Seven had mainly organized activation but with frequent episodes of uniform activation (consistent preferable activation), whereas 4 had frequent episodes of activation with focal spread (focal preferable activation). Recordings in patients with the inconsistent preferable activation pattern commonly showed random re-entry; this was less frequent in the patterns of consistent and focal preferable activation. There were few recorded complete re-entry circuits. The median fibrillation cycle length was 146 msec in patients with the inconsistent pattern, 159 msec in those with the consistent preferable activation pattern, and 165 msec in those with the focal preferable activation pattern. The mean conduction velocity during uniform activation was 64cm/sec for patients with the inconsistent pattern,

67cm/sec for those with the consistent preferable activation pattern, and 83 cm/sec for those with the focal preferable activation pattern. Neither of these measurements was significantly different between groups.

*Conclusions.*—Patterns of right atrial free wall activation vary significantly in chronic atrial fibrillation. Some research subjects show disorganized activation with multiple coexisting action waves, whereas others have mainly organized activation with either large re-entry circuits or repetitive action of an unknown mechanism and focal spread.

▶ The importance of this paper is that we continue to learn about the many aspects of atrial fibrillation. This paper suggests still different potential mechanisms for atrial fibrillation. What is certain is that there is no 1 single mechanism of atrial fibrillation. Complete mapping of the atria in patients is what is really needed. This is still very difficult to do, so we must learn from small bits of data such as those obtained in this study. Nevertheless, for this editor, it serves to reinforce the notion that empiric ablation procedures to try to cure atrial fibrillation in patients are fraught with all the uncertainties that relate to mechanism. Once we understand mechanism, the application of potentially curative ablative techniques seems more likely to have hope for effective treatment.

**A.L. Waldo, M.D.**

---

**Histological Substrate of Atrial Biopsies in Patients With Lone Atrial Fibrillation**
Frustaci A, Chimenti C, Bellocci F, et al (Università Cattolica del S Cuore, Rome; Università La Sapienza, Rome)
*Circulation* 96:1180–1184, 1997                                    6–39

---

*Introduction.*—The origin of lone atrial fibrillation, a common clinical syndrome, remains unknown. The literature does not reveal atrial biopsy or postmortem studies. The condition occurs without clinically evident abnormalities. To study the atrial histologic substrate and its relationship to biventricular histologic findings, right atrial and biventricular endomyocardial biopsies were performed on 12 patients with paroxysmal lone atrial fibrillation refractory to conventional antiarrhythmic therapy.

*Methods.*—There were 10 men and 2 women with lone atrial fibrillation (mean age, of 32 years) who had endomyocardial biopsies of the right atrial septum and of the 2 ventricles performed. Eleven patients with Wolff-Parkinson-White syndrome were used as controls, and endomyocardial biopsy specimens from the right atrial septum were used for comparison. Two-dimensional Doppler echocardiography; cardiac catheterization; coronary angiography; and hormonal, virologic, and electrophysiologic studies were performed on all the patients.

*Results.*—All lone atrial fibrillation biopsy specimens, an average of 2.8 per patient, showed abnormalities, whereas all tests and controls were normal. Severe hypertrophy with vacuolar degeneration of the atrial myocytes and ultrastructural evidence of fibrillolysis, occupying more than 50% of the areas assessed morphometrically, was found in 2 patients. Lymphomononuclear infiltrates with necrosis of the adjacent myocytes was found in 8 patients. Nonspecific patchy fibrosis was found in 2 patients. Three patients had abnormal biventricular biopsy specimens.

*Conclusion.*—In all patients with lone atrial fibrillation, abnormal atrial histology was found in multiple biopsy specimens. In 66% of patients, it was compatible with a diagnosis of myocarditis. In 17% of patients, it was compatible with a diagnosis of localized cardiomyopathy. In 17% of patients, it was compatible with patchy fibrosis. In 75% of patients, the pathologic changes were found only in atrial septal biopsy specimens, not in biventricular biopsy specimens. The cause remains unknown.

▶ Once again, this study serves to emphasize how little we really know about the underlying substrate in atrial fibrillation. The notion that myocarditis is associated with two thirds of the patients with lone atrial fibrillation is quite striking. The implications for therapy are obvious, but most important, a systematic approach to this problem may now be warranted.

**A.L. Waldo, M.D.**

---

**Hemodynamic Effects of an Irregular Sequence of Ventricular Cycle Lengths During Atrial Fibrillation**
Clark DM, Plumb VJ, Epstein AE, et al (Univ of Alabama, Birmingham)
*J Am Coll Cardiol* 30:1039–1045, 1997                                                  6–40

---

*Introduction.*—Several detrimental effects on cardiac hemodynamic are caused by atrial fibrillation. In a study of atrial fibrillation conducted in dogs, it was found that cardiac output was reduced with an irregular, as compared with a regular, paced ventricular rhythm. The independent effects on hemodynamic data of slowing or regularizing the ventricular rate are unknown, although catheter ablative techniques modify the rate and rhythm for patients with rapid ventricular rates. In patients with atrial fibrillation, the independent hemodynamic effects of an irregular sequence of ventricular cycle lengths was determined.

*Methods.*—There were 16 patients with atrial fibrillation. The right ventricular apex electrogram was recorded onto frequency-modulated tape during intrinsically conducted atrial fibrillation at a mean rate of 102 ± 22 beats/min. There were 3 pacing modes chosen in a randomized sequence after atrioventricular node ablation. The modes were ventricular demand pacing at 60 beats/min; ventricular demand pacing at the same average rate as during intrinsically conducted atrial fibrillation; and ventricular demand pacing during ventricular triggered pacing, in which the pacemaker was triggered by playback of the frequency-modulated tape recording of the right ventricular apex electrogram, previously recorded during intrinsically conducted atrial fibrillation at 102 ± 22 beats/min.

*Results.*—An irregular sequence of RR intervals increased pulmonary capillary wedge pressure when compared with ventricular demand pacing at the same average rate (17 ± 7 vs. 14 ± 6 mm Hg). There was also decreased cardiac output (4.4 ± 1.6 vs. 5.2 ± 2.4 L/min) and increased right atrial pressure (10 ± 6 vs. 8 ± 4 mm Hg).

*Conclusion.*—Adverse hemodynamic consequences that are independent of heart rate are produced by an irregular sequence of RR intervals.

▶ It has been suggested that the irregular RR interval during atrial fibrillation has adverse hemodynamic consequences. This paper documents some of these changes and advances the field. What is really needed is a study examining the regularization of ventricular rate with ventricular pacing compared with similar rates with variable RR intervals.

**A.L.Waldo, M.D.**

---

**Adenosine-induced Atrial Arrhythmia: A Prospective Analysis**
Strickberger SA, Man KC, Daoud EG, et al (Univ of Michigan, Ann Arbor)
*Ann Intern Med* 127:417–422, 1997                                      6–41

*Background.*—Adenosine has proven to be a safe and effective treatment for paroxysmal supraventricular tachycardia (PSVT). Clinical experience with the compound has suggested that it may induce atrial fibrillation and flutter; however, the existence and frequency of this effect has not been rigorously explored. The frequency of atrial arrhythmias induced by adenosine, in the treatment of PSVT, was evaluated in this prospective study.

*Methods.*—Electrophysiologic evaluation was performed on 200 patients with PSVT in order to determine the mechanism of the arrhythmia, and 12 mg of adenosine was administered as an intravenous bolus to each patient. Patients were observed for termination of tachycardia and occurrence of additional atrial or ventricular arrhythmias.

*Results.*—Adenosine administration terminated PSVT in 198 patients (99%), and induced atrial fibrillation in 24 patients (12%), of whom 2 also developed atrial flutter. Induced atrial arrhythmias began a mean of 6.3 seconds following PSVT termination and were preceded by atrial premature complexes in 100% of patients experiencing atrial fibrillation and/or flutter, compared with 58% of patients not experiencing induced atrial arrhythmias. Atrial fibrillation or flutter was accompanied by atrioventricular block in 20 patients and a prolonged P-R interval in the remaining 4. Preexcited atrial arrhythmias occurred in 6 patients with accessory pathways capable of anterograde conduction, and 1 patient with atrial fibrillation also developed preexcited atrial flutter. Spontaneous resolution to sinus rhythm occurred in 16 patients, with cardioversion required in 8 patients. Gender, age, cycle length of PSVT, isoproterenol use in PSVT initiation, length of the atrioventricular block cycle, or the R-R interval preceding atrial fibrillation were not predictive of induced atrial arrhythmia.

*Conclusions.*—The intravenous administration of 12 mg of adenosine for termination of PSVT is associated with a 12% incidence of atrial fibrillation. In situations in which the mechanism of PSVT is unknown and Wolff-Parkinson-White syndrome has not been ruled out, adenosine administration should be performed only in settings in which resuscitation equipment is readily available, because of there is a risk of preexcited rapid ventricular response during atrial fibrillation.

▶ The importance of this paper is for the administering physician to realize that about 1 in 8 patients given adenosine will develop atrial fibrillation. This is of some consequence, particularly if the patient presents with presumed atrioventricular reciprocating tachycardia (AVRT) or atrioventricular nodal re-entry tachycardia (AVNRT) for the first time. If the underlying substrate happens to be Wolff-Parkinson-White syndrome, one must be prepared for a small but very important incidence of development of very rapid ventricular response rates to the induced atrial fibrillation because of antegrade conduction over the accessory atrioventricular connection. This has been well reported in the past, and has been reported in previous YEAR BOOKS OF CARDIOLOGY. It should not be forgotten that adenosine is not something to give willy-nilly, particularly the first time one sees a patient. One must be prepared to defibrillate the patient promptly should atrial fibrillation with complications develop.

**A.L. Waldo, M.D.**

## Ventricular Arrhythmias

**Relation Between *Amiodarone* and *Desethylamiodarone* Plasma Concentrations and Ventricular Defibrillation Energy Requirements**
Daoud EG, Man KC, Horwood L, et al (Univ of Michigan, Ann Arbor)
*Am J Cardiol* 79:97–100, 1997                                         6–42

*Objective.*—There have been conflicting reports on the effect of amiodarone on the ventricular defibrillation energy requirement for implantable cardioverter-defibrillator (ICD) systems. Results of a prospective, controlled study assessing the relation between plasma concentrations of amiodarone and desethylamiodarone (DEA) and the acute defibrillation energy requirement in patients undergoing implantation of a nonthoracotomy ICD are presented.

*Methods.*—Results of electrophysiologic testing, performed in 102 consecutive patients undergoing ICD implantation, showed that 40 patients had inducible ventricular tachycardia and 62 did not. In the former group, 19 patients received 1,800 mg/day amiodarone for 10 days, and 21 received a mean amiodarone dose of 396 mg/day for an average of 7 months. The latter group did not receive amiodarone for 3 months before implantation. Plasma concentrations of amiodarone and DEA were determined on the morning of implantation.

*Results.*—The mean defibrillator energy requirement for the amiodarone-treated group was significantly higher than the requirement for the group not receiving amiodarone (22 vs. 17 J). Significantly more amiodarone-treated than non–amiodarone-treated patients required energies in excess of 25 J (55% vs. 24%). There were no significant differences in plasma DEA or amiodarone concentrations between patients with an energy requirement greater than 25 J and those with a requirement less than 25 J. The number of patients with a defibrillation energy requirement of 10 J or less was similar for amiodarone-treated patients and those not receiving amiodarone. There was no correlation between the defibrillation energy requirement and amiodarone, DEA, or amiodarone plus DEA concentration; duration of amiodarone therapy; daily dose of amiodarone; or duration of therapy times the daily dose.

*Conclusion.*—Amiodarone and DEA plasma concentrations less than 1 mg/L have an adverse effect on defibrillation energy requirements, increasing them by 23%.

▶ This article serves to remind us that although amiodarone is perhaps our most effective drug in treatment of ventricular arrhythmias, when used concomitantly with an implantable defibrillator, it may present real problems. In fact, it is one of the reasons why clinicians ought to consider other drugs first, unless there is NYHA Class IV heart failure or the left ventricular ejection fraction is less than 25. If possible, the standard drug would be sotalol because it is effective, it is a beta blocker, and it improves defibrillation threshold.

**A.L. Waldo, M.D.**

## A Comparison of Antiarrhythmic-Drug Therapy With Implantable Defibrillators in Patients Resuscitated From Near-Fatal Ventricular Arrhythmias

Zipes DP, for the Antiarrhythmics Versus Implantable Defibrillators (AVID) Investigators (Univ of Washington, Seattle)
*N Engl J Med* 337:1576–1583, 1997                                    6–43

*Objective.*—Patients who have survived ventricular arrhythmias are at risk of recurrence. A randomized multicenter clinical trial (AVID) evaluated whether implantable defibrillators or antiarrhythmic drugs are more effective in reducing mortality in these patients.

*Methods.*—Patients resuscitated from near-fatal ventricular fibrillation (45%) or sustained ventricular tachycardia with syncope or with an ejection fraction of 0.40 or less (55%) were implanted with a cardioverter-defibrillator ($n = 507$) or received class III antiarrhythmic drugs (amiodarone or sotalol) ($n = 509$). The 2 groups were 78% and 81% male and 87% and 86% white, respectively. The average age was 65. The outcome was overall mortality.

*Results.*—There were fewer deaths in the defibrillator group ($n = 80$) than in the drug group ($n = 122$). An overwhelming number of patients in the drug group were on amiodarones (95.8%). Over the average 18-month follow-up period, the crude death rates were 15.8% in the defibrillator group and 24.0% in the drug group. Unadjusted survival rates at 1, 2, and 3 years were 89.3%, 81.6%, and 75.4% for the defibrillator group and 82.3%, 74.7%, and 64.1% for the drug group, respectively. The decreases in death rate for the defibrillator group at 1, 2, and 3 years were 39%, 27%, and 31%, respectively. The percentages of defibrillator patients who were shocked at 3 months and at 1, 2, and 3 years were 36%, 68%, 81%, and 85% for patients with ventricular tachycardia and significantly lower at 15%, 39%, 53%, and 69% for patients with ventricular fibrillation.

*Conclusion.*—Patients with ventricular arrhythmias treated with implantable defibrillators have improved overall survival when compared with similar patients treated with amiodarone or solatol above.

▶ This is the first trial done prospectively which definitively establishes that in a head-to-head therapeutic confrontation, the implantable cardioverter defibrillator performs better than antiarrhythmic drug therapy in preventing mortality. The implications of this study will need to be sorted out over time, but it established what many intuitively thought. Nevertheless, we now have clear information in this secondary prevention study to establish the efficacy and superiority of the implantable defibrillator over drug therapy in the patients at risk.

**A.L. Waldo, M.D.**

---

**Defibrillators Are Superior to Antiarrhytmic Drugs in the Treatment of Ventricular Tachyarrhythmias**
Böcker D, Block M, Borggrefe M, et al (Westfälische Wilhelms-Univ, Münster, Germany; Inst For Arteriosclerosis Research, Münster, Germany)
*Eur Heart J* 18:26–30, 1997                                              6–44

---

*Objective.*—Comparison studies of implantable defibrillators vs. antiarrhythmic drugs as the treatment of choice for patients are being conducted. The evidence currently available for the superiority of implantable cardioverter-defibrillator therapy over antiarrhythmic drugs is presented.

*Best antiarrhythmic drug therapy.*—A meta-analysis and the Cardiac Arrest in Seattle: Conventional versus Amiodarone Drug Evaluation (CASCADE) study demonstrated that class-I antiarrhythmic drugs increase mortality.

*Treatment with implantable cardioverter-defibrillators.*—Retrospective comparisons, direct mortality comparisons in a control population, prospective randomized trials, and nonrandomized data support the efficacy of implantable cardioverters-defibrillator (ICD) therapy.

*Comparison of ICD-therapy to treatment with amiodarone or d,l-sotalol.*—The Cardiac Arrest Study Hamburg (CASH), Canadian Implantable Defibrillator Study (CIDS), and Antiarrhythmias Versus Implantable Defibrillators (AVID) prospective randomized trials are comparing the efficacy of ICDs with either d,l-sotalol or amiodarone at decreasing mortality. The prematurely terminated Multicenter Automatic Defibrillator Impantation Trial (MADI) demonstrated a 50% to 60% reduction in mortality in the study arm using the ICD.

*Conclusion.*—Both retrospective and prospective studies demonstrate the superiority of the ICD over class-I antiarrhythmic drugs. There is also evidence that ICDs decrease mortality when compared with class-III antiarrhythmic drugs, including sotalol and amiodarone.

▶ This short review is recommended to the reader because it puts into perspective some of the issues commented upon in other papers presented in this YEAR BOOK OF CARDIOLOGY. It succinctly makes the case for the implantable cardioverter defibrillator in the treatment of overt or potentially life-threatening ventricular arrhythmias.

**A.L. Waldo, M.D.**

---

**Prophylactic Use of Implanted Cardiac Defibrillators in Patients at High Risk for Ventricular Arrhythmias After Coronary-Artery Bypass Graft Surgery**
Bigger JT, Jr, for the Coronary Artery Bypass Graft (CABG) Patch Trial Investigators (Good Samaritan Hosp, Los Angeles; Sequoia Hosp, Redwood City, Calif; Univ of Louisville, Ky; et al)
*N Engl J Med* 337:1569–1575, 1997                                           6–45

---

*Objective.*—Implanted defibrillators lower overall mortality in patients with sustained ventricular tachyarrhythmias who have an increased risk of sudden death. A positive signal-averaged ECG (SAECG) identifies the presence of a substrate likely to support ventricular tachyarrhythmias in patients with a prior myocardial infarction.The effect on survival of prophylactic implantation of a cardiac defibrillator at the time of Coronary artery bypass graft surgery in patients with left ventricular dysfunction and a positive SAECG was evaluated (the CABG Patch Trial).

*Methods.*—In 37 clinical centers over a period of 5 years, 900 patients (141 female), aged less than 80 years, with a left ventricular ejection fraction of under 0.36 and an abnormal SAECG were randomly allocated to receive ($n = 446$) or not to receive ($n = 454$) an implanted defibrillator at the time of Coronary artery bypass graft surgery. Patients were examined every 3 months for an average of 32 months. Overall mortality was the outcome. The treatment groups were compared statistically.

*Results.*—During the follow-up period, there were 101 deaths (71 cardiac) in the defibrillator group and 95 (72 cardiac) in the control group. Kaplan-Meier survival analyses showed no benefit of defibrillator implantation.

*Conclusion.*—Prophylactic implantation of cardiac defibrillators in high-risk patients identified by low LVEF and a positive SAECG at the time of coronary artery bypass graft surgery did not improve survival.

▶ The CABG Patch Trial was a primary prevention trial with results different from MADIT I. MADIT I clearly showed that in patients with a previous myocardial infarction, left ventricular dysfunction, and nonsustained ventricular tachycardia—if sustained ventricular tachycardia could be induced in the EP laboratory but induction could not be suppressed by procainamide—the implantable defibrillator was superior to conventional drug therapy (principally amiodarone) in preventing deaths. Why then was the CABG Patch Trial neutral in outcome? It is not entirely clear, but to this editor, it does emphasize the importance of treating ischemic heart disease with the best therapy available—in this trial with coronary artery bypass graft surgery—to prevent ischemia. Nevertheless, it really points to the need to have good risk markers so that the patients who have the best hope of benefiting from a particular form of therapy get that therapy. Such a high risk marker was nonsustained ventricular tachycardia in patients with a previous myocardial infarct, depressed ventricular function, and inducible ventricular tachycardia that is not suppressed by procainamide (MADIT I).

**A.L. Waldo, M.D.**

---

## Quantitative Overview of Randomized Trials of Amiodarone to Prevent Sudden Cardiac Death

Sim I, McDonald KM, Lavori PW, et al (Stanford Univ, Calif)
*Circulation* 96:2823–2829, 1997                                    6–46

---

*Objective.*—Half of patients with clinically evident heart disease die of sudden death. Findings from randomized clinical trials of amiodarone have been inconsistent. A meta-analysis was performed on all amiodarone trials to determine if amiodarone reduced total mortality or if sudden death was selectively reduced depending on patient population and study design.

*Methods.*—Fifteen oral amiodarone trials, 3 months or more in duration, published between January 1985 and March 1997, were analyzed for total mortality, cardiac death, and sudden death. Subgroup analyses using the hierarchical Bayes linear model were performed to determine if some subgroup trial results were systematically different from the other subgroup trial results.

*Results.*—There were 2,936 amiodarone patients and 2,928 controls. Compared with controls, amiodarone patients had a significantly lower total mortality (19.2% vs. 16.5%), significantly lower cardiac mortality (16.4% vs. 13.2%), and a significantly lower sudden death rate (9.6% vs. 6.9%). Noncardiac mortality was similar between groups. Amiodarone reduced mortality in all 3 categories similarly in subgroups of patients with myocardial infarction, with heart failure, and with left ventricular dysfunction. There was a nonsignificantly greater mortality reduction in trials that included only patients with evidence of arrhythmia. Total mortality was significantly lower in "usual care" trials and in trials with active controls than in placebo controlled trials (OR 0.58 vs. OR 0.73 vs. OR 0.90).

*Conclusion.*—Amiodarone significantly reduced total mortality, cardiac mortality, and sudden death rate in patients with myocardial infarction, with heart failure, and with left ventricular dysfunction. Small sample sizes and type of control used rather than type of patient enrolled explain the inconsistencies in randomized trials.

▶ This meta-analysis would suggest that amiodarone does have a weak positive effect on outcome that can only be garnered from a meta-analysis of 15 randomized trials. For this editor, the principal implications still remain in the use of amiodarone in the treatment of atrial fibrillation in patients with ventricular dysfunction. The data more and more suggest that the implantable cardioverter defibrillator is the first line of treatment to prevent sudden cardiac death or arrhythmic mortality in patients with ventricular dysfunction. Of interest, however, is another meta-analysis which should be published soon that suggests that a combination of amiodarone with beta-blocker therapy may be a very important and effective drug combination. We await those data.

**A.L. Waldo, M.D.**

---

**Adenosine-sensitive Ventricular Tachycardia: Right Ventricular Abnormalities Delineated by Magnetic Resonance Imaging**
Markowitz SM, Litvak BL, Ramirez de Arellano AR, et al (Cornell Univ, New York)
*Circulation* 96:1192–1200, 1997                                                    6–47

---

*Introduction.*—Patients with ventricular tachycardia (VT) and no clinically evident heart disease have been examined by means of endomyocardial biopsy, signal-averaged ECG, and MRI to determine previously undetected abnormalities. These reports have conflicting results regarding the mechanisms of arrhythmogenesis. The primary defect in adenosine-sensitive VT has not been determined. Echocardiography and cardiac catheterization have limited sensitivity in detecting abnormalities in right ventricular (RV) structure and function; MRI may be more sensitive in imaging the RV. A homogeneous population of 14 patients with idiopathic adenosine-sensitive VT underwent MRI screening to determine abnormalities in RV structure and function.

*Methods.*—All antiarrhythmic agents were discontinued before electrophysiologic studies were performed. Fourteen patients with adenosine-sensitive VT (3 paroxysmal sustained VT and 11 right ventricular outflow tract [RVOT]) underwent detailed activation and pace mapping to determine the focal origin of VT and guide ablation. Eleven patients underwent radiofrequency ablation. Patients and healthy, age- and sex-matched controls underwent an identical MRI protocol at a mean of 11 months after initial ablation procedure.

*Results.*—The origin of VT was RVOT in 10 patients, RV apex in 1, and left ventricular septum in 3. Nine of 9, 10 of 10, and 6 of 7 patients, respectively, undergoing signal-averaged ECGs, RV echocardiography, and left ventriculography and coronary angiography had normal findings, compared with abnormal MRI scan results in 10 of 14 patients. Abnormal MRI findings included focal thinning (6 patients), fatty infiltration (4), and wall motion abnormalities of the RV (4). The most frequent site of abnormalities by MRI was the RV free wall. The correlation between the site of MRI abnormalities and the origin of VT was poor. Thinning of the RV wall was detected in 1 control.

*Conclusion.*—These findings question the specificity of MRI-defined fatty deposition, wall thinning, and abnormal wall motion in the diagnosis of arrhythmogenic RV dysplasia. The functional significance of MRI findings in this patient cohort is unknown.

▶ This study is of interest because it looks systematically at 1 particular aspect of the right ventricular outflow tachycardia syndrome, namely, those patients with adenosine-sensitive ventricular tachycardias. The fact that there is such a heterogeneous group is surprising to this editor. It serves to remind us that we have much more to learn about this arrhythmia and its treatment. There are real implications for this with regard to the various therapies used, including radiofrequency ablation.

**A.L. Waldo, M.D.**

---

**Idiopathic Right Ventricular Outflow Tract Tachycardia: A Clinical Approach**

Lerman BB, Stein KM, Markowitz SM (Cornell Univ, New York)
*PACE* 19:2120–2137, 1996                                                    6–48

---

*Introduction.*—Most cases of ventricular tachycardia (VT) originate from the left ventricle and occur in patients with structural heart disease. In a growing number of cases, however, VT is being detected in patients with no evidence of structural heart disease. In approximately 80% of these patients, VT originates from the region of the right ventricular outflow tract (RVOT). The clinical manifestations and management of idiopathic RVOT tachycardia are reviewed.

*Classification.*—Nearly all forms of idiopathic VT can be differentiated by response of the arrhythmia to programmed stimulation and to adenosine, verapamil, and propranolol. Nearly all forms are catecholamine facilitated. At the study institution, 90% of RVOT tachycardia results from adenosine-sensitive VT—either nonsustained, repetitive monomorphic VT or paroxysmal, exercise-induced, sustained VT. Features of both of these syndromes may be present in a single patient.

*Two Predominant Phenotypes of Adenosine-Sensitive VT.*—Repetitive monomorphic VT generally occurs at rest and is characterized by frequent ventricular extrasystoles, ventricular couplets, and salvos of nonsustained monomorphic VT with intervening sinus beats. In contrast, paroxysmal, exercise-induced VT is sustained and usually precipitated by exercise, exertion, or stress. Previous studies support the view that both forms reflect disparate clinical manifestations of an identical cellular mechanism, cyclic adenosine monophosphate–mediated triggered activity.

*Diagnostic Considerations.*—Some patients are relatively resistant to adenosine and may require higher-than-usual doses ($\geq$ 18 to 24 mg) to assess VT sensitivity. Although termination of VT in response to adenosine is usually quite clear, a transient overdrive suppression of VT by sinus tachycardia could lead to diagnostic error. It is thus important to observe ventriculoatrial block or sinus slowing at the time of VT termination. Other diagnostic dilemmas are possible.

*Clinical Manifestations.*—Men and women are equally affected by RVOT tachycardia. Most patients at the study institution are aged 30 to 50. Those with paroxysmal, sustained VT often have tachycardia during exercise, anger, or mental stress. As many as one third of patients with repetitive monomorphic VT may be free of symptoms. Those with symptoms often report palpitation and dizziness; frank syncope develops in 10% of patients with VT.

*Diagnosis and Treatment.*—The ECG, echocardiography, and exercise testing are inadequate for diagnosis, and results of cardiac catheterization have been variable. Some studies have considered the results of Holter monitoring, signal-averaged ECG, MRI, and endomyocardial histology. The preferred treatment is an antiarrhythmic agent, with a β-blocker as the first choice. The RVOT tachycardia is responsive to all classes of antiarrhythmics and shows a more favorable response than does VT caused by structural heart disease. Ablation is also successful, because the tachycardia focus is discrete, well circumscribed, and accessible. In the differential diagnosis, it is important to rule out arrhythmogenic right ventricular dysplasia.

▶ This is simply a lovely review that puts together much information and many ideas in an understandable format. It is highly recommended to the reader.

**A.L. Waldo, M.D.**

## Antiarrhythmic Effects of Increasing the Daily Intake of Magnesium and Potassium in Patients With Frequent Ventricular Arrhythmias

Zehender M, for the MAGICA Investigators (Universitätsklinik Freiburg, Germany)
*J Am Coll Cardiol* 29:1028–1034, 1997                    6–49

*Introduction.*—Experimental and clinical trials have indicated that low plasma concentrations of potassium and magnesium increase the risk of induction, facilitation, or aggravation of ventricular tachyarrhythmias (VTs). Treatment interventions have been focused on the prevention of electrolyte depletion. A large series of consecutive patients with frequent and stable VTs were evaluated in a double-blind, randomized, placebo-controlled trial to determine the potential antiarrhythmic benefit of increasing the daily recommended dietary intake of magnesium and potassium by 50% over a 3-week treatment period.

*Methods.*—Three hundred and seven patients with left ventricular ejection fraction of more than 25% and normal levels of potassium and magnesium were enrolled from 20 European cardiology centers. Patients underwent an extensive diagnostic work-up, then entered a placebo-controlled 1-week run-in period. They were reassessed. Then 232 patients with more than 720 ventricular premature beats (VPBs)/24 hr on repeat Holter monitoring were randomized to 3 weeks of either active treatment with daily oral magnesium-DL-potassium-DL-hydrogenaspartate daily (6 mmol magnesium; 12 mmol potassium) or placebo. Patients were reassessed at completion of 21 days of active or placebo treatment.

*Results.*—Patients with active treatment had a significant median decrease in VPBs by $-17.4\%$. The suppression rate was 2.4 time higher for the active treatment group, compared with the placebo group. The likelihood of a 60% or 70% or greater suppression rate was significantly greater for the active treatment group than for the placebo treatment group.

*Conclusion.*—This is the first known trial to report controlled data on the antiarrhythmic effect of oral administration of magnesium and potassium salts in patients with frequent and stable ventricular arrhythmias. With a 50% increase in the recommended daily dietary intake of magnesium and potassium for 3 weeks, a moderate, but significant, antiarrhythmic effect was observed. This therapeutic regimen had no effect on repetitive tachyarrhythmias or patients' symptoms.

▶ This multicenter trial is of interest because of the suggestions from many quarters that magnesium may be a very important antiarrhythmic agent for the treatment of ventricular arrhythmias. This study really shows that it isn't. However, the reader is reminded that in the treatment of torsades de pointes associated with prolonged Q-T interval, intravenous magnesium therapy may be critical because it will prevent runs of torsades de pointes, giving the clinician time to treat the offending cause. That usually means gaining time to permit washout of an offending drug or to administer of potassium.

**A.L. Waldo, M.D.**

**Disturbed Connexin43 Gap Junction Distribution Correlates With the Location of Reentrant Circuits in the Epicardial Border Zone of Healing Canine Infarcts That Cause Ventricular Tachycardia**
Peters NS, Coromilas J, Severs NJ, et al (St Mary's Hosp, London; Columbia Univ, New York)
*Circulation* 95:988–1996, 1997                                        6–50

*Introduction.*—A canine model of myocardial infarction was used to examine the hypothesis that disorganization of gap-junctional intercellular coupling is a cause of arrhythmogenic nonuniformity of anisotropic conduction in the early phase after infarction, before fibrotic scarring. Investigation of the hypothesis involved determination of connexin43 (Cx43) gap-junctional organization in regions of the infarct epicardial border zone (EBZ) in which reentrant circuits that caused sustained ventricular tachycardia (VT) were mapped.

*Methods.*—Six anesthetized mongrel dogs underwent 2-stage ligation of the left anterior descending coronary artery 5 to 10 mm from its origin. Four days later, the EBZs overlying infarcts in 3 dogs with inducible VT and 3 dogs in which VT could not be induced were mapped with a high-resolution electrode array and systematically examined with standard histology and confocal immunolocalization of Cx43, the principal gap-junctional protein.

*Results.*—Extensive infarction of the anterior and lateral left ventricle developed in all 6 animals after left anterior descending coronary artery occlusion. Mean thickness of the EBZ was significantly less in hearts with VT (538 µm) than in hearts without VT (840 µm). The EBZ myocardium exhibited a notable disruption of gap-junctional distribution at the interface with the underlying necrotic cells, and Cx43 labeling was abnormally arrayed longitudinally along the lateral surfaces of the cells. The disrupted Cx43 labeling extended part of the way to the epicardial surface in the EBZs of all hearts. Normal Cx43 gap-junctional distribution, consisting of a transversely oriented pattern, was present in myocytes of the subepicardial myocardium from the noninfarcted posterior wall. Only hearts with inducible VT were found to have disorganization extending through the full thickness of the surviving layer at sites that correlated with the location of central common pathways of the figure-of-8 reentrant VT circuits.

*Conclusion.*—Early postinfarct remodeling is indicated by the finding of profound alterations of Cx43 gap-junctional distribution in the surviving infarct-related myocytes 4 days after infarction and before the occurrence of fibrotic healing. Changes in gap-junctional organization in the setting of myocardial remodeling may be causally related to enhanced arrhythmogenicity.

▶ This study further reveals the complexity of reentrant circuits associated with myocardial infarction. The reader is also reminded that most of the electrophysiologic investigations that we conduct deal with membrane properties of cardiac tissue. There is as yet no electrophysiologic study that can be used clinically which identifies disturbances in cell-to-cell (connexin-gap junction) properties. These are undoubtedly very important mechanistically and also in terms of how drugs effect conduction at this critical point between cells.

**A.L. Waldo, M.D.**

---

### Spontaneous Ventricular Tachycardia Treated by Antitachycardia Pacing

Nasir N Jr, and the Cadence Investigators (Texas Arrhythmia Inst, Houston)
*Am J Cardiol* 79:820–822, 1997                                        6–51

---

*Objective.*—Whether acceleration of pacing within single bursts (autodecremental or ramp pacing) or burst pacing is more effective for treating ventricular tachycardia (VT) has not been definitively established. Results of a retrospective study of outcomes and complication rates for patients receiving the Cadence V-100 are presented.

*Methods.*—The records of 434 patients (384 men), aged 14 to 90 years, receiving the Cadence V-100 between July 1989 and March 1994 for organic heart disease and having documented VT events during the follow-up period, were reviewed for outcome and complications. A successful outcome was defined as termination of VT by pacing. Parameters evaluated included adaptive percentage of initial burst cycle length, number of programmed bursts, use of scan pacing, use of autodecremental pacing, and number of programmed stimuli per burst.

*Results.*—Patients had 22,339 episodes during an average follow-up period of 758 days. Of these, 21,003 (94%) were successfully terminated, 1023 (4.6%) were not terminated, and 313 (1.4%) were accelerated. Episodes not terminated were successfully treated by cardioversion or high-voltage defibrillation. Accelerated episodes were successfully treated by high-voltage defibrillation. Mean VT cycle lengths for episodes terminated successfully, episodes not terminated, and accelerated episodes were 395, 390, and 347 ms, respectively. Antitachycardia pacing ranges of 6 to 10 and 11 to 15 stimuli per burst were successful in 94% and 96% of patients, respectively. At 16 to 20 stimuli per burst, the antitachycardia pacing success rate dropped to 77%. Acceleration occurred in less than 2% of episodes and was independent of the number of bursts. There was no difference in success, failure, and acceleration rates with or without autodecremental pacing and with or without scanning. The success rate for patients programmed in the 81% to 85% range was significantly lower than for those programmed in the 71% to 75% range (94% vs. 99%).

*Conclusion.*—Although this study was not randomized, the results with this large patient population show that 94% of spontaneous VT episodes are successfully terminated by the Cadence V-100 device, and fewer than 2% of episodes are accelerated.

▶ The value of antitachycardia pacing as part of the implantable cardioverter defibrillator (ICD) should not be overlooked. It saves patients unpleasant shocks, provides effective therapy, and may be a reason to use class I antiarrhythmic drugs in association with the ICD. Class I drugs will slow the spontaneous ventricular tachycardia rates into a range where antitachycardia pacing is quite effective. And then the ICD provides a safety net should the antitachycardia pacing inadvertently precipitate a faster ventricular tachycardia or ventricular fibrillation.

**A.L. Waldo, M.D.**

---

**Predictors of Long-term Survival in Patients With Malignant Ventricular Arrhythmias**
Gomes JA, Mehta D, Ip J, et al (CUNY; Thoracic Cardiovascular Inst, Lansing, Mich; Morristown Mem Hosp, Madison, NJ; et al)
*Am J Cardiol* 79:1054–1060, 1997                                                                    6–52

---

*Introduction.*—The management of patients with malignant ventricular arrhythmias has improved substantially in the last decade with the use of new drugs, surgery, and the implantable cardioverter-defibrillator (ICD). The most important predictors of survival from cardiac mortality, the impact of congestive heart failure (CHF) on therapy, and the natural history of patients treated by current therapeutic modalities were evaluated in 369 patients with malignant ventricular arrhythmias.

*Methods.*—Of the 369 patients, 74% had coronary artery disease (CAD), 19% had cardiomyopathy, and 7% had no evident heart disease. Therapeutic approaches were as follows: 221 drug therapy, 47 arrhythmia surgery, and 75 ICD.

*Results.*—At a mean follow-up of 30 months (1–101), 26 of 66 deaths from cardiac causes were sudden. Multivariate analysis indicated that the most significant variables of survival from cardiac mortality were CHF class, ejection fraction, and the use of drug therapy; in patients with CAD, CHF class and ejection fraction; and in patients with cardiomyopathy, CHF class and sustained ventricular tachycardia on Holter monitoring. Survival rates from cardiac death in patients with CHF class III and IV, compared with patients with CHF class I and II, were significantly lower in patients who received drug therapy, marginally significant from 20–40 months in patients with an ICD, and nonsignificant in patients who underwent arrhythmia surgery. Patients with ICD had a better expected survival than patients who had arrhythmia surgery or drug therapy (82%, 69%, and 65%, respectively).

*Conclusion.*—Congestive heart failure class was the most significant independent predictor of survival from cardiac mortality in patients with malignant ventricular arrhythmias. The therapeutic approach influenced survival, depending on the CHF class. Patients in CHF class III and IV who underwent arrhythmia surgery or had an ICD had a better expected survival than patients on drug therapy. The negative impact of antiarrhythmia therapy was pronounced in patients with CHF class III and IV.

▶ This large experience from a very good group of electrophysiologists serves well to emphasize the importance of treatment of heart failure to favorably affect the prognosis in treatment of ventricular arrhythmias. More and more studies recognize that it is heart failure that has an association with proarrhythmia as well as an adverse outcome ultimately for the patient. We are doing so much better at treating heart failure these days that it seems obvious that this therapy would be aggressively applied. Nevertheless, this study documents how really important it is to treat the heart failure in patients with malignant ventricular arrhythmias.

**A.L. Waldo, M.D.**

---

**Nonsustained Ventricular Tachycardia in Severe Heart Failure: Independent Marker of Increased Mortality due to Sudden Death**
Doval HC, for the GESICA-GEMA Investigators (Instituto del Corazón del Hosp Italiano, Buenos Aires, Argentina)
*Circulation* 94:3198–3203, 1996                                                  6–53

---

*Introduction.*—Mortality remains extremely high in patients with congestive heart failure, and approximately 40% of deaths occur suddenly. Ventricular tachycardia and fibrillation appear to be frequent mechanisms of death in patients with severe heart failure. A homogeneous group of patients was studied to determine the independent prognostic value of nonsustained ventricular tachycardia (NSVT) on total mortality and its relation to the death mechanisms.

*Methods.*—The study enrolled 516 patients from December 1989 through March 1993; 173 patients (33.5%) had NSVT as determined by 24-hour Holter recordings. To be included in the study, patients had to be stable and in an advanced functional capacity with adequately treated advanced chronic heart failure and marked left ventricular systolic dysfunction. None were receiving anti-arrhythmic treatment, had concomitant serious associated clinical diseases, or a history of sustained ventricular tachycardia or ventricular fibrillation. Follow-up continued for 2 years.

*Results.*—At the end of the study period, 5 patients with NSVT and 14 without NSVT were lost to follow-up; follow-up was terminated in 4 patients with and 12 without NSVT who underwent cardiac transplantation. With an average follow-up of 13 months, 193 of 516 patients had died (37.4%)—87 (50.3%) with NSVT and 106 (30.9%) without NSVT. Independent predictors of the presence of NSVT in the 24-hour Holter monitoring were increased furosemide dose, decreased systolic blood pressure, increased serum creatinine level, faster heart rate, and Chagas' dis-

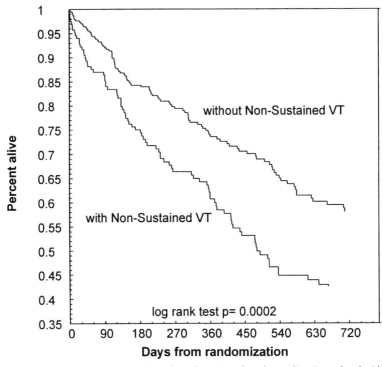

FIGURE 1.—Nonsustained ventricular tachycardia (*VT*) and total mortality. (Reproduced with permission, from Doval HC, for the GESICA-GEMA Investigators: Nonsustained ventricular tachycardia in severe heart failure: Independent marker of increased mortality due to sudden death. *Circulation* 94:3198–3203, 1996. Copyright 1996 by the American Heart Association.)

ease as the cause of heart failure. The presence of NSVT increased total mortality (Fig 1), with a relative risk (RR) of 1.69; the RR for sudden death was 2.77 with NSVT. Progressive heart failure death was also increased in the NSVT group (20.8% vs. 17.5% for those without NSVT). Treatment with amiodarone did not affect mortality in the NSVT group. Quantitative analysis of 24-hour Holter recording showed that couplets had a similar RR to that of NSVT for both total mortality and sudden death.

*Conclusion.*—Nonsustained ventricular tachycardia was confirmed to be an independent marker for increased overall mortality and sudden death in patients with congestive heart failure. The absence of NSVT and ventricular repetitive beats in a 24-hour Holter may identify patients with a low probability of sudden death.

▶ This reworking of the GESICA data is of interest because it emphasizes once again that nonsustained ventricular tachycardia is a very important independent marker of an increased risk for sudden death. However, that does not translate into a fact that suppression of the nonsustained ventricular tachycardia is an end point. In addition, in the GESICA trial, most of the patients had non-ischemic cardiomyopathy. It would really have been nice to have compared these data with something like MADIT, which went on to do an end-point study and evaluate the patient in that way. Nevertheless, as we have emphasized this year once again, it is important to use as many risk stratifiers as possible to identify the patient most likely to benefit from therapy because so many therapies have important risks.

**A.L. Waldo, M.D.**

## Pacing

**Atrial Pacing Leads Following Open Heart Surgery: Active or Passive Fixation?**
Connelly DT, Steinhaus DM, Handlin L, et al (Saint Luke's Hosp, Kansas City, Mo)
*PACE* 20(Pt I):2429–2433, 1997                                                  6–54

*Introduction.*—In patients with previous open heart surgery who require permanent atrial or dual chamber pacing, active fixation leads have often been used because of concerns about lead displacement. To establish cardiopulmonary bypass, the right atrial appendage is often amputated during open heart surgery. Patients with previous open heart surgery were evaluated for the acute and chronic performance of implanted active and passive fixation atrial leads.

*Methods.*—There were 78 patients who were paced after open heart surgery, of whom 38 had active fixation atrial leads placed, 28 had passive fixation steroid-eluting leads, and 12 had passive leads without steroid-eluting properties. These patients were compared with 76 patients who were paced without previous cardiac surgery.

*Results.*—Compared with all passive fixation leads, lead impedance and threshold were significantly higher for active fixation leads. In all 3 groups, sensed P wave amplitudes were similar at implantation. In the patients with active fixation leads compared with those with passive fixation leads, sensed P wave amplitudes were significantly lower and atrial pacing thresholds were significantly higher at follow-up. In 1 of 40 patients (2.5%) with a passive fixation lead, loss of sensing occurred, and in 6 of 38 patients (16%) with active fixation leads, loss of sensing occurred. In 2 patients with active fixation leads and in 1 with a passive fixation lead, atrial lead displcement occurred. Atrial lead performance was similar in the control and experimental groups.

*Conclusion.*—It is appropriate to implant a passive fixation atrial lead when permanent atrial or dual-chamber pacing is necessary in patients with prior open heart surgery, except on the infrequent occasions when a stable atrial position cannot be obtained.

▶ This well-done study is very reassuring regarding passive fixation of atrial leads in patients who have undergone open heart surgery. In the end, perhaps the best way to interpret this study is that one should do what makes the most sense.

**A.L. Waldo, M.D.**

---

**Interference With Cardiac Pacemakers by Cellular Telephones**
Hayes DL, Wang PJ, Reynolds DW, et al (Mayo Clinic, Rochester, Minn; New England Med Ctr, Boston; Univ of Oklahoma, Oklahoma City; et al)
*N Engl J Med* 336:1473–1479, 1997                                      6–55

---

*Introduction.*—European studies have suggested that cellular telephones can interfere with implanted pacemakers. In the United States, in vitro studies have shown the potential for such interference. A multicenter trial was performed to assess the incidence of interference with pacemakers by cellular phones, and the clinical risk arising from such interference.

*Methods.*—The prospective, crossover, double-blind study included 980 patients with implanted cardiac pacemakers. Each patient was tested with 5 types of hand-held cellular telephones in random order, including 1 analogue and 4 digital phones. In the test mode use for each phone, the phones were programmed to transmit at maximal power, thus simulating the worst-case scenario. Furthermore, 1 phone was tested during actual use. During testing, each patient underwent ECG monitoring with the phone over the ipsilateral ear and in a series of maneuvers directly over the pacemaker. When any interference occurred, it was classified as to type and clinical significance.

*Results.*—A total of 5,233 tests were performed, 20% of which caused any type of interference and 7.2% of which caused symptoms. Clinically significant interferences occurred in 6.6% of tests. Clinically significant interference never occurred with the phone held normally over the ear. The rate of definitely clinically significant interference was only 1.7%, and this occurred only with the phone held over the pacemaker. Dual-chamber pacemakers showed interference in 25.3% of tests, compared with 6.8% for single-chamber pacemakers. The interference rate was 28.9% to 55.8% for pacemakers without feed-through filters, compared with 0.4% to 0.8% for those with feed-through filters.

*Conclusions.*—Cellular telephones can interfere with pacemaker function. However, clinically significant interference does not occur with the phone placed over the ear, as during normal use. Cellular phones should not be placed over the pacemaker, and should not be carried in a pocket close to the pacemaker when turned on.

▶ More data on the potential interference with pacemakers by cellular telephones. The bottom line is simple and patients should really understand it. Hold the telephone properly to your ear, and there is nothing to worry about.

**A.L. Waldo, M.D.**

## Is Mode Switching Beneficial? A Randomized Study in Patients With Paroxysmal Atrial Tachyarrhythmias

Kamalvand K, Tan K, Kotsakis A, et al (Guy's and St Thomas' NHS Trust, London)
*J Am Coll Cardiol* 30:496–504, 1997                                 6–56

*Introduction.*—In the past, a history of atrial tachyarrhythmias was a relative contraindication to implantation of dual-chamber pacemakers. In an attempt to extend the indications for dual-chamber pacing to patients with a history of atrial tachyarrhythmias, several manufacturers have recently developed different mode-switching algorithms, which should protect the patient from rapid ventricular rates. In patients with a history of atrial tachyarrhythmias, a comparison of dual-chamber universal rate-responsive mode pacing and dual-chamber universal rate-responsive mode with mode switching was made. These were compared with standard upper rate behavior and single-chamber ventricular-inhibited rate-responsive pacing.

*Methods.*—A dual-chamber universal rate-responsive mode with mode-switching pacemaker was implanted in 48 patients with a mean age of 64 years. In a randomized crossover design, the pacemakers were programmed to mode switching, conventional upper rate behavior, and single-chamber ventricular-inhibited rate-responsive pacing for 4 weeks each. Throughout the study, all patients used a patient-activated electrocardiographic recorder. Inappropriate mode switching and inappropriate tracking of atrial tachyarrythmias were studied to determine their incidence and the contributing factors. A determination was also made as to whether there were differences in patients' preferences for the different mode-switching algorithms by having patients complete 3 symptom questionnaires.

*Results.*—Objectively and subjectively, the mode switching was better than the single-chamber ventricular-inhibited rate-responsive mode. The mode-switching method was significantly better perceived by patients compared with the conventional upper rate behavior mode. The preferred pacing period was the mode-switching method. During the single-chamber ventricular-inhibited rate responsive mode, 33% of patients had early termination because of adverse symptoms. This occurred in 19% of patients with the conventional upper rate behavior mode and only 3% of those in the mode-switching mode. The mode-switching mode was preferred by more patients with a fast mode-switching device than a slow one, but no patient with a fast mode-switching device chose the single-chamber ventricular-inhibited rate responsive mode. The mode-switching mode was also preferred in the subgroup of patients who had atrioventricular node ablation.

*Conclusion.*—In patients with paroxysmal atrial tachyarrhythmias, dual-chamber universal rate-responsive mode with mode switching was the pacing mode of choice. Inappropriate mode switching and tracking of atrial tachyarrythmias was very uncommon with optimal programming.

▶ This study confirms this editor's long-held prejudice. Mode switching is superior to DDDR with conventional upper rate behavior and VVIR in patients with a history of atrial tachyarrhythmias.

**A.L. Waldo, M.D.**

**Failure of Automatic Mode Switching: Recognition and Management**
Ellenbogen KA, Mond HG, Wood MA, et al (McGuire VA Med Ctr, Richmond; Royal Melbourne Hosp, Victoria, Australia; Univ of Rochester, NY)
*PACE* 20:268–275, 1997                                                     6–57

*Background.*—Many patients with sick sinus syndrome have alternating periods of supraventricular tachyarrhythmia and bradycardia. Dual-chamber pacing is considered to be the optimal pacing mode in such cases but can result in tracking of paroxysmal supraventricular tachyarrhythmias, leading to a rapidly paced ventricular response rate. To prevent this problem, automatic mode switching (AMS) was incorporated into pacemaker devices. The 7 reported cases show that failure to mode switch may occur when the atrial signal during tachycardia is of insufficient amplitude to be sensed, or when the atrial signal periodically occurs in the atrial blanking period.

*Methods.*—The patients had undergone implantation of the Telectronics Meta DDDR 1254 (Telectronics Pacing Systems, Englewood, Colo). Sick sinus syndrome and paroxysmal atrial flutter or fibrillation were present in all cases. Failure to mode switch was noted during routine evaluation of the device or when patients reported palpitations. Six of the 7 patients were taking anti-arrhythmic drugs. With the Meta DDDR 1254, AMS occurs when the device specifically detects 5 or 11 atrial events with a cycle length shorter than the atrial tachycardia detection interval.

*Results.*—In all but 1 of the 7 cases, failure to mode switch was not the result of an inadequate atrial electrogram amplitude during atrial tachyarrhythmias. Six patients had sufficient atrial electrogram amplitude during atrial flutter to be detected at the programmed atrial sensitivity; the remaining patient (patient 2) had intermittent undersensing of atrial electrograms during atrial fibrillation. Antiarrhythmic drugs had slowed the length of the atrial cycle in patients taking these agents. All pacemakers were reprogrammed to restore reliable mode switching during recurrences of atrial tachyarrhythmia. Initial restoration of appropriate mode switching was achieved by shortening the atrioventricular interval or by prolonging the atrioventricular interval and the postventricular atrial refractory period. In patient 2, AMS failed as a result of low electrogram amplitude and atrial signals occurring during blanking period and was restored by reprogramming atrial sensitivity and atrioventricular interval.

*Conclusion.*—Patients with paroxysmal atrial flutter who are taking an antiarrhythmic drug that slows atrial cycle length require careful pacemaker programming when the Telectronics Meta DDDR 1254 is implanted. Several steps that can enhance the AMS function of this device are presented.

▶ This study emphasizes the importance of drug effects on mode-switching patients with pacemakes that have automatic mode switching. It is important to remember that some drugs, namely the class IIIs (not amiodarone), do not slow the atrial rate, so this might be another reason to consider them. The presently available drug is sotalol. Other drugs such as dofetilide will be coming along.

**A.L. Waldo, M.D.**

---

**A Study Comparing VVI and DDI Pacing in Elderly Patients With Carotid Sinus Syndrome**
McIntosh SJ, Lawson J, Bexton RS, et al (Royal Victoria Infirmary, Newcastle Upon Tyne, England)
*Heart* 77:553–557, 1997                                6–58

---

*Introduction.*—Carotid sinus syndrome is an important but commonly overlooked cause of syncope and presyncope, especially in the elderly. Cardiac pacing stops syncope in about 90% of patients with cardioinhibition. A significant number, particularly those with a single ventricular system, continue to experience residual presyncope symptoms. The hemodynamic effects of single chamber ventricular demand (VVI) pacing was compared with that of dual chamber demand (DDI) pacing in 30 elderly patients with carotid sinus syndrome to determine whether VVI pacing is adequate for this subgroup of patients.

*Methods.*—Patients over age 60 years underwent dual chamber pacemaker implantation, then were randomized to 2 three-month periods of VVI and DDI pacing. Responses to vasodepression during carotid sinus massage, pacemaker effect, postural blood pressure measurements, and response to head-up tilt were assessed after each 3-month pacing mode.

*Results.*—In 11 and 2 patients, respectively, profound hypotension developed during upright carotid sinus massage under VVI pacing and DDI pacing. The upright pacemaker effect was significantly greater in VVI spacing than in DDI pacing. Both pacing modes were similar in postural blood pressure measurements and response to head-up tilt. Eleven patients withdrew from VVI pacing because of intolerance. The 14 remaining patients did not express a preference as pacing mode. No patients preferred VVI pacing. Patients who were withdrawn from VVI pacing were significantly older, more likely to be female, and more likely to have orthostatic hypotension with pacing DDI pacing.

*Conclusion.*—Elderly patients with carotid sinus syndrome were more likely to experience symptomatic hypotension after VVI pacing. The optimum mode of pacing for individual elderly patients cannot be determined by simple cardiovascular tests before pacing.

▶ Elderly patients with carotid sinus syndrome are not common. However, once again, atrial pacing is superior to ventricular pacing alone. The increased cost is virtually always worth the investment, in this editor's judgment.

**A.L. Waldo, M.D.**

## Clinical Presentation of Endocardial Pacing Lead Malfunction
Helguera ME, Maloney JD, Fahy GJ, et al (Cleveland Clinic Found, Ohio; Timken Mercy Med Ctr, Canton, Ohio)
*Am J Cardiol* 78:1297–1299, 1996                                             6–59

*Introduction.*—The high incidence of failure in some endocardial pacing lead models has caused concern. Because little information is available on the clinical presentation of endocardial lead failure, researchers reviewed the medical records of a group of patients with leads implanted at the study institution.

*Methods.*—During the period under review, 1,474 patients with a mean age of 64 years had 2,444 endocardial pacing leads implanted. The leads represented 123 different models from 9 manufacturers. Polarity was unipolar in 49%, bipolar coaxial in 47%, and bipolar noncoaxial in 4%. Mean duration of follow-up was 33 months; patients with less than 1 month of follow-up were excluded to avoid analysis of lead malfunction related to peri- and post-operative complications.

*Results.*—During the follow-up period, there were 398 deaths, none of which were documented as having been caused by lead malfunction. Fatal lead malfunction, however, would probably appear as a case of sudden death, and malfunction could only be confirmed by an electrocardiogram at the time of death or a postmortem lead analysis. Documented lead malfunction did occur in 54 leads (54 patients). The 34 ventricular and 20 atrial lead failures occurred at a mean of 37 months after implantation. Most patients (63%) experienced only mild symptoms or were asymptomatic and had the malfunction detected during routine pacemaker check. More definite symptoms that occurred in the remaining 20 patients suggested hemodynamic compromise. Patients with severe symptoms were more likely to have ventricular rather than atrial lead failure, and those who were pacemaker dependent were more likely to have syncope or near syncope at the time of lead failure. Most patients (75%) with severe symptoms before pacemaker implantation had severe symptoms at the time of lead malfunction. No association was found between severity of symptoms at the time of lead malfunction and age, gender, time since lead implant, total time since first pacemaker implant, or lead characteristics (model, manufacturer, insulation material, or polarity).

*Conclusion.*—Although no deaths were attributed to pacemaker lead malfunction in this patient group, 37% of those with lead malfunction experienced syncope or near syncope. Several patient subgroups were identified as being at high risk for hemodynamic compromise in the event of pacing lead malfunction.

▶ The editor recommends this short review of the experience in almost 1,500 patients.

**A.L. Waldo, M.D.**

---

**Transtelephone Monitoring for Pacemaker Follow-up 1981–1994**
Platt S, Furman S, Gross JN, et al (Montefiore Med Ctr, Bronx, NY; Albert Einstein College of Medicine, Bronx, NY)
*PACE* 19:2089–2098, 1996                                                    6–60

---

*Introduction.*—Patients with implanted pacemakers must be monitored to ensure proper functioning of the system and identify problems before malfunction occurs. Transtelephonic monitoring (TTM), introduced in 1971, allows frequent rate determinations and timely detection of impending power-source depletion. With ECG transmission capability, electrode function can also be evaluated. The accuracy of TTM in detecting pacemaker pulse-generator malfunction, battery depletion, and lead failure was examined in a review of the records of patients whose conditions were followed with TTM between October 1981 and March 1994.

*Methods.*—At the study institution, TTM is conducted by pacemaker center staff who provide transducers to patients, instruct patients in their use, operate the receivers, enter data, generate reports, and refer physicians. The magnet rate taken as the beginning rate is obtained 1 month after implantation, when the cell powering the pulse generator has warmed to body temperature. Each group of transmissions by a single patient was categorized as a cycle and classified as open (one that ends without a pacemaker-related procedure), closed (one that ends with a pacemaker procedure for management of malfunction), or continuing (no cycle-ending event; patient condition is still being followed). The TTM records of 2632 patients were analyzed and provided 3291 cycles, 2127 open, 433 closed, and 731 continuing. The median number of TTM contacts performed per cycle was 19.

*Results.*—A total of 331 procedures were indicated by TTM; 279 were elective (impending depletion) and 52 were urgent (30 for unexpected depletion and 22 for lead failure). There were 102 procedures performed without TTM indication, 17 for urgent reasons and 85 for nonurgent reasons. Forty-one of the non–TTM-indicated elective procedures were for recall; 15 of the non–TTM-indicated urgent procedures were related to lead malfunction. In no case did TTM follow-up fail to detect battery depletion. Overall, 0.4% of contacts yielded a procedure. During the first 2 years of monitoring, 75% of all secondary interventions occurred within

2 months after implantation and were performed for lead malfunction. For months 3 through 24, the rate of secondary interventions was 0.005 per month.

*Conclusion.*—Findings in this group of patients confirm that TTM is a simple and highly effective technique of pacemaker follow-up. Although 75% of patients in this study either died or were no longer available for follow-up while being monitored with TTM, no deaths were known to be pacemaker related.

▶ This enormous experience of transtelephonic monitoring for pacemaker follow-up is worthy of reading. It only reinforces the recommendation that this remain a standard part of our pacemaker follow-up.

**A.L. Waldo, M.D.**

---

**Energy Parameters in Cardiac Pacing Should be Abandoned**
Barold SS, Strokes K, Byrd CL, et al (Univ of Rochester, NY; Medtronic Inc, Minneapolis; Broward District Hosp, Fort Lauderdale, Fla)
*PACE* 20:112–121, 1997                                                    6–61

---

*Objective.*—Despite the limited information provided by energy pacing parameters, many are still being used to express the cardiac pacing threshold. Interrelationships between pacing thresholds, safety margins, and battery longevity are discussed.

*Basic Electrical Concepts.*—Pacemaker charge (Q) is the product of current (I) and time (T) ($Q = IT$), and energy is the product of voltage (V) and Q ($E = VQ = VIT$).

*Telemetered Data of Output Pulse.*—Whereas output energy of older pacemakers must be estimated, newer pacemakers can measure I, Q, and T, making possible the derivation of pacing impedance (R), charge, or energy.

*Battery Capacity: Charge vs. Current vs. Energy.*—Although there is no agreement on whether current (charge) or energy is the better measure of battery longevity, it is easier to determine the charge and the average rate at which it is used.

*Programmability of Energy.*—Programmable output is not available. In any case, it would not be as practical as programming voltage output.

*Calculation of Battery Longevity.*—Longevity (in years) = $Q/(I_C + I_L)8742$, where $I_C$ is the current used by the pulse generator circuit and $I_L$ is the current delivered through the lead-tissue circuit.

*Energy Strength-Duration Curves.*—Whereas these curves show that the energy threshold is high when pulse durations are short, voltage thresholds are high, and the charge is low, construction of these curves has no clinical value.

*Pitfalls in Threshold Measurement.*—The energy threshold does not directly relate to voltage or pulse duration values at the threshold.

*Safety Margins for Pacing: Voltage vs. Energy.*—Whereas voltage is directly related to safety margins, energy is not.

*Conclusion.*—Energy parameters are not directly related to threshold values in cardiac pacing and should not be used to express the pacing threshold.

▶ Again, a recommended review for the readership. It will help you brush up on your pacing principles.

**A.L. Waldo, M.D.**

# Subject Index

## A

Abciximab
　with coronary angioplasty in long-term
　　protection from myocardial
　　ischemic events, 128
Ablation
　radiofrequency catheter
　　of atrial fibrillation, 452
　　of atrial fibrillation, paroxysmal, right
　　　and left atrial ablation, 454
　　of atrial fibrillation produced by focal
　　　source, 453
　　of atrial fibrillation with dilated
　　　cardiomyopathy, 443
　　of atrial flutter, 452
　　of atrial flutter, common, 452
　　of atrioventricular nodal reentrant
　　　tachycardia, origin of junctional
　　　rhythm during, 461
　　His bundle, followed by ventricular
　　　rate-responsive pacing, exercise
　　　capacity after, 456
　　Maze, video-assisted thoracoscopic
　　　and cardioscopic (in pig), 460
　　in tachycardia, idiopathic right
　　　ventricular outflow tract, 490
Acadesine
　effects on myocardial infarction, stroke,
　　and death following coronary
　　bypass surgery, 156
Acebutolol
　long-term effects on sexual function,
　　277
Adenosine
　-induced atrial arrhythmia, 482
　IV, for intentional asystole during
　　endoluminal thoracic aortic surgery
　　without cardiopulmonary bypass,
　　421
　-sensitive ventricular tachycardia, MRI
　　of right ventricular abnormalities
　　in, 488
Adhesion
　molecules, cell, upregulation in chronic
　　heart failure, 50
Adipose
　tissue, production of plasminogen
　　activator inhibitor type 1 by, 252
Adolescents
　athletes, high school, at risk of sudden
　　cardiac death, screening of, 309
　diet and blood pressure in, 255
　renal failure in, chronic, cardiac
　　troponin T elevation in, 215

Aerobic
　capacity peak, in severe congestive heart
　　failure, exercise training enhances,
　　67
　exercise, regular, effect on elevated
　　blood pressure in postmenopausal
　　women, 263
Age
　aortic valve disease and, calcific, 4
　aortic valve replacement for stenosis
　　and, in adults, 8
　atrial size in hypertensives and, left, 246
　heart donor, and accelerated allograft
　　coronary artery disease, 418
　-related blood pressure changes,
　　hemodynamic patterns of, 231
　-specific incidence rates of myocardial
　　infarction and angina in women
　　with systemic lupus erythematosus,
　　204
　stroke risk and ventricular dysfunction
　　after myocardial infarction and,
　　112
Aging
　effects on left ventricular relaxation, 58
Alcohol
　cocaine-induced myocardial ischemia
　　and infarction and, 81
　-induced myocardial damage detected
　　by indium-111 monoclonal
　　antimyosin antibodies, spectrum of,
　　36
　injection in septal reduction for
　　hypertrophic obstructive
　　cardiomyopathy, outcome, 43
　intake
　　moderate daily, cardioprotective effect
　　　of, 268
　　very low, as protection from coronary
　　　disease, 37
Allograft
　(See also Transplantation)
　aortic valve replacement (see Aortic,
　　valve, replacement, homograft)
　pulmonary, as interposition graft in
　　orthotopic pulmonic valve
　　replacement, 428
American Heart Association
　recommendations for prevention of
　　bacterial endocarditis, 23
Amiodarone
　in atrial fibrillation, 442
　　efficacy, safety, and determinants of
　　　conversion with, 446

Biopsies
atrial, histological substrate of, in
patients with lone atrial fibrillation,
480
Birthplace
mortality from cardiovascular causes
and, in blacks, 180
Biventricular
repair
of conotruncal anomalies associated
with aortic arch obstruction, 329
*vs.* single ventricle repair in
congenital heart disease, 317
Blacks
coronary revascularization in, 175
hypertension prevalence in, 240
mortality among
from cardiovascular causes, related to
birthplace, 180
excess, 182
Bleeding
after allograft aortic valve replacement
for complex endocarditis, 401
postoperative, no effect of
intraoperative autologous blood
donation on, 378
Block
heart, after allograft aortic valve
replacement for complex
endocarditis, 401
Blood
donation, autologous intraoperative,
preserves red cell mass but does not
decrease postoperative bleeding,
378
flow
myocardial, in hypertension, effect of
enalapril *vs.* verapamil on, 291
pulmonary venous, in functional
single ventricle heart after operative
aortopulmonary shunt *vs.* superior
cavopulmonary shunt, 356
loss in reoperative cardiac surgery,
tranexamic acid reduces, 376
pressure
ambulatory, *vs.* clinic, in predicting
treatment-induced regression of left
ventricular hypertrophy, 228
arising, correlation with left
ventricular mass, 249
changes, age-related, hemodynamic
patterns of, 231
control in hypertensives, 269
diet and, in children and adolescents,
255
effect of antioxidant supplement on,
oral, 261
effect of dietary patterns on, 259

effect of potassium on, oral, 262
elevated, in postmenopausal women,
effect of regular aerobic exercise
on, 263
high (*See also* Hypertension)
high, prevention, detection,
evaluation and treatment, sixth
report of the Joint National
Committee on, 221
high, young adults with
predisposition to, impaired
microvascular dilatation and
capillary rarefaction in, 239
measurement, conventional or
ambulatory, antihypertensive
treatment based on, 227
nocturnal, effects of controlled-onset
extended-release verapamil on, 289
normality, ambulatory and home, in
elderly, 224
role in cognitive impairment, in
elderly, 244
stem cell transplantation, autologous, in
cardiac amyloidosis, 47
Bosetan
in heart failure, chronic (in rat), 52
Brain
natriuretic peptide, plasma
in heart failure, effect of digitalis on,
60
prognostic role in chronic heart
failure with left ventricular
dysfunction, 53
Bridge
experience with long-term implantable
left ventricular assist devices, 414
Bundle of His
ablation followed by ventricular
rate-responsive pacing, exercise
capacity after, 456
Bypass
cardiopulmonary, "on-pump," coronary
artery bypass grafting with, and
three-day discharge, 382
coronary, 154
aortic atheroma related to outcome
but not numbers of emboli during,
385
with aortic valve replacement for
stenosis, 8
after esophagostomy, bilateral
thoracotomy and inferior
sternotomy for, 389
graft obstruction after, stent
placement *vs.* balloon angioplasty
for, 149
high-risk, intraoperative
echocardiography in, 371

# Author Index